Palliative Care for Chronic Cancer Patients in the Community

Michael Silbermann
Editor

Palliative Care for Chronic Cancer Patients in the Community

Global Approaches and Future Applications

Springer

Editor
Michael Silbermann
Middle East Cancer Consortium
Haifa
Israel

ISBN 978-3-030-54525-3 ISBN 978-3-030-54526-0 (eBook)
https://doi.org/10.1007/978-3-030-54526-0

This Springer imprint is published by the registered company Springer Nature Switzerland AG
The registered company address is: Gewerbestrasse 11, 6330 Cham, Switzerland

In memory of the late Professor Ora Gilbar, whom we miss so much—a pioneer in Psycho-Oncology, a distinguished researcher, and a founder of home-care services for cancer patients in Israel.

For my friend and mentor Professor A. Hari Reddi who was so catalytic in my scientific journey and from whom so much was learned and shared.

For my associate in MECC for over 22 years, Mrs. Genoveba Breitstein.

Foreword

As we speak today, 41 million people die every year from a non-communicable disease including cancer, tragically 70% of patients who die prematurely are from the developing world.

After the landmark meeting on September 11, 2019 at the UNHLM on NCDs, finally the plight of the 40 million souls dying from NCDs was acknowledged. As a result of that historic meeting, we now have ammunition to face this epidemic head on, with an overarching target of reducing mortalities from NCDs by 25% by the year 2025. Since then, governments have adopted 11 targets, which focus mostly on prevention.

While prevention and early detection efforts *are* the cornerstone to stem future cases of NCDs, what can we do about the 41 million people who need treatment and palliation *right now*? What about the millions of cancer patients silently suffering with pain and disability NOW?

The only way to fully understand and internalize the value and urgency of palliative care is when you become the unfortunate witness of its absence. It is when you become a mere bystander and a spectator to a loved one's face, grimacing with pain for hours on end, day and night, without having the tools to stop the excruciating pain. This is when you truly understand that palliative care is not some luxury treatment that one would choose to adopt or not, it is an emergency need, part and parcel of treatment, and most importantly a human right.

So why is there such a severe shortage of palliative care in Low-Middle-Income Countries (LMICs)? The issue is certainly not only due to a lack of resources as many would imagine. All countries, even those in the LMICs, are capable of creating and implementing effective cost-effective palliative care strategies and procure the "essential package of palliative care and pain relief list" as launched by the lancet commission report, and virtually every single government is capable of procuring morphine and other opioid drugs. Yes, there are challenges in the shortage of qualified personnel, limited technological capacity, and the merits and shortcomings of hospitals versus homecare settings and other issues. But at its core, *money is not the main obstacle: political will and bureaucracy is.*

Palliative Care for Chronic Cancer Patients in the Community: Global Approaches and Future Applications offers a much-needed account of the current state of global palliative care in the community – the good, the bad, and, especially, the hopeful.

This extraordinary compendium, with chapters form 46 countries, edited by Professor Michael Silbermann, tells the remarkable stories of palliative care—from grass-root efforts by volunteers in resource-constrained countries such as India to the full integration of palliative care in high-resource countries such as the United Kingdom, New Zealand, and Australia.

What is so unique about this book is that it captures the enormous range and diversity of palliative care efforts: some led by nurses (Iran), some led by governments (Turkey), and many led by local charities and non-governmental agencies. Readers of this textbook can also learn about the challenges of a government-led palliative care initiative in the post-genocide era in Rwanda or the attempts to provide palliative care services in the conflict zones of Iraq, Palestine, and Sudan. Contextual issues requiring cultural sensitivity in Afghanistan, Latin America, and the Middle East present a real picture of both the exceptional leadership and environmental hardships that palliative care advocates face in their journeys forward.

Each of the 61 chapters in the book tells a narrative of the country's own experience, thus creating a source of on-the-ground information outlining the barriers, challenges, and successes as individual efforts progress. Many reports in the book point toward real change and hope as they relate to healthcare providers becoming empowered advocates for their patients. There are high expectations for the role of nurses to continue to grow. Educating and engaging patients, and the families in their care, has had a measurably positive impact on outcomes.

This is the first textbook to assemble such an archival resource detailing the activities of community palliative care throughout the world, and the credit goes to Professor Michael Silbermann for bringing all the authors together, both virtually by means of this text and personally through his advocacy for advancing palliative care services in resource-constrained settings.

The collaborative spirit of this book gives voice to the incredible vision, tenacity, and resilience of the teams of professionals and their supporters who work in palliative care, particularly those who work in the community. In addition, it underscores that all future efforts can only be successful with the concerted and continuous commitments of governments, academics, and NGOs across and within national boundaries.

A big thank you to Professor Silbermann and all the contributors in this book for hearing the cries of pain of all patients from all over the world and for amplifying and transmitting their voices to all decision makers—that no one should have to bear unspeakable pain at a time when we have all the tools for effective palliation at our disposal.

HRH Princess Dina Mired
President – Union for International Cancer Control (UICC)
Amman
Jordan

Preface

On September 23, 2019, heads of state and governments assembled at the United Nations and reaffirmed the 2030 Agenda for Sustainable Development and strongly recommitted to achieve universal health coverage by 2030, with a view to scaling up the global effort to build a healthier world for all [1].

As a clinical discipline, palliative care relies on the collaboration of professionals such as nurses, physicians, and social workers who have a fundamental role in running the team. Furthermore, primary care personnel have a central function in this arena—the term "primary care" includes family physicians, medical specialists, pediatricians, geriatricians, general practitioners, nurses from a variety of settings (homecare, community care), social workers, pharmacists, physiotherapists, occupational therapists, and volunteers [2].

In the community, this requires a cooperative approach between the primary care and the palliative care specialists, both within the community and among experts in the hospital. With the aging of the population, patients suffer multiple comorbidities and, consequently, there is an increasing demand for palliative care specialist support [2].

Primary care practitioners with core competencies in palliative care and with access to specialist palliative care teams should manage most patients and families.

To date, physicians in the community feel ill-prepared to deal with patients with palliative care needs due to the lack of training in pain and symptom management as well as psychological issues regarding patients and their family caregivers. Thus, the most urgent need is to train physicians, nurses, and social workers in the community to be able to practice basic palliative care principles.

One critical element that must be available to support caregivers is access to skilled homecare nursing 24/7. Utilizing other providers, such as paramedics trained in palliative care, could fill some of the voids where round-the-clock home visits are not feasible [2].

Palliative care RNs have a pivotal role in community palliative care services. Not only do they treat, advise, and help with treatment planning, they also assist in coordinating appropriate and timely care in the various institutions where the patients and families wish the care to take place.

In straightforward situations, the palliative care nurse may simply advise the primary care physician after consulting with a palliative care specialist. In a recent Canadian Expert Consensus White Paper, the authors recommend staffing a palliative care team in the community—recommendations that are applicable in many developed countries, but not yet in the developing world. It is the profession's obligation to ensure equitable availability of palliative care for rural and other vulnerable populations [3].

Lest we forget, the goal of palliative care is not just to save lives, but to also alleviate suffering. Yes, suffering is difficult to measure and even harder to understand, yet alleviating the suffering (be it physical or emotional) should guide us throughout.

In many cases of chronic cancer, the initial step in alleviating patients' suffering is pain control. All those working in the field have experienced how unrelenting, agonizing pain impacts individuals and families and the magnitude of the hardship it engenders.

Unfortunately, there is very limited access to medication for moderate and severe pain, particularly in low- and middle-income countries. The Lancet Commission on Palliative Care and Pain Relief estimates that less than two percent of opioids (morphine, oxycodone, fentanyl) needed for palliative care patients are provided in low-income countries [4]. Under-treatment of severe pain is reported in more than 150 countries, accounting for about 75 percent of the world's population. At least five billion people live in countries affected by the crisis of underconsumption and more than 18 million die annually with untreated, excruciating pain [5]. Lack of availability and limited access to opioids creates profound global health inequity and threatens the capacity of many countries to achieve Universal Health Coverage—the 2030 Agenda for Sustainable Development promises to leave no one behind.

In recent years, the increased non-medical usage of opioids has posed an alarming public health risk, and to safeguard the rational use of these medicines, local authorities must empower healthcare professionals to prescribe, dispense, and administer them according to the individual medical needs of patients; this is especially important at the level of the primary healthcare system.

The problem of non-medical consumption of opioids underscores the importance of implementing basic mandatory training for all healthcare professionals, specifically family physicians and internal medicine specialists in the community. The recently released 2019 World Drug Report confirms that "most of the morphine found in illicit markets originates from illicitly produced opium and only small quantities of morphine are likely to be diverted from licit manufactures to illicit markets" [6]. Accordingly, this year, the World Health Organization (WHO) came out with a new "WHO Guidelines for the Pharmacological and Radiotherapeutic Management of Cancer Pain in Adults and Adolescents" [7].

As already mentioned, in the greater part of the world, there is an urgent need for basic palliative care services in the community; one important reason for this is the insufficient awareness of palliative care among primary healthcare providers as well as the extreme shortage of palliative care specialists in the region.

More recently, an innovative intervention—Project Extension for Community Healthcare Outcomes–Palliative Care in Africa—was conducted in several sub-Saharan countries [8]. One of the important things learned was the necessity to reach out to the primary care providers in the community and to develop the curriculum and best practices based on local palliative care requirements. Also, local caregivers gained confidence in titrating opioids for pain control, using non-opioid analgesics appropriately, and learned to address communication issues related to end-of-life care.

In Summary

While inhabitants of developing countries comprise most of the global population, there are still significant barriers to providing community palliative care services to patients with chronic diseases. These include limitations of available workforce, lack of palliative care education, and differences in cultural competencies. We are confident that by expanding access to palliative care in these areas, pain and symptom management will improve and provide better patient and caregiver satisfaction along with diminishing the occurrence of potentially aggressive end-of-life care [9]. How to improve access remains an important issue and, in recent years, new frameworks have been developed to evolve strategies such as telehealth, community-academic partnerships, and, above all, more training for community professionals.

Haifa, Israel Michael Silbermann

References

1. Political declaration of the high-level meeting on universal health coverage. "Universal health coverage: moving together to build a healthier world". Co-facilitators' text (REV.4), 12 July 2019.
2. Henderson JD, Boyle A, Herx L, Alexiadis A, Barwich D, Connidis S, Lysecki D, Sinnarajah A. Staffing a specialist palliative care service, a team-based approach: expert consensus white paper. J Palliat Med. https://doi.org/10.1089/jpm.2019.0314.
3. Khan CP, Praver S, Lesch JK, DiGioia K, Gaglio B, Daugherty S, Clauser SB, Arora NK. Comparative clinical effectiveness research focused on community-based delivery of palliative care: overview of the patient-centered outcomes research institute's funding initiative. 22 August 2019. https://doi.org/10.1089/jpm.2019.0370.
4. Knaul FM, Farmer PE, Krakauer EL, et al. Alleviating the access abyss in palliative care and pain relief – an imperative of universal health coverage: the lancet commission report. 2018;391:1391–1454.
5. Connor SR, Sepulveda MC editors. Global atlas of palliative care at the end of life. London: UK/Geneva CH: WHPCA/WHO; 2014. Available at https://www.who.int/nmh/Global_Atlas_of_Palliative_Care.pdf.
6. UNODC. The world drug report 2019. https://wdr.unodc.org/wdr2019/prelaunch/WDR19_Booklet_3_DEPRESSANTS.pdf.
7. Development of WHO guidelines for the management of cancer pain in adults. https://www.who.int/ncds/management/palliative-care/cancer_pain_guidelines/en/.
8. Yennurajalingam S, Amos CE, Weru J, Opare-Lokko E, Arthur JA, Nguyen K Extension for community healthcare outcomes-palliative care in africa program: improving access to quality palliative care. J Global Oncol. 2019. https://doi.org/10.1200/JGO.19.00128.
9. Conlon MS, Caswell JM, Santi SA, Ballantyne B, Meigs ML, Knight A, Earle CC, Hartman M. Access to palliative care for cancer patients living in a northern and rural environment in Ontario, Canada: the effects of geographic region and rurality on end-of-life care in a population-based decedent cancer cohort. Clinical medicine insights: oncology. Available at: https://www.ncbi.nlm.nih.gov/pmc/articles/PMC6378418/2019.

Acknowledgments

When the Middle East Cancer Consortium (MECC) was established in 1996, it created a regional cancer registry network, which was then lacking in the Middle East. Very soon it became apparent that about 70 percent of all cancer patients in the region saw a physician for the first time when their illness had already reached Stage III or IV, which, for most patients, was critical as it would be too late for any curative treatment.

Unfortunately, at that time, palliative care was not practiced in most countries; the situation has increasingly improved throughout the years in major cancer centers and university hospitals such as the King Hussein Cancer Center in Amman, Jordan; the National Cancer Institute in Cairo, Egypt; the Rabin Beilinson Medical Center in Israel; the A.Y. Ankara Oncology Education and Research Hospital in Turkey; and Tawam Hospital in the United Arab Emirates. There were only a few countries that had developed palliative care services in the community: Cyprus (Cyprus Anti-Cancer Society and the Cyprus Association of Cancer Patients and Friends), Israel (Clalit Health Care Services, Sabar Health), and, more recently, Palestine (the Al-Sadeel Society for Palliative Care) and Turkey (the Pallia-Turk project). Realizing this critical situation, especially in the community, MECC embarked on regional training programs focusing on primary healthcare professionals (physicians, nurses, social workers, pharmacists, and volunteers).

It was evident that there was an unmet need for improving access to palliative care services in the community offering support to patients and their caregivers living with advanced illnesses. Furthermore, as the proportion of older adults in the population continues to grow, the urgency for more innovative health care services to meet this growing demand increases. Our goal has been to ensure that vulnerable and at-risk populations have equitable access to palliative care.

We were not surprised to discover a great interest in our activities in countries beyond the Middle East, as we had trainees in our training courses (especially nurses) from Turkey, Lebanon, Israel, Palestine, Jordan, Egypt, Sudan, Morocco, Algeria, Uganda, Iraq, Iran, Saudi Arabia, Sultanate of Oman, United Arab Emirates, Qatar, Yemen, Pakistan, and Cyprus. These training courses were conducted in close association with the American Society of Clinical Oncology (ASCO) and the American Oncology Nursing Society (ONS). These ongoing fruitful activities were supported by the National Cancer Institute at the NIH, Bethesda, Maryland, and by local governments and NGOs. MECC would not have accomplished these achievements without the exceptional support of Donna E. Shalala, Former Secretary of Health and Human Services during the Clinton Administration (1993–2000) whose ongoing encouragement helped us overcome the regional political conflicts.

The issue of caring for chronic cancer patients in the community still poses a genuine problem in Africa, Asia, some European countries, and Latin America; as palliative care moves beyond the inpatient hospital setting to outpatient community settings, our teams in the Middle East (along with other colleagues from all five continents) decided to publish a new book on the topic. I am grateful to Springer Nature for giving us the opportunity to bring together ideas, views, and suggestions concerning these matters.

We hope that this comprehensive book will serve as a useful resource for all those interested in developing proper community treatment centers and facilities, each in his or her own country, including clergy, clinicians, health system leaders, and policy makers. The authors, representing both developed and developing countries, provide valuable information on this yet unsolved grave problem. We would have no book without the drive, endurance, good will, and collaboration of all the authors. I would like to thank each one again, as it is due to their ongoing endeavors that patients and their families around the world are the recipients of these important services upon returning home from the hospital. We know that most cancer patients prefer to spend the end-of-life period at home in their community, and it is our urgent task to create the optimum conditions for a restful passing in comfort and privacy, surrounded by their beloved family members and friends.

Michael Silbermann
Middle East Cancer Consortium
Haifa, Israel

Contents

Contributors

Maihan Abdullah, MD National Cancer Control Program, Ministry of Public Health, Kabul, Afghanistan

Loai Mohammad Abu-Sharour, RN, MSN (hon), PhD Faculty of Nursing Al-Zaytoonah University of Jordan, Amman, Jordan

Meera Agar, MBBS [Hons], MPC, PhD IMPACCT – Improving Palliative, Aged and Chronic Care through Clinical Research and Translation – Faculty of Health, University of Technology Sydney, Sydney, NSW, Australia

South Western Sydney Clinical School, University of New South Wales, Sydney, NSW, Australia

Ingham Institute for Applied Medical Research, Sydney, NSW, Australia

Feranindhya Agiananda, MD Department of Psychiatry, Awal Bros West Hospital, Jakarta, Indonesia

Sheikh I. Ahamed, PhD Department of Computer Science, Marquette University, Milwaukee, WI, USA

Matthew J. Allsop, PhD Leeds Institute of Health Sciences, University of Leeds, Leeds, UK

Julio Ancochea, MD PhD Pneumology, La Princesa University Hospital, Madrid, Spain

Autonomous University of Madrid, Madrid, Spain

Tiara Aninditha, MD Department of Neurology Cipto Mangunkusumo General Hospital, Faculty of Medicine Universitas Indonesia, Jakarta, Indonesia

Tolganai Ansatbayeva, MD Almaty Oncology Center, Kazakh Institute of Oncology and Radiology, Almaty, Republic of Kazakhstan

Jemma Arakelyan, MD Department of Oncology, Yerevan State Medical University, Yerevan, Armenia

Chemotherapy Department of Adult Solid Tumors, Hematology Center after Prof. R. Yeolyan, Yerevan, Armenia

Muhammad Shamvil Ashraf, MD Indus Health Network and Consultant Pediatric Oncology, The Indus Hospital, Karachi, Pakistan

Wilson Astudillo-Alarcón, MD Paliativos Sin Fronteras / Palliative without Borders, San Sebastián, Spain, Spain

Ayfer Aydin, RN, PhD Faculty of Nursing, Koç University, Istanbul, Turkey

Asmaa El Azhari, MD Palliative Care Department, Mohammed VI Center for the Treatment of Cancers, UHC Ibn Rochd Casablanca, Casablanca, Morocco

Lodovico Balducci, MD H. Lee Moffitt Cancer Center and Research Institute, Tampa General Hospital, Tampa, FL, USA

Samira Beiranvand, PhD Department of Nursing, Student Research Committee, School of Nursing and Midwifery, Ahvaz Jundishapur University of Medical Sciences, Ahvaz, Iran

Imane Benlekbir, MSC Psychology, Education Science, Rabat, Rabat Salé Zamour Zeir, Morocco

Jeannine Brant, PhD, APRN-CNS, AOCN, FAAN Billings Clinic Cancer Center and Collaborative Science & Innovation Department, Billings, MT, USA

Bruna Burmeister, MD, MSc Universidade Católica Portuguesa, Institute of Health Sciences, Centre for Interdisciplinary Research in Health (CIIS), Portuguese Observatory for Palliative Care, Lisbon, Portugal

Linda Marisol Bustamante, MD National Unit of Pediatric Oncology, Guatemala, Guatemala

Fatma Betul Cakir, MD Bezmialem Vakif University Medical Faculty, Pediatric Hematology-Oncology, Istanbul, Turkey

Maria Minerva P. Calimag, MD, PhD Faculty of Medicine and Surgery, The Research Center for Social Science and Education and The Research Center for the Health Sciences, University of Santo Tomas, Manila, Philippines

Manuel Luís Vila Capelas, RN, MSc, PhD Universidade Católica Portuguesa, Institute of Health Sciences, Centre for Interdisciplinary Research in Health (CIIS), Portuguese Observatory for Palliative Care, Lisbon, Portugal

Lynna Chandra, BEc Rachel House (Yayasan Rumah Rachel), Jakarta, Indonesia

International Children's Palliative Care Network, Assagay, South Africa

Haris Charalambous, BM, MRCP (UK), FRCR (UK) Bank of Cyprus Oncology Center, Nicosia, Cyprus

Aleksandra Ciałkowska-Rysz, MD, PhD Clinical Department of Palliative Medicine, Medical University of Lodz, ŁódŹ, Poland

Nada Cicmil-Sarić, MD Clinical Center for Oncology and Radiotherapy, Clinical Center of Montenegro, Podgorica, Montenegro

Geraldine Damanhuri, CNS Comboni College of Science and Technology, Khartoum, Sudan

Amos Deogratius Mwaka, MD Department of Medicine, School of Medicine, College of Health Sciences, Makerere University, Kampala, Uganda

Renata Dobrila-Dintinjana, PhD, MD Department of Radiotherapy and Oncology, Clinical Hospital Center Rijeka, Rijeka, Croatia

Myrna A. A. Doumit, PhD, RN, FAAN Alice Ramez Chagoury School of Nursing, Lebanese American University, Beirut, Lebanon

Julia Downing, RN, PhD Palliative Care Education and Research Consortium, Kampala, Uganda

Department of Medicine, School of Medicine, College of Health Sciences, Makerere University, Kampala, Uganda

International Children's Palliative Care Network, Assagay, South Africa

Joanne Droney, FRCP, PhD The Royal Marsden and Royal Brompton Palliative Care Service, The Royal Marsden NHS Foundation Trust, London, UK

Catherine D'Souza, MbChB, MRCP, BSC South Canterbury Hospice and District Health Board, Timaru, New Zealand

Cameroon Baptist Convention and Hospice Africa, Bamenda, Cameroon

Mary L. Dunne, MD Supportive Care Medicine, Nuvance Health, Poughkeepsie, NY, USA

Distinguished Careers Institute, Stanford University, Stanford, CA, USA

Sofia Amado Durão, MD, MSc Universidade Católica Portuguesa, Institute of Health Sciences, Centre for Interdisciplinary Research in Health (CIIS), Portuguese Observatory for Palliative Care, Lisbon, Portugal

Hematology and Marrow Transplantation Service – Centro Hospitalar Lisboa Norte, Lisbon, Portugal

Elizabeth Namukwaya, MA, PhD Palliative Care Education and Research Consortium, Kampala, Uganda

Department of Medicine, School of Medicine, College of Health Sciences, Makerere University, Kampala, Uganda

Dina Bell Esther Hortense Murielle, MD Bonassama District Hospital, Douala, Littoral, Cameroon

Samaher Abdulrazzaq Fadhil, MD, FICMS and CABP (ped), FICMS Children Welfare Teaching Hospital, Medical City, Baghdad, Iraq

Azam Shirinabadi Farahani, PhD, RN Pediatric Nursing Department, School of Nursing & Midwifery, Shahid Beheshti University of Medical Sciences, Tehran, Iran

Maria Paz Fernández-Ortega, PhD, MSc, RN, Psych Institut Català d'Oncologia and University of Barcelona, Barcelona, Spain

Rita Cunha Ferreira, MD, MSc Universidade Católica Portuguesa, Institute of Health Sciences, Centre for Interdisciplinary Research in Health (CIIS), Portuguese Observatory for Palliative Care, Lisbon, Portugal

Home Palliative Care Team of ACES Lisboa Ocidental/Oeiras, ARSLVT, Lisbon, Portugal

Regina M. Fink, PhD, APRN-CNS, AOCN, CHPN, FAAN Division of General Internal Medicine, Department of Medicine, School of Medicine, University of Colorado, Aurora, CO, USA

Laura Galiana, PhD University of Valencia, Valencia, Spain

Shereen Gamaluddin, MD Centra Health Palliative Care Service, Lynchburg, VA, USA

Hasanein H. Ghali, MD Department of Pediatrics, College of Medicine, University of Baghdad, Children Welfare Teaching Hospital, Medical City, Baghdad, Iraq

Marin Golčić, MD Department of Radiotherapy and Oncology, Clinical Hospital Center Rijeka, Rijeka, Croatia

Sandra Gomez, MD, FAAHPM Department of Palliative Care and Rehabilitation Medicine, M.D. Anderson Cancer Center, University of Texas, Houston, TX, USA

Mohamed Ahmed Hablas, MD Palliative Care, Gharbiah Cancer Society, Tanta, Egypt

Ramzi R. Hajjar, MD Department of Internal Medicine, Geriatric Medicine Service, American University of Beirut Medical Center, Beirut, Lebanon

Gamal Abdul Hamid, PhD, MD Clinical Laboratory and Hematology Faculty of Medicine, University of Aden, Aden, Yemen

Maryam Al Harrasi, RN, PhD College of Nursing, Sultan Qaboos University, Muscat, Oman

Iman Al Hashmi, RN, PhD College of Nursing, Sultan Qaboos University, Muscat, Oman

Theresa Huntley, RN, MA, MSW, LICSW Department of Oncology, Pediatric Cancer and Blood Disorders Program, Children's Hospitals and Clinics of Minnesota, Minneapolis, MN, USA

Rana Istambouly, MD, PhD PHD student in health management, Université Paris-Est, IAE Gustave Eiffel, Creteil, France

Member of the national scientific committee for palliative medicine (SFAP), Paris, France

Member of the scientific committee of Center for Investigation and Research in Organizational Resilience (CIRERO), Paris, France

President and founder of the association of early palliative medicine (MEDPALLIAP), Paris, France

Eric Kabisa, MPH Rwanda Palliative Care and Hospice Organization, Kigali, Rwanda

Johnblack Kabukye, MBChB, MSc Uganda Cancer Institute, Kampala, Uganda

Dilyara Kaidarova, MD, PhD Kazakh Institute of Oncology and Radiology, Kazakhstan Association of Oncologists, National Academy of Sciences, Almaty, Republic of Kazakhstan

Nune Karapetyan, MD, MPH Department of Oncology, Yerevan State Medical University, Yerevan, Armenia

Chemotherapy Department of Adult Solid Tumors, Hematology Center after Prof. R. Yeolyan, Yerevan, Armenia

Senaida Keating, MD Virginia Tech Carilion School of Medicine, Roanoke, VA, USA

Veterans Affairs Medical Center, Salem, VA, USA

Rejin Kebudi, MD Pediatric Hematology-Oncology, Oncology Institute, Istanbul University & Istanbul Medical Faculty, Istanbul University, Istanbul, Turkey

Necla Kenar, PhD Department of Physics, Faculty of Arts and Science, Kocaeli University, Izmit-Kocaeli, Turkey

Mohamad H. Khleif, PhD Al-Sadeel Society for Palliative Care for Cancer and Chronic Diseases, Bethlehem, Palestine

Kye Y. Kim, MD Department of Psychiatry and Behavioral Medicine, Virginia Tech Carilion School of Medicine, Roanoke, VA, USA

Carilion Roanoke Memorial Hospital Palliative Care Service, Roanoke, VA, USA

Carilion Center for Healthy Aging, Roanoke, VA, USA

Aleksandra Kotlińska-Lemieszek, MD, PhD Department of Palliative Medicine, Poznan University of Medical Sciences, Poznan, Poland

Suresh Kumar, MB, BS, DA, MA Institute of Palliative Medicine, WHO Collaborating Center for Community Participation in Palliative Care and Long Term Care, Kozhikode, Kerala, India

Gulnara Kunirova, DPsy Kazakhstan Association for Palliative Care (KAPC), Together Against Cancer Foundation, International Association for Hospice and Palliative Care (IAHPC), Almaty, Republic of Kazakhstan

Junko Kusunoki, RN, PHN, MNSc Graduate School of Nursing, Chiba University, Chiba, Japan

Hyun Soo Lim, PhD Department of Electric and Electronic Engineering, Faculty of Technology, Sakarya University of Applied Science, Serdivan-Sakarya, Turkey

Department of Biomedical Engineering, School of Medicine, Chungnam National University, Daejeon, South Korea

Richard R. Love, MD Department of Computer Science, Marquette University, Milwaukee, WI, USA

Tim Luckett, PhD IMPACCT – Improving Palliative, Aged and Chronic Care through Clinical Research and Translation – Faculty of Health, University of Technology Sydney, Sydney, NSW, Australia

Tomoko Majima, RN, PhD Graduate School of Nursing, Chiba University, Chiba, Japan

Annamaria Di Mari, MD Medical Oncology Unit, Umberto I Hospital – RAO, Siracusa, Italy

Mohja Marhoom, MBBS Sudan Medical Specialization Board, Khartoum, Sudan

Jhon Comba Miranda, MD Department of Pathology, Hospital Univeristario Donosti, San Sebastián, Guipúzcoa, Spain

Leila Khanali Mojen, PhD, RN Medical-Surgical Nursing Department, School of Nursing & Midwifery, Shahid Beheshti University of Medical Sciences, Tehran, Iran

Narine Movsesyan, MD Department of Anesthesiology and Intensive Care, Yerevan State Medical University, Yerevan, Armenia

Mary Ann Muckaden, MD, MSc Department of Palliative Medicine, Tata Memorial Center, Mumbai, India

Olive Mukeshimana, MD, Dip Kibagabaga District Hospital, Kigali, Rwanda

Mark Donald Mwesiga, MMS, MSc Palliative Care Association of Uganda, Kampala, Uganda

Esther W. Nafula, MD, MPall HCG-CCK Cancer Centre, Nairobi, Kenya

Eve Namisango, PhD African Palliative Care Association, Kampala, Uganda

Cicely Saunders Institute, King's College London, London, UK

Sophia Nestoros, MD, MSc Cyprus Anti-Cancer Society, Nicosia, Cyprus

Scholastique Ngizwenayo, SW Kibagabaga District Hospital, Kigali, Rwanda

Najia Niazi, MA The Cancer Center at Jumhuriat Hospital, National Cancer Control Program, Ministry of Public Health, Kabul, Afghanistan

Huda Al-Noumani, RN, PhD College of Nursing, Sultan Qaboos University, Muscat, Oman

Christian R. Ntizimira, MD, MSc City Cancer Challenge Foundation, Kigali, Rwanda

Jonathan Odilo, MD Universitas Indonesia Hospital, Faculty of Medicine Universitas Indonesia, Jakarta, Indonesia

Amparo Oliver, PhD University of Valencia, Valencia, Spain

Tomoko Otsuka, RN, PhD Graduate School of Nursing, Chiba University, Chiba, Japan

Srivieng Pairojkul, MD Karunruk Palliative Care Center, Faculty of Medicine, Khon Kaen University, Khon Kaen, Thailand

Musa Pakteen, BSc The Cancer Center at Jumhuriat Hospital, National Cancer Control Program, Ministry of Public Health, Kabul, Afghanistan

Jane Phillips, BAppSc, PGDipHlthProm, PhD IMPACCT – Improving Palliative, Aged and Chronic Care through Clinical Research and Translation – Faculty of Health, University of Technology Sydney, Sydney, NSW, Australia

Sergey Postovsky, MD Pediatric Hematology Oncology and Bone Marrow Transplantation Division, Ruth Rappaport Children's Hospital, Rambam Health Care Campus, Haifa, Israel

Richard A. Powell, BA, MA, MSc MWAPO Health Development Group, London, UK

Maryam Rassouli, PhD, RN Cancer Research Center, Shahid Beheshti University of Medical Sciences, Tehran, Iran

Daniela Respini, PhD Associazione Mareluce Onlus, Siracusa, Italy

Heather Richardson, RGN, MHM, PhD St Christopher's Hospice, London, UK

Julia Riley, MRCGP, FRCP, MD Institute of Global Health Innovation, Imperial College, London, UK

The Royal Marsden and Royal Brompton Palliative Care Service, The Royal Marsden NHS Foundation Trust, London, UK

Silvia Rivas, MD Palliative Care Program, National Unit of Pediatric Oncology, Guatemala, Guatemala

Damiano Rizzi, PhD Department of Psychology, Soleterre Foundation – Policlinico San Matteo, Pavia, Italy

Fabrizio Romano, MD Medical Oncology Unit, Umberto I Hospital – RAO, Siracusa, Italy

David Rudilla, PhD Pneumology, La Princesa University Hospital, Madrid, Spain

Air Liquide Healthcare, Madrid, Spain

Suleiman Al Sabei, RN, PhD College of Nursing, Sultan Qaboos University, Muscat, Oman

Nasreen Muhammad Saleem, MD Section of Palliative Medicine, Department of Oncology, The Aga Khan University Hospital, Karachi, Pakistan

J. Antonio Salinas-Martin, PhD Department of Radiation Oncology, CHUSC – Hospital Universitario de La Candelaria, Santa Cruz de Tenerife, Spain

Libby Sallnow, MBBS, MRCP, PhD Central and North West London NHS Foundation Trust & St Christopher's Hospice, London, UK

Tânia dos Santos Afonso, RN, MSc, MNurs, PhD Universidade Católica Portuguesa, Institute of Health Sciences, Centre for Interdisciplinary Research in Health (CIIS), Portuguese Observatory for Palliative Care, Lisbon, Portugal

Hospital Palliative Care Support Team – Hospital Professor Doutor Fernando Fonseca, Lisbon, Portugal

Aurelio Saraceno, PhD Azienda Sanitaria di Siracusa, Siracusa, Italy

Ana Sofia Simões, RN, MSc Universidade Católica Portuguesa, Institute of Health Sciences, Centre for Interdisciplinary Research in Health (CIIS), Portuguese Observatory for Palliative Care, Lisbon, Portugal

Home Palliative Care Team & Hospital Palliative Care Support Team – Instituto Português de Oncologia de Lisboa, Francisco Gentil, Lisbon, Portugal

Henry R. Sofyan, MD Department of Neurology Cipto Mangunkusumo General Hospital, Faculty of Medicine Universitas Indonesia, Jakarta, Indonesia

Arva Paramaniaga, Jakarta, Indonesia

Zemilson Bastos Brandão Souza, MD Department of Oncology, Palliative Care and Pain Management, ACSC-HSJ/UNACON-Ministry of Health, Rio de Janeiro, Brazil

Scharlotte Spencer, DNP, APRN FNP-C ACHPN Memorial Hermann Healthcare System, Chamberlain College of Nursing, Humble, TX, USA

Adam Sterman, MD, FAAP Department of Pain Medicine, Palliative Care and Integrative Medicine, Children's Hospitals and Clinics of Minnesota, Minneapolis, MN, USA

Christi Stewart, MD Carilion Roanoke Memorial Hospital Palliative Care Service, Roanoke, VA, USA

Virginia Tech Carilion School of Medicine, Roanoke, VA, USA

Carilion Center for Healthy Aging, Roanoke, VA, USA

Kyriakos Stylianides, MD Cyprus Association of Cancer Patients and Friends (PASYKAF), and Supportive Care Unit Bank of Cyprus Oncology Center, Nicosia, Cyprus

Gevorg Tamamyan, MD, MSc, PhD The Pediatric Cancer and Blood Disorders Center of Armenia, Hematology Center after Prof. R. Yeolyan, Yerevan, Armenia

Department of Pediatric Hematology and Oncology, Yerevan State Medical University, Yerevan, Armenia

Lili Tang, MD Department of Psycho-Oncology, Peking University Cancer Hospital & Institute, Beijing, China

Carla Marinho Teves, Teves Psyc, MSc Universidade Católica Portuguesa, Institute of Health Sciences, Centre for Interdisciplinary Research in Health (CIIS), Portuguese Observatory for Palliative Care, Lisbon, Portugal

Ying Pin Toh, MBBS, MRCPCH Rachel House (Yayasan Rumah Rachel), Jakarta, Indonesia

Asia Pacific Hospice Network, Singapore, Singapore

Julio César de la Torre-Montero, PhD, MSN, CNS, BSN, RN Oncology Nursing Care and Palliative Care, Comillas Pontifical University, Madrid, Spain

Paolo Tralongo, MD Medical Oncology Unit, Umberto I Hospital – RAO, Siracusa, Italy

Gonca Tuncel-Oguz, MD Palliative Care Clinic, Department of Anesthesiology, Dr. A.Y. Ankara Oncology Education & Research Hospital, University of Health Sciences, Ankara, Turkey

Blaise Uhagaze, MD, MPH Rwanda Palliative Care and Hospice Organization, Kigali, Rwanda

Sandra Urusaro, RN Partners in Health/Inshuti Mu Buzima, Kigali, Rwanda

Claudia Valenzuela, MD Pneumology, La Princesa University Hospital, Madrid, Spain

Autonomous University of Madrid, Madrid, Spain

Patricia Valverde, PhD National Unit of Pediatric Oncology, Guatemala, Guatemala

Muhammad Atif Waqar, MD Section of Palliative Medicine, Department of Oncology, The Aga Khan University Hospital, Karachi, Pakistan

John K. Weru, MD Department of Medicine, Aga Khan University Hospital, Nairobi, Kenya

Myriam Weyl-Ben-Arush, MD Pediatric Hematology Oncology and Bone Marrow Transplantation Division, Ruth Rappaport Children's Hospital, Rambam Health Care Campus, Haifa, Israel

Carolyn White, NP, MSc Centra Health Palliative Care Service, Lynchburg, VA, USA

Phyllis Whitehead, PhD, APRN/CNS, ACHPN, RN-BC Carilion Roanoke Memorial Hospital Palliative Care Service, Roanoke, VA, USA

Virginia Tech Carilion School of Medicine, Roanoke, VA, USA

Basma Al-Yazidi, RN, PhD College of Nursing, Sultan Qaboos University, Muscat, Oman

Part I

North America: USA

The Role of the Palliative Care Team in Keeping Pediatric Oncology Patients at Home

Theresa Huntley and Adam Sterman

Epidemiology of Pediatric Oncology

The incidence of pediatric cancers (age 0–19) has been relatively stable over the past 40 years. As of 2016, there are 19.3 new cases of childhood cancer per 100,000 children per year in the United States. The most common childhood cancers in descending order are central nervous system (CNS) neoplasms (including benign brain tumors), leukemia, lymphomas, soft tissue sarcomas, germ cell and gonadal neoplasms, thyroid carcinomas, malignant bone tumors, neuroblastomas, and renal tumors. Due to advances in cancer-directed therapies as well as improvements in supportive care measures, the mortality rates have significantly declined. In the mid-1970s, the 5-year survival for pediatric cancer was only 62%, but is currently up to 86%. The largest improvements were seen in leukemia (45% 5-year survival up to 86%) and non-Hodgkin's lymphoma (45% 5-year survival up to 90%). However, cancer remains the leading cause of death due to a medical condition in the pediatric population, second only to deaths from accidents and other forms of violence. The most common childhood cancer-related deaths are from leukemia, CNS tumors, and bone/joint tumors [16].

T. Huntley (✉)
Department of Oncology, Pediatric Cancer and Blood Disorders Program, Children's Hospitals and Clinics of Minnesota, Minneapolis, MN, USA
e-mail: theresa.huntley@childrensmn.org

A. Sterman
Department of Pain Medicine, Palliative Care and Integrative Medicine, Children's Hospitals and Clinics of Minnesota, Minneapolis, MN, USA
e-mail: Adam.Sterman@childrensmn.org

Broader Aspects of Pediatric Palliative Care

"Palliative care" refers to the active total care of a patient's body, mind, and spirit and therefore strongly complements the whole patient's psychosocial care. Historically, the term referred to care specifically directed to patients at the end of life. The current definition is more holistic, beginning when illness is diagnosed and continuing regardless of whether or not the child is receiving disease-directed therapy [14, 21]. Palliative care has the potential now to be flexible and inclusive, allowing the care to be patient-centered and family-focused, meeting the patient literally and figuratively where they are. The changing perception from end of life to care along the continuum provides access to patients and families most in need. Children with complex and/or life-limiting illness can be engaged without requiring anyone – clinicians, patients or families – to discuss a potential dying process, change a code status to DNR, or give up access to life-prolonging therapy [10]. Pediatric palliative

M. Silbermann (ed.), *Palliative Care for Chronic Cancer Patients in the Community*,
https://doi.org/10.1007/978-3-030-54526-0_1

care (PPC) has emerged as both an approach and a medical subspecialty focused on improving the quality of life of individuals and families facing challenges associated with life-threatening illness through prevention and relief of suffering [14]. This expertise and philosophy is increasingly being incorporated into standard oncology care for both adults and kids. It is appropriate at any age and at any point in a serious illness and can be delivered together with curative treatment [3].

The Interdisciplinary Team

For a group of people to become a team, they must share a common purpose, be strongly committed to the achievement of specific tasks, and value teamwork through which they expect to accomplish more by their cooperation [12].

A fully staffed Palliative Care Consultation Team (PCCT), at minimum, comprises a physician, an advanced practice nurse, a master's prepared social worker, and a chaplain. Other members of the PCCT ideally include child life specialists, psychologists, nurse care coordinators, home care nurses, integrative medicine practitioners, pharmacologists, rehab therapists, expressive therapists (music/art therapists), and bereavement specialists. All bring experience in palliative care, share an appreciation for collaboration, and approach their colleagues with humility and respect for each discipline's expertise. This expertise includes excellent communication and interpersonal skills, which brings a biopsychosocial-spiritual approach to the care. At the center of the team's evolving plan are the patient, the patient's family, and their values, beliefs, and needs [10].

The PCCT functions differently from the traditional multidisciplinary healthcare team. In medical care, teams are described as existing along a continuum from unidisciplinary (several members within a single discipline), multidisciplinary (a reactive model with ad hoc membership that uses a consultative format), to interdisciplinary (members are identified as working together proactively, often without shared leadership and decision-making authority), to transdisciplinary (in which members create a shared team mission, benefit from role overlap, and have integrated responsibilities, training, and leadership.) [17].

In a tertiary acute care teaching hospital, teams tend to be primarily interdisciplinary, as are many palliative care teams. The PCCT often functions somewhere between interdisciplinary and transdisciplinary structures, possibly flowing back and forth depending on the task at hand, and the membership and stage of development of the team [17].

In contrast to most interdisciplinary and multidisciplinary medical team models, members of a transdisciplinary palliative care team represent their own discipline as well as the team itself. A well-functioning team can divide the workload when necessary to ensure all patients/families are seen and referrals responded to in a timely manner [17].

Symptom Management

Children with cancer, especially during the last months of life, have been reported to suffer from a number of different symptoms [18, 19]. These symptoms can be managed by the PPCT, hopefully leading to more time spent at home and out of the hospital. The top three symptoms leading to suffering are discussed below. In addition to physical symptoms, they suffer from psychosocial issues such as anxiety, depression, and social isolation. They also suffer from existential distress, even young children.

Pain is one of the most distressing symptoms experienced by pediatric oncology patients. Children of all ages are able to experience pain, which is most appropriately managed by a multimodal approach [13]. Non-pharmacologic modalities should be universally utilized in conjunction with medications. Data support the use of many integrative therapies including progressive muscle relaxation, hypnosis, acupuncture, massage, healing touch, and music therapy [1]. The route of administration and formulation of the medication is important to take into account; for example, young children would find it more difficult to swallow pills. When choosing from pharmacological therapies, one should start with non-opioid basic analgesia in order to minimize opioid-induced side effects (Table 1). However, opioids remain the pillar of cancer pain management (Table 2). A way to safely

Table 1 Basic analgesia for children older than 6 months

Medication (route of administration)	Pediatric dose	Maximal dose	Dosing interval	Comment
Acetaminophen/Paracetamol				
Acetaminophen/ Paracetamol (PO/ PR)	10–15 mg/kg	6–24 months = 60 mg/ kg/day > 2 years: 90 mg/kg/ day [max. 650 mg Q6h]	Q6h	
Acetaminophen/ Paracetamol (IV)	<10 kg = 7.5 mg/kg	30 mg/kg/day	Q6h	Due to high cost, ONLY if enteral rectal or oral administration contraindicated; re-evaluate daily
	1–2 years = 15 mg/kg;	60 mg/kg/day	Q6h	
	>2 years (<50 kg) = 15 mg/kg	75 mg/kg/day	Q6h	
	>13 years (>50 kg) = 1000 mg	4000 mg/day	Q6h	
Non-steroidal anti-inflammatory drugs (NSAIDs)				
Ibuprofen (PO)	5–10 mg/kg	400–600 mg/dose (2400 mg/day)	Q6h	
Ibuprofen-Sodium (PO) 256 mg tablet = 200 mg ibuprofen	5 (-10) mg/kg	200–(400) mg/dose	Q6h	Fast-acting compared to regular ibuprofen: onset after 10 minutes, lasts longer, and only half dose required
Ketorolac (IV)	6–24 months = 0.25 mg/kg	30 mg/dose	Q6h	Recommend dosing no longer than 5 days
	>2 years = 0.5 mg/kg	30 mg/dose	Q6h	Recommend dosing no longer than 5 days
Naproxen (PO)	5–6 mg/kg	250–375 mg/dose	Q12h	
COX-2 inhibitor				
Celecoxib (PO)	1–2 mg/kg	100 mg	Q12–24 hours	If classic NSAIDs contraindicated; safety and efficacy has been established only in children 2 years of age or older and for a maximum of 6 months of treatment in JRA

Friedrichsdorf S, 11th Annual Pediatric Pain Master Class, Minneapolis, MN (June 2018): With Permission
IV intravenous, *PO* by mouth (or enterally via gastric/jejunal tube), *PR* rectally, *Q6h* every 6 hours, *Q8h* every 8 hours, *Q12h* every 12 hours, *Q12–24h* every 12–24 hours

Table 2 Opioid starting doses for children with acute pain older than 6 months

Medication (route of administration)	Pediatric dose	Maximal dose	Dosing interval	Comment
Partial μ-receptor agonists ("weak opioid")				
Tramadol (PO, SL, PR)	0.5–1 mg/kg/dose (max 2 mg/kg/dose)	25–50 mg (max. 100 mg)/dose	Q4–6h	Analgesic ceiling effect: max. 8 mg/kg/day (>50 kg: max. of 400 mg/day)
Full μ-receptor agonists ("strong opioids")				
Morphine (PO, SL, PR)	0.15–0.3 mg/kg	7.5–15 mg/dose	Q4h	
Morphine (IV, SC)	0.05–0.1 mg/kg	2.5–5 mg/dose	Q4h	
Oxycodone (PO, SL, PR)	0.15–0.3 mg/kg	7.5–15 mg/dose	Q6h	Oxycodone can be administered every 6 hours due to longer half-life; alternatively may be given every 4 hours: 0.1–0.2 mg/kg Q4h (max. 5–10 mg Q4h)
Fentanyl (IV, SC, SL, transdermal, buccal)	0.5–1 mcg/kg	25–50 mcg	n/a	Due to short half-life, consider starting continuous infusion 0.5–1 mcg/kg/hour (max. 50 mcg/hour), if scheduled analgesia required
Hydromorphone (PO, SL, PR)	40–60 mcg/kg	2000–3000 mcg (= 2–3 mg)	Q4h	
Hydromorphone (IV, SC)	10–20 mcg/kg	0.5–1 mg	Q4h	
Multi-mechanistic full μ-receptor agonists ("strong opioid")				
Methadone (PO, PR, SL)	0.05–0.1 mg/kg	2.5–5 mg	Q8–12h	Methadone should not be prescribed by those unfamiliar with its use! Its effects should be closely monitored for several days, particularly when it is first started and after any dose changes
Methadone (IV, SC)	0.04–0.08 mg/kg	2–4 mg	Q8–12h	Whereas in pediatrics due to high bioavailability about 80% of the enteral dose appears to be the equianalgesic IV dose (e.g., 1 mg PO = 0.8 mg IV), adult recommendations suggest 50% conversion (e.g., 1 mg PO = 0.5 mg IV)

Friedrichsdorf S, 11th Annual Pediatric Pain Master Class, Minneapolis, MN (June 2018): With Permission
Dosing range: Younger children with smaller pain start on the lower end of the range, older children with severe pain start on the higher end of the dosing range; doses will then be titrated to effect
Maximum per kg dose capped at 50 kg body weight
For strong opioids: Rescue ("breakthrough" or "PRN") dose = 10% of total daily dose
IV intravenous, *PO* by mouth (or enterally via gastric/jejunal tube), *SL* sublingual, *PR* rectally, *Q4h* every 4 hours, *Q6h* every 6 hours, *mg* milligram, *mcg* microgram

administer opioids, when necessary, is via a patient-controlled analgesia (PCA) (Table 3). PCAs are pumps that can administer medications at a continuous rate, as well as deliver an additional bolus dose of the medication. The bolus is activated by a nurse, parent, or, when old enough, usually age 6 or 7, by the patient. Adjuvant analgesia can be added for opioid-sparing intent or for difficult to control pain, like in neuropathic pain (Table 4). For neonates and infants, medication doses must be adjusted due to their immature metabolism (Table 5).

Cancer-related fatigue is one of the most common symptoms reported in the pediatric population. The cause is multifactorial including anemia, poorly controlled symptoms, side effects from medications, cancer-directed therapies, and deconditioning. Management should include adequate control of symptoms, exercise/physical therapy, and medications when appropriate, with

Table 3 Starting doses for patient (or nurse)-controlled analgesia (PCA) pumps for children in acute pain older than 6 months

PCA dose	Max. PCA dose (for patients >50 kg)	Continuous infusion (basal rate)	Max. continuous infusion (for patients >50 kg)	Lock-out time	Number of max. boluses
Morphine					
10–20 mcg/kg	500–1000 mcg (= 0.5–1 mg)	10–20 mcg/kg/hour	500–1000 mcg (= 0.5–1 mg)/hour	5–10 minutes	4–6 boluses/hour
Fentanyl					
0.5–1 mcg/kg	25–50 mcg	0.5–1 mcg/kg/hour	25–50 mcg/hour	5–10 minutes	4–6 boluses/hour
Hydromorphone					
2–4 mcg/kg	100–200 mcg	2–4 mcg/kg/hour	100–200 mcg/h	5–10 minutes	4–6 boluses/hour

Friedrichsdorf S, 11th Annual Pediatric Pain Master Class, Minneapolis, MN (June 2018): With Permission

Dosing range: Younger children with smaller pain start on the lower end of the range, older children with severe pain start on the higher end of the dosing range

Doses will then be titrated to effect with escalation usually in (33-) 50% increments both for continuous and PCA bolus dose

PCA dose usually = continuous infusion (might differ in individual patients)

Maximum per kg dose capped at 50 kg body weight

Consider adding low-dose naloxone infusion 0.5–2 mcg/kg/hour (max. 25–100 mcg/hour) to treat potential opioid-induced side effects, such as pruritus, nausea, constipation, urinary retention, hallucinations etc.

Table 4 Adjuvant analgesia for infants, children, and adolescents

Medication (route of administration)	Pediatric dose	Max. dose (for patients >50 kg)	Dosing interval	Comments/side effects
Gabapentinoids				
Gabapentin (PO)	6 mg/kg (titrated up to 24 mg/kg)	300 mg (titrated up to 1200 mg) TID	TID	In school children may start at lower doses to reduce risk of initial sedation Can NOT be administered rectally (missing active transporter = no absorption) Infants <1 year: 4.5 mg/kg/dose Q6h (titrated to effect to max. of 18 mg/kg/dose)
Pregabalin (PO)	1 mg/kg (titrated up to 6 mg/kg)	50 mg (titrated up to 300 mg) BID	BID	Rotation from gabapentin, if distressing side effects or inadequate analgesia CanNOT be administered rectally (missing active transporter = no absorption) In school children may start at lower doses to reduce risk of initial sedation No data for infants
Alpha-agonists				
Dexmedetomidine (IV)	0.2 (titrate to max. 2) mcg /kg/hour	10 (titrate to max. 100) mcg /hour	Continuous infusion	
Clonidine (PO, transdermal)	1–3 mcg/kg	50–150 mcg	Q4–6h	Transdermal application usually 1:1 conversion to total daily enteral dose
NMDA-channel blocker				
Low-dose ketamine (IV)	1 mcg/kg/minute [= 60 mcg/hour] (titrated to 5 mcg/kg/minute [= 300 mcg/hour])	3 mg/hour (titrated to 15 mg/hour)	Continuous infusion	Conversion to PO ketamine 1:1 (i.e., divide total daily dose by 6 and administer Q4h PRN or scheduled)

(continued)

Table 4 (continued)

Medication (route of administration)	Pediatric dose	Max. dose (for patients >50 kg)	Dosing interval	Comments/side effects
Tricyclic antidepressants (TCA)				
Amitriptyline (PO)	0.1 mg/kg (titrated to max. 0.5 mg/kg)	5 mg (titrated to max. 25 mg)	QHS	Despite the name, medication NOT potent as an antidepressant Consider EKG to rule out QTc-prolongation Tertiary amine TCA; stronger anticholinergic side effects (including inducing sleep) than nortriptyline For infants >3 months
Nortriptyline (PO)	0.1 mg/kg (titrated to max. 0.5 mg/kg)	5 mg (titrated to max. 25 mg)	QHS	Despite the name, medication NOT potent as an antidepressant Consider EKG to rule out QTc-prolongation For infants >3 months

Friedrichsdorf S, 11th Annual Pediatric Pain Master Class, Minneapolis, MN (June 2018): With Permission
IV intravenous, *PO* by mouth (or enterally via gastric/jejunal tube), *PR* rectally, *TID* three times per day, *BID* twice per day, *Q6h* every 6 hours, *Q8h* every 8 hours, *Q12h* every 12 hours, *Q12–24 h* every 12–24 hours, *NMDA* N-methyl-D-aspertate, *QHS* once at night

Table 5 Analgesia for neonates and Infants 0–6 months of age

Drug	Route	Pediatric dose (age)	Maximal dose	Dosing interval
Basic analgesia				
Ibuprofen[a]	PO	5–10 mg/kg (infants 3–6 months)	40 mg/kg/day	6–8 hours
Acetaminophen	PO, PR	5–10 mg/kg (neonates 0–30 days) 10 mg/kg (infants 1–3 months) 10–15 mg/kg (infants 3–6 months)	20–40 mg/kg/day 40 mg/kg/day 40–60 mg/kg/day	4–6 hours (maximum 4 doses/day)
Acetaminophen[b]	IV	<10 kg = 7.5 mg/kg	30 mg/kg/day	6 hours
Opioids				
Morphine	PO/PR/SL	0.075–0.15 mg/kg (neonates 0–30 days)		6 hours
		0.08–0.2 mg/kg (infants 1–6 months)		4–6 hours
Morphine[c]	IV/SC[d]	0.025–0.05 mg/kg (neonates 0–30 days)		6 hours
		0.1 mg/kg (infants 1–6 months)		6 hours
		Infusion (with PCA bolus of same dose): 0.005–0.01 mg/kg/hour (neonates 0–30 days) 0.01–0.03 mg/kg/hour (infants 1–6 months)		
Fentanyl[c]	IV/SC[d]	1–2 mcg/kg (neonates and infants 0–12 months)		2–4 hours
		Infusion (with PCA bolus of same dose): 0.5–1 mcg/kg/hour (neonates and infants 0–6 months)		
Oxycodone	PO/PR/SL	0.05–0.125 mg/kg (infants 1–6 months)		4 hours

Adapted from: World Health Organization [20]
[a]For infants <3 months, consult Pain Service
[b]ONLY if rectal or oral administration contraindicated; re-evaluate daily
[c]The intravenous doses for neonates are based on acute pain management and sedation dosing information. Lower doses are required for non-ventilated neonates
[d]Administer IV slowly over at least 5 minutes

methylphenidate most commonly used in pediatrics [13].

Dyspnea, which occurs more frequently and intensely toward the end of life, is another distressing symptom. Opioids, usually at lower doses than those needed for analgesia, and anxiolytics such as benzodiazepines, as well as use of blowing air from a fan, are effective [13].

School Issues

School attendance plays several important roles in the lives of children and families. Education is future-oriented; attending school as a child is similar to an adult going to work [4]. Children understand their "job" is to learn, grow, and become. When routine participation is disrupted, it can be unsettling, leaving them wondering what their future may hold. Helping children remain engaged in learning—albeit it in a different format—can provide a sense of security in abnormal circumstances.

"Next to the family, school is the most important social institution in the lives of many children." [4]. It is the place where relationships with peers are developed and maintained. Finding creative ways for children to remain connected to their friends is important. This can be difficult as children living with cancer are often experiencing things incomprehensible to their classmates. Parents and staff can be instrumental in addressing this issue. They can help kids to share their story with a group of friends or classmates in a meaningful way. They can also facilitate activities tailored to promote social connection, while accommodating to any limitations.

Children and adolescents may find comfort in establishing relationships with others on a similar journey. They share a common understanding and encounter empathy. They may also face the inherent reality of having a friend relapse and die. This can exacerbate their sense of uncertainty regarding their illness and contribute to a sense of guilt if their condition is relatively stable and their friend's is not.

For the child who wants to attend school, preparation and planning are essential. Things to consider include the following: (1) Does the school have appropriate staff to address medical needs that may arise? (2) Have accommodations been made to assist the child in navigating the classroom and school? (3) Has school administration informed other students and their parents of the situation in a thoughtful manner? (4) If the child is receiving hospice care, is there a need for an out-of-hospital DNR order? While a DNR status is generally understood and honored in the hospital and hospice setting, it is rarely supported for children in school or other community settings. Under the Education for All Handicapped Children Act (Public Law 94-142), all children are guaranteed the right to be in the classroom. The question of "What is in the best interest of the individual child?" must be balanced against the interests of others in the situation, such as the school community [5]. Collaborating proactively with school personnel—the nurse in particular—will help to ease anxiety as all involved will have a clear understanding of the detailed plan. They will be prepared to act in the best interest of the child, providing appropriate comfort care rather than unintentionally implementing life-sustaining measures.

Financial Issues

Historically, health care professionals caring for children with life-threatening or life-limiting conditions had few options for treatments covered by Medicaid. Parents in all but a few states had been faced with choosing between curative therapy and hospice services. The Affordable Care Act—signed into law March 23, 2010, by President Obama—enacted a new provision termed the "Concurrent Care for Children" Requirement. This provision is critical for those children and their families seeking a combination of disease-modifying and palliative care services.

Concurrent care (CC) is a dual focus program for children with serious life-limiting conditions up to age 21 years. These conditions are such that life expectancy would be 6 months or less without curative or life-prolonging treatment or interventions. Children with Medicaid insurance or a participating insurance company qualify for this benefit. It allows them to receive curative therapy and life-prolonging treatment concurrent with home-based supportive care focused on pain and symptom management, which improve the child's and family's quality of life.

While states cannot provide fewer services than stipulated by Medicaid, they are free to increase the scope of services paid for by Medicaid and to expand the number of children who might be eligible for them. These options are available at a state's discretion and must be approved by the Centers for Medicare & Medical Services. If a state wants to provide more expansive services and eligibility, there are two basic mechanisms for implementation: (1) a state plan amendment and (2) a Medicaid waiver.

Different Settings of Care at End of Life

Choosing the location for end-of-life care is an important decision for patients and their families. There are, however, limited options for where end-of-life treatment in the pediatric patient population can occur. The majority of deaths of children with chronic conditions in the United States occur in the hospital [6]. Besides the hospital and home settings, there are few other sites available. Relative to children with other chronic conditions, children with cancer are more likely to die at home. Multiple factors are involved in determining the ideal location for end-of-life care, including patient/family preference and resource availability. Children living with end stage cancer frequently have significant care needs. The expertise and support of a specialized PCCT been shown to lead to improved outcomes at end of life in the pediatric oncology patient population [15].

A. **The Hospital:** During the course of cancer treatment, children spend a large amount of time in the hospital and develop close relationships with staff [2]. Thus, many people feel most comfortable staying in the hospital when their condition deteriorates. Though hospitals may not be the most pleasant location, they do possess an abundance of resources, including a variety of specialists, medications, and equipment. If there is concern regarding difficulty in pain control, the hospital setting may be ideal for finding the correct medication regimen. A child's end of life is commonly preceded by a serious treatment or cancer-related complication, which frequently brings them to an intensive care unit. Once it is determined that a patient is actively dying, ideally they would be transferred out of the ICU to the Oncology unit where they are cared for by familiar staff.
B. **Home:** Many families and patients would prefer to spend the remaining time of a child's life in the comfort of their home. A child may appreciate the familiar surroundings and serenity away from the frequent disruptions of the hospital staff. This allows for more privacy, intimacy, and autonomy in decision-making on the part of the family and child. Outpatient palliative care teams assist with end-of-life care at home, which include specialized visits at home by the palliative care team. These services can be managed through a hospital-based palliative care team, community medical practice, or hospice-based agency. Although not all geographic areas have access to a pediatric hospice program, some adult hospices are willing and able to care for pediatric patients, ideally in conjunction with a pediatric provider [2].
C. **Free-Standing Palliative and Respite Care Facilities:** There are very few free-standing facilities that offer inpatient palliative and end-of-life care for children. Families commonly use these facilities for respite care to afford parents and caregivers a short break from the stresses of the day-to-day care of the patient. This type of service is more prevalent in the United Kingdom, whereas in the United States, there are Ryan House in Phoenix, Arizona; George Mark Children's House in San Leandro, California; Exceptional Care for Children in Newark, Delaware; and Crescent Cove in Brooklyn Center, Minnesota [5].

Barriers/Challenges and Strategies to Address Them

Providing care to children with cancer and their families can be rewarding beyond measure. It is not, however, without challenge. Some of the barriers can include (1) withholding information given a desire to protect the child and family; (2) a delay in the palliative care service being invited to collaborate with the primary oncology team; (3) lack of sufficient availability and access to pediatric palliative care; and (4) language and/or cultural barriers [8].

The following story, derived from an amalgamation of actual patient/family situations, serves to illustrate some of the issues identified and ways to address them.

Sarah, the second oldest of four children, was diagnosed with Ewing sarcoma at age 16 years. Her parents are originally from Somalia and the children are American-born. The father and children are bilingual; mother requires an interpreter for more than basic interactions. The family was informed regarding the nature of Sarah's disease and agreed to proceed with treatment with the curative intent. The family is Islamic and states a belief in Allah as the sole deity. They shared their understanding that death is not something to fear; rather they take comfort in knowing that Allah determines the timing of one's life and death.

During initial conversations with Sarah and her parents, there were typically multiple extended family members present. Although Sarah's father and other family offered to provide interpretation for mom, our hospital policy of accessing trained interpreters for medical discussions was explained. The family verbalized understanding and interpreters were utilized consistently. While Sarah was included in most conversations, there were occasions when one or both parents asked to speak privately with the healthcare team.

Sarah is a bright student, eager to learn and happy to be in the classroom with her peers. Initially, treatment was tolerated reasonably well, and Sarah and her parents entertained the idea that she could attend school on a somewhat consistent basis. An educational plan with appropriate accommodations was developed and implemented. As the demands of treatment began to take a toll, Sarah and her parents realized that the majority of her academic learning would have to occur outside of the traditional classroom. A tutor was assigned and became a strong advocate in supporting Sarah's academic goals. School administration was receptive to Sarah attending intermittently when physically able to do so. This served to facilitate ongoing social and emotional connections.

Sarah was able to complete treatment and had no evidence of disease for a period of time. She and her family developed a familiar routine hopeful that Sarah's cancer would remain in their collective past. A routine follow-up scan determined otherwise. Her disease had recurred and was metastatic. Although devastated, the family again embraced the goal of cure. The PPCT was introduced and the family declined their services. Sarah experienced significant side effects from the intense treatment and was frequently in and out of the hospital, at times for extended admissions. Her mother was no longer employed outside the home and dad attempted to work, struggling to meet financial obligations. Sarah's siblings visited with limited frequency and parents stressed the importance of them maintaining their schedules. The extended family, while still available, had less flexibility to be present given their responsibilities.

Sarah's disease continued to progress. Members of each team explained the benefits of the PPCT and the family agreed to their involvement. Therapy directed at cure was discontinued and a new plan was developed. Chemotherapy was intended to stabilize the disease while providing a positive quality of life. Sarah was able to spend more time at home where she received nursing care. The family benefited from the addition of the child life specialist who worked with Sarah's siblings at home. Sarah enjoyed going to school, and her teachers and classmates welcomed her presence. Sarah, although committed to graduating with her class, struggled to complete the required work.

Sarah developed a life-threatening infection necessitating an extended hospitalization. Her respiratory functioning became compromised, and she was transferred to the intensive care unit.

The gravity of Sarah's condition was emphasized and the goals of care reviewed. Her parents disagreed regarding the interventions presented and several extended family members close to Sarah and her parents came forward to be with them. Her father was hopeful Sarah would improve following recovery from the infection; her mother verbalized an evolving understanding that Sarah's body was failing and unlikely to survive. The parents struggled as they faced decisions regarding her care. An older relative was asked by the parents to participate in ongoing discussions with the healthcare team.

As Sarah's condition continued to decline, she asked questions regarding it. Her parents, while previously inclined to include Sarah, requested that medical information be discussed outside the room. Sarah, noticing this change, began to share her concerns with her nurses. She also talked openly with her tutor who had remained an important person in her life. Sarah expressed a desire to graduate and the tutor worked together with school administration to have a high school diploma awarded.

As Sarah's parents debated whether or not to proceed with intubation, the staff described their increasing distress as they experienced Sarah growing weaker and struggling to breathe. Both parents voiced concern that to not intubate would interfere with Allah's timing. They requested spiritual care, and a leader from their community was arranged to meet with the family and then together with the healthcare team. Staff, meanwhile, shared Sarah's understanding of her circumstances and disclosed her stated desire to return home. Ultimately, the decision was made to not have Sarah intubated. In accordance with her wishes, Sarah was taken home, where she received hospice services. She died there several days later surrounded by her parents and siblings.

References

1. Bardia A, Sood A, Barton DL, Loprinzi CL. Integrative medicine in symptom management and palliative care. In: Abrams DI, Weil A, editors. Integrative oncology. New York: Oxford University Press; 2009. p. 470–6.
2. Bergstraesser E, Flury M. Care at the end of life for children with cancer. In: Wolfe J, Jones BL, Kreicbergs U, Jankovic M, editors. Palliative Care in Pediatric Oncology. Cham: Springer International Publishing; 2018. p. 218–26.
3. Blanco JMC, Jones E. The interdisciplinary oncology team and the role of palliative care consultation. In: Wolfe J, Jones BL, Kreicbergs U, Jankovic M, editors. Palliative care in pediatric oncology. Cham: Springer International Publishing; 2018. p. 45–7.
4. Bluebond-Langner M, Langner RW. Impact of cancer on the child, parents, siblinghs and community. In: Wolfe J, Jones BL, Kreicbergs U, Jankovic M, editors. Palliative care in pediatric oncology. Cham: Springer International Publishing; 2018. p. 21–2.
5. Carroll JM, Wright JL, Frankel LR. Settings of care. In: Wolfe J, Hinds PS, Sourkes BM, editors. Textbook of interdisciplinary pediatric palliative care. Philadelphia: Elsevier Saunders; 2011. p. 64–72.
6. Feudtner C, Feinstein JA, Satchell M, Zhao H, Kang TI. Shifting place of death among children with complex chronic conditions in the United States, 1989–2003. JAMA. 2007;297(24):2725–32.
7. Lindley LC. Health care reform and concurrent care for terminally ill children: a policy analysis. J Hosp Palliat Nurs. 2011;13(2):81–8.
8. Mack JW, Hinds PS. Practical aspects of communication. In: Wolfe J, Hinds PS, Sourkes BM, editors. Textbook of interdisciplinary pediatric palliative care. Philadelphia: Elsevier Saunders; 2011. p. 179–88.
9. Mary J, Labyak Institute for Innovation. Continuum briefing on pediatric palliative care. Alexandria: National Hospice and Palliative Care Organization; 2012. Available from https://www.nhpco.org/wp-content/uploads/2019/04/Continuum_Briefing.pdf
10. Mulkerin CM. Palliative Care Consultation. In: Altilio T, Otis-Green S, editors. Oxford textbook of palliative social work. New York: Oxford University Press; 2011. p. 43–4.
11. National Hospice and Palliative Care Organization website: Concurrent Care for Children. Available from https://www.nhpco.org/palliative-care-overview/pediatric-palliative-and-hospice-care/pediatric-concurrent-care/concurrent-care-for-children/
12. Papadatou D, Bluebond-Langner M, Goldman A. The Team. In: Wolfe J, Hinds PS, Sourkes BM, editors. Textbook of interdisciplinary pediatric palliative care. Philadelphia: Elsevier Saunders; 2011. p. 55–6.
13. Postovsky S, Lehavi A, Attias O, Hershman E. Easing of physical distress in pediatric cancer. In: Wolfe J, Jones BL, Kreicbergs U, Jankovic M, editors. Palliative care in pediatric oncology. Cham: Springer International Publishing; 2018. p. 120–38.
14. Rosenberg AR, Wolfe J, Jones B. Palliative care for children with cancer and their families. In: Abrams AN, Muriel AC, Wiener L, editors. Pediatric psychosocial oncology: Textbook for multidisciplinary care. Cham: Springer International Publishing; 2016. p. 244.

15. Schmidt P, Otto M, Hechler T, Metzing S, Wolfe J, Zernikow B. Did increased availability of pediatric palliative care lead to improved palliative care outcomes in children with cancer? J Palliat Med. 2013;16(9):1034–9.
16. SEER Cancer Statistics Review 1975–2016, National Cancer Institute. Sections 28. Childhood Cancer by Site: Incidence, Survival and Mortality. Available from https://seer.cancer.gov/csr/1975_2016/results_merged/sect_28_childhood_cancer.pdf.
17. Stark D. Teamwork in palliative care: An integrative approach. In: Altilio T, Otis-Green S, editors. Oxford textbook of palliative social work. New York: Oxford University Press; 2011. p. 415–7.
18. Wolfe J, Grier HE, Klar N, Levin SB, Ellenbogen JM, Salem-Schatz S, et al. Symptoms and suffering at end of life in children with cancer. N Engl J Med. 2000;342(5):326–33.
19. Wolfe J, Orellana L, Ullrich C, Cook EF, Kang TI, Rosenberg A, et al. Symptoms and distress in children with advanced cancer: prospective patient-reported outcomes from the PediQUEST study. J Clin Oncol. 2015;33(17):1928–35.
20. World Health Organization (1998) WHO definition of palliative care for children. Available from https://www.who.int/cancer/palliative/definition/en/
21. World Health Organization (2014) WHO definition of palliative care. https://www.who.int/cancer/palliative/definition/en/

Information Technology Tools for Palliative Care for Populations

Richard R. Love and Sheikh I. Ahamed

Imagination at scale is our only recourse. [1]

For most patients in the world needing end-of-life symptom-addressing palliative care, providers are not available or accessible, health systems are weak, and the quality and efficacy of the interventions received, if any, are likely to be low [2, 3]. Seventy to 80% of cancer deaths are accompanied by severe pain [4]. Pain is also a major symptom in patients dying of other common non-communicable diseases [5]. As an example, in Nepal, estimates for 2012 based on mortality data are that pain at the end of life was an issue for 67% of patients dying of cardiovascular disease (CVD) and 67% of patients dying of chronic obstructive pulmonary disease (COPD), and experts opined that these figures may be low [6]. Thus, approaches to palliative care in the community focusing on cancer are clearly going to be relevant for larger numbers of patients suffering from more common CVD and COPD syndromes.

In the face of always-limited resources and perhaps less than compelling data regarding the favorable impact of palliative care, communities, caregivers, and certainly patients globally suffer [2, 3]. The Lancet Commission has highlighted the details of the problems and broad policy matters, and that in fact, relatively rather limited financial resources are projected to be necessary to have a major impact [2]. However, the Commission has offered rather sparse insight into the individual patient palliative care delivery challenges that follow from use of technologies, employed business models, and organization of medical care. The Commission does talk about the concept of competencies among needed health-care professionals, de-emphasizing specific professions, calls for expanded roles of general and community nurses in palliative care, and emphasizes the need for services linkages, but specific models for doing these things are not widely discussed or described, and the potentially major roles of information technology (IT) tools as enablers in these critical areas are not explored [2]. Perhaps, to a far-too-great extent, we believe that we understand what the problems of implementing such concepts are, and what the models for care should be, when in fact global challenges, broad loco-regional issues, and appropriate social change models are dominant determinants of any greater success in global palliative care [7]. Stepping back, as we have stated in our chapter opening sentence, we suggest that we should frame the central problems as weak primary health-care systems (provider-centered instead of patient-centered) in which patients have no or very limited access to providers (the major specific loco-regional issue) and limited

R. R. Love (✉) · S. I. Ahamed
Department of Computer Science, Marquette University, Milwaukee, WI, USA
e-mail: sheikh.ahamed@marquette.edu

M. Silbermann (ed.), *Palliative Care for Chronic Cancer Patients in the Community*,
https://doi.org/10.1007/978-3-030-54526-0_2

ability to provide patient-specific/tailored (i.e., precision medicine), and critically, effective symptom interventions (the area where focus on social change models is much called for). Availability of morphine itself, while critical, as the Lancet Commission and the Economist analysis state, is not by itself enough [2, 3]. In the face of these, the major care "models" are firstly, dizzyingly academic and comprehensive (there are suggested to be eight domains for palliative care) with completely impractical, overwhelmingly complex, and lengthy patient care guidelines [5, 8] and secondly, community, in contrast to health system-organized, with an astonishing breadth of critical and needed activities [9, 10]. There appears to be a disconnect between these models and the two central problems in general palliative care identified above. Importantly, the first-line critical challenge is limiting the physical and mental suffering of all individual patients. Who can do this and what can they do? The focus for this chapter is on information technology (IT) tools, but context is everything, and so in part 1 of this communication, the focus is on palliative care barriers and metrics, patient-centered care models, details of current and ideal health service models, and elements of disruptive innovation, which set the stage for the exposition that follows in part 2, of the significant roles and promise of IT tools in delivering high-quality, affordable palliative care across all populations in alternative health-care delivery models.

Part 1: Palliative Care in the Context of Global Health Services

Current Framing of the Problem(S) in Delivering Palliative Care to all in Need

Two aforementioned major communications have sought to frame the challenges of better global palliative care—the Lancet Commission and The Economist Quality of Death Index project [2, 3]. Their major conclusions are important for what they say and do not say. The Lancet Commission takes a very global, international top-down, mostly policy approach in its analysis, highlighting six major issues, implying that addressing these might successfully improve palliative care (Table 1) [2].

Table 1 Barriers explaining neglect of palliative care globally (Lancet Commission, 2)

Opiophobia and focus on prevention of non-medical use of narcotics
Health outcome measures that ignore pain and suffering
Dearth of interventions
Medical focus on cure
Limited public advocacy
General neglect of non-communicable diseases in low- and middle-income countries

In the context of broad palliative care activities globally, these Table 1 points prompt the following take-home practical messages:

1. As noted above, availability of morphine is critical, but complex psychosocial and dysfunctional health systems issues often prevent its specific availability and use in practice. Getting our clinical practice houses in order for palliative care is critical if morphine is to be appropriately used.
2. Palliative care-focused health outcome measures are available; they are broadly underused. The use of tools for symptom assessment is an absolutely central issue in the development of high-quality care for all, and this subject will be majorly addressed later here.
3. The interventions concern is important; the major site of critical interventions however is the patient–provider interaction.
4. The fourth, fifth, and sixth listed barrier circumstances in Table 1 are not easily and rapidly addressable.

The Economist project developed a methodology for assessing quality of palliative care across countries [3]. In its second analysis, it summarizes specific indicators of higher-quality palliative care by its measures, again by implication, suggesting that addressing these issues is critical to improving palliative care (Table 2).

Table 2 National indicators of higher-quality palliative care. (2015 Quality of death index of the Economist, 3)

National policies addressing palliative care
Higher levels of public spending
Patient care subsidies
Extensive training of health professionals
Availability of opiate drugs
Public awareness

Focus on these indicators prompts a different and second set of take-home practical messages:

1. Unquestionably, there are national policies that are critical to better public palliative care; those with respect to morphine are the prime example. This said, the practice of clinical medicine is a complex psychosocial activity, changes in which are remarkably difficult to achieve with "top-down" national policy approaches. Impactful social change models are field-practice-focused.
2. The spending and patient care subsidies needs are poorly justified when they are not associated with specific clinical practice interventions and systems.
3. The repeated calls for increased training of palliative care specialists and all primary care health providers is first an unrealistic approach to the growing population needs; no country will ever be able to train adequate numbers of such providers. Further, it is not at all clear that this is the most efficient way of making skilled providers more widely available.

As noted above, what is missing from these barrier and indicator summaries is discussion of the organization of medical care—which so powerfully impacts what happens to individual patients worldwide—and the role of information technology in palliative care.

Broad Perspectives: Doctor/Provider-Centered Versus Patient-Centered Care and Premises for Current and Ideal Health Service Models

The specific needs and wishes of patients needing palliative care at the end of life bring attention to the major differences between by far the most common doctor provider-centered systems globally and patient-centered systems. In Table 3, the first three of the eight principles of patient-centered medical care should lead to activities that tend to be far less emphasized in doctor-centered care.

Table 3 Eight principles of patient-centered medical care [11]

Access to care
Physical comfort
Coordination and integration of care
Respect for patient preferences
Information and education
Emotional support
Involvement of family and friends
Continuity and transition

In doctor-centered medical care, the expectation is that the patient will come to the practitioner for help—aka "solutions", while in patient-centered palliative care, because of the very circumstances of patients with high symptom burdens, patients and families need the care to come to them. The organization of medical care globally is dominantly doctor-centered in this respect. And this model prevails in the face of limited provider numbers and often distant-from-patients in sites of service provision.

While surprising and illogical, there is far too little focus in patient encounters on the details of physical symptoms; providers simply do not seek such data with regularity [12]. Considerable further evidence on this issue will be presented below.

Finally, specifically with respect to palliative care, model systems for coordination and integration of care are rare, again because the optimal and dominant site of care is the patient's home, not providers' offices or hospitals where the personnel resources (if there are any) for such activities are present.

While here we have started with the broad concept of patient-centered care and its application to palliative care, another perspective is to consider the basic premises of medical care as currently practiced globally, and those that might characterize an ideal medical system, because many issues in such a review are basic to getting to how we can better address palliative care. In his enlightening volume Turning the world upside down, Nigel Crisp highlights current common and ideal premises [13]. In Table 4, we have summarized his ideas in modified ways.

These premises touch on some issues already considered above: public health versus individual patient focus—another view of the access issues; Hospital-physician office-centered care; and National/Federal—"top" down—solutions. This table also highlights premises critical in developing better palliative care services. Specifically,

- The issue of professionalism. Unlike in many other businesses where the specific tasks have been carefully identified and technicians have been trained to carry out these tasks, in medical care, there has been considerable resistance to delegation of care tasks to non-professionals. As has been suggested above, this position simply cannot stand if we are to achieve better palliative care for populations.
- The issue of site of accountability. With the dominance of a business model for medicine globally, the place of basic medical and palliative care as a human right has been shoved aside.
- The issue of appropriate business models; while the unsustainability of current high-income country models is evident and recognized, a focus on public health-promoting business models is still lacking.
- Finally, the need for potentially disruptive change in our health-care models is accepted, but not happening rapidly, and when and where major changes occur, they are not widely noted [14].

Table 4 Critical premises for a twenty-first century health model for populations contrasted with those currently operative in many high-income countries[a]

Ideal model	Current high-income country models
Start by understanding society	Start with descriptive data on diseases
Public health-focused	Individual patient-focused
Community and outpatient-centered	Hospital or doctor's office-centered
Non-professionalized approach	Deeply professionalized approach
Locally defined solutions, with reliance on local skills	National or federal solutions
Supportive of, complements, supplements, and strengthens primary health system	Primary health system is peripheral
Accountable to community	Accountable to business owners
Belief in co-dependence with other institutions globally as partners	Focus on independence
Deep beliefs in fairness, accountability, and transparency	Deepest focus on disease outcomes
Business models need to be defined	Business models are flawed
Constantly redesigning itself	Fixed models
Complementary central community issue activities are critical	Health care is an independent activity

[a]Summarized, supplemented, and modified from 13

Reframing Solutions: Disruptive Innovation

How can we become focused and pull out of this foregoing discussion a blueprint for taking concrete actions to develop better palliative care systems more rapidly? Christensen has provided the critical framework in his work on disruptive innovation [15]. The key elements are presented in Table 5.

Considering the first element, we need to standardize our processes, making them rule-based, simpler, affordable, and effective. Otherwise stated, we need to break down the "care" in palliative care into specific tasks, and crucially, bring to bear information "technological enablers" to make successful completion of tasks possible.

Table 5 The key elements of disruptive innovation solutions for health care [15]

Simplifying technology
Business model innovation
Value networks

These general premise statements beg formulation of premises, specifically for palliative care systems. In part 2 of this chapter to follow, we summarize the critical general premises and use Christensen's key elements for disruptive solutions, which well frame the crucial roles that information technology hardware and new software tools can play in definitions of more widely applicable and effective palliative care services.

Part 2: Information Technology Tools and Creation of Local High-Quality Palliatve Care Service Models

Practical Ground Rules for Achievable Progress

The foregoing discussion strongly suggests that we should approach improving palliative care service for populations by the following:

- Focusing first on specific measures to increase and improve patient–provider interactions.
- Acknowledging that financial resources and evidence for benefits are limited, and therefore taking local step-by-step experimental approaches.
- Designing whatever local innovations we develop, in light of the need to contribute to the gradual development of ideal health services models (Table 4).
- Focusing on symptom management, recognizing that physical comfort is the sine qua non of successful palliative care, whose key metric is pain.
- Developing business models which facilitate access for all, are patient-centered in providing home care, and are affordable.
- Organizing our services simply and in ways that encourage coordination and integration of component personnel.
- While making every effort in integration and liaisoning with existing local resources, limited as they may be, recognizing that we need to develop specific "solutions shops" for palliative care [15] (similar to specialty facilities in cataract surgery, cardiovascular disease, cancer, and other specialized surgery).

The unavoidable core conclusions is that the need is to develop capacity to take solutions to patients in their homes, and secondly, to have "centers," "solution shops," to process and act on patient cases [15]. Palliative end-of-life care of adequately high quality to make a difference is specialty care. The expectation that it is possible to have adequate specialists and all primary care providers available for the infrequently needed provision of such care at a given point in time in specific communities is unrealistic. What is new are information technology tools to address these challenges and needs efficiently and effectively.

Element #1: Simplifying Technology [15]

Following Christensen's framework, we need to first break down the components of the patient–provider palliative care process into specific routine tasks, and crucially, bring to bear on these information technology "enablers" to make successful completion of the tasks possible (Table 6).

What are the information technology "enablers" to allow operational efficiencies in accomplishing these tasks? The widespread availability and use of cell phones and the internet and worldwide web now provide the hardware infrastructure for software tools for efficient and precise conduct of these tasks (Table 7). The first part of the discussion then is how these tasks can be well completed; who and how these tasks can be done then follows.

IT Software Tool #1: Messaging and Social Media

Tasks 1, 2, and 3 in Table 6 concern "awareness" or making sure that all patients and families in need in communities know how to access local resources for help in palliative care situations. While computer access and thus worldwide web access using search engines may be limited for many citizens in low- and middle-income countries, cell phones are now available almost universally. In Nepal, there are as many cell phones

Table 6 The patient-level provider/health system task list

1. Make patients and family members aware of specific contact people/resources locally they can call on for palliative care assistance
2. Reach out to seek local community members in need of palliative care
3. Inform patients and families in need of palliative care of a process for their getting such help through local resources
4. Provide patients with a symptom questionnaire to describe repeatedly their physical discomforts and their intensities
5. Work with patients and families to create moderately detailed summaries of patients' active medical conditions
6. Create palliative care center capacity to provide services in circumstances when patients and families cannot be physically present in the center
7. Create palliative care center capacity to provide affordable, symptom-targeted, high-quality interventions to patients and families based on symptom reports and medical summaries
8. Create palliative care centers with expandable front-line palliative care clinical specialist capacity to receive, analyze, clarify, and better specify symptom reports and medical summaries
9. Establish business practices and mechanisms for payment for the local- and center-specific services and share this information with families in need

Table 7 Information technology software tools for completing major patient–provider palliative care tasks

Cell phone and internet social media materials and messages
Cell phone and web-based platform symptom questionnaires
Web-based basic medical summary electronic health record
Cell phone or internet-facilitated virtual caregiver–patient visits and sharing of personal patient and family educational materials (telemedicine)
Web-based automated decision-making algorithms for symptom management and machine learning refinements of these based on clinical management symptom report data

as there are people. While the fraction of cell phones that are smartphones varies widely across countries, many phones have multiple features. Broadly, messaging systems such as SMS (short message services) are widely available and provide a basic mechanism for addressing tasks 1–3 in local communities. Such mechanisms are low cost and direct and engage recipients effectively; they can reach large and geographically distant populations. Text messaging generally has been favorably impactful in health activities and in effecting specific behavioral change [16, 17]. While the greater experience has to date been in high-income country settings, digital tools have been effective in improving treatment for tuberculosis in Africa [18].

When social media sources are accessible, often among adult children of older adults in need of palliative care, internet websites, Twitter, Facebook, and Instagram can provide podcasts, links, videos, and photos. An in-country system we are developing in Nepal provides such an example and will be further discussed below (homepalliativecare Nepal.net). Increasing data, again admittedly from high-income country settings, suggest that social media tools can be significantly and favorably impactful in health [19, 20].

IT Software Tool #2: Symptom Questionnaires

The absolute central focus of palliative care has to be on patient symptoms and their minimization. Our major metric for palliative care is pain [2]. Thus, Task 4 in Table 6 is a, if not the major issue in palliative care, for we cannot manage impactful symptoms whose nature and intensities are not clearly defined.

Assessment of symptoms has been increasingly accomplished by use of symptom questionnaires. As the scope of outcomes from patient interventions is obviously greater than that of only symptoms, including more global measures such as "quality of life," disability-adjusted life-years of survival, and of course overall survival, the term patient reported outcomes (PROs) has been used, particularly by palliative care specialists, to describe all such measures [21]. Here we have chosen to use the more understandable basic term—symptom questionnaires—because for major clinical purposes, we wish to focus on management of patients' symptoms, and not on additional outcomes measures, and the instruments we believe are critical deal only with symptoms.

For a long time, the use of symptom questionnaires has been seen by clinicians as a burden, whose time-consuming and impractical applications were poorly justified by any obvious benefit. It has been assumed by clinicians that they can more efficiently acquire such critical data directly from questioning patients, when this is simply not the case. The situation has very much changed over the last decade, such that symptom questionnaires are now seen as a key tool in patient-centered care, and nowhere is this tool more central than in palliative care, particularly that component focusing on physical symptoms. An additional issue for some clinicians has been uncertainty regarding the validity of data from symptom questionnaires. Three general developments have put these validity concerns to rest. First, the use of multiple instruments has been shown to provide the same picture—thus providing external validity. Second, careful analyses of clusters of answers in symptom questionnaires have shown internally consistent results, providing internal validity data. Third, and really the most compelling development, has been new results of clinical trials demonstrating clear improvements in "hard" patient outcomes associated with symptom questionnaire use (emergency room visits, hospitalizations, survival) [22, 23]. The now-documented benefits are outlined in Table 8.

There are a number of well-validated symptom questionnaires tailored to different clinical situations. Recent authors have emphasized the easy usability of symptom questionnaires. It should be noted that adding or possibly subtracting a question or two to an established, validated instrument should hardly be challenged. Our own symptom questionnaire is presented here in Table 9 [35]. This instrument was created to serve cancer patients in low- and middle-income countries where symptoms consequent to treatment toxicities are uncommon.

What is key now is that the benefits of symptom questionnaires have been demonstrated and magnified by placing these instruments on cell phone and web-based platforms [22–24, 27, 29, 30, 32–34]. The use of these software IT tools clearly provides multiple benefits, specifically for both patients and providers (Table 8). For patients, what is really important is engaging them in the central issues of their medical conditions. Patient hopelessness and suffering are in part addressed by this engagement per se [38]. For providers, the previous excess burdens associated with the use of these questionnaires as paper tools have been removed; it is possible to make comprehensive and specific repeated patient symptom data easily accessible for both

Table 8 Benefits of use of symptom questionnaires [6, 12, 21–34]

Provide data justifying palliative care service needs
Facilitate accessibility of patients to care providers
Prompt clinicians to increase attention to symptom management
Improvement in symptom control with increased adherence to interventions
Provide richer, multiple metric data than those for only pain and its intensity
Enhancement of patient–clinician communication
Increased patient satisfaction
Empowerment of patients and families with increased participation in care
Suggested improved quality of life and increased survival
Suggested more effective in particular in lower socio-economic groups with less computer literacy
Essentially technology enablers, allowing precision medicine

Table 9 The Marquette Symptom Assessment Survey (MarqueSAS) [35]

Nausea[a]
Tiredness[a]
Depression[a]
Anxiety[a]
Drowsiness[a]
Appetite[a]
Well-being[a]
Shortness of breath[a]
Current pain[a]
In the last 24 hours: Worst level of pain[b]
Lowest level of pain[b]
Usual level of pain[b]
Constipation
Quantity of sleep
Quality of sleep

[a]From the Edmonton Symptom Assessment Survey [36]
[b]From the Brief Pain Inventory [37]

providers and patients. While a review of all of the new data justifying the statements in Table 8 is beyond the practical scope of this chapter, the work reported over the last 15 years in the listed references provides strong support for these summary conclusions. Clearly, we need more data, particularly data on application of these symptom data tools in low-resource settings. In this context, we can share our own experience.

We developed a cell phone (android and IOS) platform-based visual and audible instructional "app" for our MarqueSAS (Table 9). We have used this in preliminary longitudinal patient populations in Bangladesh, and in a one-time assessment cross sectional study in over 1000 patients with advanced cancers presenting to tertiary care centers in Bangladesh and Nepal [24, 35]. What was remarkable was that all of the patients were able to easily and quickly answer the questionnaire items, even patients who were illiterate; they all essentially said they would be comfortable using this "app" to report repeatedly on their symptoms. We have now moved on to developing a Nepalese website and physician web-app to receive and organize patient symptom reports and provide a menu of written and video interventions, which can be sent to patients' cell phones or patient or family email sites (homepalliativecareNepal.net). Our cell phone symptom questionnaire "app" named NAPCare is available for free at https://play.google.com/store/search?q=napcare.

As the last bullet point in Table 8 states, the use of symptom questionnaires with IT tools allows higher-quality "precision" symptom management medicine, and this technology enabler can be made available to essentially everyone.

IT Software Tool #3: Basic Medical Summary Electronic Health Record

Besides having past and current broad patient symptom data, central to providing adequately high-quality palliative care to make a difference is having a sufficiently detailed summary of major relevant and active individual patient medical diagnoses and problems (Task 5 in Table 6). In Table 10, we suggest what such a summary should cover. The challenge here is to get in one place for patients, and local and sometimes distant center providers to see, the information critical to making, together with symptom data, patient-tailored palliative care management recommendations. All-too-frequently, clinicians are either working with inadequate basic patient status information or are spending excess time searching (again and again) for key information. Creating this summary is too often seen as an overwhelming burden, when in fact paraprofessional medical technicians can be trained to do this task remarkably well. Putting such a summary into some kind of web-based system associated with a center (as discussed below) creates essentially an electronic medical record summary, which can be easily amended, but most importantly easily accessed and used.

Our assumptions in defining the specific items in this list are the following. First, our major patient population is that of patients with malignancies. Here then the primary cancer site, the state of clinically evident and potentially symptom-causing regional and metastatic disease needs to be clarified. The later Table 10 item on details of common symptoms is listed because disease involvement at specific anatomic sites

Table 10 Components of basic palliative care patient medical summary

Primary cancer site
Dominant or potentially life-threatening loco-regional or distant cancer metastatic site
Secondary loco-regional or distant cancer metastatic site
Cardiac disease
Ischemic heart disease
Congestive heart failure
Other cardiac disease
Chronic obstructive pulmonary disease
Diabetes mellitus
Cerebrovascular disease
Other major health problem
Any medication causing allergic or major adverse reaction
Details of common symptoms
Patient's major health concern

needs to be stated if the pathophysiology of patient's symptoms is to be appropriately understood. An example: Writing the word bone under "Dominant.... distant cancer metastatic site," can only be helpful if the particular anatomic sites known to be affected are identified. Having to make assumptions that metastatic cancer lesions cause particular symptoms, without some specific objective symptom data, leads to interventions that are too often ineffective.

Other common non-communicable diseases are listed in this medical summary table only to acknowledge their active presence (often existing because the general population of patients with major malignancies is older and therefore likely to be so afflicted), and because in advanced stages, these common conditions and their management must temper optimal symptom management.

Finally, this table lists "Patient's major health concern" because far too often providers make assumptions about what bothers patients most (even in the face of good symptom questionnaire data), when an uncommon physical or a mental or other domain issue is in fact most important to an individual patient (Table 3).

In summary, after a symptom questionnaire, the second critical mini-database necessary for high-quality palliative care is an electronic summary medical record. Here we are not asking for a complete re-creation of a patient's medical history and listing of all of his/her problems; rather, we are insisting that good care cannot be given without an adequately detailed summary of current major active medical problems. Use of these two basic instruments with IT facilitated means is central to the development of affordable, widely available, and as stated high-quality effective, palliative care. Their regular use essentially "standardizes the process" [15].

IT Software Tool #4: Cell Phone or Internet-Facilitated Virtual Caregiver–Patient Visit Programs

Task 6 in Table 6 is the provision of virtual palliative care center service capacity. The concept and necessity of palliative care centers will be approached below as a business model matter, together with the payment model challenges of non-visit care. Here, we wish to highlight the powerful capacity of new cell phone and internet systems to allow "virtual" (i.e., not face to face physically) patient and family visits with providers. Historically, the organization of medical care has not placed major value on patients' time and the indirect costs of provider office- and hospital-based care. With palliative care, the "site of care" issue comes very much to the fore. The downsides of office/hospital-based care have been too long ignored. One example from our own data illustrates how our current systems sadly contribute to patient suffering. In our cross sectional study in outpatient tertiary care facility clinics in Dhaka, Bangladesh and Kathmandu, Nepal, patients reported that their current pain levels were higher than their usual pain levels, presumably because of the discomforts and symptom-alleviating disruptions associated with getting to a tertiary care facility [24].

Duffy and Lee have recently well described why in-person health care should be "option B" [39]. They emphasize, and this is particularly applicable to palliative care, that development of virtual care systems should be an explicit goal, and we agree. Further, as they write, the burden should be on the providers to develop such systems.

Cell phone and internet-based conferencing capacities are now multiple: for the former WhatsApp and I-phone Facetime, and for the latter Skype, Zoom, and Gotomeeting. Telemedicine programs are increasing and remarkably successful [40]. In the two general component services model we have been alluding to heretofore (and will expand upon below) i.e., local community palliative care specialists and palliative care centers, the experience with telemedicine services has not unexpectedly been that over time the skills and capacities of the local providers increase with decreased dependence on the centers [41]. There is a desperate need to develop such local country and community prototypes in palliative care—the basic IT tools are available.

IT Software Tool #5: Web-Based Automated Decision-Making Algorithms

The central critical activity in palliative care is providing appropriate patient-symptom-tailored effective interventions. The major emphasis in better addressing this task for populations has been on training of all health-care providers and on increasing the numbers of palliative care specialists [3]. As has been suggested at the beginning of this chapter, creation of different kinds of palliative care specialists/technicians may offer an alternative and more realistic approach; the nature of these specialists will be further discussed below. Our current patient–provider care loops are woefully "black box" (from symptoms to interventions), and adequately high-quality care is so dependent on high levels of training for the providers. The purpose of Table 6 has been to spell out the specific tasks to make the processes of individual patient care transparent and thus more effectively addressable.

What has been missing from the discussions however has been the role that creation of patient symptom management automated artificial intelligence-facilitated decision-making systems can play in efficiently and productively meeting this care demand, and this is critical Task 7 (Table 6 above).

Bell has summarized the significant potential of such software systems, and Kamdar and Mooney have provided recent detailed examples of these in palliative care [27, 29]. Asch et al. have described how such systems can meaningfully contribute to the creation of better health system operations [42].

The breadth of symptoms and the basic evidence about useful interventions are well summarized by Kelley (5, suppl). Mooney et al. demonstrated how such multi-symptom-addressing applications might work, while Kamdar et al. focused on pain management [27, 29]. In addressing the development of algorithms for malignancies, it is clear that definition of optimal baseline interventions for the same symptom might differ by cancer type, and symptom site, and thus, key input data for individual patients will be that from his/her basic medical summary in addition to her symptom questionnaire information. For example, lumbo-sacral vertebral bone pain associated with multiple myeloma might be approached differently than similar site pain associated with metastatic lung cancer. Decision trees, which allow recognition of very treatable symptom causes such as infection or bronchospasm in the case of lung cancer, are important. What needs to happen now is to create and share initial patient symptom management dynamic algorithms and accumulate significant experience with these and their impacts on symptom intensities to use machine learning to refine algorithm specifics. This kind of software tool then can be used by palliative care specialists first at centers to define quickly a selection of potential interventions, which can then, based on "exception" individual patient information, be directed to the patient.

This type of symptom management tool capacity will be critical to extending high-quality palliative care to greater number of patients through paraprofessional providers. The essentials of the model we are proposing are presented in Fig. 1.

Element #2: Business Model/Health System innovation to Routinize Critical Elements of Palliative Care [15]

As has been stated in earlier discussions, we propose that instead of emphasizing palliative care expertise and training throughout health-care systems, the central activities of palliative care should be carried out in centers for palliative care (Task 8, Table 6). Such a model for high-quality palliative care services is no different than those successfully developed and promoted for eye cataract care [43]. The core argument is that such centers can deliver high-quality, cost-effective care because in essence, in employing Christensen's simplification technology model and standardized processes, they can care for larger numbers of patients [15, 42]. What we have proposed above in the discussion of such centers as tele-medicine operations is that they

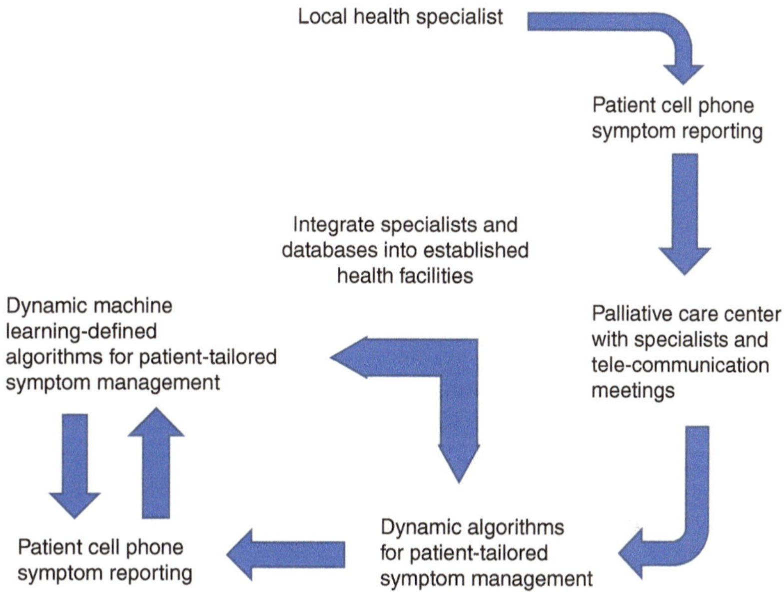

Fig. 1 Putting IT all together: Health system changes with increased palliative care paraprofessionals and IT tools

are planned as true centers, that is providers of regional, not just local use, expertise.

The second critical component of our disruptive innovation model is paraprofessional palliative care specialists locally and in centers. They may come from different health-care backgrounds—nursing or pharmacy primarily—and maybe attached to different local health-care organizations. The principle tasks for these specialists were defined in #s 1–6 in Table 6, and it is primarily for these tasks that their training should be targeted. Their work now can productively be carried out with the five software tools we have discussed in detail above. In some sense, we are talking about local navigators for patients and families in need of palliative care. First, they are the point people for awareness about palliative care resources and systems (Tasks 1–3, Table 6). Next, they become experts in facilitating patient access to a cell phone-based symptom questionnaire and teaching patients how to use this tool (Task 4), Finally, they work with the patient and family to establish the necessary medical summary (Task 5). Heretofore, training in palliative care has been majorly about biology, physiology, and interventions, when such information can only be well used by providers who are engaged in this kind of care every day. Training for these five tasks is completely different and absolutely manageable to create a new type of health-care specialist. The concept of local community health-care workers with specialty focus has been of course broadly applied in maternal and child health with enormous success. Over time, the local specialists will become more involved in Task 6—interaction with palliative care centers—and tele-medicine conferencing and then logically with implementation of intervention recommendations.

Paraprofessional palliative care specialists at palliative care centers can have focused capacity to receive, analyze, clarify, and better specify symptom reports and medical summaries (Task 8). These specialists are the front-line professionals for face to face or virtual patient/family visits (Task 6) and use of software management algorithms to define and work to implement appropriate interventions (Task 7). Discussions of use of "technicians" in such capacities often get bogged down over concerns about the nuances and details of patients' specific circumstances, which appropriately define better targeting of interventions, and the need for "super specialists" to therefore provide such care. We believe that we can build into the initial algorithms necessary "exception management" flags, and that in fact over time, nursing paraprofessional palliative care specialists in centers can become experts in carrying out these tasks.

With palliative care centers, and local and in-center paraprofessional palliative care specialists, the third essential component of such a model system is, of course, finances (Task 9, Table 6). While payment systems have been in high-income country settings the perceived major barrier to implementation of such a disruptive model of care with tele-medicine service at its core, in fact these are becoming increasingly manageable and accepted by patients and families, particularly when the specifics of the care system are engaged in and transparent to these consumers—the repeated use of a symptom questionnaire; the creation of a medical summary; the convenience of tele-medicine virtual visits; the focus on patient's major health concerns and physical symptoms [39]. Efficient, patient-symptom-tailored care using the software tools we have emphasized here can be inexpensive for patients and families, even when they are paying the direct costs completely themselves. Electronic payment systems can be facilitating; in-person visits by family members to palliative care centers (as for prescriptions) can allow use of the usual outpatient visit charging mechanisms; and over time, governmental and non-governmental organizational support for local paraprofessionals and palliative care centers can be expected with demonstration of operational efficacy and patient outcome data.

Element #3: Value Networks [15]

While it is implicit in the foregoing discussion of the two health system components—palliative care centers and local palliative care specialists—that these must work well together for a successful palliative care model, Christensen emphasizes that in such innovated systems, it is vital for all stake-holders to recognize coherent value in each component.

We need to convince providers of the value of all parts of the system:

- Ease of administration.
- Ease of access.
- Ease of understanding.
- Guidance to action.
- Confidence of quality and security.

in order to promote a strong widespread desire to use the system.

Summary

We have proposed a theory and general medical system practice-grounded approach to accelerating improvement of palliative care for patients in widely different health systems. Our approach is "bottoms up" focusing on innovation that needs to happen at the local patient–provider encounter level. We envision potential for leap-frogging the challenges that prevent many systems now from developing better palliative care efforts. Almost universal cell phone and web-internet capacities now provide the hardware infrastructure for use of information technology software tools in five critical areas for palliative care: increasing local patient and family awareness, symptom questionnaires, basic medical summary, virtual patient visits, and algorithms for tailored symptom management. Employment of these tools within a palliative care-niche model with local paraprofessional specialists and palliative care centers can offer "public health palliative care." Imagining at scale and experimenting with such software tools and palliative care organizational models is the way forward [1, 7]. Models will evolve over time.

References

1. Ledgard J. In: Taub B, editor. Jonathan Ledgard believes imagination could save the world: New York: The New Yorker; 2019.

2. Knaul FM, Farmer PE, Krakauer EL, et al. Alleviating the access abyss in palliative care and pain relief—an imperative of universal health coverage: The Lancet Commission report. Lancet. 2018;391:1391–454.
3. The Economist Intelligence Unit. The 2015 quality of death index: ranking palliative care across the world: London: The Economist; 2015.
4. Cleary J, Gelband H, Wagner J. Cancer pain relief. In: Cancer disease control priorities 3. Washington, D.C.: The World Bank; 2015.
5. Kelley AS, Morrison RS. Palliative care for the seriously ill. New Engl J Med. 2015;373:747–55.
6. Swarbrick EM, Pietroni MAC, Munday DM. The need for palliative Care in Adults in Nepal: projections based on modeling mortality data. Indian J Palliat Care. 2019 Jan-Mar;25(1):41–5. https://doi.org/10.4103/IJPC.IJPC_177_18.
7. Love RR. Improving cancer outcomes in low- and middle-income countries. J Global Oncology. https://ascopubs.org/doi/full/10.1200/JGO.19.00297
8. https://www.nccn.org/professionals/physician_gls/pdf/palliative.pdf
9. Kumar S. Models of delivering palliative and end-of-life care in India. Curr Opin Support Palliat Care. 2013;7:216–22. https://doi.org/10.1097/SPC.0b013e3283610255.
10. Downing J, Grant L, Leng M, Namukwaya E. Understanding models of palliative care delivery in sub-Saharan Africa: learning from programs in Kenya and Malawi. J Pain Symptom Manag. 2015;50:362–70.
11. https://www.oneviewhealthcare.com/the-eight-principles-of-patient-centered-care/
12. Au E, Loprinzi CL, Dhodaptkar M, et al. Regular use of verbal pain scale improves the understanding of oncology inpatient pain intensity. J Clin Oncol. 1994;12:2751–5.
13. Crisp N. Turning the world upside down the search for global health in the 21st century. London: Royal Society of Medicine Press; 2010.
14. Emanuel EJ. Prescription for the future: the twelve transformational practices of highly effective medical organizations. Public affairs. New York: Perseus Books; 2017.
15. Christensen C, Grossman JH, Hwang J. The innovator's prescription. A disruptive solution for health care. New York: McGraw-Hill; 2009.
16. Hall AK, Cole-Lewis H, Bernhardt JM. Mobile text messaging for health: a systematic review of reviews. Annu Rev Public Health. 2015;36:393–415.
17. Cole-Lewis H, Kershaw T. Text messaging as a tool for behavior change in disease prevention and management. Epidemiol Rev. 2010;31(1):56–69.
18. Yoeli E, Rathauser J, Kimenye MK, et al. Digital health support in treatment for tuberculosis. Lett N Engl J Med. 2019;381:986–7.
19. Laranjo L, et al. The influence of social networking sites on health behavior change: a systematic review and meta-analysis. J Am Med Inform Assoc. 2014;22(1):243–56.
20. Loh IH, et al. Implementation of text-messaging and social media strategies in a multilevel childhood obesity prevention intervention: process evaluation results. Inquiry. 2018;55:0046958018779189.
21. Kotronoulas G, Kearney N, Maguire R, et al. What is the value of the routine use of patient-reported outcome measures toward improvement of patient outcomes, processes of care, and health services outcomes in cancer care? A systemic review of controlled trials. J Clin Oncol. 2014;32:1480–501.
22. Basch E, Deal AM, Kris MG, et al. Symptom monitoring with patient-reported outcomes during routine Cancer treatment: a randomized controlled trial. J Clin Oncol. 2015;34:557–65.
23. Denis F, Basch E, Stephans A-L, et al. Two-year survival comparing web-based symptom monitoring vs routine surveillance following treatment for lung Cancer. JAMA. 2019;321(3):306–7.
24. Love RR, Ferdousy T, Paudel BD, et al. Symptom levels in care-seeking Bangladeshi and Nepalese adults with advanced cancer. J Global Oncology. 2016;3(3):257–60.
25. Cleeland CS, Portenoy RK, Rue M, et al. Does an oral analgesic protocol improve pain control for patients with cancer? An intergroup study coordinated by the Eastern Cooperative Oncology Group. Ann Oncol. 2005;16:972–80. https://doi.org/10.1093/annonc/mdi191.
26. García-Pérez L, Libertova R. A systematic review of specialised palliative care for terminal patients: which model is better? Palliat Med. 2009;23:17–22.
27. Kamdar M, Centi AJ, Agboda S, et al. A randomized controlled trail of a novel artificial intelligence-based Smartphone application to optimize management of cancer-related pain. J Clin Oncol. 2019;37(Suppl Abs 11514)
28. Ballantyne JC, Sullivan MD. Intensity of chronic pain—the wrong metric? New Engl J Med. 2015;373:2098–9.
29. Mooney K, Beck SL, Wong B, et al. Automated home monitoring and management of patient-reported symptoms during chemotherapy: results of the symptom care at home RCT. Cancer Med. 2017;6:537–46.
30. Jensen RE, Snyder CF, Abernethy AP, et al. Review of electronic patient-reported outcomes systems used in cancer clinical care. J Oncol Pract. 2014;10:e215–22.
31. Bennett AV, Jensen RE, Basch E. Electronic patient-reported outcome systems in oncology clinical practice. CA Cancer J Clin. 2012;62:337–47.
32. Marshal J, Wiebe LA, Isenstein H, et al. J Clin Oncol. 2019;37(suppl; abstr e 23119)
33. Vikas P, Gilbertson-White S, Saeidzadeh T, et al. J Clin Oncol. 2019;37(suppl; abstr e2315)
34. Anand S, Walling AM, DAmbruoso SF, et al. J Clin Oncol. 2019;37(suppl; abstr e18312)
35. Love RR, Ahamed SI. The Marquette palliative care system. In: Mollaoglu M, editor. Palliative care: IntechOpen, London: Open Access Publishing; 2019.
36. Bruera E, Kuehn N, Miller MJ, et al. The Edmonton symptom assessment system (ESAS): a simple

method for the assessment of palliative care patients. J Palliat Care. 1991;7:6–9.
37. Cleeland CS, Ryan KM. Pain assessment: global use of the brief pain inventory. Ann Acad Med Singap. 1994;23:129–38.
38. Cassel EJ. The nature of suffering and the goals of medicine. New Engl J Med. 1982;306:639–45.
39. Duffy S, Lee TH. In-person health care as option B. New Engl J Med. 2018;378:104–6.
40. https://echo.unm.edu/
41. Bell D, Gachuhi N, Assefi N. Dynamic clinical algorithms: digital technology can transform healthcare decision-making. Am J Trop Med Hyg. 2018;98:9–14.
42. Asch DA, Nicholson S, Berger ML. Toward facilitated self-service in health care. New Engl J Med. 2019;380:1891–3.
43. https://en.wikipedia.org/wiki/Aravind_Eye_Hospitals

Models of Community-Based Palliative Care

Scharlotte Spencer and Sandra Gomez

The Community Palliative Care Interdisciplinary Team

"Palliative care is a complex field including medical, ethical, psychological, social, existential, and emotional dimensions" [12, 13]. In Sweden, indications are that as interdisciplinary teams communicate their varied assessments, the outcome of patient care is greater due to the collaboration, expertise, and knowledge of the team members [13]. Staffing a community-based palliative care teams is based on the needs of the patients and families served, the resources available, and the future goals and growth of the program. There are several models of community palliative care in existence that can vary in staffing ratios, interdisciplinary team members, funding, legal structure and other factors. At the core of all the different models is the goal to improve the quality of life of the patients and their families by providing access to specialized professionals.

S. Spencer (✉)
Symptom Management Consultants, Prairie View A&M Univesity, Humble, TX, USA
e-mail: Scharlotte@supportivemedicine.net

S. Gomez
Department of Palliative Care and Rehabilitation Medicine, M.D. Anderson Cancer Center, University of Texas, Houston, TX, USA
e-mail: sandra@supportivemedicine.net

In Canada, the Canadian Society of Palliative Care Physicians (CSPCP) recommends starting a program with a registered nurse who is overseen by a palliative care physician [11]. In the United States, community-based palliative care (CBPC) ideally consists of a physician, nurse, social worker, and chaplain. The focus is expert assessment and management of pain and other symptoms, assessment and support of the patient's and caregiver's needs, and the coordination of care with the primary care physician and oncologist caring for the patient. The care is based on the individual patient's needs and not the prognosis associated with the disease.

The nurse-led model utilizes **registered nurses** or **nurse coordinators** empowered to practice at top-of-license. This leads to direct patient advocacy, care coordination, and education as the core responsibilities of the registered nurse on the interdisciplinary team. The nurse also provides immediate and ongoing assessment of patient and family needs. In this nurse-led model, the registered nurse is often the first to meet the patient and families. They assess the patients for physical symptoms and psychosocial needs and arrange family meetings. The registered nurse then brings this information back to the team and triages the services of other disciplines.

As the psychosocial expert on the team, the **social worker** focuses on the family interactions, assesses and supports coping mechanisms, and

M. Silbermann (ed.), *Palliative Care for Chronic Cancer Patients in the Community*,
https://doi.org/10.1007/978-3-030-54526-0_3

evaluates the social determinants of health. In addition, the social worker on the team identifies and facilitates access to resources and mediates family and social conflicts. Many social workers who practice palliative care hold a master's degree in social work, and Licensed Community Social Workers (LCSW) can be an integral addition to the care of patients when issues of mental and emotional health are of concern. There are currently certification programs for palliative care social workers as well as registered nurses.

Chaplains are the professionals on the team who are tasked to provide spiritual care for patients and families enrolled in CBPC. In the hospital setting, professional chaplains may be required to hold a board certification or added qualifications. In the community palliative care environment, these qualifications may not be as strict and there is more variation in qualifications and formal training. Nevertheless, training is essential in order to provide quality palliative care and support a patient facing a serious and life-threatening illness, particularly if the patient is at end of life. The spiritual assessment includes active listening, using a set of questions to engage and assess the patient's spiritual needs, and meeting with family members in the patient's home or environment that they call home. Chaplains also educate patients and families on community resources and help facilitate continuity with the patient's faith community and other spiritual sources of support. The work of the chaplain is interfaith and does not have to focus on a particular faith-based practice or organized religion; the focus is on the spirituality of the patient. Many community programs are unable to fund the chaplain position due to current models of reimbursement, and so, often this is a missing component of many programs. There are innovative collaborations between community palliative care programs and local hospices to mutually fund a chaplain position, and hospital-supported community palliative care programs may cross train acute care chaplains to fill this role. In some community models, the chaplain and social worker often meet with the patient together; this is done since many patients are debilitated and families are exhausted. The two disciplines find it synergistic to work closely together and jointly assess the psychosocial issues in the same initial visit so that the patient does not have to repeat their "story" more than once. Then the two disciplines decide how to best support the patient at their individual level of expertise.

Palliative medicine in the United States became a subspecialty designated in 2006 by the American Board of Medical Specialties (ABMS) as an advance level practice that focuses on the total care of patients with serious illness. **The community physician** component of the interdisciplinary practice of palliative care comprises physicians with specialized training in pain and symptom management. "The physician, as the director of the team, focuses on the illness trajectory, prognosis, and medical treatments" [3]. They provide direct patient care and provide oversight and collaboration with any nurse practitioners or physician assistants on the team. Due to the high volume of community patients who need this care and the limited availability of physicians who provide community-based palliative care, **Advanced Practice Providers** (nurse practitioners or physician assistants) increase the capacity and accessibility to provide this specialized care.

A study published in the *New England Journal of Medicine* suggested that early use of palliative care improved life expectancy by more than 2 months, improved quality of life, and reduced cost for people with metastatic lung cancer [2].

Transitions of Care from Acute Care to Community

The two primary acute care models in the United States are consultation services and palliative inpatient units. Hospital-based palliative care teams have grown and 63% of all US hospitals reported having a palliative care team in 2011 [1]. A consultation service in the hospital setting typically consists of a physician as the medical director and one or more of the interdisciplinary team members. A Palliative Care Unit (PCU) is a specialty unit providing care to palliative care patients in a hospital setting. Patients are admitted to the PCU when they need inpatient management of intense personal or symptomatic distress or have family members who are in severe distress. Each inpatient unit has specific criteria for admission. In comparison to many similar units around the country, most models require distinct goals-of-care criteria for admission or transfer [14].

With data collection in the United States, the efficacy of the program over time demonstrated a large improvement in quality-of-care by identifying patients' goals and aligning them with the plan of care, which leads to improved clinical outcomes. Palliative care programs have shown a reduction in cost for both hospitals and payers with the identification of patient and family goals. This is due, in part, to identifying and providing healthcare resources and transitioning to the appropriate level of care that meets the needs of the patients [4]. With hospital-based palliative programs in place, a decrease in hospital resources and emergency room and ICU utilization is seen, resulting in cost reduction. In a large healthcare system in Texas, a palliative care program reduced the 30-day readmission rate of seriously ill patients by half (from 18% to 9%) with the use of an interdisciplinary palliative care team [15].

As the acute care palliative programs identified patients who benefited from palliative care in the hospital systems, the need for transitioning these patients back into the community grew. Palliative care patients discharged into the community have complex post-discharge needs. Community-based models of palliative care focus on guiding principles and core competencies of community-based programs. The core competencies are described as follows:

- Identification of the target population.
- Goal-based care plans.
- Team-based care.
- Caregiver training.
- Attention to social determinants of health.
- Symptom management.
- Medication management.
- Transitional care.
- Ability to measure value for accountability and improvement.

Adopting these competencies is the standard of a high-quality community-based palliative care program for all patients with serious illness [4].

Identification of the Target Population

To have a successful and sustainable program, care should be taken to initially focus limited resources on high areas of impact. One way this can be achieved is to properly identify patients in need of palliative services who would benefit from the interventions available. For example, an Accountable Care Organization (ACO) that data mines their patient population and identifies patients who could benefit cannot have an impact on a patient who is a resident of a nursing home if they do not have the ability to perform nursing home visits or collaborate with the nursing home. Proper patient identification can be performed in various ways. Examples of ways to identify patients can include, but are not limited to, screening tools that utilize diagnosis; functional status; emergency room readmission; hospital admissions; and lack of documented advance care planning (ACP) as some of the criteria. Data mining of high-risk populations for readmission and high mortality is becoming more available as data scientists help large health systems position themselves to be able to abstract this data and ACOs gain expertise as they study their population.

Having an interdisciplinary team that includes physical, emotional, and spiritual support experts is defined as **team-based care.** Family and caregivers are also important stakeholders in the care of the patient and thus are considered part of the team. This leads to a more comprehensive and holistic approach to care in the community. Team-based care has the added advantage that it not only focuses on the care of the patient but also if nurtured by the leadership of the program can place a high level of importance on the well being of the team members themselves. Self-care and resilience are seen in programs that have active leaders championing teams' well-being, and this can lead to decreased turnover in staff members and less compassion fatigue and burnout [16]. A particular challenge that community programs face is team member isolation. Hospital-based teams, by the nature of their location, are exposed to other medical professionals and healthcare givers on a daily basis. Community program team members, particularly those who are home-based, can often work without the daily physical interaction with other colleagues. This can add a different level of stress not experienced by palliative care teams working in the acute care setting, clinic, or long-term care. This should be taken into account when interviewing potential hires and in developing strategies to support current employees. One innovative way to help with this challenge is the utilization of current technologies to allow teams that may be geographically spread out to feel more connected by using video technology to hold team huddles and conferences. Program leaders can also identify specific areas to focus on to improve team well being and team connectivity, for example, by holding retreats or regularly scheduled meetings where team members can be brought into one venue to increase team cohesiveness. This addition of focus to include the well being of providers and adding a fourth dimension to the Triple Aim movement has been referred to as the Quadruple Aim [20].

Community-based palliative care is often provided at home and the day-to-day care is provided by family and or caregivers. Caregivers are defined as a family member or paid helper who provides support. It is important that they are provided **caregiver training** to ensure that the patient is receiving optimal support. The palliative care team often collaborates with home health agencies to ensure that patients, families, and caregivers receive training for tasks provided in the home. Some examples include proper medication administration, tube feeding, wound care, assistance with activities of daily living, and proper utilization of equipment in the home. One of the most important parts of caregiver training is the ability to identify and convey any problems or concerns to the medical team and palliative care team. Identifying a change in the physical, emotional, or spiritual condition of the patient and explaining those needs to the team are core competencies.

Social determinants of health have been defined by the Centers for Disease Control and Prevention (CDC) as "conditions in the places where people live, learn, work, and play [that] affect a wide range of health risks and outcomes" (www.cdc.gov). Some examples include poverty, mental illness, unsafe living conditions, low literacy, limited or no access to food and water, and lack of transportation. Social determinants of health are identified as major influences on a patient's inability to remain in the community resulting in unwanted emergency room and hospital visits. They are a universal challenge to delivering healthcare in many parts of the world.

Palliative care team members receive specialized training in **communication skills** that help them educate patients and their **support system** regarding specific diseases and their progression. These skills allow team members to further help educate family members and caregivers on medication administration and risk versus benefit of treatment options. A growing field is community healthcare workers who are often non-medical trained personnel who reside in the community setting where the patient lives and can be trained to provide focused education. This new addition of labor force is being utilized by innovative palliative care teams to increase their work force. Any member of the palliative care team can be trained to facilitate family meetings where the patient's goals of medical care are clarified, and advance care planning is conducted. Proper training allows each individual to practice at top-of-license. In the meetings, the team ensures that the **goal-based care plan** is specific to patient and family wishes. The team ensures that proper documentation is completed and provided to the patient, caregiver, and their oncologist and primary care physician. These documents include a medical power of attorney, living wills, and out-of-hospital do-not-resuscitate (DNR) forms where legally required. Some states have specific documents such as physician orders for life-sustaining treatment (POLST) or medical orders for life-sustaining treatment (MOLST) forms, which are medical orders signed by a licensed provider based on that state's legal requirement.

Emergency department visits and unwarranted hospital admission can often be a result of unfavorable **symptom management** related to the chronic disease exacerbation. Palliative care team members are trained to identify and address symptoms such as pain, difficulty breathing, agitation, constipation, nausea, and other symptoms that patients are unable to control alone in the community. This is done with specialized **medication management** that focuses on decreasing side effects, adherence to regiment, financial access, and education on medication uses. The success of these action plans partly depends on the 24/7 phone access patients and families get from community programs. A goal of palliative care in the community is to provide patients with a serious illness **access** to quality care in their home setting and, when that home setting changes, the team provides transitional care with thorough handoff to the care team in the setting that is now identified with providing the level of care needed [4].

The guided principles discussed in Cohn et al. derive from the National Consensus Project for Quality palliative care. These principles include patient/family-centered care; shared decision making of patient goals; comprehensive, coordinated care; accessibility; and to provide value [4]. **Patient/family-centered care** is defined as support of the patient and the family goals combined as a unit. The care should be centered around the values of the family as a unit. **Shared decision making of patient goals** is led by a plan of care that originates from patients' beliefs and preferences. A comprehensive initial assessment is completed to identify and clarify the goals and key players in the care of the patient. **Comprehensive, coordinated care** is necessary to accommodate the complex needs of patients with serious illnesses. The needs can vary from home health support, meal delivery services, medication assistance, caregivers, emotional support to respite care. Palliative care teams in the community are valuable in assisting patients and families in filling these gaps in care. In recent years, the value of the program has been observed by payers and has been included in value-based healthcare models. The programs must **provide value** and show cost saving through shared savings, bundled payments, risk saving, and readmission penalties [4].

Palliative Care in Ambulatory Settings

The Oncology Clinic

An article published in the Journal of Clinical Oncology recommends that cancer patients newly diagnosed or living with advanced cancer should have palliative care services offered concurrent with cancer treatment and as early as possible if not at time of diagnosis [5]. Models of providing palliative care in the oncology clinic may include providing access to a member of the interdisciplinary team such as a palliative physician or advance practice provider in the clinic. It is encouraged to introduce the palliative care team (PCT) to the patient as early in the disease process as possible, as encouraged by the literature. The focus of the PCT physician or advance practice provider in the oncology clinic is to provide expert level symptom management to minimize symptom burden of the disease. These symptoms, if not managed, have the potential to delay the treatment plan created by the patient's oncology team. In models where other members of the PCT such as nurses, social workers, or chaplains are available, the care can be more interdisciplinary. This team approach to provide care focuses on relationship building and to provide not only support for symptom burden but psychosocial and spiritual support. There are models where only a social worker with special training in palliative care is available. The social worker focuses on the psychosocial factors and can be the person tasked with initiating the advance care planning discussions that benefit most patients. Since advance care planning is not the process of simply discussing code status but rather to identify patient's goals, expectations, and values, this is a conversation very well suited to this member of the team who is then practicing at top-of-license.

Goal setting begins by ensuring that patients and families understand the plan and options that were presented by their oncology team and have good lines of communication with all members of the healthcare team. The American Society of Clinical Oncology guidelines reports that integrating palliative care services into routine care of patients with advanced cancer improves patient satisfaction, reduces depression, and improves quality of life. It also reduces the use of chemotherapy at end of life for patients and increases enrollment and length of stay in hospice [5].

Primary Care Clinics

Core competencies and principles of high-quality community palliative care remain the same in every setting where palliative care services are provided. Each setting has a unique need that is the focus of their palliative care program. Community-based palliative care is beginning to emerge in the primary care setting but finding a comprehensive palliative care team in a primary care setting is still rare at the time of this publication. Hurdles include the limited time allotted for the office visit with primary care providers, reimbursement for social workers and chaplains in a primary care setting, and lack of understanding of how to utilize palliative care in a primary care practice. Most settings involve a primary care physician who has received palliative care training and sees patients with palliative care needs within his or her primary care patient panel. An area of opportunity is teaching primary care providers additional skills in pain and symptom management and communication skills. These are core competencies that primary care clinicians should have in order to better care for patients with a serious or chronic illness. Integrating a goals-of-care discussion in an office visit and identifying high symptom burden from a serious illness are two examples of additional interventions that can help provide improved quality of life for patients in the primary care setting [17]. An even more focused area is advance care planning, which is now reimbursable by the Centers for Medicare & Medicaid Services (CMS) and many commercial insurance plans in the United States that pay for voluntary advance care planning (ACP) under the Medicare Physician Fee Schedule (PFS) and the Hospital Outpatient Prospective Payment System (cms.gov).

Palliative Care Outpatient Clinic

Interdisciplinary specialist palliative care in stand-alone clinics remains the gold standard for ambulatory palliative care [6]. Palliative care clinics have shown the greatest impact on multiple patient and caregiver outcomes as the program is not integrated into other specialty clinics. Fewer resources are required in other models; however, they may not be able to provide the same level of comprehensive palliative care [6]. Patients are referred to palliative care clinics by acute hospital palliative teams, oncology clinics, and other specialty providers. Most often, these clinics are managed and funded by hospital systems as they have found value in post-acute care follow-up. Patients seen in the hospital with palliative care needs that are not home-bound are candidates to be referred to the palliative care clinic, thus providing continuity of care. When patients are no longer physically able to receive services in the clinic, they can be transitioned to a home program when this is available.

Home Visits

As palliative care continues to prove its value in patient care, it is seen in more hospital settings and specialty clinics. A variety of specialty clinics such as oncology, congestive heart failure, left ventricular assisted device (LVAD), nephrology, and amyotrophic lateral sclerosis (ALS) clinics have invested in this service. When patients of these specialty clinics are no longer capable of leaving their home as a result of disease progression, palliative care can be provided in their homes: private homes, personal care homes, or assisted living facilities. Qualifications to receive palliative care services in the home are set by the entity providing the care. An assessment is performed by a team member during the initial visit to identify the needs of the patient and families. The patient's need for symptom management, advance care planning, community resources, and spiritual or psychosocial support is assessed and discussed with the other members of the interdisciplinary team. Based on the assessment, one of the team members is assigned to the patient for follow-up [8]. Most importantly, the palliative care team ensures that patient's family and primary providers are updated on patients' plan of care.

Home Health and Hospice Models

Several Medicare-Certified home health agencies also operate Medicare-approved hospice programs. Likewise, Medicare-approved hospices operate community palliative care programs [7]. Both entities have developed innovative programs to meet gaps in care faced by seriously ill patients but both programs face problems in reimbursement for this care by traditional payment models. These models of community-based palliative care (CBPC) are attractive to patients since there is no need to end curative treatments and patients can continue to pursue aggressive and curative treatments. Most of the home health CBPC programs admit patients who meet the Medicare eligibility criteria for home health and have a prognosis of one year or less, or meet other screening criteria such as functional decline, high symptom burden, or have declined hospice services [18]. This allows the home health to recover some of the cost of their operations.

Hospice programs that house a CBPC do not admit those patients to hospice; these programs often fund their own operations, and a few have developed value-based contracts with payers or other entities to fund the program cost. Hospice programs providing CBPC often refer to these programs as "bridge" programs, as they seek to meet the gap between hospice eligibility and lack of services for seriously ill patients. Once there is decline and the patient becomes hospice eligible with a prognosis of 6 months or less, if the disease follows its normal course and the patient chooses comfort care, the patient can be offered this service. Many agencies cross train staff so that the patient can be seen by the same team and not have to transition to different providers.

Palliative Care in Long-Term Acute Care (LTAC) and Skilled Nursing Facilities (SNF)

There are emerging models of palliative care in the LTAC and SNF setting. As with other CBPC programs that utilize physicians and advance practice providers, the consulting physician or non-facility employed advance practice provider are the only members of the palliative team whose time is usually reimbursable by traditional payment models. Innovative programs have been able to develop value-based agreements with payers to get reimbursement for the interdisciplinary members of the team. Composition of teams can vary but some of these programs cross train their nursing and social work staff to meet the needs of the program. Chaplains are becoming increasingly more available in these settings. Studies have shown that the palliative care teams in long-term care have been effective in reducing emergency department visits and depression. The programs have also promoted more appropriate care resulting in more favorable clinical outcomes toward the resident's end of life [19].

Palliative Care in Rural Areas

According to the American Telemedicine Association, telehealth saves patients', providers', and payers' money when compared to traditional care [10]. Telemedicine in palliative care can provide resources that can improve patient outcomes and prevent avoidable use of healthcare resources. With telemedicine, palliative care patients can receive frequent assessment and support, access to a team member that can be used to prevent escalation of symptoms and crisis, receive education, information, and assist with in home management improving outcomes. Access to healthcare in rural areas is limited by structural, financial, personal, and cultural barriers. These barriers also play a major role in access and delivery of palliative care to seriously ill patients. Providing palliative care in the rural setting brings about its own challenges as well. Some examples of these challenges are funding, lack of clinicians, windshield time, and state regulations [9]. To bridge the gap, telemedicine is used to improve access in rural and underserved areas.

Advance Care Planning in the Community

As medicine continues to evolve, more and more options of care are presented to patients living with serious illness. Discussing patients' goals are a vital part of the patient's care plan. Advance care planning (ACP) is a discussion among patient, provider, family, and care team to clarify patient-centered goals of care. These conversations assess and provide clarification and understanding of disease process for patients and families. Patients are provided the opportunity to express their wishes regarding their medical care to their medical team and family. The medical team also provides the patient with benefits and risk of therapy options and aligns them with patient's goals. During this conversation, patients are encouraged to designate someone who can honor their decision when they are unable. It is also explained that the plan of care may change and will be frequently reassessed. While completion of legal documents such as directives to physicians, medical power of attorney, physician orders for life-sustaining treatment (POLST, and medical orders for life-sustaining treatment (MOLST), out-of-hospital do not resuscitate forms are important to physically document patient's wishes; the most important part of the advance care planning is the conversation itself.

Palliative care team members receive specialized training to facilitate advance care planning conversations. They also educate other providers on how to effectively carry out the conversation. As this can be uncomfortable for some or time consuming, a variety of tools have been created to guide the conversations. Advance care planning can occur in any community-based setting.

Sample Palliative Care Screening Tool

Please complete on adult patients prior to patient being seen by provider.

Patient receives 1 point in each section for any yes answer.

MPOA/AD section do not receive a score

Points	
/1	In the last 30 days, have you been admitted to the hospital? Y / N In the last 30 days, have you had an ER visit? Y / N If so, how many visits? ________________ Reason why: ________________
/1	Are you currently, or in the past 24 hours have you, experienced uncontrolled: Pain Dyspnea Nausea/vomiting Diarrhea/constipation Anxiety/depression Fatigue

/1	Are you currently having difficulty with: Stress/coping Medication access Transportation to medical visits Access to meals Assistance with activities of daily living at home
/1	Would you like to request spiritual or emotional support? Y / N
Total: /4	
Do you have a medical power of attorney (MPOA)? Y/N advance directives (AD)? Y/N If already in place, is there a copy in patient files? Y/ N Name and relation of MPOA ________________________________	
Created by Scharlotte Spencer DNP, APRN, FNP-C, ACHPN	

Patient with 3 or more points: Consider palliative care referral
Patients with 0–2 points: Re-evaluate on next visit

References

1. Morrison RS. Models of palliative care delivery in the United States. Curr Opin Support Palliat Care. 2013;7:2.
2. Temel JS, et al. Early palliative care for patients with metastatic non–small-cell lung cancer. N Engl J Med. 2010;363:733–42. https://doi.org/10.1056/NEJMoa1000678.
3. The National Coalition for Hospice and Palliative Care Clinical Practice Guidelines for Quality Palliative Care, 4th edn.
4. Cohn, J., J. Corrigan, J. Lynn, D. Meier, J. Miller, J. Shega, and S. Wang. 2017. Community-based models of care delivery for people with serious illness. NAM perspectives. Discussion paper, National Academy of Medicine, Washington, DC. https://doi.org/10.31478/201704b.
5. Ferrell B, Temel J, Temin S, Alessi E, Balboni T, Bash E, Firn J, Paice J, Peppercorn J, Phillips T, Stovall E, Zimmermann C, Smith T. Integration of palliative care into standard oncology care: American society of clinical practice guideline update. J Clin Oncol. 2016;35:96–112.
6. Hui D. Palliative cancer care in the outpatient setting: which model works best? Curr Treat Options in Oncol. 2019;20(2) [17]:35–62.
7. Meier D, Bowman B, Collins K, Dahlin C, Twohig JS. Palliative care in the home; a program design. Center for advancing palliative care.
8. Bhavsar NA, Bloom K, Nicolla J, Gable C, Goodman A, Olson A, Harker M, Bull J, Taylor DH. Delivery of community-based palliative care: findings from a time and motion study. Journal of Palliative Medicine. 2017; 20(10):1120–26.
9. Temple KT. Community-based palliative care: scaling access for rural populations. The Rural Health Hub. 2018;19(2):130–9.
10. Head B, Schapmire T, Zheng Y. Telemedicine in palliative care: a systematic review of patient-reported outcomes. J. Hosp Palliat Nurs. 2017;19:1318–23.
11. Henderson J, Boyle A, Herx L, Alexiadis A, Barwich D, Connidis S, Lysecki D, Sinnarajah A. Staffing in a specialist palliative care service, a team approach: expert consensus white paper. J Palliat Med. 2019;22:1148–51.
12. O'Connor NR. Palliative Care Office Hours for Patients with Hematologic Malignancies: An Innovative Model for Symptom Management and Education. J Palliat Med. 2017;20(10):1148–51 https://doi.org/10.1089/jpm.2017.0091. Epub 2017 May 24. PMID: 28537777.
13. Klarare A, Hagelin C, Fürst C, Fossum B. Team interactions in specialized palliative care teams: a qualitative study. J Palliat Med. 2013;7:60–4. https://doi.org/10.1089/jpm.2012.0622.
14. Drury L, Baccari K, Fang A, Moller C, Nagus I. Providing intensive palliative care on an inpatient unit: a full-time job. J Adv Pract Oncol. DSouza MJ, Center of palliative care National Seminar 2018 poster presentation on Quality improvement. 2016.
15. D'Souza M. Supportive medicine reducing readmissions: Center for Advancing Palliative Care; 2018.
16. Yates S. Physician stress and burnout. Am J Med. 2020;133(2):160–4.
17. Ahia C, Blais C. Primary palliative care for the general internist: integrating goals of care discussions into the outpatient setting. Ochsner J. 2014 Winter;14(4):704–11.
18. Labson M, et al. Innovative models of home-based palliative care. Cleve Clin J Med. 2013;53(5):874–88.
19. Comart J, et al. Palliative care for long-term care residents: effect on clinical outcomes. The Gerontologist. Ann Fam Med 2014;12(6):573–6.
20. Bodenheimer T, Sinsky C. From triple to quadruple aim: care of the patient requires care of the provider. Ann. Fam. Med. 2014;12(6):573–6. https://doi.org/10.1370/afm.1713.

Role of the Nurse in the Palliative Care Community

Jeannine Brant and Regina M. Fink

Introduction to Palliative Care

Palliative care is a person/family-centered approach that focuses on the physical, functional, psychological, social, practical, and spiritual consequences of a serious illness [17]. When offered early in the serious illness trajectory, palliative care has been shown to improve quality of life; decrease symptom burden; facilitate advance care planning by ensuring health care is concordant with patient and family caregiver goals, values, and preferences; and increase survival [1, 7, 16, 36]. Nurses play a paramount role in the palliative care community around the world, a variety of settings, and in diverse roles. This chapter highlights the role of the nurse in the delivery of palliative care.

Palliative Care in Various Settings

Palliative care may be delivered in primary, secondary, or tertiary settings (Fig. 1) [23, 31, 39]. All health-care providers, including nurses, should be able to offer primary palliative care to patients and family caregivers. Primary palliative care includes employing basic pain and symptom management strategies and discussing goals of care in a variety of settings from community hospitals to remote villages around the world. Tertiary palliative care is characteristically provided at tertiary or quaternary academic medical centers by an interdisciplinary team (physician, nurse, social worker, and spiritual care provider). Many of these institutions provide both inpatient and outpatient palliative care consultation, have an inpatient palliative care unit or designated hospice beds, and have access to a palliative home care program. Interprofessional health-care team members in these academic settings, including expert nurses, are often engaged in research and educate other professionals about palliative care through fellowship programs and mentoring. Secondary palliative care, envisioned as a "bridge" between primary and tertiary PC, can be offered by specialist clinicians in community, rural, and other underserved settings.

Hospital-based inpatient palliative care programs, usually located in tertiary or quaternary centers, should be recognized as they have changed the quality of care seriously ill patients receive and end-of-life care should they die during the hospitalization. Improved standards of care, policies and processes, and outcomes' measurement are key to the provision of quality palliative care. The Joint Commission's Palliative

J. Brant (✉)
Billings Clinic Cancer Center and Collaborative Science & Innovation Department, Billings, MT, USA
e-mail: jbrant@billingsclinic.org

R. M. Fink
Division of General Internal Medicine, Department of Medicine, School of Medicine, University of Colorado, Aurora, CO, USA
e-mail: regina.fink@cuanschutz.edu

M. Silbermann (ed.), *Palliative Care for Chronic Cancer Patients in the Community*,
https://doi.org/10.1007/978-3-030-54526-0_4

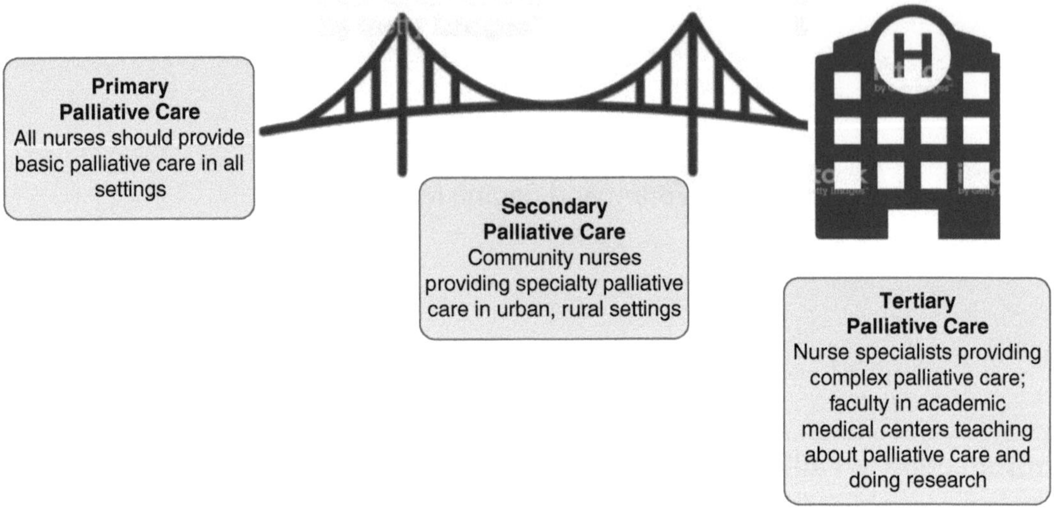

Fig. 1 Primary, secondary, tertiary palliative care: the role of the nurse

Care Certification is intended to distinguish hospital inpatient programs demonstrating exceptional patient- and family-centered care and focuses on optimizing the quality of life for those with serious illnesses [37].

While quality inpatient palliative care is important, it is ideal for patients and their family caregivers to spend the majority of their time outside of the hospital with only an occasional need to be seen by a palliative care specialist. An outpatient team or service can prove helpful, if available, to see patients who are transitioning from hospital to home and have difficulties managing symptoms or emergency needs. Having robust relationships with various community agencies such as home hospice and palliative care can prevent hospital admissions. Having access to freestanding hospice facilities, skilled hospice care within long-term care, and assisted living facilities are other options for those patients who can no longer be cared for by family caregivers in the home setting. In rural communities, home hospice care may not be an option. Visits from nurses employed by community health nursing agencies may be available; however, nurses with palliative care expertise may be scarce. Using telehealth to connect nurses in these settings to tertiary care nursing experts may be the best solution. Regardless of the setting, nurses should be equipped in a variety of roles to deliver palliative care. A description of the various roles is included below.

Nursing Roles

The American Nurses Association along with the Hospice and Palliative Nurses Association recently convened a work group to examine the role of nurses in the provision of palliative care. The report was a Call for Action for nurses to lead and transform palliative care through clinical practice, education, research, and health-care policy [5]. Nurses, being the largest health-care workforce, have an imperative to contribute their holistic and patient/family-centered care to provide quality palliative care. A recent qualitative meta-synthesis found that "Being Available" and "Being Present" were key themes depicting nurses' palliative care roles. Nursing presence is a sacred gift that can be given to patients and family caregivers in times of greatest need.

Nurses' roles in palliative care are diverse and far reaching. They span from the bedside of a patient in a hospital setting, to remote villages with minimal resources, and into classrooms and research labs. They may even be the only health-care resource available in some settings [10].

Table 1 Various nursing roles in palliative care

Nursing role	Role description	Primary palliative care responsibilities
Bedside nurse	Provide direct patient care in the hospital setting	Pain and symptom management as prescribed Communication between disciplines for seamless care delivery Patient/family communication and support Advocacy
Ambulatory nurse	Provide direct patient care to patients in the outpatient setting, such as a clinic, a telephone triage center, or infusion center	Patient/family education Early detection of uncontrolled symptoms and problems Patient/family communication and support
Nurse navigator	Coordinate care from the time of diagnosis through treatment and/or the disease trajectory	Health-care appointment coordination Patient/family education Patient/family communication and support
Case manager	Consult with patients for needs regarding care transitions, community health, and costs of care	Assist in care transitions and with home health or hospice referrals Mobilize community resources as needed Inform about costs of care and treatments
Community health nurse	Provide direct care to patients in the home, school, or long-term care facility	Pain and symptom management in the home or community setting Communication with the physician regarding care needs Patient/family education Patient/family communication and support
Advanced practice nurse	A nurse practitioner, clinical nurse specialist, or certified nurse midwife who has advanced skills in nursing and hold an advanced practice degree	Lead palliative care efforts in some settings Deliver palliative care as a health-care provider Provide disease-modifying treatment Provide pain and symptom management Facilitate advanced care planning and discussion of goals of care
College of nursing faculty	Assistant, associate, or professor at a college of nursing who is responsible for palliative care education of the nursing work	Palliative care curriculum development Palliative care education of the nursing workforce
Nurse scientist	PhD or DNP prepared nurses within a university or health-care setting who conduct palliative care research, quality improvement, and/or promote evidence-based practice	Encourage the use of evidence-based practice in palliative care Discover new knowledge to expand nursing science of palliative care

Table 1 includes a summary of nursing roles in palliative care with further discussion below. The most common roles are listed, although many roles such as patient/family caregiver education and support and advocacy are cross-cutting to some degree across nursing roles.

Bedside Nurses

Seriously ill patients who require hospitalization are often the sickest and most vulnerable. They are in the hospital because they require 24-hour nursing care. Control of pain and other deleterious symptoms is paramount and the focus of palliative care in the hospital setting [12]. Within the clinical setting, nurses are called to improve pain and symptom management through comprehensive assessment, and prompt management through the delivery of both pharmacologic and nonpharmacologic interventions. The goal is to manage symptoms quickly and effectively so that patients can spend more time at home, if preferred. Nurses may need to advocate for patient comfort and easy access to supportive medications [28].

Hospitalized patients may also be in crisis, with progressive disease, medical emergencies, and uncontrolled symptoms. This can often be the reason for hospitalization; admission to the intensive care unit (ICU) is not uncommon. Disease progression and changes in physical status may warrant a change in the goals of care. These events lead to important conversations, and nurses should be well-equipped in communicating with patients and family caregivers during these crises to ensure goal-concordant care. A survey of 598 ICU nurses found that the majority (88%) engaged in conversations about prognosis, goals of care, and palliative care [6]. Nurses perceived these conversations as important role functions that are critical to quality care.

Because palliative care requires specialized training and skills, some hospitals are providing focused training for bedside nurses. One model hospital in Florida, the USA, has initiated an advanced training program for a select group of nurses. The Palliative Care Resource Nurse is embedded on the nursing unit to provide patient advocacy, discuss goals of care, and help patients discuss advance directives [20]. As hospitals become more focused on palliative versus curative models of care, these nurse-based resources are likely to soar.

Ambulatory Care Nurses

Nurses are key members of the health-care team in ambulatory care settings. Roles include telephone triage, patient education, and provision of infusion therapies such as chemotherapy and blood products [40]. Patients receiving ambulatory care are often more stable than hospitalized patients but have ongoing needs for optimal control of pain and symptoms [28]. Nurses in this setting should ensure optimal quality of life while keeping the patient out of the hospital setting. Early identification for palliative care is another role. Nurses are often the first to recognize uncontrolled pain or symptoms or psychosocial distress, which could warrant a palliative care referral [18].

Ambulatory palliative care programs are also growing and provide an important extra layer of support for many patients. Ambulatory care nurses or advanced practice nurses (APNs) often serve on these teams, providing navigation or coordination of care, which will be further described later. Communication is also important in this role in lieu of discussions about advanced directives and advanced care planning as patients receiving ambulatory care are often well enough to discuss care preferences and personal goals of care [22]. It is important that nurses are equipped and trained to have these discussions when opportunities arise.

Nurse Navigators

Nurse Navigators are often referred to as guides, who walk patients and family caregivers through the care trajectory, from diagnosis through treatment. Because of the relationship established with the patient and family caregiver early in the course of a disease, establishing rapport and trust is often a tremendous benefit when discussions about supportive and palliative care emerge. Nurse navigators serve a variety of palliative care roles including symptom relief, communicating with patients and families about goals of care, and facilitating care transitions with a change in health status. They can also continue to be in touch with families during bereavement [21]. Being a coordinator of care was a top theme identified in one qualitative meta-synthesis of the nurse's role in palliative care [33].

One model program for palliative care navigation is the Billings Clinic Cancer Center, located in Billings, Montana, in the USA. The palliative and supportive care navigator is the link between the ambulatory palliative care team and the patient. The navigator schedules patients for visits with providers, attends palliative care meetings to provide input into care, conducts follow-up phone calls to assess for symptom improvement following palliative care interventions, and fields all phone calls coming into the palliative care service line. Patients and families report high satisfaction with the ability to access palliative care through a known nurse navigator.

Case Managers

Nurses serve as case managers in a variety of settings including hospitals, clinics, and even insurance companies. Their role is to facilitate coordination of care, care transitions (e.g., from the inpatient hospital setting to home with hospice care), equal access to care, and appropriate use of health-care resources [27]. While these roles are emerging in many health-care settings, opportunity exists for these nurses to be engaged in palliative care and population health management. Patients should have access to a care manager and be informed about how these nurses can support their care. Determining pre-authorization of payment for procedures and medications to advocating for community services, care managers can help support patients and families along the care continuum.

Community Health Nurses

Community health nurses provide palliative care in homes, schools, and in long-term care facilities around the world. A recent survey of 532 home health nurses from 29 countries found that most of the work performed is palliative. Duties included health maintenance, patient and family education, and shared decision-making [10]. In many remote communities, nurses may be the only available health-care professionals, thereby their roles are expansive and of utmost importance. Millions of patients around the globe are living with serious and life-threatening conditions, requiring palliative care. Nurses can close this gap in rural and remote areas [25]. Diligent pain and symptom management, communication with the physician and other team members, communication about advanced directives and goals of care, education about self-care, and emotional support are all important roles of the community health nurse. One qualitative analysis reported four themes that reflected strategies nurses use when providing palliative care in the home: (1) adjusting care around the home environment, (2) helping patients and families discover a balance between self-care, independence, and safe care, (3) guiding patients and family members with changes needed for optimal palliative care at home, and (4) using the time at home to reflect, recuperate, and prepare for end of life [3].

Children experiencing chronic diseases and life-threatening illnesses require palliative care in a variety of settings. One goal for children is to keep them in school to normalize their life as much as possible. While some acute illnesses arise at school, most school nurses spend much of their time providing palliative care. Children with diabetes, cystic fibrosis, and cancer can require supportive care during the school day, and the school nurse is a valuable community health nurse in this setting [2].

Long-term care facilities are common in the USA and their availability is growing in many countries around the world. It is estimated that approximately 40% of all US deaths will occur in long-term care facilities by 2030. Nurses and aides are often the primary care givers within these facilities, providing ongoing palliative care. Older adults comprise the greatest numbers of residents in these facilities, who often have multiple comorbid or life-threatening conditions deeming the majority of these patients eligible for palliative care. Unfortunately, palliative care is often lacking in these facilities. Increasing access to palliative care and improving symptom management, communication, and advanced care planning is critical given the growing need of these facilities [35].

Advanced Practice Nurses

Advanced practice nurses (APNs) including nurse practitioners, clinical nurse specialists, and even nurse midwives play an essential role in the provision of palliative care [30, 32]. While not recognized in all countries around the world, their presence is growing as physician shortages grow more expansive. APNs can be a cost-effective as well as an excellent resource for patients in need of palliative care. Their holistic model of care is focused on disease-modifying care, evidence-based pain and symptom management, expert communication, education, and compassionate end-of-life care [19]. Nurse-led primary palliative care clinics are rapidly emerging in outpatient settings [13].

As noted, with the vast palliative care needs around the globe, APNs are one solution to alleviate care shortages and close the gap on unmet palliative care needs. In order to equip APNs, significant education and skills are needed. According to a 2017 survey of 556 APNs, 41% perceived that their palliative care training and education was inadequate. Existing programs need to better incorporate palliative care curricula and developing programs should heed to these recommendations [30].

College of Nursing Faculty

Despite palliative care education and training programs, the number of qualified nurse providers remains limited. Major gaps in palliative care access exist for most patient populations in community settings. Nursing Professors and other Nursing Educators have a tremendous responsibility in educating the nursing workforce about palliative care. The needs are diverse, ranging from training APNs in resource-rich countries to training generalist nurses in resource-poor countries [8]. For undergraduate education, the American Association of Colleges of Nursing identified 17 competencies that undergraduate nursing students should achieve by the time they graduate. These are listed in Table 2 [4, 14].

The End-of-Life Nursing Education Consortium (ELNEC)-Core curriculum is one notable program that has been disseminated around the world to over 19,500 nurses in more

Table 2 Competencies necessary for nurses to provide high-quality care to patients and families facing serious illness

1. Promote the need for palliative care for seriously ill patients and their families, from the time of diagnosis, as essential to quality care and an integral component of nursing care.
2. Identify the dynamic changes in population demographics, health-care economics, service delivery, caregiving demands, and financial impact of serious illness on the patient and family that necessitate improved professional preparation for palliative care.
3. Recognize one's own ethical, cultural, and spiritual values and beliefs about serious illness and death.
4. Demonstrate respect for cultural, spiritual, and other forms of diversity for patients and their families in the provision of palliative care services.
5. Educate and communicate effectively and compassionately with the patient, family, health care team members, and the public about palliative care issues.
6. Collaborate with members of the interprofessional team to improve palliative care for patients with serious illness to enhance the experience and outcomes from palliative care for patients and their families and to ensure coordinated and efficient palliative care for the benefit of communities.
7. Elicit and demonstrate respect for the patient and family values, preferences, goals of care, and shared decision-making during serious illness and at end of life.
8. Apply ethical principles in the care of patients with serious illness and their families.
9. Know, apply, and effectively communicate current state and federal legal guidelines relevant to the care of patients with serious illness and their families.
10. Perform a comprehensive assessment of pain and symptoms common in serious illness using valid, standardized assessment tools and strong interviewing and clinical examination skills.
11. Analyze and communicate with the interprofessional team in planning and intervening in pain and symptom management using evidence-based pharmacologic and nonpharmacologic approaches.
12. Assess, plan, and treat patients' physical, psychological, social, and spiritual needs to improve quality of life for patients with serious illness and their families.
13. Evaluate patient and family outcomes from palliative care within the context of patient goals of care, national quality standards, and value.
14. Provide competent, compassionate, and culturally sensitive care for patients and their families at the time of diagnosis of a serious illness through the end of life.
15. Implement self-care strategies to support coping with suffering, loss, moral distress, and compassion fatigue.
16. Assist the patient, family, informal caregivers, and professional colleagues to cope with and build resilience for dealing with suffering, grief, loss, and bereavement associated with serious illness.
17. Recognize the need to seek consultation (i.e., from advanced practice nursing specialists, specialty palliative care teams, ethics consultants, etc.) for complex patient and family needs.

than 85 countries [15]. The modules include both didactic lectures as well as group interaction and discussion. The curriculum has been embedded into undergraduate nursing courses [26] and a graduate ELNEC program exists to educate APNs [14, 29] and educate masters and doctorate nursing practice students in primary palliative care.

Another nationally acclaimed model is one that started with a collaboration between the Middle Eastern Cancer Consortium (MECC), the Oncology Nursing Society (ONS), and the Oman Cancer Association (OCA). The training comprised four parts: Foundations, Advanced Concepts, Leadership, and Research in Palliative Care. The course engages participants using Liberating Structures (ref), which encourage participation by all attendees to brainstorm and develop individualized solutions to local problems [11, 24, 34]. Both ELNEC and this course encourage a "Train the Trainer" approach to increase spread of palliative care philosophy and principles.

A way for hospice and palliative care nurses to be recognized for their palliative care expertise and knowledge is to be certified through the Hospice and Palliative Nurses' Certification Corporation [26]. Competency-based specialty nursing certification is offered to advanced practice nurses, registered nurses, pediatric palliative nurses, nursing assistants, and those caring for patients experiencing perinatal loss. Palliative care preparation courses are offered through the Hospice and Palliative Nurses' Association and many colleges of nursing.

Nurse Scientists

Nurse Scientists provide the conduit for the discovery of new knowledge for the provision of palliative care. High-quality research is essential to build the science around pain and symptom management. While a multitude of options exist, over 65% of patients with advanced cancer and 55% of patients after cancer treatment [38] continue to suffer from pain. Other symptoms are also in need of better management [9]. The management of pain and symptoms is complex and will require nurse scientists to test educational, technological, and multimodal approaches to improve management. Better understanding of patient and caregiver perspectives will be important to gain progress in this area of research [28].

Additional palliative care research topics include best approaches to discuss advance care planning with patients from diverse cultures and backgrounds, better understanding of the complex interplay between health-care systems, health-care professionals, patients, and families, and identifying best approaches to educate patients and family caregivers about palliative care. Nurse-led models of care should further be explored as well, which examine outcomes as well as costs of care. These studies will all require multi-system study approaches. Finally, compassion fatigue and burnout of the nursing workforce are on the rise, and research should consider best approaches to sustain and improve the health of nurses who provide palliative care [5].

Barriers

While nurses work in a variety of roles in primary, secondary, and tertiary palliative care, some barriers exist that prevent quality palliative care, education, and research. First, nurses may not be fully equipped to deliver palliative care due to a lack of preparation and experience. Undergraduate and continuing education of palliative care should be fully supported by nursing leaders across all health-care settings and within every country around the world. Improving the palliative care knowledge of nurses will tremendously expand palliative care access around the globe. Second, nurses may not be practicing at their full scope due to restrictions in prescribing or care within their states or countries. Nurses should advocate for health-care policy that advances the scope of nursing so that patient access to palliative care can be fully expanded and available. Nurses should have a seat at the table to discuss care preferences, goals and care, and advance care plans with patients and families along with other palliative care responsibilities.

Third, nurses report care disparities that result in moral distress. Nurses need to advocate for appropriate pain and symptom management and optimal palliative care and support one another during these crises, in order to alleviate patient and family pain and suffering [5].

Future Directions

Nurses have the ability to both lead and transform palliative care around the globe. As the largest health-care workforce, nurses are often the only ones "present" and "available" to meet the complex physical, psychological, social, and spiritual needs of patients and families who need palliative care. The holistic approach of nursing is conducive to palliative care, and the future is bright, and yet as a profession, nursing will need to better prepare and educate nurses to meet the large demand for palliative care in the future. Education should include didactic material, but most important, it should include simulation to practice skills, discuss case studies, and shadow expert clinicians who can serve as role models. The knowledge of palliative care can be built in a classroom, but the art of palliative care must be through experiential learning and patient engagement.

Permission to reprint these competencies is under consideration.

https://www.aacnnursing.org/Portals/42/ELNEC/PDF/New-Palliative-Care-Competencies.pdf

References

1. Ahluwalia SC, Chen C, Raaen L, Motala A, Walling AM, Chamberlin M, et al. A systematic review in support of the National Consensus Project Clinical Practice Guidelines for quality palliative care, fourth edition. J Pain Symptom Manag. 2018;56(6):831–70. Retrieved from https://www.ncbi.nlm.nih.gov/pubmed/30391049. https://doi.org/10.1016/j.jpainsymman.2018.09.008.
2. Akard TF, Hendricks-Ferguson VL, Gilmer MJ. Pediatric palliative care nursing. Ann Palliat Med. 2019;8(Suppl 1):S39–48. Retrieved from https://www.ncbi.nlm.nih.gov/pubmed/30180727 http://apm.amegroups.com/article/view/20026/22765. https://doi.org/10.21037/apm.2018.06.01.
3. Alvariza A, Mjornberg M, Goliath I. Palliative care nurses' strategies when working in private homes-a photo-elicitation study. J Clin Nurs. 2020;29(1–2):139–51. Retrieved from https://onlinelibrary.wiley.com/doi/abs/10.1111/jocn.15072. https://doi.org/10.1111/jocn.15072.
4. American Association of Colleges of Nursing. End-of-Life Nursing Education Consortium (ELNEC). 2019. Retrieved from https://www.aacnnursing.org/ELNEC
5. American Nurses Association. Call for action: nurses lead and transform palliative care. 2017. Retrieved from https://www.nursingworld.org/~497158/global-assets/practiceandpolicy/health-policy/palliativecare-professionalissuespanelcallforaction.pdf
6. Anderson WG, Puntillo K, Boyle D, Barbour S, Turner K, Cimino J, et al. ICU bedside Nurses' involvement in palliative care communication: a multicenter survey. J Pain Symptom Manag. 2016;51(3):589–96.e582. https://doi.org/10.1016/j.jpainsymman.2015.11.003.
7. Bakitas M, Lyons KD, Hegel MT, Balan S, Brokaw FC, Seville J, et al. Effects of a palliative care intervention on clinical outcomes in patients with advanced cancer: the project ENABLE II randomized controlled trial. JAMA. 2009;302(7):741–9. Retrieved from https://www.ncbi.nlm.nih.gov/pubmed/19690306. https://doi.org/10.1001/jama.2009.1198.
8. Bassah N, Seymour J, Cox K. A modified systematic review of research evidence about education for pre-registration nurses in palliative care. BMC Palliat Care. 2014;13:56. Retrieved from http://www.ncbi.nlm.nih.gov/pubmed/25859159 https://www.ncbi.nlm.nih.gov/pmc/articles/PMC4391725/pdf/12904_2014_Article_248.pdf. https://doi.org/10.1186/1472-684X-13-56.
9. Brant JM. Palliative care for adults across the cancer trajectory: from diagnosis to end of life. Semin Oncol Nurs. 2010;26(4):222–30. Retrieved from http://www.ncbi.nlm.nih.gov/pubmed/20971403 http://ac.els-cdn.com/S0749208110000495/1-s2.0-S0749208110000495-main.pdf?_tid=5b591a7e-5d7d-11e5-a563-00000aacb35d&acdnat=1442523049_50b6bfb35d52e416120bc59f82dc7a53. https://doi.org/10.1016/j.soncn.2010.08.002.
10. Brant JM, Fink RM, Thompson C, Li YH, Rassouli M, Majima T, et al. Global survey of the roles, satisfaction, and barriers of home health care nurses on the provision of palliative care. J Palliat Med. 2019;22(8):945–60. Retrieved from https://www.ncbi.nlm.nih.gov/pubmed/31380727. https://doi.org/10.1089/jpm.2018.0566.
11. Brant JM, Newton S, Maurer MA. Pain Management in the Middle East: building capacity with global partners. Oncol Nurs Forum. 2017;44(4):403–5. Retrieved from http://www.ncbi.nlm.nih.gov/pubmed/28632244. https://doi.org/10.1188/17.ONF.403-405.

12. Campbell ML. Caring for dying patients in the intensive care unit: managing pain, dyspnea, anxiety, delirium, and death rattle. AACN Adv Crit Care. 2015;26(2):110–20. ; quiz 121–12. Retrieved from https://www.ncbi.nlm.nih.gov/pubmed/25898878 http://acc.aacnjournals.org/content/26/2/110.long https://aacnjournals.org/aacnacconline/article-abstract/26/2/110/15038/Caring-for-Dying-Patients-in-the-Intensive-Care?redirectedFrom=fulltext. https://doi.org/10.1097/NCI.0000000000000077.
13. Feldenzer K, Rosenzweig M, Soodalter JA, Schenker Y. Nurses' perspectives on the personal and professional impact of providing nurse-led primary palliative care in outpatient oncology settings. Int J Palliat Nurs. 2019;25(1):30–7. Retrieved from https://www.ncbi.nlm.nih.gov/pmc/articles/PMC6410708/pdf/nihms-1015627.pdf. https://doi.org/10.12968/ijpn.2019.25.1.30.
14. Ferrell B, Malloy P, Mazanec P, Virani R. CARES: AACN's new competencies and recommendations for educating undergraduate nursing students to improve palliative care. J Prof Nurs. 2016;32(5):327–33. Retrieved from http://www.ncbi.nlm.nih.gov/pubmed/27649590. https://doi.org/10.1016/j.profnurs.2016.07.002.
15. Ferrell B, Malloy P, Virani R. The end of life nursing education nursing consortium project. Ann Palliat Med. 2015;4(2):61–9. https://doi.org/10.3978/j.issn.2224-5820.2015.04.05.
16. Ferrell BR, Temel JS, Temin S, Smith TJ. Integration of palliative care into standard oncology care: ASCO clinical practice guideline update summary. J Oncol Pract. 2017;13(2):119–21. Retrieved from https://www.ncbi.nlm.nih.gov/pubmed/28972832. https://doi.org/10.1200/JOP.2016.017897.
17. Ferrell BR, Twaddle ML, Melnick A, Meier DE. National Consensus Project Clinical Practice Guidelines for quality palliative care guidelines, 4th edition. J Palliat Med. 2018; https://doi.org/10.1089/jpm.2018.0431.
18. Fitch MI, Fliedner MC, O'Connor M. Nursing perspectives on palliative care 2015. Ann Palliat Med. 2015;4(3):150–5. Retrieved from http://www.ncbi.nlm.nih.gov/pubmed/26231811. https://doi.org/10.3978/j.issn.2224-5820.2015.07.04.
19. George T. Role of the advanced practice nurse in palliative care. Int J Palliat Nurs. 2016;22(3):137–40. https://doi.org/10.12968/ijpn.2016.22.3.137.
20. Glover TL, Turpening P, Garvan C, Kittelson S. The palliative care resource nurses pilot survey: a descriptive report of their primary palliative care role and educational needs. J Palliat Med. 2018;21(2):128–9. https://doi.org/10.1089/jpm.2017.0526.
21. Hauser J, Sileo M, Araneta N, Kirk R, Martinez J, Finn K, et al. Navigation and palliative care. Cancer. 2011;117(15 Suppl):3585–91. Retrieved from https://www.ncbi.nlm.nih.gov/pubmed/21780093 https://acsjournals.onlinelibrary.wiley.com/doi/full/10.1002/cncr.26266. https://doi.org/10.1002/cncr.26266.
22. Head BA, Song MK, Wiencek C, Nevidjon B, Fraser D, Mazanec P. Palliative nursing summit: nurses leading change and transforming care: the Nurse's role in communication and advance care planning. J Hosp Palliat Nurs. 2018;20(1):23–9. https://doi.org/10.1097/njh.0000000000000406.
23. Kamal AH, Maguire JM, Meier DE. Evolving the palliative care workforce to provide responsive, serious illness care. Ann Intern Med. 2015;163(8):637–8. Retrieved from https://www.ncbi.nlm.nih.gov/pubmed/26258800. https://doi.org/10.7326/M15-0071.
24. Kav S, Brant JM, Mushani T. Perspectives in international palliative care. Semin Oncol Nurs. 2018;34(3):284–93. Retrieved from https://www.ncbi.nlm.nih.gov/pubmed/30122428. https://doi.org/10.1016/j.soncn.2018.06.009.
25. Mayer DD, Winters CA. Palliative Care in Critical Rural Settings. Crit Care Nurse. 2016;36(1):72–8. Retrieved from https://aacnjournals.org/ccnonline/article-abstract/36/1/72/3515/Palliative-Care-in-Critical-Rural-Settings?redirectedFrom=fulltext. https://doi.org/10.4037/ccn2016732.
26. Mazanec, P. G-Cares: graduate competencies and recommendations for educating nursing students in primary palliative care. 2019. Retrieved from https://advancingexpertcare.org/ItemDetail?iProductCode=APRNWEBGCARES
27. Mazanec P, Lamb G, Haas S, Dahlin C, Mooney A, LaFond D. Palliative nursing summit: nurses leading change and transforming care: the Nurse's role in coordination of care and transition management. J Hosp Palliat Nurs. 2018;20(1):15–22. https://doi.org/10.1097/njh.0000000000000413.
28. Paice JA, Battista V, Drick CA, Schreiner E. Palliative nursing summit: nurses leading change and transforming primary palliative care: Nursing's role in providing pain and symptom management. J Hosp Palliat Nurs. 2018;20(1):30–5. https://doi.org/10.1097/njh.0000000000000405.
29. Paice JA, Ferrell BR, Virani R, Grant M, Malloy P, Rhome A. Appraisal of the graduate end-of-life nursing education consortium training program. J Palliat Med. 2006;9(2):353–60. Retrieved from https://www.ncbi.nlm.nih.gov/pubmed/16629565. https://doi.org/10.1089/jpm.2006.9.353.
30. Pawlow P, Dahlin C, Doherty CL, Ersek M. The hospice and palliative care advanced practice registered nurse workforce: results of a National Survey. J Hosp Palliat Nurs. 2018;20(4):349–57. https://doi.org/10.1097/njh.0000000000000449.
31. Quill TE, Abernethy AP. Generalist plus specialist palliative care--creating a more sustainable model. N Engl J Med. 2013;368(13):1173–5. Retrieved from https://www.ncbi.nlm.nih.gov/pubmed/23465068 https://www.nejm.org/doi/pdf/10.1056/NEJMp1215620. https://doi.org/10.1056/NEJMp1215620.
32. Salamanca-Balen N, Seymour J, Caswell G, Whynes D, Tod A. The costs, resource use and cost-effectiveness of clinical nurse specialist-led

interventions for patients with palliative care needs: a systematic review of international evidence. Palliat Med. 2018;32(2):447–65. Retrieved from https://www.ncbi.nlm.nih.gov/pmc/articles/PMC5788084/pdf/10.1177_0269216317711570.pdf. https://doi.org/10.1177/0269216317711570.
33. Sekse RJT, Hunskar I, Ellingsen S. The nurse's role in palliative care: a qualitative meta-synthesis. J Clin Nurs. 2018;27(1–2):e21–38. Retrieved from https://onlinelibrary.wiley.com/doi/full/10.1111/jocn.13912. https://doi.org/10.1111/jocn.13912.
34. Sheldon LK, Brant JM, Hankle KS, Bialous S, Lubejko B. Promoting cancer nursing education, training and research in countries in transition. In: Silbermann M, editor. Cancer care in countries in transition. Geneva: Springer; 2016. p. 473–94.
35. Stephens CE, Hunt LJ, Bui N, Halifax E, Ritchie CS, Lee SJ. Palliative care eligibility, symptom burden, and quality-of-life ratings in nursing home residents. JAMA Intern Med. 2018;178(1):141–2. Retrieved from https://www.ncbi.nlm.nih.gov/pubmed/29159368 https://jamanetwork.com/journals/jamainternalmedicine/article-abstract/2663850 https://jamanetwork.com/journals/jamainternalmedicine/articlepdf/2663850/jamainternal_stephens_2017_ld_170060.pdf. https://doi.org/10.1001/jamainternmed.2017.6299.
36. Temel JS, Greer JA, Muzikansky A, Gallagher ER, Admane S, Jackson VA, et al. Early palliative care for patients with metastatic non-small-cell lung cancer. N Engl J Med. 2010;363(8):733–42.
37. The Joint Commission. Palliative care certification. 2019. Retrieved from https://www.jointcommission.org/accreditation-and-certification/certification/certifications-by-setting/hospital-certifications/palliative-care-certification/
38. van den Beuken-van Everdingen MH, Hochstenbach LM, Joosten EA, Tjan-Heijnen VC, Janssen DJ. Update on prevalence of pain in patients with Cancer: systematic review and meta-analysis. J Pain Symptom Manag. 2016;51(6):1070–1090 e1079. Retrieved from http://www.ncbi.nlm.nih.gov/pubmed/27112310. https://doi.org/10.1016/j.jpainsymman.2015.12.340.
39. von Gunten CF. Secondary and tertiary palliative care in US hospitals. JAMA. 2002;287(7):875–81. Retrieved from https://www.ncbi.nlm.nih.gov/pubmed/11851580. https://doi.org/10.1001/jama.287.7.875.
40. Wiencek C, Coyne P. Palliative care delivery models. Semin Oncol Nurs. 2014;30(4):227–33. Retrieved from https://www.ncbi.nlm.nih.gov/pubmed/25361874 https://www.sciencedirect.com/science/article/abs/pii/S0749208114000643?via%3Dihub. https://doi.org/10.1016/j.soncn.2014.08.004.

Understanding the Impact of Community-Based Palliative Care

Phyllis Whitehead, Senaida Keating, Shereen Gamaluddin, Carolyn White, Christi Stewart, and Kye Y. Kim

Introduction

In the past century, medicine has changed and advanced more than at any other point in history. Innovative treatments, earlier diagnostic capabilities, and improvements in clinical and surgical techniques have changed previously terminal diseases, such as certain cancers, coronary artery disease, and HIV care from "death sentences" to chronic disease states. The population is living longer than ever before, and the average life expectancy has increased from 53.5 years in 1919 to 78.3 years in 2019 [1]. With the advancements in treatments for previously terminal conditions, more Americans are now living with chronic serious illnesses for longer periods of time. Not only are there often associated symptoms of the disease itself, but often treatments for these chronic disease states have significant and debilitating side effects. These serious illnesses often impact quality of life (QOL), comfort, and function. Dealing with serious illness for prolonged periods of time can threaten an individual's and family's financial stability, dignity, comfort, and even rob a person of their identity.

Palliative medicine was formally approved by the American Board of Medical Specialties as a subspecialty in 2006, but the practice of palliative medicine can be dated back far earlier. Palliative medicine as a subspecialty focuses on the management of pain, symptoms, and stress for those living with a serious chronic disease. It provides

P. Whitehead
Carilion Roanoke Memorial Hospital Palliative Care Service, Roanoke, VA, USA

Virginia Tech Carilion School of Medicine, Roanoke, VA, USA
e-mail: pbwhitehead@carilionclinic.org

S. Keating
Virginia Tech Carilion School of Medicine, Roanoke, VA, USA

Veterans Affairs Medical Center, Salem, VA, USA

S. Gamaluddin · C. White
Centra Health Palliative Care Service, Lynchburg, VA, USA

C. Stewart
Carilion Roanoke Memorial Hospital Palliative Care Service, Roanoke, VA, USA

Virginia Tech Carilion School of Medicine, Roanoke, VA, USA

Carilion Center for Healthy Aging, Roanoke, VA, USA
e-mail: castewart1@carilionclinic.org

K. Y. Kim (✉)
Carilion Roanoke Memorial Hospital Palliative Care Service, Roanoke, VA, USA

Carilion Center for Healthy Aging, Roanoke, VA, USA

Department of Psychiatry and Behavioral Medicine, Virginia Tech Carilion School of Medicine, Roanoke, VA, USA
e-mail: kykim@carilionclinic.org

M. Silbermann (ed.), *Palliative Care for Chronic Cancer Patients in the Community*,
https://doi.org/10.1007/978-3-030-54526-0_5

an interdisciplinary focus and layer of support for patients and their families. Palliative medicine as an adjunct to standard medical care has been shown to improve quality of life and reduce emergency department and hospital utilization, and in some cases even prolong life expectancy. Palliative medicine, unlike hospice medicine, is appropriate at all points in chronic disease states, from the time of diagnosis, throughout the course of treatment, through end-of-life care, and even for families in bereavement support. The type of services and support that palliative medicine can provide may change and increase with disease progression over time, but unlike hospice care, palliative medicine can and should be provided concurrently with disease treatment through all points of management for chronic serious illness.

Palliative medicine provides a team-based approach to patient care to allow comprehensive assessment of patient needs and address care across a variety of domains. These include: (a) control of pain, symptoms, and side effects of treatments; (b) caregiver support; (c) social support; and (d) spiritual support. Addressing these domains can lead to improvement in pain and symptom management and relief of psychological, emotional, and spiritual suffering. Family and caregiver support is also paramount in the field of palliative medicine, including referrals to local community resources as indicated to allow better, more individualized care for patients in their preferred environment, whether that be home, long-term care, or group home settings. Palliative care provides communication about goal setting in the face of chronic disease management and can help to align patient and provider expectations with the reality of living with a serious illness. Team-based care is usually provided by physicians/providers, nurses, social workers, and chaplains, but also possibly including dieticians, counselors/psychologists, pharmacists, therapists (physical, occupational, or speech), and volunteers [2].

Due to the extensive needs and volume of patients and the lack of sufficient numbers of trained palliative specialists, it is imperative that aspects of palliative care be addressed by all providers. Primary palliative care can be provided by primary care providers and specialists without formal training in palliative medicine. Primary palliative care involves identification and basic management of symptoms of pain and suffering. It may also involve basic management of depression and anxiety often associated with chronic disease states. Providers can also engage patients and families in basic discussions of prognosis, code status, and goals of treatment. Specialized palliative medicine, also known as secondary palliative medicine, would be delivered by providers with specialty level training in palliative care, such as specialty certification or fellowship. These specialized practitioners can provide focus and management on refractory symptoms and/or complex depression, anxiety, grief, and existential suffering. They can also assist in conflict resolution regarding treatment plans and goals of care within families, between medical staff and families, and between treatment teams. Tertiary palliative medicine is indicated for patients with the most complex supportive care needs and is usually provided in an inpatient or academic center [3].

Throughout this chapter, the field of palliative medicine will be further explored at the community level—at national, state, and local levels—including barriers, resources, and opportunities for growth within the field.

Defining Hospice and Palliative Care

The terms palliative care and hospice care are often used interchangeably for one another, yet there is a significant difference between the two patient services. The National Hospice and Palliative Care Organization (NHPCO) clearly states that "palliative care is not hospice care: it does not replace the patient's primary treatment being received (See Fig. 1). It focuses on the pain, symptoms and stress of serious illness most often as an adjunct to curative care modalities." [4] The National Cancer Institute's definition of palliative care is defined as care given to improve the quality of life of patients who have a serious or life-threatening diseases, such as cancer. Palliative care is an approach to care that addresses the person as a whole, not just their dis-

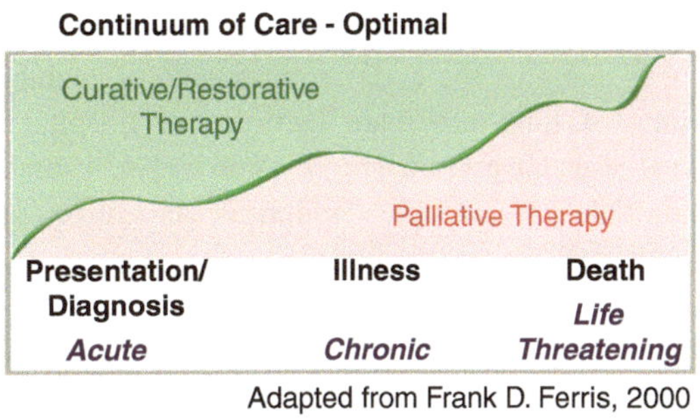

Fig. 1 Continuum of care—optimal. (Center to Advance Palliative Care 2019)

ease. The goal is to prevent or treat, as early as possible, the symptoms and side effects of the disease and its treatment, in addition to any related psychological, social, and spiritual problems [5]. Hospice care, on the other hand, is defined by NHPCO as care focusing on the pain, symptoms, and stress of serious illness during the terminal phase. The terminal phase is defined by Medicare as an individual with a life expectancy of 6 months or less if the illness, disease, or condition runs its typical course [4]. The critical differences between palliative care and hospice care are the time limitation and not pursuing aggressive interventions in hospice. Whereas hospice care is provided when life expectancy is 6 months or less, palliative care has no time limitation and may be elected to manage secondary symptoms resulting from treatments of an illness from which recovery is a possible, but not guaranteed, prognosis.

Hospice Challenges

A goal of hospice has been to utilize a multidisciplinary team approach to patient care and needs. Addressing a patient's emotional and psychosocial needs is as important as their physical needs. For this to be successful, hospice requires a group of providers, healthcare professionals, and caregivers to coordinate care. Until recently, any measure and reporting of the quality or success of that care was not required. The Affordable Care Act of 2010 mandated the initiation of a quality reporting program for hospices (HQRP) [4]. Mandated reporting creates a necessary initiative to develop quality standards within hospice, which in turn can translate into improved patient care [6].

The Department of Health and Human Services (HHS) utilized the Measure Applications Partnership (MAP) to help initiate this strategy. MAP consists of 60 organizations representing diverse interests and was convened in 2011 by the National Quality Forum (NQF) to provide guidance on measures for use in performance-based payment, public reporting, and other quality improvement programs [6].

The areas of focus for assessment for hospice coincide with essential needs for successful hospice implementation and care.

- Access and Availability of Services
- The average hospice length of stay continues to be less than 6 weeks. Measures would focus on when patients and family initially become aware of hospice services, the timeliness of care initiation once a patient has opted to utilize hospice services, as well as the accessibility to the healthcare team on a 24-hour basis.
- Patient- and Family-Centered Care
- Educating and providing support to patients and caregivers so they understand the scope of services provided, including spiritual, physical, and psychological care.
- Goals and Care Planning
- Establishing patient and family goals with regard to the care of the patient and assessing if these are being met.
- Care Coordination
- Hospice care is now often given across multiple settings. Measures help track potential breakdowns in care or communication concerns that occur in transitions. The average Medicare hospice enrollee is in the home for 56% of the time, an assisted living facility for 11% of the time, and a nursing home for 17% of the time [7].
- Provider Competency
- Ensures that the patient is cared for by a qualified healthcare team appropriately trained to provide hospice care. Physical aspects of care including management of pain, dyspnea, and

constipation are assessed using a standardized scale. Psychological and psychiatric aspects of care such as anxiety, depression, delirium, and behavioral disturbances are evaluated as well.

- Appropriateness/Affordable Care
- Assesses if patients are successful in avoiding unwanted trips to the hospital and/or unwanted medical procedures.

Utilizing these quality measures can create an opportunity to continually evaluate if care is appropriate, high-quality, patient-centered, and coordinated across providers. Though the primary goal of hospice has remained the same, hospice has undergone changes in the last decade. The use of hospice services has increased by 50% over the past decade [2]. The primary hospice diagnosis has also changed, moving from a primarily cancer as an admitting diagnosis to a variety of diseases including dementia, respiratory, and Parkinson's disease. As the demographics of hospice continue to change, care implementation will also need to be adapted to meet patient and family needs [8].

While having a reporting standard of quality is important, assessing and translating those measures to a personal, community level is also imperative. Communities now often include hospice needs as part of their community health need assessments. This specifically takes into account information such as the demographics of the population. Age, race, cultural preferences, as well as socioeconomic factors are important to understanding your specific population and their needs. The health status of the community, including the number of individuals using tobacco products, certain environmental exposures, or stress level is also important to take into consideration. Understanding care resources including hospital centers, physician and provider availability, and specialty services can impact how you coordinate or deliver care.

As hospice grows and its utilization increases, where and how to care for these patients also come into question. Many patients are not living out their days at home, either because they do not have caregiver support or because they do not meet requirements of a hospital or inpatient unit. This is where residential hospices can come into play. Since residential hospices do not need to meet many of the code requirements or regulations of long-term care facilities or hospitals, they often have a much more comfortable, serene, homelike atmosphere, which is appealing to many patients and families [9].

While hospice covers the medications, equipment, and nursing services, the room and board costs are typically not covered. Those expenses are often covered by the patient or family paying a daily room-and-board rate out of pocket. This can sometimes be subsidized by an endowment fund or other donations.

Palliative Care Challenges

Access to palliative care options in the United States, and the care itself, has made significant gains in the last two decades. According to 2018 Palliative Care Growth Snapshot issued by the Center to Advance Palliative Care (CPAC), the prevalence of hospitals (50 or more beds) with a palliative care team increased from 658 to 1831—a 178% increase from 2000 to 2016. The rise in prevalence of palliative care in US hospitals has been steady over the last 16 years. In 2000, less than one-quarter of US hospitals (658) had a palliative care program, compared to three quarters (1831) in 2016. The unremarkable increase, however, has occurred at centralized medical facilities in urban areas that serve a community so long as the members of that or nearby communities can access the hospital to receive palliative care. Rural areas are less likely to have access to palliative care services where populations are disproportionately older, poorer, and more likely to have a range of chronic illnesses than their urban counterparts [10].

A survey conducted in California in 2011 found that while the majority (53%) of California's acute hospitals offered inpatient palliative care services, only about 18% offered outpatient palliative care [6]. A 2018 analysis by Kathleen Kerr of data collected in California indicates that statewide, there is only a 52% inpatient palliative care (IPPC) sufficiency and only a 40% community-based palliative care (CBPC) [11]. The significance of sufficiency data from California is that as of 2014, the California Department of Health Care Services (DHCS) is required to expand community-based palliative care services to Medi-Cal beneficiaries [11].

The costs, the relative newness of the formal recognition of palliative care, and misunderstanding of palliative care by those who could benefit from it serve as roadblocks for the expansion of community-based palliative care outpatient programs. Costs affect both providers and patients and/or their insurance providers. Although studies have shown the benefits gained through the use of community-based palliative care, including statistically significant 20% reduction in total medical costs, 38% reduction in ICU admissions, 33% reduction in hospital admissions, and 12% reduction in hospitals days [2], the fee-for-service does not adequately support the significant amount of time spent by an interdisciplinary team with patients and families [9].

To date, there are only a few models or examples of how a palliative care service can break even in a fee-for-service billing context, regardless of setting, and persuasive arguments are required for hospital or health plan subsidies. For patients, not all palliative care options are covered by Medicare or Medicaid, resulting in them paying out of pocket or simply forgoing the care. Many insurance plans cover some palliative care services, such as pain management. Many Medicare, Medicaid, and private insurance plans offer scant or no coverage of home visits, coordination of care, wound care, social and spiritual counseling, 24-hour hotlines, advanced care planning, or family support. Most of the insurance coverage is for patients who are hospitalized or in hospice care [12]. Most often, palliative care is provided to the geriatric group who are typically on fixed incomes.

Formalized and Board-recognized palliative medicine is relatively new to healthcare. It was only as recent as 2006 when the American Board of Medical Specialties (ABMS) approved the creation of Hospice and Palliative Medicine (HPM) as a subspecialty of 10 participating boards [13]. Although it has been shown that the expansion of palliative care providers is on the rise and the number of Accreditation Council for Graduate Medical Education (ACGME)-approved Hospice and Palliative Care Fellowship Program slots has jumped from 283 in 2013–2014 to 413 for 2018–2019, only 87% of the slots are filled. Only in 2016 did the Joint Commission establish a community-based palliative care (CBPC) certification that recognizes home health and hospice organizations that provide top caliber community-based palliative care to patients and families in their home (primary place of residence) [14]. Compounding the issue of the requirements resulting from the rapid expansion of palliative care is the misunderstanding and poor messaging of palliative care in general. Overall, 9 of 10 adults in the United States have little or no knowledge of palliative care and still more physicians are unaware that their own institutions offer it [15]. Berry Medical institutions themselves often combine palliative care medicine with geriatric care medicine, as is the case with the University of Texas, the University of Chicago, and The George Washington University, to name a few, which can lead patients to associate palliative care with geriatric care. Further compounding the difficulty of correctly branding palliative care is the frequent association of palliative medicine as hospice or end-of-life care, and studies of patients with cancer suggest that many initially associate palliative care with hospice and death and/or dying [15].

Financial Issues

There are many challenges to community based palliative care programs. These programs are often "stand alone," providing care for the most complicated, ill patients who live at home. They are doing so without the support of a facility or programs such as hospice. As most community-based programs are not affiliated with or part of an integrated health system, their services cannot be subsidized [16]. The traditional form of Medicare fee-for-service is not sustainable when trying to support the services of a multidisciplinary team, which is the hospice care model. Reimbursement for physicians and advance practice registered nurses is inadequate considering the time required to effectively manage these complex patients. Additionally, the Medicare system does not financially reimburse healthcare providers such as registered nurses, social workers, bereavement counselors, and the administrative staff needed for an effective advanced illness management program [16].

Staffing Issues

Access to healthcare services is critical to achieving or maintaining health, yet those who live in rural areas face a variety of access barriers. There is no single definition of a rural area. One general definition is a geographical area not neighboring a city or town with insufficient healthcare resources, not greatly populated, with predominance of medically underserved patient populations [21]. It is especially important for those residents in rural areas to have access to hospice and palliative services as it can improve the quality of life for those of all ages who are dealing with serious, life-limiting illnesses. Unfortunately, the less populated a county or area, the higher the degree of poverty and less likelihood of a hospice agency to provide those services [1].

Residents in rural areas often encounter general barriers to healthcare that limit their ability to obtain the care they need. These residents must have sufficient access to appropriate health services, and those services must be available, affordable, and obtainable in a timely manner. Even if services are available in the community, there can be many other factors that could limit a resident's ability to access these services [17]. This section will look at these barriers that rural residents often face today.

In order for rural residents to utilize appropriate healthcare services, they must have the following:

- Financial means to pay for services
- Means to reach and use those services
- Confidence in their ability to communicate with providers
- Trust that they can use those services without compromising their privacy
- Belief that they will receive quality care [17].

Those individuals without health insurance have less access to healthcare services, especially in rural areas. A US Census Bureau Report found that the proportion of populations living outside a metropolitan area without any type of health insurance coverage was 9.2% in 2017, compared to 8.8% in metropolitan areas [18].

According to the National Advisory Committee on Rural Health and Human Services, even rural residents who have Medicare may have limited access to hospice care [19]. This is very problematic since rural people tend to be older, sicker, and have lower incomes than their urban counterparts. The use of hospice services by Medicare beneficiaries has increased overall since 2000 in all locations, but hospice is still more available and used more often in urban areas. According to the Hospice Services chapter in the 2019 Report to Congress, Medicare Payment Policy, as of 2017, there were a total 878 rural hospices, down from a peak of 945 in 2007, with a decline of 2.6% from 2016 to 2017 alone. Therefore, in 2017, only 20% of all hospices in the United States were located in rural areas. The Report also notes that although the number of rural hospices has decreased, the percentage of rural Medicare decedents using hospice services has increased over this same period. [20]

Providing hospice and palliative care in rural areas can involve many challenges. In a 2013 phone survey of 53 rural hospice directors and key staff members from 47 states, the most important issues identified included the following:

- Financial issues, such as reimbursement and operating costs
- Rural factors, such as population changes, economics, culture, and geography
- Federal regulations and policies, such as requirement for face-to-face visits for recertification of hospice patients
- Workforce issues, such as challenges in recruiting and retaining staff, and staff burnout
- Relationships with other healthcare providers and competition for resources and patients
- Technology issues, such as limited access to Internet and connectivity problems [21].

Not just the elderly and poor have difficulty in getting appropriate care in rural areas. Another subset of patients that has great difficulty in accessing hospice and palliative care in the rural communities are those in the (lesbian, gay, bisexual and transgender) LGBT community. Lack of healthcare provider training/education in lesbian, gay, bisexual, and transgender cultural competence may greatly diminish access to providers. Even those culturally competent providers may exhibit microaggressions when providing care to the LGBT patient, especially in socio-politically conservative areas. Microaggressions are those everyday verbal, nonverbal, and environmental slights, snubs, or insults, whether intentional or unintentional, which communicate hostile, derogatory, or negative messages to target persons based solely on their marginalized group membership [10]. In a study of healthcare providers in rural Tennessee, many of the interviewed providers felt they were competent to provide LGBT patient care, but they did describe behaviors and attitudes that likely contributed to inequities of care in those communities [22].

Palliative care has its own set of challenges. Although hospice is covered by Medicare and many other insurance plans as a benefit, palliative care typically is not [22]. Palliative care can be utilized at any time in the course of a chronic life-limiting illness. Optimally, it should be offered at the time of diagnosis, once clinical decline from the illness begins, and when the patient begins to experience treatment failures. This is especially difficult in rural populations due to the multiple issues outlined in this section. It can be generally stated that living in rural communities is negatively associated with hospice and palliative services as these patients often exhibit poorer health status and greater need for care [1].

One answer to the difficulty in accessing palliative care could potentially be the use of telemedicine. While this can often be easily utilized in urban areas, it is frequently difficult to access in rural areas. Some of the difficulties encountered can include the following:

- Limited access to high-speed internet
- Limited access to smartphones
- Credentialing and licensing of telehealth providers
- Reimbursement issues
- Sustainability
- Malpractice concerns as some policies do not cover telehealth
- Transportation, as some telehealth services still require patients to travel to participate in live video consultations
- Interoperability, in which some telehealth programs may have issues with secure methods to access and share medical information
- Mistrust of technology and healthcare in genera
- Lack of provider utilization if they lack interest or ability to effectively interact by video [22].

Clinician Self Care and Staff Challenges in Rural Areas

Some of the many challenges faced by the rural hospice and palliative care workforce are outlined in the report of Perspectives of Rural Hospice Directors [17]. The challenges include the following:

- Heavy workloads and provider shortages
- Wearing multiple hats
- Limited options for training
- Coping with fear and anger among patients and families who are having difficulty accepting their loved ones' illness or injury
- Emotional stress of caring for dying patients with whom they may have close relationships
- Safety concerns related to traveling to remote areas
- Low retention rates
- Physical stress
- Lower salaries in rural areas
- Potentially only part-time hours available due to financial constraints of rural agencies
- Scheduling concerns where staff may work alone and without adequate support
- Fewer options of medications and medical equipment in rural pharmacies
- Ongoing opioid crisis in rural areas may limit opioid use or choice.

Provider shortages are fairly typical in rural areas and encompass primary care and all specialties. Nurse practitioners (NPs), clinical nurse specialists (CNSs), and physician assistants (PAs) often fill the provider role in rural communities due to physician shortages [23]. Although these advanced practice providers partially fill the gap, rural communities continue to struggle. Additionally, shortages of trained hospice and palliative providers are a common theme in rural areas. All of these provider roles are often inadequately prepared for the care of terminally ill patients [24]. These providers can often be uncomfortable with talking to their patients and families about palliative and hospice referrals due to the lack of specialized training opportunities. Another issue is the limited scope of practice for NPs, CNSs, and PAs in certain states. Statutory laws often hinder NPs, CNSs, or PA from referring or admitting a patient to hospice. This can delay or defer access to services if these providers must defer a hospice referral to a physician. At this time, only physicians can certify that a patient has a terminal illness with a prognosis of less than 6 months and admit that patient to hospice. This can severely limit hospice care in those rural areas with very limited numbers of physicians [1]. Another provider issue can be overconfidence in their ability to manage a patient's symptoms and disease trajectory, which again delays or defers utilization of hospice or palliative services.

Another challenge is the limited options for education. End-of-life care is often not comprehensively taught in most undergraduate, graduate, or medical schools. Though this is slowly changing, it is still a major issue in the rural areas as opposed to urban areas where the majority of new medical school graduates tend to work. As chronic and terminal diseases progress, acute deterioration and symptom management can be more complex than providers are initially prepared to manage independently [25]. When providers are not adequately prepared to manage these conditions, patients suffer. This is especially true in rural communities.

The emotional stress of caring for patients at end of life can be especially difficult for providers and employees of hospice and palliative care agencies in rural communities. Many of those caring for patients are local to their communities and often know them personally. The boundary between professional and personal can become blurred and emotional. The fear of losing a loved one or personal friend can create a sense of urgency, a desire to continue curative treatments even when they are no longer effective, and result in discounting a patient's wish to focus on quality of life instead of quantity [1]. This situation becomes more difficult when providers and caregivers cannot accept reality and prognosis, either based on close relationship, fear, lack of education, or difficulty in communication of facts.

Often providers are uncomfortable or unable to have frank conversations with their patients about the specific disease process and prognosis, as well as all those services potentially available and provided by hospice or palliative care [26]. These hospice and palliative referrals can sometimes be perceived as negative options and can be seen as giving up, both by providers and families. Though these perceived negative options are seen in both urban and rural areas, they are more prevalent in rural areas. Rural patients and families tend to be less trusting of the medical establishment due to their limited education and increased poverty [23]. They can also be "more likely to think they are not getting equal treatment and that providers who discuss treatment withholding or withdrawal are doing so to save money." [23]. This can be especially true in the African American communities.

Safety concerns in rural areas are different from those in urban areas. Those providers and caregivers traveling to remote areas have their own set of concerns. Providers and staff often have to travel great distances alone as they have to cover large service areas. This can be especially difficult or dangerous in bad weather. It can be a financial burden due to lower salaries, rising gas costs, and wear and tear on personal vehicles. It is also an emotional stress to be alone without support from colleagues in dealing with those patients at end of life and those with difficult symptom management needs. Cell phone service is often sporadic and unreliable in remote areas, leaving hospice and palliative staff without the ability to call for assistance if needed.

The ongoing opioid crisis can affect care in rural areas. Recent opioid legislation and increasing scrutiny from federal and state agencies have created multiple barriers for providers and patients to obtain adequate pain relief. These challenges can include prescription limitations, practitioner fear of litigation, and need for frequent face-to-face provider visits for refills and monitoring [27]. Rural communities suffer disproportionately from lack of opioid prescribers, shortages of opioid medications, and reluctance of providers to prescribe in those areas most affected. There is often a stigma associated with the use of opioids from providers, patients, family members, and caregivers.

Even at end of life, there is continuing stigma and fear surrounding the use of opioids. It is imperative that providers and nurses caring for patients at end of life in rural communities stay up-to-date on current regulations, opioid availability in their area, and education needs of their patients with respect to opioid use.

Ethical Issues Considerations

Ethical challenges exist in the community setting as in inpatient settings. Clinicians may experience ethical dilemmas such as the lack of surrogate decision makers, advance care planning for serious ill patients who lose capacity to make their own medical decisions, and palliative sedation. When these ethical issues arise, it is important to have access to a bioethicist and/or bioethics committee to assist in determining the most appropriate ethical course of action.

It is important to understand the following ethical principles. Autonomy is acknowledging the moral right of every capable individual to choose and follow his or her own plan of life and actions. Palliative care clinicians should always integrate shared decision-making with patients and their families/loved ones. Self-determination is crucial when appropriate, evidence-based medical interventions are clearly presented to patients and their loved ones.

Clinicians should consider the following questions when determining the ethically appropriate course of action [28]:

- Has the patient been informed of benefits and risks?
- Informed consent: does documentation matter ... Legally?
- Is the patient mentally capable and legally competent?
- If mentally capable, what are the patient's preferences?
- If lacking capacity, has the patient expressed prior preferences?
- Who is the appropriate surrogate?
- Is the patient unwilling or unable to cooperate with medical treatment?

Medical decision-making capacity is determined by evaluating the following items [28]:

- Comprehension and understanding of one's medical conditions
- Evaluation of the benefits and risks of the intervention and the consequences of refusing the intervention
- Selection of realistic alternative options of interventions
- Ability to communicate one's thoughts, questions, and concerns
- Psychiatry may be needed to verify if clinicians do not feel patients have medical decision-making capacity. It is important to know your agency or facility's policy for determining medical decision-making capacity.

Additionally, clinicians should be familiar with the legal hierarchy of designated decision makers. The process varies from locality to locality. If an advance directive or guardianship documentation does not exist, then the next of kin is spouse, majority of adult children (includes adopted children), both parents, majority of siblings, and so forth.

Beneficence is to do the right thing. It is the act of charity, mercy, and kindness with a strong connotation of doing good to others including moral obligation. Nonmaleficence is defined as doing no harm. Medical futility is a common problem that occurs many times at end of life. It is defined as medically unnecessary, nonbeneficial healthcare interventions usually related to end-of-life care. Restricted quality of life (QOL, severely compromised QOL and/or profoundly diminished QOL are factors associated with futility. The following questions should be considered [28]:

- Are the interventions in question recommended and indicated?
- What are the medical teams recommending?
- Is there consensus among the medical teams?
- What is the prognosis with and without treatment?
- What has been communicated to the patient and/or family?
- How do we determine QOL for our patients?
- Are there biases in determining QOL?
- Is this suicide if someone chooses to die?

Moral distress occurs when an individual's moral integrity is seriously compromised, either because one feels unable to act in accordance with core values and obligations, or attempted actions fail to achieve the desired outcome [29]. Moral injury is a new way of looking at burnout. It is the inability to provide high-quality care and healing related to complexities of healthcare. Moral injury focuses on system issues, whereas burnout implies poor individual resiliency and coping skills. Moral injury may lead to clinicians feeling wounded, disengaged, and learned helplessness. Moral residue is an aspect of moral distress. It is the residue that remains that can be damaging to the self and one's career, particularly when morally distressing episodes repeat over time.

Palliative sedation is defined as "when terminally ill, conscious patients experience intolerable symptoms that cannot be relieved by expert palliative care, palliative sedation involves administering sedatives and non-opioid medications to relieve suffering in doses that may induce unconsciousness, but not death." [30]. Palliative sedation is used more commonly to relieve severe physical symptoms such as dyspnea, pain, nausea, and delirium and more rarely in patients with existential suffering [30]. Ethicists, numerous healthcare professional organizations, and the US Supreme Court has sanctioned palliative sedation therapy as an acceptable means of relieving suffering in the last days of life [30]. Palliative sedation is not euthanasia or assisted suicide.

A concern has emerged regarding whether it is ethically appropriate to sedate dying patients in such a way to intentionally make them unconscious to alleviate symptoms when all possible treatments have failed until they die [31]. Clinicians may struggle with potentially eliminating the patient's opportunity to live their last days with their children and family and secondly with accelerating their death. Despite frequent reports of palliative sedation, there have not been any studies to find a correlation between palliative sedation and the hastening of death [31]. Of particular debate is the use of palliative sedation to treat existential suffering. For example, if a patient has a prognosis of greater than two weeks, requires sedation that prevents oral intake, and refuses artificial hydration and nutrition, many experts feel palliative sedation may become a contributing cause of death. Mental health and spiritual care experts should be consulted to treat existential suffering prior to initiating total palliative sedation and to foster closure activities. It is imperative to incorporate the interdisciplinary team in assessing the patients' suffering and communicating with the patient, family, and other healthcare clinicians. [31]

Justifying ethical principles for palliative sedation include dignity, respect for autonomy, beneficence, nonmaleficence, and double effect. Having access to bioethicists and bioethics committees is essential in providing medically and ethically appropriate care.

Mental Health Challenges

Palliative care, designed to improve patients' QOL, often plays an important role in end-of-life care for those with advanced illnesses and their families [32]. In view of its care practices, the

World Health Organization further clarifies the core features: "Palliative care—integrates the psychological and spiritual aspects of patient care." [33]. Most palliative care practitioners are keenly aware that the psychological distress of patients and their families can be a challenging clinical aspect, but the presence of psychiatric clinicians in this field previously has been limited. Various barriers that interfere with proper recognition and treatment of psychiatric problems at end-of-life care have been addressed in recent years. Some of them are related to professional factors, such as the belief among palliative care clinicians that they themselves could adequately address psychological distress, or lack of confidence among psychiatrists about their ability to be of value in caring for patients near the end of life.

Practice patterns with the field of psychiatry may have hindered the field's involvement as well, because the emergence of palliative care coincided with the movement of psychiatry toward increasing reliance on psychopharmacology and away from psychotherapeutic modes of care. System-level factors, including funding structures that have been unfamiliar or inadequate to compensate psychiatry providers, may have been barriers [34, 35]. Although some of the barriers mentioned above still exist, the concept of palliative care psychiatry has been steadily evolving and maturing over the years. Several academic centers currently include psychiatrists on their palliative care services [36]. The American Psychiatric Association reports on formally integrating mental health services into hospice settings in one major community-based hospice care program [37].

Potential roles of the psychiatrist in caring for patients at the end of life are multiple. They can be (1) diagnosis and treatment of psychiatric disorders, (2) understanding psychodynamics and dysfunctional coping, (3) consultation on psychopharmacology, (4) assessment of decision-making capacity, (5) recognizing and treating staff stress, (6) facilitating effective team work and identifying team dysfunction, (7) bereavement care, (8) integrating developmental considerations into treatment plans, (9) psychiatric education for palliative care staff, and (10) research [8]. In view of psychopharmacological contributions to the patient care, psychiatrists may review the appropriateness of medications, especially various psychotropic agents [38]. In an ideal model, mental health professionals such as psychiatrists, psychologists, and social workers should be included in a palliative care team. Each team member can make contributions to psychopharmacological intervention, cognitive-behavioral therapy, grief intervention, and mindfulness, etc.

As mental health professionals continue to evolve into an expert discipline in palliative care, there should be also more efforts to promote research in challenging areas, such as palliative care for patients with serious mental disorders, substance abuse disorders, personality disorders, delirium, dementia with neuropsychiatric symptoms, depression, anxiety, and desire to hasten death. In particular, it would be clinically valuable to know more about the relationship of mental health issues with pain.

Opportunities for Growth

Palliative care services are beginning to be successfully integrated into ambulatory clinics and home health agencies [39]. Another opportunity is partnering with managed care plans and local Area on Agency Aging offices and other elder service agencies. It is critical to target the most vulnerable individuals such as low-income ethnic and racial minorities. Experts continue to call for innovative models to deliver community-based palliative care to address these and other gaps in care. Because service agencies serve over 90% of elders with multiple chronic conditions including cancer, many have functionality deficits and report poorer health compared to older adults who do not receive these services [39–41].

Other studies provide further evidence to encourage adoption of community based palliative care specialists across multiple serious illnesses/conditions [42]. These findings should encourage policy makers and service providers to target delivery of palliative care services to all people who could benefit, not just those with cancer [42, 43].

Furthermore, chronically ill patients in rural areas face challenges in accessing palliative care due to poverty, lack of insurance, and transportation [44]. Rural communities would greatly benefit from community-based palliative care programs. Culturally informed community-based palliative care services including patient navigators should be developed for Latinos, Asian, and African descendants [45].

Another vulnerable population is that of individuals with mental health disorders. People with schizophrenia were half as likely to enroll in community-based specialist palliative care and were half as likely to be admitted to hospital in the last year of life compared to people without schizophrenia who had a similar sociodemographic profile [42]. This presents an excellent opportunity to design community based palliative care programs that can address the unique challenges of people with mental illnesses.

Community-based palliative care services are associated with reduced use of costly hospital care, health system cost savings, reduced EOL care costs, increased hospice utilization with improved care patient satisfaction, and increased likelihood of death occurring out of the hospital [2, 40, 46–49]. As based upon the WHO's concept of palliative care, CBPC should be accessible to the entire community [47].

Future research should examine which aspects of the specialist palliative care teams contribute most to reducing health system costs using multilevel regression models and should assess the impact of these teams on informal caregiver costs [50].

Conclusion

Patients with serious illnesses prefer to receive care and die at home, yet the end-of-life period is characterized by high levels of acute care utilization, in-hospital deaths, and healthcare costs [10, 51, 52].

More intensive training, including didactic classes, shadowing of clinicians, case studies, and continuing education, would help to improve EOL skills in some key areas. These include understanding the concept of community-based palliative care and need for greater focus on emotional issues at the end of life and distinguishing between what constitutes an emergency versus the natural dying process and conveying this information to patients and families [44, 53–55].

As the healthcare entities move to a more patient-centric healthcare delivery system tied across the community, community based palliative care programs are well positioned to bridge across the continuum of care settings and deliver a person-centered interprofessional approach to people dealing with serious illnesses and conditions [48, 51, 52, 56].

Care that is primarily driven by values, goals, and preferences of seriously ill individuals and their family members may result in more compassionate, affordable, sustainable, and high-quality care [2].

References

1. Teddler T. Analysis of common barriers to rural patients utilizing hospice and palliative care services: an integrated literature review. J Am Assoc Nurse Pract. 2017;29:356–62. https://doi.org/10.1002/2327-6924.12475.
2. Program C, Yosick L, Crook RE, et al. Effects of a population health community-based palliative care Program on cost and utilization. J Palliat Med. 2019;XX(Xx):1–7. https://doi.org/10.1089/jpm.2018.0489.
3. Pashikanti L, Von AD. Impact of early mobilization protocol on the medical-surgical inpatient population: an integrated review of literature. Clin Nurse Spec. 2012;26(2):87–94. https://doi.org/10.1097/NUR.0b013e31824590e6.
4. Palliative care versus hospice. nhpco.org/wp-content/uploads/2019/04/PalliativeCare_VS_Hospice.pdf. Published 2019.
5. Parr JD, Zhang B, Nilsson ME, et al. The influence of age on the likelihood of receiving end-of-life care consistent with patient treatment preferences. J Palliat Med. 2010;13(6):719–26. https://doi.org/10.1089/jpm.2009.0337.
6. Beresford L, Kerr K. Next generation of palliative care: community models offer services outside the hospital; 2012.
7. Hunt LJ, Covinsky KE, Yaffe K, et al. Pain in community-dwelling older adults with dementia:

results from the National Health and aging trends study. J Am Geriatr Soc. 2015;63(8):1503–11. https://doi.org/10.1111/jgs.13536.
8. Teno JM, Gozalo PL, Bynum JPW, et al. Change in end-of-life care for Medicare beneficiaries: site of death, place of care, and health care transitions in 2000, 2005, and 2009. JAMA. 2013;309(5):470–7. https://doi.org/10.1001/jama.2012.207624.
9. Inker JK. Home and community-based palliative care: best practices and resources for providers; 2018.
10. Lakin JR, Benotti E, Paladino J, Henrich N, Sanders J. Interprofessional work in serious illness communication in primary care: a qualitative study. J Palliat Med. 2019;XX(Xx):1–13. https://doi.org/10.1089/jpm.2018.0471.
11. Kerr K. Narrowing the Gap; 2018.
12. Ollove M. Why some patients aren't getting palliative care. Stateline Article. //www.pewtrusts.org/en/research-and-analysis/blogs/stateline/2017/07/10/why-some-patients-arent-getting-palliative-care. Published 2017.
13. Program data. American Academy of Hospice and Palliiative Medicine. //aahpm.org/certification/subspecialty-certification. Published 2019.
14. The Joint Commission. Community based palliative care certification.
15. Finlay E, Rabow M, Buss M. Filling the gap: creating an outpatient palliative care program in your institution. Am Soc Clin Oncol. 2018;
16. Barnato AE. Challenges in understanding and respecting patients' preferences. Health Aff. 2017;36(7):1252–7. https://doi.org/10.1377/hithaff.2017.0177.
17. Perspectives of rural hospice directors. https://ruralhealth.und.edu/projects/health-reform-policy-research-center/pdf/perspectives-of-rural-hospice-directors-march-2015.pdf. Published 2015.
18. Health insurance coverage in the United States. https://www.census.gov/content/dam/Census/library/publications/2018/demo/p60-264.pdf. Published 2017.
19. Hunnicutt JN, Tjia J, Lapane KL. Hospice use and pain management in elderly nursing home residents with cancer. J Pain Symptom Manag. 2017;53(3):561–70. https://doi.org/10.1016/j.jpainsymman.2016.10.369.
20. 2019 Report to Congress Medicare Payment Policy; 2019.
21. Lynch S. Hospice and palliative care access issues in rural areas. Am J Hosp Palliat Med. 2013;30(2):172–7. https://doi.org/10.1177/1049909112444592.
22. Patterson JG, Jabson Tree JM, Kamen C. Patient education and counseling. Rural Hosp Palliat Care. 2019; https://doi.org/10.1016/j.pec.2019.06.003.
23. Artnak KE, McGraw RM, Stanley VF. Health care accessibility for chronic illness management and end of life care. J Law Med Ethics. 2011;39(2):140–50. https://doi.org/10.1111/j.1748-720.
24. Hospice and Palliative Nurses Association, Dahlin C, Lynch MT. Core curriculum for the advanced practice hospice and palliative registered nurse: Hospice and Palliative Nurses Association; 2013.
25. Fink RM, Oman KS, Youngwerth J, Bryant LL. A palliative care needs assessment of rural hospitals. J Palliat Med. 2013;16(6):638–44.
26. Love AW, Liversage LM. Barriers to accessing palliative care: a review of the literature. Prog Palliat Care. 2014;22(1):9–19.
27. Foxwell AM, Uritsky T, Meghani SH. Opioids and cancer pain management in the United States: public policy and legal challenges. Semin Oncol Nurs. 2019;35(3):322–6.
28. Jonsen AR, Siegler M, Winslade WJ. Clinical ethics: a practical approach to ethical decisions in clinical medicine. 8th ed. New York: McGraw-Hill; 2015.
29. Ulrich CM, Grady C, Hamric AB, Berlinger N. Response to "Nurses at the table: nursing, ethics, and health policy". Nurs Outlook. 2017;65(2):142. https://doi.org/10.1016/j.outlook.2017.01.010.
30. Elie D, Marino A, Torres-Platas SG, et al. End-of-life care preferences in patients with severe and persistent mental illness and chronic medical conditions: a comparative cross-sectional study. Am J Geriatr Psychiatry. 2018;26(1):89–97. https://doi.org/10.1016/j.jagp.2017.09.018.
31. Beller EM, van Driel ML, Mcgregor L, Truong S, Mitchell G. Palliative pharmacological sedation for terminally ill adults. Cochrane Database Syst Rev. 2015;(2017, 6):373–4. https://doi.org/10.1002/14651858.CD010206.pub2.
32. Morrison RS, Meier D. Palliative care. N Engl J Med. 2004;350(25):2582–90.
33. Malec M, Shega JW. Pain management in the elderly. Med Clin North Am. 2015;99(2):337–50. https://doi.org/10.1016/j.mcna.2014.11.007.
34. Shuster JL, Higginson IJ. Hospice and palliative care: a psychiatric perspective. In: Chochinov HM, Breitbart W, editors. Handbook of psychiatry in palliative medicine. 2nd ed. New York: Oxford University Press; 2009. p. 3–10.
35. Fairman N, Hirst JM, Irwin SA. Psychiatry in palliative care. In: Clinical manual of palliative care psychiatry. 1st ed; 2013.
36. Meier EA, Gallegos JV, Montross-Thomas LP, Depp CA, Irwin SA, Jeste DV. Defining a good death (successful dying): literature review and a call for research and public dialogue. Am J Geriatr Psychiatry. 2016;24(4):261–71. https://doi.org/10.1016/j.jagp.2016.01.135.
37. Kasl-Godley JE, King DA, Quill TE. Opportunities for psychologists in palliative care: working with patients and families across the disease continuum. Am Psychol. 2014;69(4):364–76. https://doi.org/10.1037/a0036735.
38. Holms H, Sachs GA, Shega JW, et al. Integrating palliative medicine into the care of person with advanced dementia: identifying appropriate medication use. J Am Geriatr Soc. 2008;56(7):1306–11.
39. Capezuti E, Gardner D. HHS Public Access. 2018;6(Suppl 1):1–6. https://doi.org/10.21037/apm.2017.03.10.Expanding.
40. Koh S-J, Kim S, Kim J, et al. Experiences and opinions related to end-of-life discussion: from

oncologists' and resident physicians' perspectives. Cancer Res Treat. 2017; https://doi.org/10.4143/crt.2016.446.
41. Bull J, Kamal AH, Harker M, et al. Standardization and scaling of a community-based palliative care model. J Palliat Med. 2017;20(11):1237–43. https://doi.org/10.1089/jpm.2017.0027.
42. Spilsbury K, Rosenwax L, Brameld K, Kelly B, Arendts G. Morbidity burden and community-based palliative care are associated with rates of hospital use by people with schizophrenia in the last year of life: a population-based matched cohort study. PLoS One. 2018;13(11):1–21. https://doi.org/10.1371/journal.pone.0208220.
43. Spilsbury K, Rosenwax L. Community-based specialist palliative care is associated with reduced hospital costs for people with non-cancer conditions during the last year of life. BMC Palliat Care. 2017;16(1):68. https://doi.org/10.1186/s12904-017-0256-2.
44. Tran QNH, Dieu-Hien HT, King IN, Sheehan K, Iglowitz M-L, Periyakoil VS. Providing culturally respectful care for seriously-ill Vietnamese Americans. J Pain Symptom Manag. 2019; https://doi.org/10.1016/j.jpainsymman.2019.03.012.
45. Morris DA, Johnson KS, Ammarell N, Arnold RM, Tulsky JA, Steinhauser KE. What is your understanding of your illness? A communication tool to explore patients' perspectives of living with advanced illness. J Gen Intern Med. 2012;27(11):1460–6. https://doi.org/10.1007/s11606-012-2109-2.
46. Mitchell G, Zhang J, Burridge L, et al. Case conferences between general practitioners and specialist teams to plan end of life care of people with end stage heart failure and lung disease: an exploratory pilot study. BMC Palliat Care. 2014;13(1):24. https://doi.org/10.1186/1472-684X-13-24.
47. Kim SN, Choi SO, Shin SH, Ryu JS, Baik JW. Development of a community-based palliative care model for advance cancer patients in public health centers in Busan, Korea. Cancer Res Treat. 2017;49(3):559–68. https://doi.org/10.4143/crt.2016.276.
48. Taub JM, Coats H, Coats C, et al. Palliative care delivery: descriptions of community-based services in Vellore, India, and Seattle, Washington. Int J Palliat Nurs. 2019;25(1):39–45.
49. Butler M, Ratner E, McCreedy E, Shippee N, Kane RL. Decision aids for advance care planning: an overview of the state of the science. Ann Intern Med. 2014;161(6):408–18. https://doi.org/10.7326/M14-0644.
50. Seow H, Salam-White L, Bainbridge D. Community-based specialist palliative care teams and health system costs at end of life: a retrospective matched cohort study. CMAJ Open. 2019;7(1):E73–80. https://doi.org/10.9778/cmajo.20180113.
51. Foglia MB, Lowery J, Sharpe VA, Tompkins P, Fox E. A comprehensive approach to eliciting, documenting, and honoring patient wishes for care near the end of life: the veterans health Administration's life-sustaining treatment decisions initiative. Jt Comm J Qual Patient Saf. 2019;45(1):47–56. https://doi.org/10.1016/j.jcjq.2018.04.007.
52. Stewart R, Dimmock A, Green M, et al. An analysis of recruitment efficiency for an end-of-life advance care planning randomized controlled trial. Am J Ho. 2019;36(1):50–4. https://doi.org/10.1177/1049909118758158.
53. Edwards J, Hooper D, Rothwell G, Kneen K, Watson J, Saurman E. A nurse practitioner-led community palliative care service in Australia. Int J Palliat Nurs. 2019;25(5):245–53.
54. Chan A, Chien I, Moseley E, et al. Deep learning algorithms to identify documentation of serious illness conversations during intensive care unit admissions. Palliat Med. 2019;33(2):187–96. https://doi.org/10.1177/0269216318810421.
55. Abdul-Razzak A, Heyland DK, Simon J, Ghosh S, Day AG, You JJ. Patient-family agreement on values and preferences for life-sustaining treatment: results of a multicentre observational study. BMJ Support Palliat Care. 2019;9(1):e20. https://doi.org/10.1136/bmjspcare-2016-001284.
56. Bullen T, Maher K, Rosenberg JP, Smith B. Establishing research in a palliative care clinical setting: perceived barriers and implemented strategies. Appl Nurs Res. 2014;27(1):78–83. https://doi.org/10.1016/j.apnr.2013.10.007.

Palliative Care Resources

Local Resources

Palliative Medicine services through Carilion Clinic. https://www.carilionclinic.org/specialties/palliative-medicine-and-supportive-care

Palliative Medicine services through Lewis-Gale. https://lewisgale.com/health-education/palliative-care-information-for-patients-and-families.dot

Palliative Medicine services through the Salem VA Medical Center. https://www.salem.va.gov/services/hospice_palliativecare.asp

Palliative Care Partnership of the Roanoke Valley http://www.pcprv.org/.

Roanoke County Local Office on Aging https://www.loaa.org/.

Local chapter of the Alzheimers Association, including lists of support groups – https://alz.org/cwva.

State Resources

Virginia Dept of Health – palliative care http://www.vdh.virginia.gov/palliative-care/

Virginia Association for Hospices and Palliative Care https://www.virginiahospices.org/.

Virginia Advance Directive for Healthcare https://www.wcch.org/Content/Uploads/Wythe%20County/files/Advance-Directive-Simple.pdf.
Virginia Academy of Elder Law Attorneys https://www.vaela.org/.

National Resources

National Hospice and Palliative Care Organization www.nhpco.org.
American Association of Hospice and Palliative Medicine www.aahpm.org.
National Hospice Foundation. https://www.nationalhospicefoundation.org/

Educational Resources for Patients and Providers

Get Palliative Care – information for patients on palliative care www.getpalliativecare.org.
Vital Talk – structured conversations for providers on how to discuss prognosis and goals of care www.vitaltalk.org
Center to Advance Palliative Care – educational courses for providers on palliative care and symptom management (requires institutional membership for some courses) www.capc.org
End of Life Nursing Education Consortium – educational courses for nurses on end of life care. www.aacnnursing.org/ELNEC
https://www.the-hospitalist.org/hospitalist/article/121673/hospice-palliative-medicine/new-community-based-palliative-care
https://www.chcf.org/publication/up-close-a-field-guide-to-community-based-palliative-care-in-california/
https://www.chcf.org/wp-content/uploads/2017/12/PDF-UpCloseFieldGuidePalliative.pdf
https://www.capc.org/about/palliative-care/
https://www.chcf.org/wp-content/uploads/2017/12/PDF-InnovativeModelsPalliativeFactSheets.pdf
https://media.capc.org/filer_public/2d/09/2d092090-5d06-4107-b4c6-851a93139ae9/capc-nhpco_webinar_slides.pdf
https://www.nhpco.org/wp-content/uploads/2019/04/PalliativeCare_VS_Hospice.pdf
http://worh.org/rural-community-based-palliative-care
https://www.cancer.gov/about-cancer/advanced-cancer/care-choices/palliative-care-fact-sheet
https://www.pewtrusts.org/en/research-and-analysis/blogs/stateline/2017/07/10/why-some-patients-arent-getting-palliative-care
https://www.capc.org/seminar/poster-sessions/novel-approach-outpatient-palliative-care-clinic-flow/
https://www.nationalcoalitionhpc.org/last-call-outpatient-palliative-care-programs-become-a-testing-site/
http://aahpm.org/about/strategic-plan
https://www.nationalcoalitionhpc.org/wp-content/uploads/2019/04/MACRA-Field-Test-Recruitment-Flyer-updated.pdf
https://www.jointcommission.org/community-based_palliative_care_certification_option_july_1_2016/
https://reportcard.capc.org/
https://www.chcf.org/publication/palliative-care-california-narrowing-gap/
https://www.capc.org/about/press-media/press-releases/2018-2-28/palliative-care-continues-its-annual-growth-trend-according-latest-center-advance-palliative-care-analysis/
https://www.sciencedirect.com/science/article/abs/pii/S0885392412004629
https://www.ruralhealthinfo.org/rural-monitor/palliative-care/
https://www.chcf.org/project/increasing-access-palliative-care-rural-california/
https://www.thoughtco.com/us-states-by-area-1435125
https://www.ncbi.nlm.nih.gov/pmc/articles/PMC3214714/
http://aahpm.org/certification/subspecialty-certification
https://csupalliativecare.org/sb-1004/
http://aahpm.org/uploads/Program_Data_122718.pdf
https://www.acgme.org/
https://med.uth.edu/internalmedicine/geriatric-palliative-medicine/
https://www.uchicagomedicine.org/conditions-services/geriatrics
https://smhs.gwu.edu/medicine/divisions/geriatrics-palliative

Dr. Phyllis Whitehead is a clinical nurse specialist with the Carilion Roanoke Memorial Hospital Palliative Care Service and Associate Professor at the Virginia Tech Carilion School of Medicine. She is a clinical ethicist and initiated the Moral Distress Consult Service at CRMH. She is certified in pain management and as an advanced practice hospice and palliative care nurse. Dr. Whitehead has done numerous presentations on pain and symptom management, opioid-induced sedation, moral distress, and patients' end-of-life preferences locally, regionally, nationally, and internationally. Her research interests include moral distress and improving communication with seriously ill patients. She has been a co-lead of the NACNS Pain Task Force and the Access to Care Workgroup and recently appointed as co-lead of the Virginia Action Coalition. She is a Distinguished Practitioner and Fellow to the Nursing Academy of the National Academy of Practice. She is a graduate of Radford University where she earned her BSN and MSN and earned her doctorate degree at Virginia Tech.

Dr. Senaida Keating is an Academic Hospitalist at the Salem VA Medical Center. She is an Associate Professor at the Virginia Tech Carilion School of Medicine and the Edward Via College of Osteopathic Medicine. She is a coauthor of the chapters "Palliative Care for Persons with Serious Mental Illness" in Palliative Care, Perspectives, Practices, and impact on quality of life, a Global View published in 2017, and "End-of-Life in Persons with Severe and Persistent Mental Illness: A Review of the Research Outcomes" in Palliative Care, The Role and

Importance of Research in Promoting Palliative Care Practices published in 2019. She completed her Internal Medicine Residency Program at Virginia Tech Carilion School of Medicine/Roanoke Memorial Hospital as well as Fellowships in Geriatric, and Palliative and Hospice Medicine. She is board-certified in Internal, Geriatric, and Palliative Medicine.

Dr. Shereen Gamaluddin is a palliative attending with the Centra Health Palliative Care Service in Lynchburg, Virginia, and the Associate Medical Director for Good Samaritan Hospice. She earned her bachelor's degree in biology from Carnegie Mellon University. She completed her medical degree at University of Pittsburgh School of Medicine and subsequent Family Medicine training at Lancaster General Hospital. After nearly 10 years of private practice, she transitioned her focus to palliative and hospice medicine, completing a fellowship at Carilion Clinic. She is board-certified in Family Medicine and Hospice and Palliative Medicine.

Ms. Carolyn White is a nurse practitioner in the palliative medicine department at Centra Health in Lynchburg, Virginia. She has been a nurse practitioner since 2009, and prior to that was a registered nurse in hospice. She received her BSN from Radford University and MSN from University of Alabama in Birmingham. Serving patients and their families during serious illness and/or end of life is her life's greatest calling and honor.

Dr. Christi Stewart is the Palliative Medicine Medical Director at Carilion Roanoke Memorial Hospital and the Hospice Medical Director at Carilion Hospice Services of Roanoke, Virginia. She completed her medical degree at the University of Pittsburgh School of Medicine and subsequent Family Medicine training at Lancaster General Hospital. She is board-certified in Family Medicine, Geriatrics, and Hospice and Palliative Medicine.

Dr. Kye Y. Kim is a Geriatric Psychiatrist at Carilion Clinic Center for Healthy Aging and is also a Professor at the Virginia Tech Carilion School of Medicine's Department of Psychiatry and Behavioral Medicine. He received his medical degree at Yonsei University College of Medicine, Seoul, South Korea. Subsequently, he finished his general psychiatry residency at the State University of New York at Buffalo and geriatric psychiatry fellowship at the University of South Florida affiliated hospitals.

Culture and Palliative Care

Lodovico Balducci

Introduction

To highlight the role of culture in delivering and receiving palliative care, I present two clinical cases.

Case 1 Father O'Malley was a 78-year-old Irish priest with hormone-resistant prostate cancer metastatic to the bone. Incapacitated by the disease to perform his parish duties, he was admitted to the hospice house. With a smile he asked the nurse practitioner in charge not to prescribe opioid around the clock, because he wanted "to join the pain of the suffering Christ, and atone for his own and his neighbor's sin." A student nurse objected that uncontrolled pain may hasten his death, and he answered that he was ready for the Lord. The hospice chaplain reminded him that a prominent prelate with terminal Parkinson's had recently asked for palliative sedation prior to his death. "Of course, I don't object to the soothing of pain and I always encouraged my parishioners to seek relief of physical and spiritual pain," responded the priest, "but I was raised to look at pain as one of my assets. My parents were farmers and had nine children. My family was poor and could barely survive and it was not unusual for us to miss a meal. Since a young age we were asked to work in the field and agricultural accidents were common. The hospital was far from our village and most of the time it was unaffordable. Our devout parents taught us to endure our pain as Christ had done with His, to deliver us from the slavery of sin. In the bank of the kingdom of God my pain is currency available to whoever wants to borrow it free of interest to pay his/her own unsolved debts and be redeemed from the slavery of sin." Impressed by this answer, the chaplain instructed us to abide with the patient's requests. Father O'Malley spent many nights awake and in prayer. He asked for opioids only when he expected visits from his parishioners as he wanted to be able to talk to them and to listen to their confessions. Some members of the staff sought counseling from Father O'Malley, during their breaks. He passed 6 weeks later surrounded by mourning parishioners and hospice staff in tears.

Comments The history of Father O'Malley highlights the difference between pain and suffering [1]. While his pain would have been excruciating for most, Father O'Malley was kind of reveling in it because he had discovered a spiritual meaning to his symptoms. Any attempts to medicate him would have caused more suffering than the pain did. This difference is basic to planning palliative care and we will visit it again in this chapter. My main interest is to describe the case as an example of hospice care success due to

L. Balducci (✉)
H. Lee Moffitt Cancer Center and Research Institute, Tampa General Hospital, Tampa, FL, USA

M. Silbermann (ed.), *Palliative Care for Chronic Cancer Patients in the Community*,
https://doi.org/10.1007/978-3-030-54526-0_6

positive interaction between the culture of the patient and that of the caregiver(s). The culture of rural Ireland in the middle of the past century in which the priest had grown up was quite different from that of hospice providers in a large American city at the turn of the millennium. As a very successful minister, he had clearly been able to embrace the culture of his new country in pastoring his flock. At the meantime, he maintained the skills to cope with physical pain he had learned in his youth, springing from an accepted, albeit not universally held, Christian interpretation of physical pain. After asking legitimate questions and consulting a chaplain (a spiritual consultant), the staff obliged the priest's unusual request. The peacefulness of the priest's death and the mourning and bereavement of the staff testified the mutual satisfaction for this approach.

Undoubtedly many factors contributed to this success including a common language and a culture based on values that are widely understood even if they are not universally shared in the USA. But I believe that Father O'Malley's ability to articulate his beliefs and defend his culture as a personal asset, more than anything else, allowed a smooth and satisfactory relation between patient and staff. He made the case that his culture was a precious gift he received from loving parents and he wished to be able to keep such jewel with him, at the time of his death, as a pledge of their love.

We may also say that the care of Father O'Malley was successful because the goals of care were clearly defined, the communication vas unhinged, the patient was able to articulate his beliefs and to convince a skeptical staff to buy them, and he took full charge of his care.

Case 2 Let's call him Jaime, the name he gave to the EMT who rescued him after he passed out while laying the foundations of a house in Southern Florida. He received two blood transfusions in the local hospital and was transferred to our cancer center with the diagnosis of acute myeloid leukemia. Jaime was a man in his early 40s, from some remote village in the Yucatan peninsula, and he was working illegally in the USA. He had reached the country crossing Mexico from South through North, landed in Texas, and had been dispatched to Florida by a network of illegal labor. His physical appearance revealed him as a native Mesoamerican or as a mestizo. Jaime understood and spoke Spanish, but his English was very rudimentary. We communicated with him partly through an interpreter. I myself am fluent in Spanish as so was the social worker assisting the medical team. Two things impressed us since the beginning: the stoicism of Jaime when faced with the diagnosis of a lethal disease and his reluctance to provide personal information or even to reveal his symptoms. When he died, we did not know whether he was married and whether he had children. When we announced to Jaime that the induction regimen had not worked, and a cure was impossible, he accepted this response without a grimace or a tear, and he did not object to a do-not-resuscitate order. He refused to see a chaplain: indeed we had no idea of what religious beliefs he held if any. When asked if he wanted for us to try to reach his family, he told us not to get involved in this personal matter. Anytime we asked how he was doing, he answered "fine" and never demanded extra-relief of chemotherapy-induced nausea and vomiting or any pain medication. I don't remember a single smile or even a single expression of feelings on his face. He reminded me of the stone masks that adorn the Maya ruins in Southern Mexico and Guatemala.

Clearly the staff, including myself, was uncomfortable in dealing with Jaime and probably Jaime was uncomfortable in dealing with us, though I am not sure there would have been a situation in which Jaime would have felt comfortable. In any case caring for Jaime was a distressing experience for a caring medical staff and sadly his passing represented a relief.

One may certainly ascribe the failure to provide palliative care to Jaime to his extreme mistrust and suspicion of Caucasian Americans, which included members of the medical profession and of the clergy, mistrust fed and confirmed by centuries of deception and exploitation. To that one may add the fear to be jailed and sent back to his country of origin given his illegitimate residence in the USA. Whatever the ultimate cause of the failure, I wish to analyze the situation according to the same parameters we used for Father O'Malley and to highlight a multistep botch. Jaime did not have an opportunity to articulate the goals of his care nor to participate in care-related decision. We communicated with Jaime the way we communicate with our middle-class patients, whose culture determines our standard patient-provider communication. This communication style involves a disclosure of the medical conditions, options, and prognosis and may be totally inappropriate in a culture where the discussion of death with a patient is considered a taboo [2] or a manifestation of disrespect [3]. Likewise the demeanor we present to our American patients might have been inappropriate for Jaime. We try to smile as a sign of emotional allegiance to the patient even if we convey painful information, but for Jaime our smile might have meant that we did not care about his disease and his death, or even that we made fun of him. While autonomy is a pillar of medical ethics, the definition of autonomy may change in different cultures. A patient who exercises his/her right to defer medical decisions to family members or the practitioner should be seen as autonomous as the patient who wishes to have all medical information and direct himself/herself all medical decisions [4]. We assumed that Jaime was a Christian, most likely of Roman Catholic persuasion, as he was Mexican. Irrespective of whether this assumption was correct, it gave us very little insight into Jaime's beliefs. I learned from the masterpiece of Octavio Paz, *The Labyrinth of Solitude* [5], that a common belief for people of Mesoamerican origin holds that the revelation of oneself is tantamount to a definitive violation of one's intimacy and is the equivalent of a psychological death. This belief may have explained as well as mistrust the reluctance of Jaime to provide personal information, and our insistence for obtaining such information might have sounded to him as a form of aggression. Likewise, the offer to see a minister might have sounded as an intrusion.

In discussing these two cases, we emphasized four aspects of patient-practitioner' interactions: treatment goals, communication, beliefs, and decision making. As it will be shown, these parameters may represent the gates from where the patient's culture emerges when approaching health care [6] and the best opportunity for the practitioner to provide culturally sensitive care.

Palliative Care and Culture

The goal of palliative care is healing, a process through which a patient comes to co-opt into his/her life the disease and its consequences, which may include mortality. While cure is possible only occasionally, healing is always possible [7–10]. Freedom from pain and suffering are essential to healing, as long as freedom is understood as lack of interference with a person's enjoyment of life, rather than as absence of pain and suffering. We underlined how excruciating physical pain was associated with personal satisfaction in the case of Father O'Malley. In addition to this, healing involves the discovery of the meaning of illness congruent with one's beliefs, expectations, and desires, in other words congruent with one's culture. We may safely affirm that healing is an individual experience obtained through a personal culture. Father O'Malley died and was healed because he received culturally sensitive care, while Jaime did not experience healing at the time of his death because such care had been impossible.

The awareness that different cultures exist around the world has made culturally sensitive care an imperative of patient-centered rather than disease-centered medicine that is of palliative care.

The initial studies of culturally congruent palliative care were conducted in population groups living in isolated areas for generations. Palliative care programs sensitive to the culture of Native Americans [11] in Canada or the indigenous population of Oaxaca, Mexico [8], resulted in increased satisfaction for patients, family caregivers, and practitioners. These studies are extremely important because they demonstrated the possibility and the effectiveness of culturally attuned palliative care. They also helped identify the elements that constitute a culture and define culture in operative terms. Properly they were designed for populations living in remote communities where a common culture was predictable and well defined.

Globalization represents a new challenge to the practitioner of palliative care who may have to deal with patients from different cultures, with little time to address, let alone to study, different communications styles and different beliefs. The cases we described may provide a clue on how to address cultural issues in the limited time allowed for a medical encounter.

Purposefully we mentioned culture several times without defining culture, to accustom the reader to the idea that culture is a fluid and poorly definable but certain reality. In the case of Father O'Malley, the effectiveness of care resulted from an approach congruent with a complex of inextricably interwoven threads including the patient's language, demeanor, beliefs, social norms, and values, rather than with a single element. We refer as culture to the unique design of the carpet resulting from the intersecting of different threads. In the case of Jaime this approach failed and so did any attempt to palliation.

After establishing that the construct of culture is fluid and dynamic, the time might have come to define culture in operative terms for the practitioner of palliative care. In several clinical studies, culture was defined as a complex of similar languages, beliefs, and values held by a population group [12–16]. Other authors [6] have specified that this complex "evolves and adapts within an ecologic and technical setting through historical, political and social forces," "provides a structure that positions its sub-group members in juxtaposition," and "provides its members a sense of safety, identity, and meaning." To this one should add the presence of several cultural subgroups within the same culture. They are supported by religious beliefs, professional vision, political and social standing, income, and living conditions. One can easily imagine how the cultures of different castes in a caste-divided society may result quite different even if language and religious beliefs are the same.

The constructs of race and ethnicity are addressed as they have been used as complements or even as equivalents of culture [6]. Race is an outdated concept based on the misconception that the *Homo sapiens* species was subdivided in four different groups whose phenotypic distinctions (such as skin color and skull shape) revealed underlying genetic distinctions [6]. Molecular genetics has shown the fallacy of this concept, and the discussion of race as such does not belong to the scientific literature. Still, some phenotypic characteristics may help the identification of an individual's culture. For example, the appearance of Jaime led us to believe that his culture was native Mesoamerican. Ethnicity has been defined as "one's sense of identity as a member of a cultural group within a power structure of a multicultural society and identified so by others within a sociohistorical context of a particular geopolitical setting [6]." Ethnicity appears as a legitimate construct. Its value in medical practice appears limited to help in identifying an individual's culture.

Based on the definition and the cautions provided, we will try to furnish a blueprint for culturally sensitive palliative care in a multicultural society.

Practical Recommendations for Culturally Sensitive Palliative Care in a Multicultural Society

The first step in addressing cultural differences includes awareness of these differences. Most practitioners may be primed to explore culture when dealing with foreign patients and patients from ethnic or religious minority. Some trigger signs (Table 1) [6] may suggest a need for cultural assessment.

When the communication appears difficult, it is important to make sure that the patient can hear and understand the language of the practitioner. Many patients may be reluctant to state they don't understand for fear of being judged or of offending the physician. Once these difficulties

Table 1 Areas of patient-provider interaction where cultural differences may emerge

Areas of patient-practitioner interaction	Trigger signs
Definition of treatment goals	Unwillingness to afford the issue Involvement of spouse, family, and friends
Communication style	Unwillingness to receive information about treatment and prognosis Facial expression poorly readable Lack or excess of emotion related to specific information Hostility toward the demeanor of the practitioner (smiles, touch) Unwillingness to disclose personal information
Beliefs	Unwillingness to discuss personal beliefs Unwillingness to talk to the chaplain Request for a special minister or guru
Decision making	Reluctance to address end-of-life decisions Involvement of family members with treatment-related decision Involvement of a minister in treatment-related decisions

have been ruled out, a discussion of goals of treatment might be illuminating.

To establish treatment goals is the first step of planning palliative care. The inability to address this issue clearly underlines cultural differences. They may include communication styles, role of the family, role of the practitioner, and interpretation of suffering [17]. Before initiating the conversation on treatment goals, it may be prudent to ask to each patient how much they know of their disease, how much they wish to know, how much their symptoms interfere with their daily life, and if they want family members present at the discussion. Since the beginning it may be useful to manifest a willingness to respect whatever limits a patient wishes to impose in the conversation. An open-ended statement such as "Most patients like to know the outcome of the diseases and make decisions related to their health care. We came to realize that everyone is different and some people prefer for their family members to be present at the discussion and sometimes even receive the information instead of them and make decisions for them. We are here to make sure you are comfortable with us, so whatever you prefer is right with us" may invite the patient to express freely his/her preference and establish a climate of trust between patient, practitioner, and palliative care team. One patient asked to be treated by me instead of the specialist to whom she had been referred, because she learned I was a practicing Roman Catholic, and for this reason she trusted that my treatment decisions would have been consistent with her beliefs and values. As in the case of Father O'Malley, some patients may consider physical pain a blessing in disguise, an atonement for their own or somebody else's sins, a challenge to their endurance capacity, and even a mystical way to become intimate with the deity or to reach a condition of inner peace. Failure to cater to these convictions will result in mutual suspicion and hostility and compromise any attempt to palliation.

Difficulties in communication may be expressed in several ways that may go from inattentiveness to open hostility. Non-verbal communication deserves special attention in populations that might have difficulties with the spoken language. Casual avoidance of physical contact may identify a culture for which touching of the patient is contraindicated. Stoicism might indicate lack of comprehension as well as unwillingness to discuss feelings outside – and sometimes even within – a family context. The opposite, disproportionate reaction to bad news may be read as unwillingness to listen or as a desire to co-opt the practitioner's compassion.

The practitioner should be aware of some general distinction in communication styles. Some cultures prefer an indirect form of communication. For example, in some Asian languages, the direct negation does not exist and a negative response to a question must occur with a periphrasis. In this culture a direct discussion of prognosis may sound inappropriate or even offensive. In some cultures the communication is preferentially non-verbal and the demeanor or the facial expressions may be more revealing than the words the patient is able to utter.

Beliefs are also reflected in communication: in some forms of Muslim and Christian culture, complaints of pain or desperation may be seen as blasphemous. Likewise, in a patriarchal type of family, a communication with the practitioner that has not been cleared with the patriarch may sound disrespectful.

In some cultures, as represented by the case of Jaime, the disclosure of one's intimacy may be considered tantamount to self-destruction.

Beliefs are part of culture and it is legitimate to investigate if the patient has any religious beliefs. The awareness of a patient's adherence to a particular religion has practical implications, such as the importance that faith has in a patient's life and the resources available in a religious community [18]. During my training in medicine, I did care for a pastor with chronic myelogenous leukemia and severe anemia in need of multiple blood transfusions. I called the local Baptist seminar and in a day we received more blood donors than we could handle. This investigation needs to be conducted with caution for two reasons. First the patient might be afraid of discrimination if he/she reveals his/her religious beliefs or lack thereof. Second one should not assume to know the person's beliefs simply because somebody reveals himself/herself as Muslim, Christian, or Jew. Each one of these religions includes different denominations and different beliefs not uncommonly at odds with each other. It may be helpful to ask the patient which roles the beliefs have in the management of the disease and in which community if any the patient is worshiping. An introduction to the investigation stating that the practitioner found in his/her practice that religious faith has been a significant help for some patients may relieve any suspicion and mistrust.

Decision making may reveal any of the cultural aspects already described, including difference in communication style, beliefs, and family structure.

In Table 2 we summarize the aspects of culture that may be relevant to patient's care.

Table 2 Cultural elements relevant to patient's care [17]

Emphasis on individualism (as is common in North America) or on collectivism (as may be the case among some Muslim, Orthodox, and Hasidic Jewish communities).
Definition of family: Extended, nuclear, and even including non-blood kinship. It is common in some Middle Eastern populations to refer to close friends as "brothers and sisters."
Roles within the family: Who is responsible for child rearing, taking care of older adults, and making financial decisions? In some African societies, the maternal uncle, rather than the father, is responsible for child rearing.
Views about marriage and other types of relationships.
Communication patterns (direct vs. indirect, relative emphasis on non-verbal communication, meaning of non-verbal gestures). For example, in some Asian languages, the word "no" does not exist and the negation is expressed in a roundabout way; in some Asian populations, a smile indicates embarrassment rather than amusement.
Religious and spiritual belief systems. The monotheistic religions of the West emphasize the unique sacredness of each human being subjected to the justice of the same god. Some of the Eastern beliefs hold that each person is assigned by the deity a social situation that is unchangeable for a person's lifetime.
Views about physicians.
Views about suffering.
Views about the afterlife.

Conclusions

From this brief review, one may draw the following conclusions:

- Culturally sensitive care is essential to the success of palliative care.
- In a multicultural society, delivery of culturally sensitive care is a new challenge, as culture is a dynamic and ever-changing construct and because of the limited time the practitioner has to become familiar with different cultures. An important dimension of this challenge is the reluctance of illegal residents in the USA and Western Europe to reveal themselves.
- Culture should not be confused with race and ethnicity, but ethnicity may be helpful to penetrate one's culture.

- Through a medical interview described in Table 1, practitioners may unearth cultural elements related to palliative care (Table 2) and plan palliative care accordingly.
- Giving the dynamic and ever-changing nature of culture, the practitioners may expect frustrations in delivering culturally based palliative care, for which experience is a more valuable teacher than any textbook.

References

1. Balducci L. Geriatric oncology, spirituality and palliative care. J Pain Symptom Manag. 2018;57(1):171–5. https://doi.org/10.1016/j.jpainsymman.2018.05.009.
2. Colclough YY. Native American Health Taboo: implications for health care clinicians. Am J Hosp Pall Med. 2017;34:584–91.
3. Bito S, Matsumura S, Singer MK, et al. Acculturation and end-life decision making: comparison of Japanese and Japanese-American focus groups. Bioethics. 2007;21:251–62.
4. Gilber R, Miola J. One size fits all? On patient's autonomy, medical decision making, and the impact of culture. Med Law Rev. 2015;23:375–99.
5. Paz O. The labyrinth of solitude. New York: Grove Press; 1961.
6. Cain CL, Surbone A, Elk R, et al. Culture and palliative care: preferences, communication, meaning, and mutual decision making. J Pain SymptManag. 2018;55:1408–19.
7. Byock I. The prospective of death at the end of life. New York: Riverhead Book; 1997.
8. Lopex Sanchez O, Nance DC. "Something born of the heart" culturally affiliated illnesses of older adults in Oaxaca. IssuMent Health Nurs. 2019;29:1–8.
9. Andrade PE, Bhattacharya J. Not cure but heal: music and medicine. Advneurobiol. 2018;21:283–307.
10. Delguadi-Guay MO. Developing a healing environment for broken souls of patients with life-threatening diseases and their caregivers. J pain Sympt Manag. 2018;55:1231–6.
11. Kelley ML, Prince H, Nadin S, et al. Developing palliative Care programs in Indigenous Communities using participatory action research: a Canadian application of the Public Health Approach to Palliative Care. Ann Pall Med. 2018;7(Suppl2):S52–72.
12. Collier MJ, Hedge P, Lee N, et al. Dialogues on the edges: ferments in communication and culture. In: Collier MJ, et al., editors. Transforming communication about culture. Thousand Oaks, California: Sage; 2002. p. 229–30.
13. Lee C. "Race" and "Ethnicity" in Biomedical research: how do scientists construct and explain differences in health? Social Sci Med. 2009;68:1183–90.
14. Cacciatore J, Thieleman K. We rise out of the cradle into the grave: an ethnographic exploration of rituals, mourning, and death on a Hutterite colony. Omega. 2014;69:357–79.
15. Prossr R, Korman D, Feinstein RA. An orthodox perspective of the Jewish end-of-life experience. Home Healthc Nurse. 2012;30:579–85.
16. Goldstein D, Thewes W, Butow P. Communicating in a multicultural society: Greek communities attitudes toward cancer in Australia. Int Med J. 2002;32:289–96.
17. Searight HR, Gafford J. Cultural Diversity at the End of Life: Issues and guidelines for family physicians. Am Family Phys. 2005;71:515–22.
18. Puchalski CM. The FICA spiritual history tool # 274. J Pall Med. 2014;17:105–6.

Part II

Latin America: Guatemala

Pediatric Hospice Experience in Guatemala: Our History

Linda Marisol Bustamante, Silvia Rivas, and Patricia Valverde

Our Location

Guatemala is a country located in Central America, which has approximately 15 million inhabitants [1] in an area of 108,800 square kilometers, with coasts to the Pacific and Atlantic Ocean, as well as borders with the countries of Mexico, El Salvador, Honduras, and Belize. In addition, we have 59.3% of the population in poverty and 23% in extreme poverty in the last census [2]. We still have high levels of illiteracy and malnutrition and high rates of maternal mortality.

It is also good to mention that we have 22 indigenous groups, each with different characteristics such as languages, worldviews, and manifestations of spirituality. Having so much diversity in the same geographic area represents a challenge for the health system that struggles to interact with different beliefs, values, and points of view that influence the health-disease process.

L. M. Bustamante (✉)
National Unit of Pediatric Oncology, Guatemala, Guatemala

S. Rivas
Palliative Care Program, National Unit of Pediatric Oncology, Guatemala, Guatemala

P. Valverde
National Unit of Pediatric Oncology, Guatemala, Guatemala

Under these circumstances, a group of private companies decide to undertake an ambitious project by opening the first pediatric cancer hospital, the National Pediatric Oncology Unit of Guatemala, (in Spanish *Unidad Nacional de Oncología Pediatrica* (UNOP)), which opened in 2000. UNOP has unique infrastructure and philosophies of care that have been sustained since the hospital opened. These include a strong supportive relationship with the foundation AYUVI, who have helped to obtain financial resources for patient care. These resources come, in different proportions, from the Ministry of Health, contributions from civil society, and various alliances in both the public and private sectors. This collaborative and enduring relationship with AYUVI has been central to UNOP's ability to remain sustainable and grow.

One of the most important premises of the work at UNOP is to provide free access to quality pediatric cancer care for any child in Guatemala; this has created the opportunity to achieve cure rates similar to those of high-income countries. The number of new patients diagnosed with cancer each year has grown to a high of 560 patients in 2019. This represents a positive impact because year after year we see patients who can resume their lives after facing the process of diagnosis, treatment, and recovery from cancer.

Another value present in the work of UNOP since its inception is the importance of interdisciplinary team care. Oncologists, nutritionists,

M. Silbermann (ed.), *Palliative Care for Chronic Cancer Patients in the Community*,
https://doi.org/10.1007/978-3-030-54526-0_7

pharmacologists, nurses, intensivists specialists, surgeons, orthopedists, psychologists, social workers, child life specialists, and volunteers all work shoulder to shoulder in coordination throughout the course of care for children with cancer.

Important Changes in Care

Five years after the opening of UNOP, under the direction of Dr. Federico Antillón and Dr. Patricia Valverde, Dr. Silvia Rivas (a pediatric intensivist) was invited to develop a clear plan of care for patients with high-risk, low-prognosis disease. The overarching goals were to create improved attention to symptom management and reduction of suffering, programs to decrease abandonment, and education of medical personnel in communication, decision-making, and coordination of other projects that impact the treatment of patients and the support of their families. A decision was made to change the name of the team (that would be charged with instituting this new plan of care) from the palliative care team to the integral medicine team. The intention was to more clearly convey the transdisciplinary nature of the care provided by the team and to make it part of care for patients from the time of diagnosis throughout the disease and treatment process. Since then, more people have been added to the team, improving attention and creating a model that includes not only the integral medicine team but also an algorithm for initiating care which was developed to ensure those patients who are most in need of intervention receive it immediately and help guide the future interventions of each team member strategically.

Below is a table illustrating both the growth in new diagnoses and the number of patients receiving care from the integral medicine team (Table 1).

Table 1 Number of new cancer diagnoses and new patients in palliative care [3]

	New diagnoses	Patients entering the palliative care program
2000	191	0
2005	298	19
2006	279	107
2007	281	94
2008	300	85
2009	274	81
2010	419	109
2011	484	87
2012	484	92
2013	497	111
2014	484	132
2015	464	140
2016	454	148
2017	535	168
2018	493	178
2019	490	151

Patients to whom we can only offer palliative care could be treated at the hospital or at home, although, due to geographical difficulties and safety/security, it was not possible to make home visits to all patients. It should be mentioned that some patients must travel 8–10 hours on the way to attend their appointments, while others travel 2 days, because transportation to leave from their villages is not available on a daily basis. Although some patients live closer to UNOP, it is not possible to make home visits because the areas in which they live are considered too dangerous. For these families, patients are monitored as closely as possible by phone, but sometimes they must return to the hospital for admission. This has created a problem with bedspace, creating daily census at the 90–100% levels. This created an especially urgent need for a designated space for palliative patients.

Dreaming of a Hospice

In 2011, a volunteer approached the integral medicine team, Ms. Myriam Aceituno, who had been very active in providing financial and logistical resources for the transfer of patients to their homes and provision of critical support for families. An architect by profession, her role had been to assist with charitable financial and personal support resources. However, her dream was to find a physical space that could address the important needs of patients at end of life. She wanted to find a place near a lake, using a space donated by a member of the Rotary Club, and use combined volunteer expertise to provide design, engineering, and medical planning for the "dream" hospice. The goal was to provide all the comforts of home in a place designed for the medical care that would meet the patients and families´ needs in the difficult moments of advanced illness.

During the initial phase of the hospice being open, a wide variety of patients with advanced illness were served. The majority were in the terminal phase of advanced illness, but others include (a) patients who had the potential to return home but need to have symptoms better controlled, (b) families at risk of caregiver fatigue, (c) patients who needed prolonged chemotherapy or antibiotics that would be difficult to manage at home but did not require hospitalization, (d) some patients with a pending diagnosis who needed lodging, and (e) families who required extra time for education to learn how to care at home for their children with complex needs.

At that time, the "Villa de la Esperanza" hospice also expanded service to non-UNOP pediatric patients with non-cancer diagnoses who required palliative care. This created an additional collaboration with another foundation and a total capacity of five beds.

In the first 2 years, the hospice served many patients, improving quality of life for patients and creating an opportunity to serve families with many needs. As in UNOP, the care was provided at no cost, one or two family members could stay 24 hours a day, and visiting hours were generally open, depending upon the patient's conditions and needs of the moment. Through the generous work of many volunteers, there were multiple group activities celebrating birthdays, Christmas and other December celebrations, and spiritual activities such as first communions, baptisms, and even marriage. End-of-life wishes of children were fulfilled, family reunions and reconciliations happened, and volunteers promoted the cause of celebrating life all the time. Many employees had never experienced working in care at end of life, and there were many learning and teaching opportunities.

Moments to Grow

In 2013 we are approached by another volunteer, Jorge Mini, who mentioned the need to open a hospice and was unaware of the existence of the "Villa de la Esperanza" hospice, but we decided to put them in contact and they materialized together a more ambitious dream. At another place of the city, they decided to build a building in which the structure was designed for the care of patients with complex diseases. This structure would have ten individual rooms, and each area would have easy access by wheelchair or if necessary by stretcher. In addition the area of the rooms would be larger with greater comfort for the patient and his family. The bathrooms were also designed to facilitate access; they were building a space based on a hospice and not adapting the existing construction to work as a hospice.

For 2 years, work continued with the foundation led by Myriam, *Ammar Ayudando* (AMMAR), who were in charge of the administrative and fundraising area, in addition to having their medical and nursing team who were the ones who gave direct care to patients under the direction of the UNOP palliative medical team. We continue these years by entering UNOP patients and patients from other centers that will need palliative care.

New Time, Multiplying the Work

In 2015, it was decided to separate the "Villa de la Esperanza" hospice who would be located in another area and would attend non-cancer child and adult patients and open their services for other hospitals of the Guatemalan health system that until now was neglected. The facilities were occupied by the Hospice "Hogar Estuardo Mini" where we would attend exclusively to UNOP patients; this represented several challenges for the team; the most important thing was to maintain in patients the continuity of care by being the same team who continued attending and getting involved in the decisions and accompanying the patients and their families; we also had to take care of obtaining resources, managing them, and improving the liaison processes between the unit and the hospice.

Learning Curves and Growth

With the influx of new patients, both hospice and non-palliative patients, a decision was made that care for the two different groups of patients would need to be separated and carried out in different locations. Several factors contributed to this decision but, by establishing a hospice specific to the UNOP patients, it became easier to unify patient care teams, manage equipment compatibility, and facilitate administration and fundraising for this high-need, rapidly growing group of patients. "Hogar Estuardo Mini" now has ten individual rooms, permanent 24-hour nursing staff, and two doctors in charge of medical care, in addition to a medical coordinator that works as the liaison between UNOP and the hospice. Nursing and kitchen staff have been increased due to demand, and the administration of fundraising and use of funds is being managed by the same foundation (AYUVI) that has helped build capacity at the UNOP (Table 2). From the time that UNOP assumed a more active role in the administration and medical care program design at "Hogar Estuardo Mini," the number of patients has grown significantly, as demonstrated in the table below.

Barriers Found along the Way

Although the integral medicine team has now been providing palliative care for several years at UNOP and the hospice, we still have barriers that we must face. The first barrier is based on the cultural misconceptions regarding admission to the hospice. These ideas arise not only from the families of the children with terminal cancer but also from the circles of influence of each family. For Guatemalans, as part of the decision-making process, extended family, the communities where they live, as well as the religious leaders often contribute to decisions made. All these actors can influence, in small and large ways, how decisions are made about treatment or a move into hospice care. Misinformation contributes to resistance to accepting hospice care as the best form of medical care and support for patients with incurable disease. For that reason, the name was changed to "Home (Hogar)." This appears to improve acceptance by some families.

Another barrier to hospice that the integral medicine team anticipated was a potential resistance to referral to hospice by the treating oncology teams. In fact, the existence of the hospice turned out to be a positive incentive for the teams to make earlier referrals. An administrative education program for all medical staff that included visits to the hospice facility and orientation to amenities and services provided helped the UNOP staff understand the benefits of the hospice. The result was an educational multiplier for the families who heard the medical staff speak positively about the hospice and the encouraged families to consider admission, reducing their fears and resistance to admission.

The economic challenges of financially supporting and staffing a pediatric hospice have been complex. However, much effort directed at finding creative ways to obtain funds has allowed the hospice to continue to operate and grow. Transparent and ethical fundraising, the involvement of people with a genuine commitment to the hospice, and the building of strategic collaborative relationships in the community have helped the hospice to continue its work.

Table 2 Admissions to the hospice per year

2015	89
2016	192
2017	245
2018	202
2019	305

Permanent Values

Beyond establishing the financial and infrastructure stability to maintain the hospice, a set of shared values remains at the core of the work done in the hospice. These values are practiced daily.

We are all one: Each family is attended without distinction regarding ethnic groups, beliefs, socioeconomic group, or any other characteristic that could bias the quality of care provided to the patients.

Bereavement: The hospice and its team members and volunteers are an institution that values life, attending to suffering in all its facets and finding together, with families, the best approach to reduce that suffering. We provide ethical care that is not just for patients with conditions in which prognosis is uncertain, but we also strive to give tools to families to survive the grieving process and move forward with their lives after the loss of their child.

Self-care: All members of the hospice team receive ongoing training in grief management, terminal care, total pain, and aromatherapy. There are specific activities designed to both address and prevent burnout and compassion fatigue, so that all staff can maintain their ability to care for both themselves and their patients over time. There is a shared understanding that the work of pediatric hospice care is difficult, that it can place staff and volunteers at risk for attrition, and that learning about and participating in activities to prevent burnout is important.

Spiritual care: Spiritual care and support of different beliefs in the spiritual domain is an important and respected part of the care provided to patients and families in the hospice. A team of volunteers is continuously available to serve the families who are going through difficult times. The population in Guatemala is mostly Catholic and Protestant, but in some cases there are leaders from the Mayan religion who attend to the spiritual needs of the family members and patients.

Children as children: We have learned that at all times the child is a child, so providing an environment that encourages and supports play, fun, and companionship helps our pediatric patients maintain their lives in childhood, despite the hard moments that they have faced and continue to experience.

Physician support: An important aspect of the success of the hospice that should be mentioned is the enthusiastic acceptance of the hospice by the oncologists and pediatricians of UNOP. Their belief in and support of the care provided at the hospice gives families more confidence when they are referred for hospice care. The involvement of the integral medicine team from the time of diagnosis, with the ongoing clinical presence in the hospice, creates a true continuity of care that is very helpful to both families and staff. This clearly impacts the decision-making process and reduces the suffering and impact of treatment of the patients.

Evaluation

One meaningful source of feedback and evaluation of the impact of our hospice comes from the bereavement meetings that are held twice a year. Families whose children have died in the hospital, in the hospice, or at home come together for grief support. The families of children who have died in hospice are more frequent attenders of the bereavement support events. Families often go to both the hospital and the hospice to express their thanks to the staff for the care their children received. We often see parents return, 1 or 2 years after their child's death, to volunteer and also become advocates in their communities for seeking help for children with cancer early after a cancer diagnosis is presented.

As described earlier, we have a small group of non-palliative patients receiving treatment that stay at the hospice. They frequently ask to be readmitted if there is space in the hospice because they feel cared for there. And although this is not the team's primary goal, there is a sense that publicity, parent and family education, and the daily work done in the hospice are contributing to a change in the mindset of the Guatemalan people about the meaning and value of hospice care.

Last Reflections

Although the resources of Guatemala are very limited, as are the resources of many countries in our region, our team believes there is no excuse for failing to provide quality care. There are only excuses that justify not caring enough to fight for what our patients need and deserve. It is important to have a dream. When you have a dream, doors will open, and projects can be achieved. Although there are countries with more resources and better laws to promote the development of palliative care, it is possible to make a precious jewel, like our hospices, in more difficult circumstances. We still have work ahead, a population to educate, patients to attend to, and projects to carry out, but we do this work with one eye on the future and both feet firmly in the present with our patients currently experiencing the struggles of life-threatening illness. We continue to fundraise and to spread the word about the value of improved quality of life even when time is short. The hospices of both "Villa de la Esperanza" and "Hogar Estuardo Mini" are both ambitious projects that have remained true to their principles and values since they opened their doors. This is the story of our dream come true and of our experience, and we hope it motivates others to make their own dreams, perhaps held for years, come true.

References

1. Guatemala IN. Censo Poblacional. Guatemala 2019.
2. Instituto Nacional de Estadistica, G. d. (201). Censo 2014. Guatemala.
3. Pediatrica UN (octubre de 2019). Informe estadistico. Guatemala, Guatemala, Guatemala.

Part III

Western Europe: France

Early Integrated Palliative Care in Oncology: Organizational Challenges and Perspectives in France

Rana Istambouly

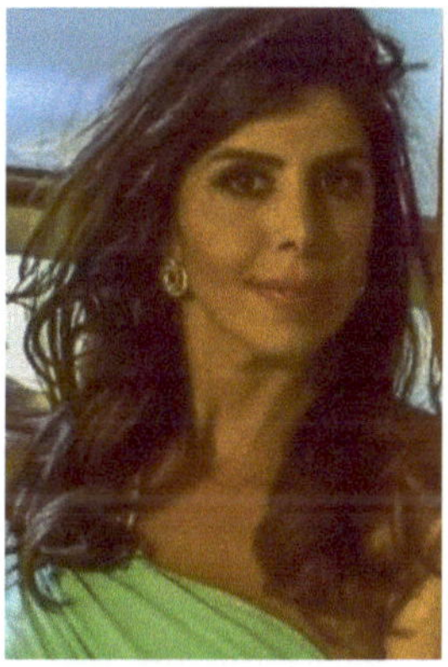

Rana Istambouly is pursuing a PhD in health management at Université Paris-Est. She earned a French State degree in nursing in 2007. She then got degrees in pain management, hypnosis and cognitive and behavioral therapy. Bridging her passion for both palliative care and management, she earned from 2013 till 2018 consecutive master's degrees in management of health institution from Gustave Eiffel's School of Management then in palliative medicine (clinic and research) from Université Paris-Descartes. From 2010 till 2018, she worked at several pain and palliative care units in France, before directing the program of palliative medicine at a university hospital in Lebanon.

After having created a consultancy, she became a trainer in France and Middle East to set up hospice and palliative home care services. She has participated actively in several international conferences and symposia. She is currently a member of the national scientific committee of the SFAP (French Society of Palliative Care) and a member of the scientific committee of CIRERO (Center for Investigation and Research in Organizational Resilience).

Introduction

Reducing the Impact and Optimizing the Quality of Life of Cancer Patients: A Global Public Health Challenge Worldwide

According to Eurostat, cancer is the second most common cause of death in the European Union, accounting for 29% and 23% of male and female deaths, respectively.

According to the GLOBOCAN database (built in 2018 as part of the IARC Global Cancer Observatory), the global cancer burden for all cancer sites combined reached 18.1 million new cases and 9.6 million deaths [1, 2]. Worldwide, one in five men and one in six women will develop cancer during their lifetime. According to the WHO, cancer is the second most common cause of death worldwide [3]. The WHO estimated an epidemiologic trend where cancer will

R. Istambouly (✉)
PHD student in health management, Université Paris-Est, IAE Gustave Eiffel, Creteil, France

Member of the national scientific committee for palliative medicine (SFAP), Paris, France

Member of the scientific committee of Center for Investigation and Research in Organizational Resilience (CIRERO), Paris, France

President and founder of the association of early palliative medicine (MEDPALLIAP), Paris, France

M. Silbermann (ed.), *Palliative Care for Chronic Cancer Patients in the Community*,
https://doi.org/10.1007/978-3-030-54526-0_8

become the fifth leading cause of death between 2016 and 2060 and, therefore, malignancies will become the leading causes of mortality around the world immediately following 2030 [1, 4].

Globally, the total number of people living with cancer that is incurable within 5 years of diagnosis is estimated at 43.8 million [4]. Moreover, these figures are expected to increase due to the aging of the population and the new therapies. The impact on the quality of life and on the professional, social, and spiritual lives of individuals and their families and the economic repercussions are increasingly significant [5–7]. Furthermore, patients are living much longer between the time of diagnosis of an incurable cancer and death due to the new therapies.

Social, Spiritual, Psychological, and Professional Impact

These patients often experience severe symptoms as well as deep emotional and spiritual suffering. Their lives are sometimes considered intolerable and their suffering unbearable for them and their families [8, 9]. According to several studies, patients continue to experience complications that often result in disability, incapacity, loss of autonomy, and serious complications that lead to significant personal, family, professional, psychosocial, and financial losses for the person with cancer and his or her entourage, who are not always well-cared for by their oncologists. Numerous reports, including a series from the Institute of Medicine (IOM), have documented the persistence of uncontrolled pain and distress in cancer patients [10]. Several other studies have reported that, despite medical advances, patients continue to experience physical, psychological, and spiritual distress.

Economic Impact

Economically, patients with advanced cancer use significant healthcare resources, and recent trends suggest that healthcare utilization rates are increasing [11, 12]. In fact, these patients often spend several days in oncology centers for treatment and symptom management and are frequently hospitalized for medical complications related to their cancer treatment [13, 14]. Hospitalizations account for a significant portion of this healthcare utilization. More than half of cancer patients are admitted to hospital at least once during their last month of life [15, 16].

A US study of 28,000 patients under the age of 65 with advanced solid tumors (lung, colon, pancreas, prostate, etc.) showed that 75% of them received at least one aggressive treatment during their last month of life [6]. The most common form of this treatment was a hospital admission, with 65% of them visiting the emergency department. However, a high proportion of them also received chemotherapy (between 24.2% and 32.6% depending on the tumor) or radiotherapy (between 5.8% and 20.6%). 25.3–31.1% of patients also underwent invasive procedures, such as biopsies. A third of them died in hospital and not at home as they wished [16, 17].

End-of-life care of cancer patients is recognized as a significant problem in oncology, and there are many published guidelines that recommend limiting the use of aggressive treatments which may be more harmful than helpful to patients at the end of life, as well as increasing the use of palliative and hospice care [18]. Despite these recommendations, several international studies report that it is increasingly common for cancer patients to receive unnecessary chemotherapy and invasive treatments at intensive care units toward the end of life [16, 17].

It is important to note that patients with advanced cancer often prefer to avoid hospitalization, particularly toward the end of life, yet many still die in hospital [19, 20]. Not only do hospital admissions not match patients' preferences, but they result in significant costs that account for more than 25% of healthcare spending, and more than half of these costs occur in the last 60 days of life due to aggressive care and overmedication. Rising healthcare costs represent a major global public health challenge affecting patients and families as well as providers who reimburse care and health systems [21, 22].

Communication between oncologist and patients seems insufficient and has serious consequences on therapeutic decision-making:

A patient's treatment journey begins with effective communication between patient and physician. Effective communication is associated with high-quality healthcare [23]. In addition, understanding a patient's treatment options, concerns, and preferences can help physicians identify misconceptions and lead to better medical decisions [24]. Sometimes treatment decisions are inconsistent with patients' priorities, needs, and expectations. For example, many patients with advanced cancer are offered systemic and aggressive treatment options even in the very advanced stages of the disease, while comfort care options are not explained.

In an analysis of difficult communication situations in cancer patients, Owen and Jeffrey described how oncologists feel guilty and have the impression that they are "abandoning" their patients during transfer to palliative care; death can be seen as a failure of increasingly sophisticated medicine and not as the natural consequence of a lethal disease. Hence, the difficulty in stopping disease-specific care lies in the risk of the physician being faced with the dilemma of either over-treating the patient or neglecting a last chance for improvement [25].

In a review of the literature regarding communication about the transition from curative to palliative care, Schofield et al. report that people with advanced disease often underestimate the extent of their illness: this may be due to misunderstanding the information given or overestimation of the prognosis by the professional [26]. However, several studies that assessed patients' knowledge when discharged from the hospital found that no more than half of them had accurate information concerning every aspect of their condition, including diagnoses, medications, and adverse treatment effects [27]. In fact, an effective communication between physicians and patients regarding treatment plans is not easy to achieve. This challenge is more pronounced in cancer patients because of the complexity of the care required. It is difficult for oncologists to relay treatment options and potential side effects in a comprehensive and effective manner, particularly with the complexities of targeted therapies and clinical trials, while at the same time taking sufficient time to ensure that the patient's understanding of his or her disease is understood and that the patient's myriad of physical, psychosocial, and spiritual needs are met. In addition, patients need support in coping with their illness, understanding their disease experience, treatment, their care goals, and their preferences for care [28, 29].

Providing patients with both cancer therapy and personalized management of their quality of life (and that of their family and friends) requires immense resources and expertise. Traditionally, oncologists have been at the center of patient care, with particular emphasis on the use of chemotherapy, radiotherapy, immunotherapy, and many other therapies to control and stabilize the progression of cancer for as long as possible. This traditional single-specialty model of care can no longer satisfactorily address all the complex needs of the patient and the concerns of those around him or her. This requires multi-expertise in various fields and resources for the coordination of care and anticipation of complications. It is, therefore, a challenge for all physicians to ensure disease management while considering patients' quality of life.

Early Integrated Palliative Care (EIPC): Evidence-Based Practice and Recommendations at the International Level

In order to better meet the complex and emerging needs of cancer patients, researchers have been studying a new approach, "early integrated palliative care" in cancer care [30, 31]. Early integrated palliative care (EIPC) is a model of personalized care in the cancer patient care pathway and a fundamental component of the cancer care trajectory [32, 33]. It is integrated into curative treatments from the time an incurable cancer is diagnosed. Initially distinguished from terminal palliative care, EIPC is a new paradigm for a model of integrated care in the management of the quality of life of cancer patients [34, 35].

According to the 2019 Lancet Oncology Commission report, at the international level, there are seven controlled, randomized, and fundamental studies published by the following teams [36]: Jordhoy et al. (2000) [37], Bakitas et al.

(2009) [38], Temel et al. (2010) [39], Zimmermann et al. (2014) [40], Bakitas et al. (2015) [41], Maltoni et al. (2016) [42], Temel et al. (2017) [43], Groenvold et al. (2017) [44], and Zimmerman et al. (2016) [45]. The benefits of early palliative care in oncology care services have been demonstrated in several multicenter, randomized trials using a variety of rigorous, quantitative, and qualitative methods. They have highlighted the many benefits of EIPC for patients, families, and healthcare professionals (summarized in Table 1) and have also demonstrated that it is economically efficient for the healthcare system.

Patients, Caregivers, and Families

Early integrated palliative care is a holistic approach that aims to meet all of the physical, psychological, and spiritual needs of the individual and family, not just at the end of life, but from the time of diagnosis of an incurable cancer [46–49]. This allows for better symptom management and improved quality of life for patients throughout the trajectory of cancer disease. Caregivers and families benefit from better support, better ongoing information, and a lighter burden [50–52].

This philosophy reinforces the person's autonomy, allows him or her to participate more actively in his or her own care, and gives people and families a sense of greater control [53]. In fact, the patients will have better access to key elements at the appropriate time and in the care setting of their choice, so that they are informed early and regularly about the range of possible treatments and their risks and benefits, as well as the prognosis [40, 42]. This allows the drafting of advance directives (which can be changed at any time) that are less threatening when a person is feeling well than when they are experiencing a crisis or imminent death.

Cancer patients do not express their questions and fears, but are generally grateful if their doctors offer to talk about these distressing issues [53]. The early palliative approach allows patients to address the questioning of what is really wrong, to define their preferences and goals, and to designate a proxy or trusted person [54]. Above all, it allows for advance care planning and readjustment of care strategies throughout the course of the illness. All this patient information should be easily accessible to anyone caring for the patient. Frank discussions about the prognosis and trajectory of the disease do not destroy people's hope; on the contrary, according to several studies, it helps them to be better prepared even if they prefer to wish for a (unlikely) cure ("what if" discussions) [54, 55]. It also appears that these types of conversations are more useful when they occur early on. EIPC may also help patients make appropriate decisions to reduce unreasonable therapies and improve their quality of life and death [56–58]. In addition, the latest trial results have shown that early palliative care, integrated with cancer care, improves coping skills, increases resilience to illness and death, and lessens symptoms of depression and anxiety [59, 60].

Health Professionals

The EIPC model is a comprehensive approach practiced by a multi-professional team that collaborates and places the patient and family at the center of care delivery. Palliative medicine has enhanced the development of interprofessional collaboration by bringing together the ideas of different disciplines or areas [61, 62]. This model responds to the many serious ethical and medical decisions necessary to manage complex situations and therapeutic strategies. Thus, it optimizes the management of patients with serious, chronic, and incurable diseases [62, 63]. EIPC addresses the complex needs of patients and prevents burnout syndrome. All healthcare professionals are largely dependent on each other in their care actions [41, 64]. Thus, they develop expertise and training adapted to each stage of the disease process.

Providing effective and appropriate palliative care is not limited to relieving patients' symptoms of discomfort. The spirit of palliative medicine goes beyond comfort and quality of life. It helps to develop ethical thinking to set benchmarks and standards that help society to make

Table 1 Synthesizing the benefits of EIPC for patients, families, health professionals, and the health system

PATIENTS	FAMILIES
✓ Better holistic care of the patient in its entirety with all its dimensions: physical, psychosocial and spiritual. ✓ Better quality of life, fewer physical symptoms. ✓ Better coping and resilience in the face of illness and death and reduced symptoms of anxiety and depression. ✓ Better autonomy and respect for one's will. ✓ Better particpation in medical decisions. The patient is at the center of care and decisions. ✓ Better understanding and communication about their illness. ✓ Better anticipation with the patient of the future of his disease, elaboration of advance care planning and antipep guidelines; ✓ Better seamless care pathway in accordance with patient's wishes. ✓ Better end-of-life care in the living environment of the patient's choice. ✓ Better survival ✓ Better satisfaction.	✓ Best accompaniment ✓ Better information about the disease ✓ Better satisfaction ✓ Best bereavement support ✓ Better communication between patient and caregiver, ✓ Better knowledge of the patient's wishes ✓ Better participation in the medical decision when the patient can no longer express him/herself
✓ Better communication and discussion between health professionals the patient and family. ✓ Better communication between professionals with different specialties. ✓ Better coordination between health professionals from different specialties. ✓ Better anticipation of complications ✓ Better treatment decisions in complex situations. ✓ Better planning of goals of care projects ✓ Better training, skills and expertise adapted to the different stages of the disease process. ✓ Better working conditions and reduced stress.	✓ Improved efficiency: Reduction in the cost of health services. Reduced duplication of procedures, unplanned hospitalizations, unnecessary admissions to emergency, intensive care and resuscitation. Reduced treatment intensity, less use of expensive and ineffective intensive interventions in the last days of life. ✓ Better utilization of health care professionals and more effective use of specialists. ✓ Better referrals to hospitals, more appropriate use of the most appropriate care ✓ Development of a system centered around the chronically ill patient by strengthening the means indispensable to his or her care around the place where he or she lives. ✓ Better access to high-quality palliative care for more people with a wider range of diagnoses.
HEALTH PROFESSIONALS	HEALTH SYSTEM

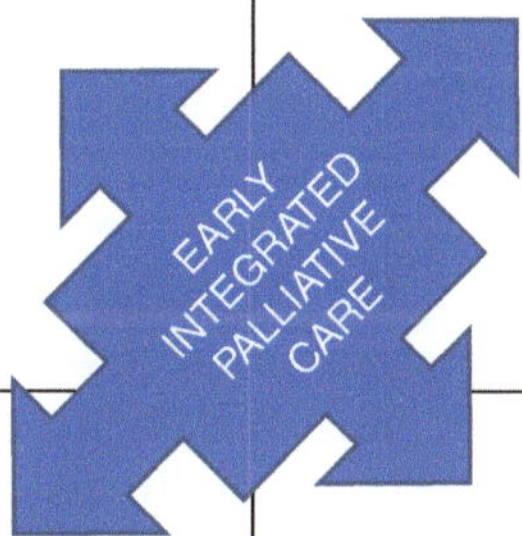

decisions and direct itself in complex cases [65–67]. It also protects the patient from unreasonable investigations and treatments by planning and anticipating care goals and by readjusting advance care planning and advance directives throughout the course of the disease [68, 69].

Several studies show that early palliative care improves coordination among professionals, making the collaboration smoother and less stressful. They also show that communication becomes more effective between cancer patients and their treating physicians, which makes for better outcomes [70].

The Healthcare System

Previous studies have shown that early enrolment in palliative care leads to greater efficiency at a lower cost, more appropriate referrals among different partners in the health system, more effective use of specialists, and better management of medical interactions [71, 72]. Some research suggests that the EIPC is not a source of cost, but rather tends to reduce end-of-life hospitalization costs and reduce the number of cases in emergency departments and intensive care units [73, 74]. Ultimately, it also reduces unnecessary hospitalizations and the use of expensive and ineffective intensive interventions in the last days of life [75, 76]. They can thus avoid unreasonable extensions of certain therapies, aggressive care, and recourse to emergency departments [77, 78].

International Recommendations of Learned Societies and the WHO

In recent years, the World Health Organization (WHO) and several learned societies, including those of oncology such as the Lancet Oncology Commission, ESMO (European Society for Medical Oncology), ASCO (American Society of Clinical Oncology), and NCCN (National Comprehensive Cancer Network), have shown a growing interest in EIPC and have recommended it [30, 36, 79–81]. The WHO's Executive Board has called upon all countries to strengthen the development of EIPC and to include it in chronic disease management. The WHO released new guidelines for integrating primary palliative care into healthcare in October 2018 [82]. The International Association for Hospice and Palliative Care (IAHPC) has designed, developed, and implemented a project to adopt, on a consensus basis, a new definition of palliative care with a focus on early and primary palliative care in the management of cerebrovascular disease [83]. Universal health coverage of early palliative care has thus become a major goal of health reform in many countries and a priority objective of the WHO [84].

Early Integrated Palliative Care in France: "From an Organizational Point of View"

In France, the number of new cancer cases diagnosed in 2018 was 382,000 (204,600 men and 177,400 women). The number of cancer deaths was estimated at 157,400 in 2018: 89,600 men and 67,800 women (compared to 84,041 men and 66,000 women in 2017) [85, 86]. Despite advanced treatments being increasingly successful in sustaining lives, the number of people with cancer and the numbers for morbidity and mortality continue to evolve. According to projections of studies for the coming decades, by 2030 cancer will be the leading cause of death. Although the survival rates of a majority of cancers (breast, prostate, colon, rectum, cutaneous melanoma, etc.) have improved, 63.5% of people suffer from sequelae derived from cancer or its treatment [87].

More and more people with cancer are having to cope with the physical effects of cancer and its treatment, which can lead to functional and cognitive impairments as well as other psychological and economic difficulties that degrade their quality of life. Cancers often result in disability, incapacity, loss of autonomy, and serious complications that weigh heavily on the quality of life of the patients and their families. They also result in significant personal, professional, psychosocial, and financial losses. According to the French National Cancer Institute (INCa), 63.5% of people suffer from the after-effects of cancer or treatment and, among those in the labor force at the time of their diagnosis, 20% are no longer working 5 years later [88].

In addition to the serious effects on quality of life, the economic consequences of cancer are colossal. According to INCa, hospitalization expenditures in 2018 for chemotherapy sessions and hospital stays will amount to nearly EUR 2.5 billion (EUR 1.27 billion for stays and EUR 1.21 billion for chemo sessions), an increase of 1.8% compared to 2017 [87]. France offered universal medical coverage to all citizens in 2014; three million people (4.4% of France's population) suffered from managed cancer (1.44 million men, 1.56 million women). The national cancer-related expenditure was EUR 16 billion, of which 6 billion was spent on primary healthcare (2.7 billion on drugs) and 9 billion on hospitals (1.6 billion on drugs) [89, 90]. Cancers are one of the largest groups of chronic diseases in terms of both patients and expenditure. While the number of patients remains stable, spending is increasing, mainly on drugs [90].

As a follow-up to World Health Assembly Resolution WHA67.19 in 2014 which recommends the development of the so-called integrated palliative care or integrated palliative approach in all health systems [91], the WHO Assembly recognized integrated palliative care as a fundamental component of integrated and person-centered care services, not as complementary or optional, and considers it a human right. According to several studies, integrated palliative care improves the quality of life, coordination of services, effectiveness, satisfaction, and efficiency of care [47, 91, 92]. Several international learned societies recommend it, and even the Lancet Oncology Commission now refers to the concept as "integrated medicine" [36].

A taxonomy-based organizational framework for integrated care would play an important role in facilitating the description and comparison of different models of integrated services useful for policy development, as well as the implementation and evaluation of integrated service models. It is recognized in the literature that integration of services is possible through a range of processes that may focus on systems, teamwork, or professional behaviors. A typology of integrated palliative care, the Rainbow Model of Integrated Care, was developed by Valentijn et al. to guide implementation and evaluate the integrated care integration strategy at three levels: macro, meso, and micro [93]. At the core of integrated care for people with multiple morbidities is the holistic understanding of the individual in his or her environment.

I use international recommendations as a basis for evaluating integrated palliative care integration processes at the macro level (system integration), meso level (organizational integration), micro level (clinical integration), and cross level – the level (functional and normative integration) with interconnected roles which contributes to integrated care (summarized in Table 2 and 3) [94–98].

Table 2 Description of main types of integration and allied integrative processes

Organizational integration	How is the organization formally structured? Leadership and governance mechanisms to provide comprehensive services to a defined population. For example, by coordinating structures, communicating, and aligning policies, rules, regulatory frameworks, etc. (meso level)
Functional integration	How are non-clinical support and back-office functions integrated? For example, key support functions that include media, policies, financial, rules, regulatory frameworks, and management and information systems structured around service delivery (micro, meso, and macro level)
Service integration	How are the clinical services offered by the organization integrated with each other? For example, the integration of different clinical services at an organizational level, such as through teams of multidisciplinary professionals (meso and micro level)
Clinical integration	At the clinical team level, is care for patients integrated in a single process both intra- and interprofessionally through, for example, the use of shared guidelines and protocols along the whole pathway of care? (micro level)

Table 3 Level management analysis

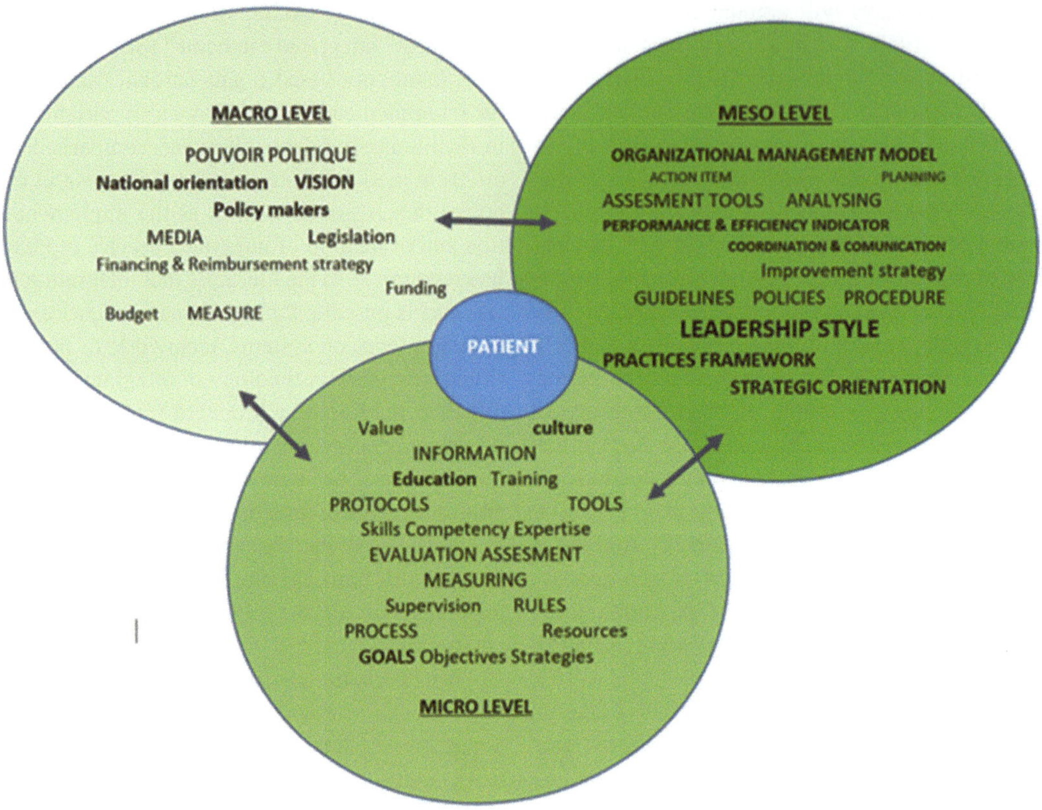

In addition, two factors are crucial in determining how successful integration is:

Normative integration	Developing shared values, culture, vision, norms, practices, and tools among organizations, professional groups, and individuals in coordinating work (micro, meso and macro levels)
Systemic integration	The coherence of rules and policies at the various levels of organization (micro, meso, and macro levels)

The Macro Level

Palliative care has political recognition and support:

Indeed, in terms of societal recognition, palliative care benefits from the unfailing support of the public authorities who are working to develop it throughout France, as evidenced by the legal and legislative facts in their favor (numerous circulars, laws, and decrees since 1986), unparalleled elsewhere in the world, granting ever greater rights and autonomy to users/patients. The creation of the French National Society for Palliative Care (SFAP) in 1990 [99] has been recognized by public authorities and has developed several national palliative care development programs (initiated since 1999). The recognition of a national resource center for palliative care (2002–2016) is currently being replaced by the National Observatory on the End of Life (2010–2015). The merger of these two entities led to the creation of a National Center for Palliative and End-of-Life Care (CNSPFV) in 2016 [100] and, recently, the launch of the national platform for national research on end of life (2018) [101] with the aim of creating a network of researchers around the social and medical realities of the end of life, supported by the Ministry of Higher Education, Research and Innovation.

Several pieces of legislation have been developed with a more end-of-life focus:

The first law of June 9, 1999, formalizes the right to palliative care as "active and continuous care practiced by an interdisciplinary team in an institution or at home" [102]. They aim to relieve pain, alleviate psychological suffering, safeguard the dignity of the sick person, and support those around him or her. Then the Act of March 4, 2002, Article L.1111-4 of the Public Health Code gives everyone the opportunity to make decisions concerning their health [103]. The refusal of treatment is one of these decisions that the doctor is obliged to accept by informing the patient about the consequences and ensuring that he/she receives the best care, whatever the decision. Secondly, the law of April 22, 2005, known as the Leonetti Law, underlines the right of patients not to be subjected to therapeutic persistence (the law speaks of "unreasonable obstinacy") [104]. And lastly, the Claeys-Leonetti Law of February 2, 2016, created new rights in favor of patients and those at the end of life [105, 106].

The national policy and strategic planning framework is oriented toward traditional palliative care and abandoning early integrated palliative care:

In fact, the model of traditional terminal palliative care is predominant and the development of early integrated palliative care seems rudimentary, according to the 2016 report of the National Center for Palliative and End-of-Life Care [107]. According to the 2018 study of the Atlas of Palliative and End-of-Life Care in France, the lack of access to PPS represents a major public health gap [108]. The 2020 report of the General Inspection of Social Affairs (IGAS) evaluating the "2015–2018 national plan for the development of palliative care and end-of-life support" points out that the latest national plan has not changed care provision despite all the international recommendations on early palliative care [109].

The media has a reduced view of palliative care: the concept of EIPC is poorly understood by the general public:

Palliative care is negatively perceived as being limited to end-of-life care. According to the HAS report, the term "supportive care" is more commonly used for cancer patients. According to a survey, nearly two out of three French people (63%) nevertheless feel they are poorly informed about palliative care [110]. When asked about the conditions of access, the content of care, or the terms of reimbursement for palliative care, only one French person in three (33%) feels well-informed (only 6% "very well informed") [109, 110]. Reports and information given on palliative care through the media are rather oriented toward end of life and early integrated hospice palliative care is rarely discussed.

Palliative care/medicine is not recognized as a medical specialty:

First of all, the discipline of palliative care has only very recently been recognized through a sub-section of the National Council of Health Universities (sub-section 4605 – clinical epistemology, then palliative medicine) chaired by Professor François Goldwasser, and end-of-life care has not penetrated other university disciplines as it has in other comparable countries even though the mission has met with oncologists, resuscitators, and geriatricians, among others, who publish in this field. Secondly, the initial training of medical students, both theoretical and practical, is insufficient and the continuing education of doctors is even more so. This observation must be qualified for nurses. According to a study conducted in 2019, palliatology is not yet a fully recognized medical specialty in its own right and lacks legitimacy in French hospitals, which blocks its use [112].

The funding and reimbursement systems are inappropriate and unsatisfactory for end-of-life care, so let's not talk about early palliative care!

The method of financing activity-based pricing (T2A) is not suitable for end-of-life care, nor is it suitable for early palliative care. Financing methods are focused on rather short-term episodes, without taking into account the entire course of care, and thus block the development of early palliative activity [109, 110, 113].

Concerning reimbursement, there is a palliative lump sum for patients with "palliative status": the team's support is reimbursed by social security and the rest by the mutual insurance company. In addition, palliative status opens the door to a series of free aids for the patient and his or her close companion. The palliative status is a status recognized by the mutual insurance company.

The T2A has led to fairly significant repercussions on the care of palliative patients: the problem concerns the T2A, activity-based pricing, which has applied to all hospital services since 2004. The principle of the T2A is to no longer pay hospitals with a global annual envelope, but according to the number and nature of acts performed for each patient, without really considering the length of hospitalization. The main objective is to encourage hospitals to shorten the length of stays in order to increase revenue. In principle, this seems rather incompatible with end-of-life care. How can we rationalize procedures for a patient for whom it has been decided not to have any more examinations or operations? What sense does it make to try to shorten hospital stays when the objective of palliative care is to accompany the patient progressively until death? This is an ethical misunderstanding [111].

Concretely, the application of T2A to palliative care means that when a patient is hospitalized in a palliative care unit between 4 and 12 days, the hospital will receive exactly the same amount from Medicare; starting on the thirteenth day, the budget allocated increases a little, but very slowly. From a strictly accounting point of view, it is therefore in their interest to discharge the patient at the end of the fourth day and to bring in another one. And that is the view of some hospital directors who have to make their hospitals profitable. This method of financing has created several early hospital discharge excesses and disruptions in care, which obviously seriously affect the quality of care [112, 113].

Although the T2A is probably the "least worst" solution for controlling healthcare spending – and it is really needed – it seems clearly inappropriate at the end of life. The challenge is to invent another system. In the meantime, we could start by better controlling budgets so that money allocated to palliative care is not used for other purposes. Above all, governments should invest more in palliative medicine. Over and above "dying well," which is fundamental for all of us, it has been clearly demonstrated that early use of palliative care makes it possible to avoid therapeutic relentlessness, such as the latest chemo which is useless and costs EUR 15,000. It is undoubtedly a better way to save money in hospital.

The Meso Level

The organization of the supply of terminal palliative care seems not to be harmonized, practitioners differ, and there is a lack of tools for early identification of palliative patients:

Several studies show differences in organization, practices, and operations among hospitals [114]. In addition, they show a lack of harmonization of protocols, scales, and tools deployed in this field, between one healthcare institution and another and even between one region and another. Currently, we are seeing the existence of several strategies and "juxtaposed" programs, and the management of palliative patients remains very compartmentalized, far from the concept of the continuum of care [116–119].

There are several scales and assessment tools specific to early palliative care that have been validated at the international level; however, they are very rarely used and inappropriate in the French context. The PALLIA-10 form is inappropriate for identifying patients in need of early palliative care. There is still no common tool to help healthcare professionals identify palliative care needs at an early stage.

The organization of palliative care services lacks monitoring and evaluation of efficiency and performance indicators, and experimentation with an organizational model for EIPC is still far from being a reality:

In the documents on the strategy and organization of palliative care supply, there are several objectives, multiple measures, and timeframes for implementation and the people responsible for these actions, but monitoring and evaluation, which are essential steps in the rehabilitation and evolution of the organization, are almost absent. Moreover, the two reports by the General Inspection of Social Affairs (IGAS) devoted to palliative care over the last 2 years have pointed out serious problems in evaluating the supply of palliative care [109, 120]. There is no clear doctrine for use or evaluation, nor are there clear indicators of the quality of "identified palliative care beds" (LISP), which are sometimes physically grouped together in quasi-hospice, sometimes isolated in this or that service, or sometimes simply virtual [120].

SFAP supported a survey conducted in 2016 by Dr. Ferrand, to assess the activity status of LISP. This survey indicated that there is a lack of criteria for evaluating nationally relevant LISP activity and the results are far from positive [121].

In general, hospital and out-of-hospital palliative care activity (at home) is very heterogeneous in quantity and quality and difficult to measure. Their impact on patients is not evaluated at all, and even indicators and criteria for evaluating the quality, efficiency, and performance of the current palliative care organization are almost nonexistent [120, 122].

The organization of palliative hospital structures is geared more toward end-of-life care and is poorly adapted to early palliative care:

In France there are three types of palliative care structures in place to receive patients in institutions: palliative care units, beds identified in hospital structures, and mobile palliative care teams (which travel to the patients' place of residence). The specifications of these structures are based on the slightly dated circular DHOS/02 n°2008-89 of March 25, 2008, relating to the organization of palliative care [123]. These circulars, job descriptions, roles, and missions have not been readapted nor evolved for early palliative care.

Moreover, the provision of palliative care in hospitals presents difficulties, and this has been documented on numerous occasions by the various reports on palliative care, all of which underline the fragility of existing data. Several studies are underway to make these data more reliable, but three aspects stand out at this stage: the overall inadequacy of the supply, its poor organization, and its very uneven distribution at the departmental and territorial levels.

The organization of the extension of a system of palliative care outpatient care in medical and social establishments and at home does not meet the needs of the population and shows significant disparities:

Several types of structure are dedicated to traveling to the home and to social medical centers: hospitalization at home services (HAD), home nursing care services (SSIAD), general practitioners, and several home networks [114]. An increasing number of mobile palliative care teams (EMSP) now have an extra-hospital activity at home and in hospices [124]. In practice, it relies mainly on the intervention of emergency services and can lead, for lack of an alternative, to hospitalization that is not always appropriate or desired [109]. In practice, it is based mainly on the use of emergency facilities and can lead, for lack of an alternative, to hospitalization which is not always appropriate or desired [109]. The vast majority of deaths occur in hospital (57%) as opposed to 25% at home and 12% in retirement homes [109, 125]. A large majority of people (85%) remain at home, the most preferred place to end their lives [110, 125].

Organization of information systems and the coordination model are informal and deficient:

Ensuring a continuous health trajectory requires good coordination between healthcare workers and a smooth transfer of information between healthcare professionals at the right time and place. Their coordination is ensured by several layers of support mechanisms for the coordination of complex health pathways.

However, institutional fragmentation and the juxtaposition of actors – attending physicians, pharmacists, nurses, SSIAD, HAD, palliative care networks, health networks, PAERPA's CTA, MAIA, territorial support platforms (PTAs), local information and coordination centers (CLICs), etc. – provide an unstable framework for the succession of actors, which is generally difficult to understand for the patient and his or her entourage and too often unsuited to the actual situation of the individual. Moreover, coordination between all these actors is carried out in an informal way and is different from one region to another. Thus, the coordination of care pathways, sometimes successfully carried out informally by a particular doctor or nurse or institution, has not yet found a level of standardization or a model that can be deployed on a larger scale [109, 126, 127].

These differences and segmentations in coordination and communication are accentuated by the limitations of information systems and the lack of centralization of the tools deployed in this field, for example shared medical records, and it is not interoperable between hospital establishments and city practitioners [118, 128].

The Micro Level

The value and vision of early integrated palliative care is confused with terminal care by health professionals: palliative care is still stigmatized:

According to several studies, the concept of early integrated palliative care is confused with terminal palliative care and poorly understood in France by patients, families, and health professionals, leaving a negative image in people's minds. Understanding of early palliative care is still too low. Palliative care for patients remains very late, including in oncology departments, although the situation varies greatly depending on the department and personality.

According to the 2015–2018 National Plan for the Development of Palliative Care and End-of-Life Support, "a still too large proportion of patients do not have access to the palliative care they need, in particular because they are identified too late" (Action 12-1 of the 2015–2018 National Plan for the Development of Palliative Care and End-of-Life Support) [128].

A national retrospective cohort study in 2019 was aimed primarily at measuring the prevalence of access to palliative care for hospitalized patients and identifying the delay between access to palliative care and death [129]. More than half of cancer patients who died within 2 years of diagnosis had access to inpatient palliative care. Furthermore, access to palliative care occurs late in the disease trajectory, often in the last month of life.

A multicenter study was conducted with patients diagnosed with metastatic cancer in five university medical centers or comprehensive cancer centers [130]. The purpose of the study was to determine the intensity of therapeutic interventions and the timing of integration of palliative care into cancer care. The overall values (min-max) of the indicators, as reported by the care facility rather than by the place of death, were 16% (8–25%) of patients received chemotherapy within 14 days prior to death, 16% (6–32%) had more than three acute care admissions, 6% (0–15%) had more than two emergency department visits, and 18% (4–35%) had more than one intensive care admission. Only half of these patients (53%) met with the palliative care team. The median time from palliative care intervention to death was 29 days.

These results are similar to those of other studies assessing the timing of the reporting of palliative care needs [131]. Notification of palliative care needs was timely (91 to 31 days before death) for 26.8% of patients and late (30 to 0 days before death) for 44.3%, and 29.4% of patients reported no palliative care needs. This means that the need for palliative care was not detected for almost one-third of end-of-life patients (29%) with metastatic lung cancer who died in hospitals. In addition, this study reports

(1) high frequencies of chemotherapy administration in the 14 days prior to death, (2) more frequent overuse in comprehensive cancer centers than in academic medical centers, and (3) higher intensity of care and medicalization in younger patients.

The study carried out by Sarradon et al. in 2019 highlights one of the obstacles encountered in promoting early palliative care in oncology in France [115]. In fact, the authors essentially wanted to point out the negative perception of oncologists toward palliative care in France. Some oncologists interviewed stated that this care should be reserved for patients with a life expectancy of less than 3 months. The vast majority of cancer patients are referred to this care too late. This reduced image masks the reality of the management of this holistic care. Some oncologists have changed the name of palliative care centers to "supportive care units" because of the stigma attached to the term. The sociological analysis of this study shows that France has adopted a palliative care model that addresses the end of life in cancer centers in France because the concept of early palliative care remains poorly understood in France by patients and families. Similarly, the practice of avoidance and reappointment also reflects the lack of understanding of this concept by health professionals.

Legislation is very poorly known by health professionals and the general public:

The report written by Professor Regis Aubry, president of the National Observatory on the End of Life (ONFV), pointed out that even after 7 years since the Leonetti Law was stipulated in 2005 (which prohibits therapeutic obstinacy), it was still unknown to a large majority of French people and was therefore rarely applied by the medical world [118].

According to several studies, the French are poorly informed about legislative and regulatory measures concerning the end of life, such as the Claeys-Leonetti Law, even though this subject is at the heart of their concerns. Only 12% know precisely what it is all about and nearly two out of three French people have never heard of it (62%) [110, 132, 133].

Concerning the anticipated directives, while making known one's wishes regarding the end of one's life is important for 92% of the French, only a minority have ever heard of the anticipated directives and 21% know precisely what they are about. Even more worryingly, among those who are aware of advance directives, only 12% have already drawn one up [110, 134].

For professionals and, even more so, for patients and their families and relatives, insufficient information on the legislation and meaning of the palliative approach is another problem. The report drawn up by the IGAS in 2019 points out that information on the Claeys-Leonetti Law (in 2016) was still too limited and there is still a great deal of educational work to be done with the general public [109].

Recommendations for good practice, procedures, protocols, evaluation tools, and quality indicators concerning the development of PPSs are very insufficiently developed:

Since 2002, the National Health Agency has recommended the use of early palliative care (EPC) in the medical management of patients with progressive incurable diseases [135]. The HAS, for its part, stresses the value of early palliative care [136]. In particular, the HAS emphasizes that "the perspective is not to separate palliative care from specific treatments for the disease and to aim for the development of a palliative culture or approach whose vocation is to integrate palliative care skills into all clinical practice and to avoid being locked into a specialized activity; it is part of the overall patient management, being both a global and individualized approach." In 2016, there were a series of publications on the trusted person, advance directives, improving hospital discharge for palliative patients, home care, and sedation and a fact sheet providing tools for identifying patients in need of palliative care and advice on how to talk to them about it.

Guidelines for advance directives (DA) and advance care planning regarding early anticipation and management of palliative patients are not widely known by healthcare professionals:

Early integrated palliative care brings a sense of ethical reflection to medical decisions that help physicians make decisions and provide direction in complex cases. On the other hand, patient autonomy and involvement in the medical decision-making process regarding their health is also emerging. It also protects the patient from unreasonable investigations and treatments, by planning and anticipating care goals with the patient by readjusting advance care planning and advance directives throughout the course of the illness [136, 137].

The physician must rely on the patient and consider the patient's preferences. Discussions should be seen as a multi-step process, to give the patient time to reflect or change his or her mind. "Advance directives" regarding end-of-life situations are the patient's wishes, expressed in writing, about what treatments or medical procedures he or she wants or does not want if one day he or she can no longer communicate after a serious accident or during a serious illness. They concern the conditions at the end of his/her life, i.e., to continue, limit, stop, or refuse the medical treatments or acts [138].

A descriptive study was carried out in 2019 among a hundred or so medical and paramedical personnel to assess the level of knowledge of this system. Only 10% of the staff were aware of the DA [133]. The majority of healthcare providers were not in favor of informing all patients in consultation or hospitalization and 44% believed that only end-of-life patients should be informed in hospital [109].

Another study reports that only 2.5% of French people wrote advance directives. The DA remains poorly understood by health professionals and the general public [110]. According to the IGAS report, deep and continuous sedation until death was still poorly understood by health professionals.

Not all palliative care professionals are properly trained or are inadequately trained in palliative care:

There is a major training deficiency. More than a third of these physicians have a university degree (DU) in palliative care or an inter-university diploma (DIU) in palliative care. Two-thirds have between 5 and 10 years of experience in palliative care and only one in ten has more than 10 years' experience [110]. Only 10% of hospital nurses have a specialized education. This percentage even falls to 2.5% for general practitioners [121].

Lack of research in EIPC; at present there is no model of early integrated palliative care that has been tested:

Currently in France there are only a few dedicated research centers, research projects, and programs on the end of life. Although publications in France have increased over the last 10 years (+28% per year between 2005 and 2016), the number is still not sufficient (an average of 26 publications per year compared to 1550 in the United States) and they are often published in international journals with a low impact factor [109].

Studies on this subject are limited to a few research centers and no randomized studies have been carried out to promote the concept of early integrated palliative care and no organizational model has been tried to date.

Lack of resources and infrastructure to develop early integrated palliative care provision (in hospital and at home) to better meet the needs of patients:

According to a SFAP "flash" survey carried out by e-mail between April and June 2018, it was estimated that about 800 doctors in France are practicing exclusively in palliative care, representing fewer than 2% of hospital practitioners. According to the SFAP survey, there is a shortage of physicians in relation to the projected workforce of the French medical order; one-third of the planned internship positions in palliative care structures would not be filled [109]. One-third of palliative care physicians would leave their structures within 5 years, and three-quarters of the teams are worried about their future renewal. Lack of candidates would be the main difficulty in recruitment [109]. There is a difficulty in recruiting trained staff because this specialty attracts very few young people.

Population satisfaction with the economic and holistic management of quality of life at the end of life:

Access to care for all, a pillar of our social protection system, is only satisfactory in the eyes of 53% of respondents in terms of end-of-life care. Despite a strong social security system, the costs of care and treatment are a source of dissatisfaction; 55% of respondents felt that support was not sufficient. The same applies to support for the families and relatives of a patient at the end of life [109].

Likewise, judgment with regard to palliative care is mixed: while there is little doubt about its effectiveness, more than three-quarters of French people (76%) consider it to be effective in alleviating suffering but insufficient for all aspects of patient care.

Caregivers in medicine and palliative care consider the patient as a whole, going beyond pathology and insisting on the importance of a holistic approach that respects the person; the WHO included spirituality in its 2002 definition of palliative care. Culture and spirituality are fundamental parts of being and both play an important role in a person's journey through life; yet they are often misunderstood and may not seem important in healthcare settings. These existential concerns become particularly critical at the end of life and to family survivors after the death [139]. Patients and families report the importance of spiritual, existential, and religious concerns throughout the cancer trajectory. Leading hospice palliative care organizations have developed guidelines that define spiritual care, show the importance of integrating it into care settings, and provide recommendations to guide the provision of spiritual services [140, 141]. The following are some of the key findings from the literature review:

In France, spiritual care is somewhat neglected and confused with religious care [142]. Attention to person-centered and family-centered oncology care requires the development of a healthcare environment that is prepared to support the religious, spiritual, and cultural practices preferred by patients and their families. These services need people who are trained in these types of care to help healthcare professionals identify, assess, and respond appropriately to spiritual need and distress.

Conclusion

Challenges, Perspectives, and Recommendations

> "You never change things by fighting the existing reality.
> To change something, build a new model that makes the existing model obsolete." – Buckminster Fuller

To conclude, the development of palliative care in France gives the impression of a case-by-case process, with fragmented responses to societal movements and not to a long-term global strategy (societal, economic, ethical, managerial, and organizational).

The French palliative movement emerged in the early 1980s from an ethical revolt, denouncing and deeming unworthy the conditions reserved for our fellow citizens at the end of life, thus challenging biomedicine in its instrumental drifts (unreasonable obstinacy, uncontrolled symptoms, therapeutic abandonment, or euthanasia) and driven by the explicit desire to change the attitude of medicine and society as a whole toward death, dying, and mourning. France was among the first countries to develop this concept and was a pioneer in this field.

Thirty years later, in 2020, France has still retained the traditional model of terminal palliative care, while other countries have successfully adapted it to meet the new challenges and needs of patients. We are far from a true integrated palliative approach as advocated by the WHO and all international learned societies. Palliative care services, "often relegated to a corner or even outside the hospital" as Didier Sicard pointed out in his 2012 report, are too often still identified primarily with places of death and situations of failure and not with places of care and quality of life.

Moreover, palliative care still remains essentially in the terminal phase, despite the value of early care [143]. Moreover, as the above assessment shows, the organizational integration of palliative care seems very weak. According to several studies, informal/formal organizational integration is fundamental to integrated care. To date there is no optimal model of integrated hospice palliative care that could be deployed at the national level, and no experimentation is underway.

These shortcomings in the current organization of palliative care provision have resulted in a loss of effectiveness, performance, and efficiency for our health system. They have led to poor coordination, anticipation, and communication and an ineffective information-sharing system.

On the one hand, this has colossal economic repercussions leading to repeated acts, unnecessary hospitalizations, and additional costs for the health system. On the other hand, it has unsatisfactory consequences for the management of patients who are often treated in "crisis situations" or late in life. The current crisis in the emergency department is one example that illustrates this observation. The vast majority of patients (two-thirds of patients) are admitted several times to the emergency department for complications related to chronic/incurable pathologies. Even more alarming is the fact that the number of patients treated in the emergency department who die in the emergency department is constantly increasing and nothing seems to be able to stem this trend. The other crisis is the movement for the demand for legalization of euthanasia and assisted suicide. Some patients can no longer bear the suffering; as the disease evolves and progresses, the impact on their quality of life worsens, and their lives are sometimes deemed intolerable and their suffering unbearable for them and their families. Those who request euthanasia or assisted suicide do not really want to end their lives, but simply want to put an end to the pain, distress, suffering, and dismay accumulated over months, if not years, by progressive illnesses. These patients want to maintain their control, autonomy, and dignity. These requests for euthanasia, for dying, and for "I can't take it anymore, let me go" are understandable requests and are the result of shortcomings in the organization and management of their quality of life while at the end of life.

Unlike the development of end-of-life palliative care, which relies on a single team providing humanitarian support at the end of life when there is nothing left to do, early integrated palliative care is based on support by teams from different cultures, skills, and specialties that must learn to coordinate and collaborate together while putting the patient at the center of the management from the time of diagnosis and throughout the disease.

The major issue facing the deployment of EIPC teams is the articulation and coordination of the two types of care (palliative and curative) throughout the course of an illness, for several months, with the palliative care component increasing when the activity of the curative team may be reduced.

Studies point out that several organizational frameworks have been developed to respond to the integration of the palliative approach. They describe that the integration of EIPC remains fragile because of its informal nature based on mutual trust and shared values, as well as its limited scope. Multidisciplinary teamwork and consultation are important components of horizontal integration. However, full integration also requires vertical, formal integration as adjacent levels in a chain of care. Segmentation of health services and late referral to palliative care prevent many patients from receiving them at the right time and place [143]. The qualitative survey was carried out by Carlos Centeno et al. in 2017 for the European Association for Palliative Care Atlas of Palliative Care in Europe with boards of directors of health systems. This study highlights that the development of integrated palliative care is diversified and lacks effective integration into the European system. Existing models in Europe are based on informal organization and this does not help to promote them on a higher national and international scale [144].

In 2019, a European study called InSuP-C aimed to study integrated practices in Europe and to make recommendations for effective integration of early palliative care [145]. This study reported that there is little consensus on which aspects of organizational integration are important and which should be prioritized. How to implement early integration is not well-defined and will certainly vary depending on the types of practices, the size and existing resources of a health system, the patient population, the patient needs, and the current level of palliative care provided by primary care physicians. The recommendations of this study focus on the implementation of an organizational framework based on processes at three levels of integration: macro, meso, and micro.

Several studies have developed recommendations on the development of early integrated palliative care and emphasize the importance of developing valid common tools needed to identify and screen the population in need of integrated palliative care at an early stage. For example, they point to the value of developing a scale of need for EIPC based on the stage of disease progression. Finally, they show the value of implementing and harmonizing good practice recommendations, protocols, and tools for monitoring and evaluating patients.

According to the 2019 report of the Lancet Oncology Commission, despite the evidence and recommendations for the early integration of EIPC in cancerology, international data demonstrate the low rate of referral of patients to EIPC. The timing of early palliative care intervention is not clearly defined. This commission reports that the content and manner of integration of EIPC are not detailed and models of integration remain poorly defined. For example, it points to the lack of international agreements on organizational standards and strategies for the development of EIPC. The commission will address the issue of an optimal organizational model as a process that includes different parts of the journey through the healthcare system, both horizontally and vertically, ensuring continuity of care and putting the patient at the center of this process. Early integration thus raises new research questions: When and how should palliative care be delivered? What is the optimal model of integrated palliative care?

"The appearance of a new activity can be analyzed as the grafting of a foreign body on a hitherto autonomous organism" (Igor Ansoff) [146]. This quote shows how crucial and potentially dangerous changes in structure are. For a new activity to be integrated, therefore, it is fundamentally a matter of defining who does what and how in the organization, while keeping the informality among employees.

This involves transforming practices and restructuring organizational patterns and looking for new ways to move forward along the patient quality-of-life continuum of care.

References

1. Ferlay J, Colombet M, Soerjomataram I, et al. Estimating the global cancer incidence and mortality in 2018: GLOBOCAN sources and methods. Int J Cancer. 2019;144(8):1941–53.
2. Allemani C, Matsuda T, Di Carlo V, Harewood R, Matz M, Nikšić M, Bonaventure A, Valkov M, Johnson CJ, Estève J, Ogunbiyi OJ. CONCORD Working Group Global surveillance of trends in cancer survival 2000–14 (CONCORD-3): analysis of individual records for 37 513 025 patients diagnosed with one of 18 cancers from 322 population-based registries in 71 countries. Lancet. 2018;391:1023–75.
3. WHO. Cancer prevention and control [WHA 58.22]. Geneva: World Health Organization; 2017.
4. Mattiuzzi C, Giuseppe Lippi G. Current cancer epidemiology. J Epidemiol Global Health. 2019;9(4):217–22.
5. Cheung WY, Le LW, Zimmermann C. Symptom clusters in patients with advanced cancers. Support Care Cancer. 2009;17:1223–30.
6. Gilbertson-White S, Aouizerat BE, Jahan T, Miaskowski C. A review of the literature on multiple symptoms, their predictors, and associated outcomes in patients with advanced cancer. Palliat Support Care. 2011;9:81–102.
7. Greer J, Jackson V, Meier D, Temel J. Early integration of palliative care services with standard oncology care for patients with advanced cancer. Am Cancer Soc J. 2013;63(5):349–63.
8. Mitchell AJ, Chan M, Bhatti H, et al. Prevalence of depression, anxiety, and adjustment disorder in oncological, haematological, and palliative care settings: a meta-analysis of 94 interview-based studies. Lancet Oncol. 2011;12:160–74.
9. Tucker-Seeley RD, Abel GA, Uno H, et al. Financial hardship and the intensity of medical care received near death. Psychooncology. 2015;24(5):572–8.
10. Pirl WF, Muriel A, Hwang V, et al. Screening for psychosocial distress: a national survey of oncologists. J Support Oncol. 2007;5:499–504.

11. Mohammed AA, Al-Zahrani O, Salem RA, Elsayed FM. Aggressive care at the end of life; where are we? Indian J Palliat Care. 2019;25(4):539–43.
12. Ho TH, et al. Trends in the aggressiveness of end-of-life cancer care in the Universal Health Care system of Ontario, Canada. J Clin Oncol. 2011;29(12):1587–91.
13. Choi Y, Keam B, Kim TM, et al. Cancer treatment near the end-of-life becomes more aggressive: changes in trend during 10 years at a single institute. Cancer Res Treat. 2015;47:555–63.
14. Ho TH, Barbera L, Saskin R, et al. Trends in the aggressiveness of end-of-life cancer care in the universal health care system of Ontario, Canada. J Clin Oncol. 2011;29:1587–91.
15. Barbera L, Seow H, Sutradhar R, et al. Quality of end-of-life cancer care in Canada: a retrospective four-province study using administrative health care data. Curr Oncol. 2015;22:341–35.
16. Chang TS, Su YC, Lee CC. Determinants for aggressive end-of-life care for oral cancer patients: a population-based study in an Asian country. Medicine. 2015;94:e460.
17. Falchook AD, Dusetzina SB, Tian F, Basak R, Selvam N, Chen RC. Aggressive end-of-life care for metastatic cancer patients younger than age 65 years. JNCI. 2017;109(9):1–6
18. Basch E, Loblaw DA, Oliver TK, et al. Systemic therapy in men with metastatic castration-resistant prostate cancer: American Society of Clinical Oncology and Cancer Care Ontario clinical practice guideline. J Clin Oncol. 2014;32(30): 3436–48.
19. Gruneir A, Mor V, Weitzen S, et al. Where people die: a multilevel approach to understanding influences on site of death in America. Med Care Res Rev. 2007;64:351–78.
20. Sahm S, Will R, Hommel G. What are cancer patients' preferences about treatment at the end of life, and who should start talking about it? A comparison with healthy people and medical staff. Support Care Cancer. 2005;13(4):206–14.
21. Bekelman JE, Halpern SD, Blankart CR, et al. Comparison of site of death, health care utilization and hospital expenditures for patients dying with cancer in 7 developed countries. JAMA. 2016;315(3):272–83.
22. Greer JA, Pirl WF, Jackson VA, et al. Effect of early palliative care on chemotherapy use and end-of-life care in patients with metastatic non-small-cell lung cancer. J Clin Oncol. 2012;30(4):394–400.
23. Zolnierek KB, Dimatteo MR. Physician communication and patient adherence to treatment: a meta-analysis. Med Care. 2009;47(8):826–34.
24. Say RE, Thomson R. The importance of patient preferences in treatment decisions – challenges for doctors. BMJ. 2003;327(7414):542–5.
25. Owen R, Jeffrey D. Communication: common challenging scenarios in cancer care. Eur J Cancer. 2008;44:1163–8.
26. Mack JW, Smith TJ. Reasons why physicians do not have discussions about poor prognosis, why it matters, and what can be improved. J Clin Oncol. 2012;30:2715–7.
27. Almalki H, Absi A, Alghamdi A, Alsalmi M, Khan M. Analysis of patient-physician concordance in the understanding of chemotherapy treatment plans among patients with cancer. JAMA Netw Open. 2020;3(3):e200341.
28. Maguire P, Faulkner A, Booth K, Elliott C, Hillier V. Helping cancer patients disclose their concerns. Eur J Cancer. 1996;32A(1):78–81.
29. Sumpio C, Knobf MT, Jeon S. Treatment complexity: a description of chemotherapy and supportive care treatment visits in patients with advanced-stage cancer diagnoses. Support Care Cancer. 2016;24(1):285–93.
30. Ferrell BR, Temel JS, Temin S, et al. Integration of palliative care into standard oncology care: American Society of Clinical Oncology clinical practice guideline update. J Clin Oncol. 2017;35(1):96–112.
31. Bauman JR, Temel JS. The integration of early palliative care with oncology care: the time has come for a new tradition. JNCCN. 2014;12(12):1763–71.
32. Hui D, Kim YJ, Park JC, Zhang Y, Strasser F, Cherny N, et al. Integration of oncology and palliative care: a systematic review. Oncologist. 2015;20:77–83.
33. Schlick CJR, Bentrem DJ. Timing of palliative care: when to call for a palliative care consult. J Surg Oncol. 2019;120(1):30–4.
34. Courteau C, Chaput G, Musgrave L, Khadoury A. Patients with advanced cancer: when, why, and how to refer to palliative care services. Curr Oncol. 2018;25(6):403–8.
35. Gärtner J, Daun M, Wolf J, von Bergwelt-Baildon M, Hallek M. Early palliative care: pro, but please be precise! Oncol Res Treat. 2019;42(1–2):11–8.
36. Kaasa S, Loge JH, Aapro M, et al. Integration of oncology and palliative care: a lancet oncology commission. Lancet Oncol. 2018;19(11):588–653.
37. Jordhoy MS, Fayers P, Saltnes T, Ahlner-Elmqvist M, Jannert M, Kaasa S. A palliative-care intervention and death at home: a cluster randomized trial. Lancet. 2000;356(9233):888–93.
38. Bakitas M, Lyons KD, Hegel MT, et al. Effects of a palliative care intervention on clinical outcomes in patients with advanced cancer: the project ENABLE II randomized controlled trial. JAMA. 2009;302:741–9.
39. Temel JS, Greer JA, Muzikansky A, Gallagher ER, Admane S, Jackson VA, et al. Soins palliatifs précoces pour les patients atteints d'un cancer du poumon non à petites cellules métastatique. N Engl J Med. 2010;363:733–42.
40. Zimmermann C, Swami N, Krzyzanowska M, et al. Early palliative care for patients with advanced cancer: a cluster-randomized controlled trial. Lancet. 2014;383:1721–30.
41. Bakitas MA, Tosteson TD, Li Z, et al. Early versus delayed initiation of concurrent palliative oncology

care: patient outcomes in the ENABLE III randomized controlled trial. J Clin Oncol. 2015;33:1438–45.
42. Maltoni M, Scarpi E, Dall'Agata M, Zagonel V, Berte R, Ferrari D, et al. Systematic versus on-demand early palliative care: results from a multicenter, randomized clinical trial. Eur J Cancer. 2016;65:61–8.
43. Temel JS, Greer JA, El-Jawahri A, Pirl WF, Park ER, Jackson VA, et al. Effets des soins palliatifs intégrés précoces chez les patients atteints de cancer du poumon et du GI: un essai clinique randomisé. J Clin Oncol. 2017;35:834–41.
44. Groenvold M, Petersen MA, Damkier A, et al. Randomized clinical trial of early specialist palliative care plus standard care versus standard care alone in patients with advanced cancer: the Danish Palliative Care Trial. Palliat Med. 2017;31(9):814–24.
45. Zimmerman C, Swami N, Krzyzanowska M, et al. Perceptions of palliative care among patients with advanced cancer and their caregivers. CMAJ. 2016;188:e217–27.
46. Vanbutsele G, Pardon K, Van Belle S, Surmont V, De Laat M, Colman R, Eecloo K, Cocquyt V, Geboes K, Deliens L. Effect of early and systematic integration of palliative care in patients with advanced cancer: a randomized controlled trial. Lancet Oncol. 2018;19(3):394–404.
47. Ewert B, Hodiamont F, van Wijngaarden J, et al. Building a taxonomy of integrated palliative care initiatives: results from a focus group. BMJ Support Palliat Care. 2016;6:14–20.
48. Jones J, Cohen R, Zimmermann C, Rodin G. Quality of life and symptom burden in cancer patients admitted to an acute palliative care unit. J Palliat Care. 2018;26(2):94–102.
49. White C, Noble S, Watson M, Swan F, Allgar V, Napier E, Nelson A, McAuley J, Doherty J, Lee B, Johnson M. Prevalence, symptom burden, and natural history of deep vein thrombosis in people with advanced cancer in specialist palliative care units (HIDDen): a prospective longitudinal observational study. Lancet Haem. 2019;6(2):9–88.
50. Kavalieratos D, Corbelli J, Zhang D, et al. Association between palliative care and patient and caregiver outcomes: a systematic review and meta-analysis. JAMA. 2016;316:2104–14.
51. Hannon B, et al. Experiences of patients and caregivers with early palliative care: a qualitative study. Palliat Med. 2017;31(1):72–81.
52. McDonald J, et al. Caregiver quality of life in advanced cancer: qualitative results from a trial of early palliative care. Palliat Med. 2018;32(1):69–78.
53. Pardon K, Deschepper R, Vander Stichele R, et al. Are patient's preferences for information and participation in medical decision-making being met? Interview study with lung cancer patients. Palliat Med. 2011;25:62–70.
54. Bakitas M, Dionne-Odom JN, Jackson L, Frost J, Bishop MF, Li Z. "There were more decisions and more options than just yes or no": evaluating a decision aid for advanced cancer patients and their family caregivers. Palliat Support Care. 2017;15(1):44–56.
55. Rietjens JAC, Sudore RL, Connolly M, et al. Definition and recommendations for advance care planning: an international consensus supported by the European Assoc. for Palliative Care. Lancet Oncol. 2017;18(9):e543–51.
56. Sudore RL, Lum HD, You JJ, et al. Defining advance care planning for adults: a consensus definition from a multidisciplinary Delphi panel. J Pain Symptom Manag. 2017;53:821–32.
57. Pautex S, Herrmann FR, Zulian GB. Role of advance directives in palliative care units: a prospective study. Palliat Med. 2008;22:835–41.
58. Maltoni M, Scarpi E, Dall'agata M, Schiavon S, Biasini C, Codeca C, et al. Systematic versus on-demand early palliative care: a randomized clinical trial assessing quality of care and treatment aggressiveness near the end of life. Eur J Cancer. 2016;69:110–8.
59. Greer JA, Applebaum AJ, Jacobsen JC, Temel JS, Jackson V. Understanding and addressing the role of coping in palliative care for patients with advanced cancer. J Clin Oncol. 2020;38(9):915–25.
60. Greer J, Jacobs J, El-Jawahri A, Nipp R, Gallagher E, Pirl W, Park E, Muzikansky A, Jacobsen M, Jackson V, Temel J. Role of patient coping strategies in understanding the effects of early palliative care on quality of life and moo. J Clin Oncol. 2018;36(1): 53–60.
61. Sargeant J, Loney E, Murphy G. Effective interprofessional teams: "contact is not enough" to build a team. J Contin Educ Heal Prof. 2008;28(4):228–34.
62. Junger S, Pestinger M, Elsner F, Krumm N, Radbruch L. Criteria for successful multiprofessional cooperation in palliative care teams. Palliat Med. 2007;21(4):347–54.
63. King JD, Eickhoff J, Traynor A, Campbell TC. Integrated onco-palliative care associated with prolonged survival compared to standard care for patients with advanced lung cancer: a retrospective review. J Pain Symptom Manag. 2016;51(6):1027–32.
64. Tartaglione E, Vig E, Lynn F. Bridging the cultural divide between oncology and palliative care subspecialties: clinicians' perceptions on team integration. Am J Hospice Palliat Care. 2017;35(7):978–84.
65. Emmerich N. Leadership in palliative medicine: moral, ethical and educational. BMC Med Ethics. 2018;19(55):2–11.
66. Shale DS. Moral leadership in medicine: building ethical healthcare organizations. Cambridge: Cambridge University Press; 2011.
67. De Panfilis L, Di Leo S, Peruselli C, et al. "I go into crisis when …": ethics of care and moral dilemmas in palliative care. BMC Palliat Care. 2019;18(70):2–8.
68. Frist WH, Presley MK. Training the next generation of doctors in palliative care is the key to the new era of value-based care. Acad Med. 2015;90:268–71.

69. Mack JW, Weeks JC, Wright AA, et al. End-of life discussions, goal attainment, and distress at the end of life: Predictors and out comes of receipt of care consistent with preferences. J Clin Oncol. 2010;28:1203–8.
70. Thomas T, Jackson V, Carlson H, Rinaldi S, Sousa A, Andrea Hansen A, Kamdar M, Jacobsen J, Park E, Pirl W, Temel J, Greer J. Communication differences between oncologists and palliative care clinicians: a qualitative analysis of early, integrated palliative care in patients with advanced cancer. J Palliat Med. 2019;22(1):41–9.
71. Obermeyer Z, Makar M, Abujaber S, et al. Association between the Medicare hospice benefit and health care utilization and costs for patients with poor-prognosis cancer. JAMA. 2014;312(18):1888–96.
72. Wu CC, Hsu TW, Chang CM, Lee CH, Huang CY, Lee CC. Palliative chemotherapy affects aggressiveness of end-of-life care. Oncologist. 2016;21(6):771–7.
73. May P, Garrido MM, Cassel JB, Kelley AS, Meier DE, Normand C, Stefanis L, Smith TJ, Morrison RS. Palliative care teams' cost-saving effect is larger for cancer patients with higher numbers of comorbidities. Health affairs (Project Hope). 2016;35(1):44–53.
74. Smith S, Brick A, O'Hara S, Normand C. Evidence on the cost and cost-effectiveness of palliative care: a literature review. Palliat Med. 2014;28(2):130–50.
75. Gunjur A. Early in-patient palliative care consultation saves costs. Lancet Oncol. 2015;16(7):321.
76. May P, Garrido MM, Cassel JB, et al. Cost analysis of a prospective multi-site cohort study of palliative care consultation teams for adults with advanced cancer: where do cost-savings come from? Palliat Med. 2017;31(4):378–86.
77. May P, Garrido MM, Cassel JB, et al. Prospective cohort study of hospital palliative care teams for inpatients with advanced cancer: earlier consultation is associated with larger cost-saving effect. J Clin Oncol. 2015;33(25):2745–52.
78. Mathew C, Hsu A, Prentice M, Lawlor P, Kyeremanteng K, Tanuseputro P, Welch V. Economic evaluations of palliative care models: a systematic review. Palliat Med. 2020;34(1):69–82.
79. WHO. Strengthening of palliative care as a component of comprehensive care throughout the life course. Resolution WHA. 2014;67:19.
80. Schrijvers D, Cherny NI, on behalf of the ESMO Guidelines Working Group. ESMO Clinical Practice Guidelines on palliative care: advanced care planning. Ann Oncol. 2014;25(S3):138–42.
81. Ferrell BR, Twaddle ML, Melnick A, Meier DE. National consensus project clinical practice guidelines for quality palliative care guidelines, 4th edition. J Palliat Med. 2018;21(12): 1684–9.
82. Dans M, Smith T, Back A, Baker JN, Bauman JR, Beck AC, Block S, Campbell T, Case AA, Dalal S, Edwards H, Fitch TR, Kapo J, Kutner JS, Kvale E, Miller C, Misra S, Mitchell W, Portman DG, Spiegel D, Sutton L, Szmuilowicz E, Temel J, Tickoo R, Urba SG, Weinstein E, Zachariah F, Bergman MA, Scavone JL. NCCN guidelines insights palliative care, version 2. J Natl Compr Cancer Netw. 2017;15(8):989–97.
83. WHO Global Conference on Primary Health Care: declaration of Astana. (2018). https://www.who.int/docs/default-source/primary-health/declaration/gcphc-declaration.pdf.
84. WHO 13th General Programme of Work (GPW 13) impact framework: targets and indicators (2018). https://www.who.int/about/what-we-do/GPW13_WIF_Targets_and_Indicators_English.pdf.
85. Bray F, BSc FJ, Soerjomataram I, Siegel R, Torre L, Jemal A. Global cancer statistics, GLOBOCAN estimates of incidence and mortality worldwide for 36 cancers in 185 countries. CA Cancer J Clin. 2018;68(6):1–31.
86. Cowppli-Bony A, Colonna M, Ligier K, et al. Épidémiologie descriptive des cancers en France métropolitaine : incidence, survie et prévalence [Descriptive epidemiology of cancer in metropolitan France: Incidence, survival and prevalence]. Bull Cancer. 2019;106(7–8):617–34.
87. INCa. (2019). https://www.e-cancer.fr/Actualites-et-evenements/Actualites/L-Institut-publie-L-essentiel-des-faits-et-chiffres-des-cancers-en-France-edition-2019.
88. INCa. (2018). La vie cinq ans après un diagnostic de cancer. https://www.e-cancer.fr/Expertises-et-publications/Catalogue-des-publications/La-vie-cinq-ans-apres-un-diagnostic-de-cancer-Rapport.
89. https://www.e-cancer.fr/Professionnels-de-sante/Les-chiffres-du-cancer-en-France/Epidemiologie-des-cancers/Donnees-globales.
90. Bousquet PJ, Lefeuvre D, Tuppin P, et al. Cancer care and public health policy evaluations in France: usefulness of the national cancer cohort. PLoS One. 2018;3(10):e0206448.
91. World Health Assembly. WHA67.19 Strengthening of palliative care as a component of comprehensive care throughout the life course. 67th World Health Assembly. 2014 Available from: http://apps.who.int/gb/ebwha/pdf_files/wha67/a67_r19-en.pdf.
92. Brazil K. A call for integrated & coordinated palliative care. J Palliat Med. 2018;21(S1):S27–9.
93. Valentijn PP, Boesveld IC, van der Klauw DM, Ruwaard D, Struijs JN, Molema JJ, Bruijnzeels MA, Vrijhoef HJ. Towards a taxonomy for integrated care: a mixed-methods study. Int J Integr Care. 2015;15:e003.
94. Fulop N, Mowlem A, Edwards N: Construire des soins intégrés: leçons du Royaume-Uni et d'ailleurs. The NHS Confederation, Londres: www.nhsconfed.org/~/media/Confederation/Files/Publications/Documents/Building%20integrated%20care.pdf.
95. World Health Organization Regional Office for Europe. (2016). Integrated care models: an overview. Health Services Delivery Programme, Division of Health Systems and Public Health, 42 p.

96. Williams P, Sullivan H. Faces of integration. Int J Integr Care. 2009;9:e100.
97. Shaw SE et al. "What is integrated care? An overview of integrated care in the NHS Research report". 2011.
98. World Health Organization. Report by the Secretariat. Sixty-Ninth World Health Assembly. Geneva: WHO; 2016. Apr 15, Framework on integrated, people-centred health services. Available at: http://apps.who.int/gb/ebwha/pdf_files/WHA69/A69_39-en.pdf?ua = 1.
99. Site de la SFAP: http://www.sfap.org/rubrique/la-sfap.
100. Site de CNSPFV: https://www.parlons-fin-de-vie.fr/qui-sommes-nous/atlas-des-soins-palliatifs-et-de-la-fin-de-vie/.
101. National platform for end-of-life research: https://www.plateforme-recherche-findevie.fr/.
102. Law no 99-477 du 9 juin 1999: https://www.legifrance.gouv.fr/affichTexte.do?cidTexte=JORFTEXT000000212121&categorieLien=id.
103. Law n° 2002-303 du 4 mars 2002: https://www.legifrance.gouv.fr/affichTexte.do?cidTexte=JORFTEXT000000227015&categorieLien=id.
104. Law n° 2005-370 du 22 avril 2005: https://www.legifrance.gouv.fr/affichTexte.do?cidTexte=JORFTEXT000000446240&categorieLien=id.
105. Law 2016-87, 2 février 2016: https://www.legifrance.gouv.fr/affichTexte.do?cidTexte=JORFTEXT000031970253&categorieLien=id.
106. Claeys A, Leonetti J. Rapport de présentation et texte de la proposition de loi créant de nouveaux droits en faveur des malades et des personnes en fin de vie. Paris: Documentation Française; 2014. http://www.assemblee-nationale.fr/14/rapports/r2585.asp.
107. CNSPFV. Activity report 2016 2017. https://www.parlons-fin-de-vie.fr/wpcontent/uploads/2018/09/CNSPFVRapportActivite2016.pdf
108. Ravanello A., Rotelli-Bihet L. Atlas des soins palliatifs et de la fin de vie en France, Première édition. Center national des soins palliatifs et de la fin de vie (CNSPFV). 2018
109. IGAS report 2020 file:///C:/Users/Utilisateur/OneDrive/Bureau/information%20epc%20france/igas%202019.pdf.
110. SFAP 2016. file:///C:/Users/Utilisateur/OneDrive/Bureau/information%20epc%20france/etude2016_findevie_fondationadrea.pdf.
111. "Soins palliatifs: un financement parfois pervers". Rev Prescrire. 2010;30(319):377.
112. Devalois B. "Tarification à l'activité: ses problèmes pour les soins palliatifs" Congrès national d'accompagnement et de soins palliatifs. 2009:23.
113. Comité consultatif national d'éthique "Avis sur les questions éthiques liées au développement et au financement des soins palliatifs – 2010." https://www.ccne-ethique.fr/fr/publications/avis-sur-les-questions-ethiques-liees-au-developpement-et-au-financement-des-soins
114. HAS, Methodological note and documentary; Summary Update on the Palliative Care Approach 2016. file:///C:/Users/Utilisateur/OneDrive/Bureau/information%20epc%20france/HAS%20%20Advance%20care%20planning.pdf.
115. Sarradon-Eck A, Besle S, Troian J, Capodano G, Mancini J. Comprendre les obstacles à l'introduction de soins palliatifs précoces pour les patients atteints de cancer en France. J Palliat Med. 2019;22(5):508–16.
116. Cnam 2018. Rapport sur les charges et produits de l'assurance maladie pour 2019: Améliorer la qualité du système de santé et maîtrizer les dépenses : propositions de l'Assurance Maladie pour 2019. Paris Cnam https://www.ameli.fr/l-assurance-maladie/statistiques-et-publications/rapports-etperiodiques/rapports-charges-produits-de-l-assurance-maladie/rapports-charges-et-produits-pour2018-a-2020/rapport-charges-et-produits-pour-l-annee-2019.php.
117. Institut Montaigne. Réanimer le système de santé; propositions pour 2017. 2016. https://www.institut-montaigne.org/ressources/pdfs/publications/reanimer_systeme_de_sante.pdf.
118. Aubry R. État des lieux du développement des soins palliatifs en France en 2010. Paris Ministère chargé de la santé 2011. http://www.sante.gouv.fr/IMG/pdf/Rapport_Etat_des_lieux_du_developpement_des_soins_palliatif s_en_France_en_2010.pdf.
119. Cour des Comptes. Les soins palliatifs : une prize en charge toujours très incomplète. Rapport public annuel 2015 de la Cour des Comptes., Paris: Cour des comptes; 2015, 221–248. https://www.ccomptes.fr/fr/publications/le-rapport-public-annuel-2015.
120. IGAS 2017 file:///C:/Users/Utilisateur/OneDrive/Bureau/information%20epc%20france/igas%20soins%20palliatifs%20a%20domicile.pdf.
121. SFAP 2016. Etude ELIPSE. http://www.sfap.org/actualite/enquete-elipse#xd_co_f=YWU1ZTgyNzYtMjljNS00YzQ3LWEyOTgtZWMzZTc5NWM1MDk0~.
122. Libération 2016, lit fantômes à l'hôpital. https://www.liberation.fr/france/2016/06/19/soins-palliatifs-a-l-hopital-des-milliers-de-lits-fantomes_1460615.
123. http://www.sfap.org/document/annexe-5-de-la-circulaire-ndegdhoso2200899-du-25-mars-2008
124. Fonds Pour les Soins Palliatifs. et Malakoff Médéric 2017. Guide régional des soins palliatifs. Occitanie.
125. Poulalhon C, Rotelli-Bihet L, Moine S, Fagot-Campagna A, Aubry R, et Tuppin P. Utilisation des soins palliatifs hospitaliers en fonction du lieu de décès et de maladie un an avant le décès en 2013: étude nationale d'observation française. BMC Palliat Care. 2018;17(1):75. https://doi.org/10.1186/s12904-018-0327-z.
126. Soins palliatifs de proximité : Axe 3, Action 12-1 & Stratégie de santé publique 2016 file:///C:/Users/Utilisateur/OneDrive/Bureau/information%20epc%20france/soins_palliatifs_de_proximite_strategie_de_sante_publique_20161117.pdf.

127. Rapport du senat, au nom de la commission des affaires sociales sur les urgences hospitalières, 2017. Les urgences hospitalières, miroir des dysfonctionnements de notre système de santé. http://www.senat.fr/rap/r16-685/r16-685_mono.html.
128. National palliative care development plan 2015–2018: https://solidarites-sante.gouv.fr/soins-et-maladies/prizes-en-charge-specializees/findevie/ameliorer-la-fin-de-vie-en-france/article/le-plan-national-soins-palliatifs-2015-2018
129. Janah A, Gauthier L, Morin L, Bousquet PJ, Le bihan C, Tuppin P, Peretti-Watel P, Bendiane MC. Access to palliative care for cancer patients between diagnosis and death: a national cohort study. Clin Epidemiol. 2019;11:443–55.
130. Colombet I, Bouleuc C, Piolot A, et al. Multicenter analysis of intensity of care at the end-of-life in patients with advanced cancer, combining health administrative data with hospital records: variations in practice call for routine quality evaluation. BMC Palliat Care. 2019;18(35):2–8.
131. Goldwasser F, Vinant P, Aubry R, et al. Timing of palliative care needs reporting and aggressiveness of care near the end of life in metastatic lung cancer: a national registry-based study. Cancer. 2018;124(14):3044–51.
132. Zeisser M, Weber JC. Lesdirectivesanticipées: unsemi-échectransitoire? Ethique Sante. 2016;13:156–63.
133. De Courson T, Sfeir C, De Guillebon G, Sanson H, Yannoutsos A, Priollet P. Advance directives in hospital practice: a matter of concern for every healthcare professional and consumer. La revue de medecine interne. 2019;40(3):145–50.
134. Barret L, Fillion S et Viossat LC. Évaluation de l'application de la loi du 2 février 2016 sur la fin de vie. 2 tomes. 2018. Paris Igas http://www.igas.gouv.fr/spip.php?article709
135. Agence Nationale d'Accreditation et d'Evaluation en Sante´ (ANAES): Modalite's de prize en charge de l'adulte necessitant des soins palliatifs. https://www.has-sante.fr/portail/upload/docs/application/pdf/txt_soins_palliatifs_recommendations_final_es_mize_en_ligne.pdf.
136. HAS, l'essentiel de la demarche palliative 2016, https://www.has-sante.fr/upload/docs/application/pdf/2016-12/mc_247_lessentiel_demarche_palliative_coi_2016_12_07_v0.pdf
137. HAS. Pourquoietcommentrédigermesdirectivesanticipées?Lesdirectivesanticipées concernant les situations en fin de vie. Guide pour le grand public. 2016. https://www.has-sante.fr/jcms/c_2722363/fr/pour-tous-comment-rediger-vos-directives-anticipees
138. HAS 2016. Haute Autorité de santé. Les directives anticipées concernant les situations de fin de vie guide pour le grand public. HAS; 2016. https://www.has-sante.fr/upload/docs/application/pdf/2016-11/da_formulaire_v2_maj.pdf
139. Ferrell B, Otis-Green S, Economou D. Spirituality in cancer care at the end of life. Cancer J. 2013;19(5):431–7.
140. Long CO. Cultural and spiritual considerations in palliative care. J Pediatr Hematol Oncol. 2011;33(Suppl 2):S96–S101.
141. Edwards A, Pang N, Shiu V, Chan C. The understanding of spirituality and the potential role of spiritual care in end-of-life and palliative care: a meta-study of qualitative research. Palliat Med. 2010;24(8):753–70.
142. François Buet. L'accompagnement spirituel de la personne en soins palliatifs. France: nouvelle cite; 2016, 116 p.
143. van der Eerden M, Csikos A, Busa C, et al. Experiences of patients, family and professional caregivers with integrated palliative care in Europe: protocol for an international, multicenter, prospective, mixed method study. BMC Palliat Care. 2014;13:52.
144. Centeno C, Sitte T, De Lima L, Alsirafy S, Bruera E, Callaway M, Foley K, Luyirika E, Mosoiu D, Pettus K, Puchalski C. White paper for global palliative care advocacy: recommendations from a PAL-LIFE expert advisory group of the pontifical academy for life, vatican city. J Palliat Med. 2018;21(10):1389–97.
145. Payne S, Hughes S, Wilkinson J, Hasselaar J, Preston N. Recommendations on priorities for integrated palliative care: transparent expert consultation with international leaders for the InSuP-C project l. BMC Palliat Care. 2019;18(32):2–8.
146. Ansoff I. Stratégie du développement d'entreprise. Paris: Editions d'Organisation; 1989.

Part IV

Western Europe: Italy

The Role of the Physician in the Community in Running the Palliative Care Interdisciplinary Team: "Thinking out Loud"

Paolo Tralongo, Aurelio Saraceno, Fabrizio Romano, Daniela Respini, and Annamaria Di Mari

Introduction and Definitions

There are no miracles, no exceptions to the laws of nature. – (Stephen Hawking: *The Grand Design*, 2010)

"Your illness is no longer susceptible to specific and effective treatments. I'm sorry, but there is nothing more we can do": this was, and perhaps still is, the phrase commonly communicated to patients and their families to state that their illness was incurable. At this point, the patient had no hope for assistance nor the possibility of receiving any hospital or home treatment. It was precisely this phrase, repeated dryly and with glacial detachment, that stimulated the birth of "palliative care," because when there is nothing more to do, there is still much to do. Palliative care (hereafter indicated as PC) was created to fill the care gap between the active therapeutic phase of poor-prognosis diseases and the patient's death, guaranteeing the active care and global assistance in the terminal phase of incurable diseases. The definition formulated by Law 38 of March 15, 2010 [1], says that PC is "the set of therapeutic, diagnostic and care interventions, aimed at both the sick person and his family, with the goal of active and total care of patients whose underlying unresponding disease is characterized by an unstoppable evolution and a poor prognosis" (Article 2, Paragraph 1a). The World Health Organization frames PC as "an approach that improves the quality of life of patients and their families who face the problems associated with incurable diseases, with the prevention and relief of suffering through early identification and by optimal pain treatment of physical, psychophysical and spiritual problems." Among the most recent definitions is the one presented in 2018 by the International Association for Hospice and Palliative Care (IAHPC): "Palliative care is the active holistic care of individuals across all ages with serious health-related suffering due to severe illness, and especially of those nearing the end of life. It aims to improve the quality of life of patients, their families and their caregivers." In the common Italian language, the term "palliative" is usually associated with the low value and uselessness of any intervention or even with the

P. Tralongo (✉) · F. Romano · A. Di Mari
Medical Oncology Unit, Umberto I Hospital – RAO, Siracusa, Italy
e-mail: tralongo@raosr.it; romano@raosr.it; dimari@raosr.it

A. Saraceno
Azienda Sanitaria di Siracusa, Siracusa, Italy

D. Respini
Associazione Mareluce Onlus, Siracusa, Italy
e-mail: mareluce@mareluce.it

M. Silbermann (ed.), *Palliative Care for Chronic Cancer Patients in the Community*,
https://doi.org/10.1007/978-3-030-54526-0_9

concept of deception and illusion, but in the Anglo-Saxon countries and in the international medical field, the term "palliative care" finds its meaning in the Latin verbum "pallium" which indicates a cloak or blanket, i.e., an object of total protection, which wraps and consoles those who suffer. According to this meaning, therefore, PC is a health and care approach that treats the patients for all of their conditions, to alleviate suffering and to meet their needs with the aim of improving their quality of life, even when it continually decreases both in quantitative terms and in terms of function. The palliative approach is global and considers the sick person as a whole, with all the physical, psychological, and spiritual components as well as with the family and social dimensions; therefore, it addresses the patient's family members as well as the caregivers as recipients of help, support, and assistance.

Legislative Procedures

Legum servi sumus ut liberi esse possimus. – (We are slaves to the laws to be free – M. T. Cicero, Rome)

Just in the last 20 years, since 1999, many regulatory directives in this area have been issued in Italy. But, as it often happens, PC was established in some Italian regions before the laws that regulated it, thanks to the free initiative of doctors, other voluntary professionals, and citizens who, sensitive to the discomfort of patients and families affected by oncological diseases, pioneered various forms of voluntary home care aimed at treating the associated symptoms of end-stage patients. The first legislative act that recognized a citizen's right to PC was the Law 39 of February 26, 1999 [2], but it was necessary to wait for the publication of the Ministerial Decree implemented on September 28, 1999 [3], to see the birth of the "National Program for the Construction of Structures for Palliative Care." In this decree there was already the far-sighted and still current concept of a NETWORK of assistance for terminal patients, consisting of "a functional and integrated aggregation of districts and hospitals, health and social services, which work in synergy with the network of social solidarity present in the territorial context, respecting the clinical-assistance autonomy of the respective components" (see Annex 1 of the Ministerial Decree of September 28, 1999). The original vision of a local network offered a variety of components, with the aim of ensuring diversified care interventions for the different health and living conditions of the patients. The forms of PC proposed in this document were (1) outpatient care, (2) integrated home care, (3) specialist home care, (4) hospitalization in the ordinary regime or day hospital, (5) residential care in residential palliative care centers, and (6) consultations and palliative assistance in hospital wards for acute care. The local network model aimed to create a convergence of forces and skills not only for health but also for social and welfare purposes and therefore tended to involve local authorities as being primarily responsible for integrating between different subjects and the so-called third sector, i.e., voluntary and private non-profit organizations. Shortly before, in 1998, it was the National Health Plan (PSN) for the 3-year period of 1998–2000 [4] courageously subtitled "A Solidarity Pact for Health" that urged the bodies of the National Health Service to provide the necessary attention to all patients suffering from end-stage pathologies, identified as weak subjects and therefore deserving of a specific and appropriate form of assistance. This population was considered to be bearers of complex and peculiar needs and the PSN established a "Solidarity Pact" in which the strengthening of assistance at various levels, including home care and psychosocial support to the patient and the family, was guaranteed. Starting from the aforementioned plan, all subsequent documents of equal value have reserved a space for palliative care in accordance with the citizen's right to access them and have implemented the organizational care model throughout the nation. Each National Health Plan, which is the main health planning tool, gives a direction to the regions and healthcare companies indicating the general rules, the objectives to be achieved, and the actions and strategies for their realization. It is not necessary to remember them all, but one may just refer to the PSN 2011/2013 [5], which dedicates an entire section to palliative care and pain therapy (page 117, B 10) and finances a series of objective projects which gives impetus and concreteness to the enhancement of home palliative care and the creation of hospices. It would become pedantic and tedious to examine all the rules that have been enacted in this period of time by the Italian government and other state or regional bodies with legislative functions, but it certainly deserves to be mentioned once again, as a milestone, the Law 38 of March 15, 2010, "Provisions to ensure access to palliative care and pain therapy" [1], which established the citizen's right to receive appropriate care and assistance during the end-of-life path and incorporated PC among the competencies of the doctors, health structures, and the National Health Service.

Among the most recent decisive legislative steps taken is the Decree of the President of the Council of Ministers (Prime Ministerial Decree) of January 12, 2017, "Definition and updating of the essential assistance levels (LEA)" [6], which includes both palliative home care and residential care in hospices among the services that the NHS guarantees and ensures for people in the terminal phase of life affected by progressive and advanced diseases, with rapid evolution and poor prognosis. An important institutional body that has guided the birth and development of palliative care in Italy is the State-Regions Conference, which translated the directives of the government and Parliament into agreements and understandings concretely achievable at the local level by all the regions and the autonomous provinces [7–9]. In order to carry out a constant, careful monitoring system for the start and development of palliative care throughout the national territory, a Technical Health Committee was created, composed of experts in palliative care (including nine doctors and one psychologist), found among the most successful professionals in the sector, and four representatives from the Ministry of Health, who work in close synergy with the General Directorate of Health Planning of the ministry itself. Among other obligations, the Ministry of Health had the task of periodically proceeding with the drafting of the Report to Parliament on the State of Implementation of Law 38 of March 15, 2010, "Provisions to guarantee access to palliative care and pain therapy." The last of these reports, relating to the 3-year period of 2015–2017 [10], shows the level reached by the organizational and welfare path of PC services in Italy, along with the numerical data relating to the structures built and the services provided, the critical issues that still slow down the flow, and the goals and the results that followed. From this report to Parliament, it can be seen how each Italian region, from Sicily [11] to Lombardy [12], already had its own decrees and specific programs implemented before 2017, which, on the one hand, favors the creation of local networks and the provision of services and, on the other hand, explains the presence of significant differences and uneven levels of assistance between the various national territories, precisely in relation to administrative decentralization and local autonomy.

Professional Roles

Lieve è l'oprar se in molti è condiviso. – (Light is the task where many share the toil – Omero)

Over the years, greater attention has been paid to the needs of the sick person and to analyzing the demands, explicit or implicit, of families and society to find the most suitable skills and conditions available in order to meet expectations. Professionals responded to this need with the goal of better defining the requirements and experimental paths required to bridge the gap of specialization in palliative care. In Italy, still no learning institution for acquiring a specialization in palliative care for doctors and other health professions has been established; therefore, in order to make up for this educational gap, there are now several post-graduate master's degrees that graduates in the various healthcare disciplines can access offering varied and specific courses for each profession.

1. As part of PC, the medical physician certainly represents the primary and indispensable figure for identifying patients' needs with relation to the state of their health and the stage of the disease; the physician defines a therapeutic plan for the multiple and complex symptoms and guides the team in disease trajectory. With the current regulations, the palliative care operative units (i.e., teams operating at home or in hospice) must be directed by a physician with documented experience and training in PC, recognized by the region of origin or with specialization in related branches such as oncology, anesthesia and resuscitation, internal medicine, hematology, geriatrics, infectious diseases, neurology, pediatrics, or radiotherapy. The PC physician and the general practitioner, who already know the patient and his/her needs, can take on the role of case managers and can monitor the health of the patient.
2. Equally important is the professional nurse, who keeps in close contact with the patient, administers the treatments, observes the patient's physical and mental state, detects the compliance and effectiveness of the treatments, evaluates any changes or the emergence of new needs, and reports findings to the other members of the team. Specific expertise in PC is required for the nurse as well as for the physician and for the other healthcare professionals on the team.
3. Psychological aspects are considered fundamental in PC to support the patient and the family during the path of illness and the difficulties that arise when caring for the sick person. A psychologist can connect between patients and healthcare providers and can facilitate communication between the family and the PC team. In addition to a specialization in psychotherapy, the psychologist must have the skills necessary to evaluate and manage the team supervisor and the teamwork of the healthcare providers to prevent the occurrence of "burn-out."
4. The social worker must work with the team to analyze the patient's personal and family history, the socio-cultural framework, and the possible presence of minors or fragile family members. The social worker must be able to offer suitable solutions to social and welfare needs, to provide information to the social welfare institute, and to carry out networking and community work.
5. The primary task of the social healthcare worker (O.S.S.) is to respond to the physical needs of the patient. The O.S.S. must possess critical thinking skills, clinical analysis, and judgment and attend and listen to emotional, psychosocial, and spiritual needs to empathize with those who suffer and to be able to communicate in a team.
6. A physiotherapist evaluates the patient's ability to recover autonomy, or at least partial autonomy, in order to carry out daily life activities and must know how to plan a physiotherapy program. The physiotherapist plans activities that help to achieve maximum possible autonomy and mobility and to modify and adapt the objectives of physiotherapy to the patient's conditions with regard to the evolution of the disease.
7. The dietician is an important part of the team; however, he/she is not always present or sufficiently valued; the dietician must collaborate with the team when evaluating the nutritional needs of the patient, providing specific indications regarding the nutritional status and food support appropriate for the state of illness and the patient's condition and educating family members in providing the appropriate nutrition for the patient.
8. The spiritual advisor's function and importance in PC are better described in the following paragraph dedicated precisely to spirituality in the context of culture and well-being.
9. The requirements of the various professionals and their respective competences have been identified and defined in the State-Regions Agreement of July 10, 2014 [9].

Home Settings

The most beautiful thing about a trip is the return home. – (Fausto Brizzi: *Cento Giorni di Felicità – 100'one hundred Days of Happiness*, 2013)

PC is best provided at home, which allows the patient and his/her family to maintain familiarity and the emotional relationships with people, animals, or objects surrounding them while avoiding long hospitalizations with all the inconveniences that may derive from them.

The DPCM Decree on Minimum Health Assistance (Prime Ministerial Decree of January 12, 2017: Definition and updating of essential levels of assistance – Art. 23 [6]) places palliative home care among the health services guaranteed by the Italian state and specifies that they must be comprised of various professional services including medical, nursing, rehabilitation, and psychological care from diagnostic testing to the supply of drugs and medical devices to preparations for artificial nutrition, when necessary.

The National Health Service wanted to establish a single system of PC home care for the entire national territory, but it has, in fact, differentiated from region to region and sometimes even among different areas within the same region. The various agreements reached by the permanent State-Regions Conference have accelerated the development of greater uniformity, but a satisfactory result which would guarantee every citizen the same level of assistance and the same type of services has not yet been reached.

Home PC is normally provided by a multiprofessional team, consisting of a palliative doctor, professional nurse, psychologist, social-health worker, physiotherapist, social worker, and general practitioner. The team is not always used in the same way in each region of Italy or in each individual case. This is due both to the different models adopted by the regions themselves and to the specific conditions and welfare needs that each individual case presents. Some healthcare institutions have an internal palliative care unit able to offer assistance at the patient's home, but, in the majority of cases, the service is entrusted to external accredited bodies which work with their own staff sometimes arising from volunteers driven by a deep sense of solidarity with the patients and their families.

Theoretically, according to the scientific and legislative directives, home care presupposes the global management of the patient and family in which the individual services of each operator are not considered, nor is the sum of the visits to the patient's home; however, there is a unified and interactive vision promoted between all of the healthcare providers on the one hand and the patient and family on the other, to provide a complete approach to the needs of the sick person as well as appropriate responses to the needs of the entire family. The patient as a person is seen as a whole entity with many components – physical, psychological, social, spiritual, etc.

The DPCM Decree on Minimum Health Assistance provides only two levels of care with regard to the patient's status: a level of basic assistance and a level of specialized assistance; the first is coordinated by the general practitioner or "free choice pediatrician" and presupposes a partial commitment on the part of the competent team, while the second is totally entrusted to the multi-professional palliative care team and requires highly skilled and complex interdisciplinary working methods.

In 2017 throughout Italy, the number of patients treated at home reached 40,849, an increase of 32.19% compared with the total number of patients treated in 2014; at the same time there was an increase in the total number of days palliative care assistance was provided at the home, which reached 326,000. Although this increase appears to be significant, the number of days of palliative care provided at home was far lower than the standard identified by Ministerial Decree 43 of 2007, Indicator 4, which was calculated taking into account that 45% of the deaths were from cancer (representing the average number of patients in home PC) multiplied by 55 days (representing the average duration of home palliative care) [13].

Hospice

> *...and this hedge, which, from so many parts*
> *of the last horizon, the sight excludes.*
> *But sitting and gazing, endless*
> *spaces beyond it, and superhuman*
> *silences, and the deepest quiet,*
> *I fake myself in my thoughts;* – (G. Leopardi: "L'Infinito," 1819)

A hospice is a social-health reception structure in which patients are welcomed, cared for, and recognized as a person entitled to all needs and rights; it is not the place where the patient goes to die, but the place where he or she can carry out end of life with dignity. In Italian legislation, further recognition of the hospice and its characteristics came from the aforementioned Prime Ministerial Decree of January 12, 2017, "Definition and updating of essential levels of assistance" (DPCM) [6], which states:

"Art. 31. Residential social and health care for people in the terminal phase of life"

1. The National Health Service within a palliative care local network guarantees people in the terminal phase of life – affected by progressive and advanced diseases with rapid evolution and poor prognosis – the integrated variety of services through the use of methods and tools based on the most advanced scientific specialized medicine, nursing, rehabilitation assistance, diagnostic testing, and psychological and pharmaceutical assistance along with the supply of preparations for artificial nutrition, social, tutelary services, and spiritual support. The services are provided by multidisciplinary and multi-professional teams in the specialized centers of palliative care hospices which, even when operating within a hospital, remain within the context of territorial social-health care. Hospices ensure medical and nursing assistance and the presence of technical assistance operators 7 days a week, 24 hours a day, and have formalized protocols for the control of pain and symptoms, sedation, nutrition, and hydration as well as formalized programs for information, communication, and support for the patient and the family, death and bereavement assistance, clinical auditing, and psycho-emotional support for the team.
2. The treatments referred to in Section 1, above, are the total responsibility of the National Health Service.

A hospice is not only a healthcare residence that provides the necessary medical care but also a place where the patient can spend his/her end of life with a familiar domestic and family model and, if possible, while maintaining residual autonomy, surrounded by people who support the patient in the best possible conditions allowed by the patient's state of health.

Generally, it is preferable for the hospice to be located in an extra-hospital structure, but even if it is intra-hospital, the hospice maintains a welcoming and familiar atmosphere with common spaces available to patients and carers and single rooms with an attached bathroom, where patients are hospitalized and where a family member or caregiver can stay. Each room is equipped to provide healthcare, but it is also equipped with private home-style furnishings, where dignified conditions are offered for the continual care of the patient and the companion.

Often hospices have a small number of beds (8–20) and are open to family members and volunteers who collaborate with the multidisciplinary team to improve the quality of life of patients. Some hospices have kitchen facilities or herbal tea available to everyone, while others have a kitchenette inside each room; in each case the aim is to create opportunities for all hospitalized patients to feel free to prepare a meal or refreshments as if they were at home. It is helpful to have an outdoor space or a garden available, where guests can relax and take pleasant walks.

The number of beds required in hospices in Italy was calculated based on the standard set by Ministerial Decree 43/2007 (1 bed for every 56 cancer patients) [13] and, at the end of 2017, there were 2777 posts with a shortage of just 244, or 8% of the total expected. It was recorded that the Italian regions of Lombardy and Lazio had the highest number of hospices and available beds, while Piedmont, Calabria, Campania, and Sicily had the most significant shortage.

While patients in hospices are mainly cancer patients, in 2017 the ratio between the number of patients who died in hospice following a diagnosis of malignancy (ICD-9 CM 140-208 codes) and the total deaths from malignancy stood at approximately 13%. There were significant inequalities between the northern and southern regions due to both the difference in the number of beds available and the socio-economic and cultural differences between the two areas. On the other hand, if we consider the total number of deaths from all causes, we find that the number of deaths in hospice was about 7% in 2017.

Reassuring data was found regarding waiting times for admission to hospices in all regions: most admissions took place within 2 days from the request, while a low number of admissions took place between 4 and 7 days from the time of the request.

Considering that the number of non-oncological patients admitted to hospice is constantly growing, the prospect of a gradual but significant increase in non-oncological pathologies requires multi-professional teams to have an equally significant update of the assessment tools, therapeutic techniques, and communication styles necessary for global management and appropriate living conditions for the changing needs and numerous variables of new patients.

Pediatric PC

Three passions, simple but overwhelmingly strong, have governed my life: the longing for love, the search for knowledge, and unbearable pity for the suffering of mankind. – (Bertrand Russell: *The Autobiography of Bertrand Russell*, 1969)

Younger patients affected by particular pathologies for which specific interventions are necessary to support specialized care, called pediatric palliative care (PPC), require careful attention to both the specialists' competence and the requirements and organization of the facilities responsible for assistance. The remarkable delicacy and complexity of the pediatric palliative environment, the greater difficulties and the emotional intensity that denotes an empathic and caring relationship between very young patients and their families, and the need for appropriate structures and conditions for children (as opposed to teenagers) have caused the development of a dedicated and satisfactory system to be slow and fragmented.

The directives issued by the Italian institutions responsible for the entire national territory indicate organizational references within a general model, in which "the care network must guarantee each child in need of pediatric palliative care the answer to its main current and evolutionary health needs and those of the family. In particular, essential actions must be guaranteed as part of the diagnostic assessment process and taking charge, with active participation in the decision-making processes of the family, and, as far as possible for age and condition, for the child" [3–7]. Point 4 of the same agreement states that "home care remains the main objective for children. Despite this, there are moments during the path of care and particular transitional conditions of families that may require a residential solution. In these cases, the place of care must be adequate to accommodate the minor as well as the staff specifically trained for pediatric palliative care."

According to the Technical Document of the Ministry of Health, implemented by the State-Regions Conference and annexed to the aforementioned agreement [7], in Italy there are, on average, about 11,000 children (between 7500 and 15,000) who are eligible for PPC and to whom the regions and healthcare facilities must guarantee an adequate and appropriate level of assistance.

The Report to the Parliament [10] found that, at the end of 2017, only 14 regions out of 20 issued a legislative or regulatory document for the creation of a regional network of services capable of responding to the needs of the local population; these findings were provided by the State-Regions Conference (CSR) of July 25, 2012 [8], and some of these focused only on pain therapy in children. In nine regions, the reference centers for pain therapy (PT) and PPC were clearly identified and the services were already activated in accordance with the organizational model envisaged, although they are still being implemented [14].

Three pediatric hospices are currently active throughout the nation; the first was built in Padua in the Veneto region in 2007; the other two are located in Basilicata and Piedmont, and five are under construction or in the activation phase in Emilia-Romagna, Liguria, Lombardy, and Tuscany.

A structured pediatric home care network in pain therapy (PT) and PPC is present in five regions: Basilicata, Friuli-Venezia Giulia, Liguria, and the autonomous provinces of Trento and Bolzano and Veneto. The structure of the PT and PPC and pediatric services in the regions of Emilia-Romagna, Lombardy, Piedmont-Valle d'Aosta, and Tuscany is unclear. Specialist and dedicated home care in PT/CPP are absent in the rest of the regions.

The number of minors being followed-up in adult PC units and PPC centers is very small in all Italian regions, especially when compared with the estimated requirements. In fact, out of approximately 11,000 eligible children, only 109 were very young patients being followed-up in the aforementioned structures and, in particular, the number of minors followed-up by the PC centers for adults was practically zero. If this last datum can be seen as a positive element in understanding the specificity of dedicated pediatric responses confirmed as necessary and optimal by more research and scientific literature, the lack of specifically activated centers and networks dedicated to pediatric PC highlights a serious lack of care responses for minors with incurable and highly complex diseases. Therefore, young patients remain in acute care units or are followed-up by their own family members at home, but do not receive any appropriate and specific type of palliative care.

The notable gaps in care are accompanied by the serious shortage of specialized training offered in the pediatric field for all of the professional figures required to constitute a multidisciplinary team; this has become the cause and, at the same time, the effect of the lack of professionals and competent bodies. It is evident that, while the PC for adults is establishing itself throughout Italy with dedicated and increasingly specialized facilities, pediatric palliative care is just in the initial stages and is currently unable to meet at least part of the actual need.

Family

My dear father, cling to my neck; I will hold you up on your shoulders;
this effort will not be heavy for me.
One danger, one salvation for both. – (Virgilio: "Eneide," v. 1152–1155)

"The show must go on" seems to be the imperative that governs habits, rhythms, logic, and intentions within society today, and this reflects on the family. In Italy, the family model tends to establish itself through the hectic society, always running to pursue affirmation of the self in all its manifestations and the subjective right to have what one wants most, searching for both psychophysical and socio-economic well-being. In this context, the disease is not only the reason for suffering, concern, and the commitment to find adequate therapeutic responses but also becomes an unexpected event that confuses and hijacks each person's routine. Families are never prepared to suffer the stress of a sudden and disruptive change such as an incurable disease or one that could become such. As understandable as this serious sense of confusion may be in the face of fearing a serious and demanding disease, families become upset because they have not considered the possibility of experiencing such a drama during the course of their lifetime and, even more, deny the inevitability of death.

The traditional family structure in Italian culture was always regarded as a nest of indissoluble affection, protection, and mutual help in good and bad times; however, the contemporary family model often assumes a new hierarchy of needs and a different scale of values. Consider, for example, households reduced to only a few members, either with separated or divorced parents or single parents with an only child who lives far away. With the complex and demanding problems that advanced and terminal disease presents, there is, therefore, a breakdown of families rather than cohesion and support between the various family members and the sick patient.

As part of PC, it is said that when a member of the family gets sick, it is the whole family that gets sick. On an emotional level, distress can be caused by the threat of separation from one's relatives due to cancer. If a family member takes on the role of caregiver, he or she must take on the full weight of the care of the patient, which sometimes causes considerable suffering and may become a real burden. This emotional load is difficult to bear. Often the consequences of caregiving on one's mental state and physical health may persist even beyond the duration of the assistance.

Like the patient, the family member is also dragged from the diagnosis into that tortuous path, officially recognized as "Kubler-Ross phases" [15], perhaps not perfectly parallel or with the same intensity, but there is sometimes excessive rationalization due to the common fears and the carer's sense of protection toward the patient.

Under these conditions, the family cannot always be a resource for the patient, nor for the team of carers, but may become the recipient of help and assistance, in need of emotional and social support, clear information, and reassurances. Patients' relatives are therefore seen in the dual role of "potential carer" and "potential patient," and the task of the different healthcare professionals is to help the family members, each according to their respective needs, to best play his or her role in the relationship with the sick relative and to protect themselves from overbearing emotions in order to be able to take care of oneself, the patient, and the rest of the family.

The Spiritual Dimension of Palliative Care

Elì, Elì, lemà sabactàni?
My God, my God, why did you abandon me? – (Vangelo secondo Matteo, 27, 46)

As a serious illness progresses, with the prospect of an end-of-life path and the possibility of death no longer deferrable, patients sometimes start to ask themselves, in a frantic and insistent way, many questions related to the meaning of their current condition or to the sense of one's whole existence, the reason for the disease or the reason for the separation from all that they love, the importance of the things they have done or the value of the sacrifices they sustained, and the futility of the projects pursued with commitment or the lightness of living the next day in an irresponsible "carpe diem."

Why me? What harm have I done to have this disease?
What will become of me and us? What will become of our past and our future?
Where do we come from? Where do we go?

The need to seek answers to these and many other questions is considered an integral part of the human dimension, and it is the spiritual yearning that pervades the existence of each person. Spirituality concerns all life, identity, values, emotional and social relationships, the ethics of the human being, and the relationship with the real and the supernatural, with the present and with the eternal.

The global care of patients, according to any palliative model and according to all scientific and regulatory indications, presupposes specific attention to the spiritual needs of the sick person; Italian legislation constantly emphasizes that the patient and family must receive assistance without ever neglecting the spiritual dimension of the human being. Public and private organizations that provide PC must ensure spiritual support and, therefore, must include a spiritual advisor among the members of the team.

Although the definition of spirituality is not always clear, it is widely accepted that it should not be simplistically confused with religiosity or belonging to a specific faith. In the same way, the distinctions among spiritual assistance, psychological support, or empathic listening can be blurred.

In light of the above reflections, it seems urgent, in Italy as in other countries, to deepen the sense of spirituality in PC and to help deal with the issues that arise and affect the patients, their families, and the carers themselves, who face daily questions regarding their own spirituality as well as being severely tested with the patient's own spiritual issues.

According to the Italian Society of Palliative Care (SICP ONLUS [16]), each team must be able to identify not only the symptoms of physical suffering but also those of inner suffering and must understand that the two require the same attention as they often coexist and enhance each other; they must be responded to adequately and with the same commitment to all needs. In particular, before proceeding to the terminal or palliative sedation of the patient, it is considered necessary for the teams to have tended to and satisfied all spiritual aspects. SICP itself recommends that particular attention be paid to the patients' need for reconciliation with themselves, with family members, and, for believers, with God.

Alongside the spiritual advisor, who primarily and specifically takes on this task, all health professionals should be prepared to talk about the profound aspects of existence and the prospect of death, not only with patients who express this need but also with family members who often ask about the reason for illness and death, while not projecting their own cultural conceptions, values, and beliefs onto them. Precisely because they are properly trained, healthcare professionals are instructed to learn how to communicate their ideas, fears, expectations, death experiences, and feelings regarding their own death, as the acknowledgment and understanding of common experiences in illness can sometimes help one to understand the meaning of life.

Volunteering

Do you want to live happily? Travel with two bags, one to give, the other to receive. – (J. W. Goethe: *Maximen und Reflexionen*, 1833)

Volunteering is encouraged and supported by Italian PC legislation, both in the home and at hospices; in fact, it completes the concept of global assistance, humanizing treatment and being available wherever carers and healthcare professionals cannot be present. Volunteers participate in the internal life of the hospice through coordinated and individualized interventions of the patients' needs, assist the staff, and promote recreational, social, cultural, and artistic activities.

The participation of volunteers in PC is not taken for granted; however, both patients and family members must be protected from any inappropriate interventions, and the volunteers themselves must be protected from painful or harmful experiences for their own emotional well-being. Therefore, it is appropriate for those who intend to carry out voluntary activities in PC to first attend a training and motivational course, at the end of which the trainers can evaluate the suitability of the volunteers to take on this role. To this end, the Italian Society of Palliative Care has developed a core curriculum [17] for volunteers who intend to serve in these areas, to acquire the skills, knowledge, and empathic abilities required.

Conclusions

In light of the subjects presented here and despite the shortcomings in some critical aspects of PC in Italy, over the past 20 years, there has been a significant increase in palliative care services, providing assistance and disseminating the acceptance of PC in social, cultural, and family contexts, as well as bringing recognition and respect to the various healthcare professionals concerned, especially by the medical community and specialized scientific organizations. This is also associated with growth on a technical-professional level and an increased variety of organizational models which can respond to the many needs of the sick and of the entire population. In all regions of Italy, there are now more or less stable and accessible forms of structures capable of ensuring adequate and appropriate PC.

PC is a new and dynamic approach to the care needs of a community, which is ever evolving and seeking appropriate resolutions for the most severe and pathological conditions. In a society where the progressive aging of the population and chronic, disabling diseases are an emerging problem, professionals and professional organizations are called upon to redefine their identity and role, to advocate for political attention and health choices, to find and implement care paths capable of supporting the health problems of the sick, to improve patients' quality of life wherever possible, and to listen to the expectations of the entire community and take responsibility for them.

The world of PC in Italy is, in reality, in strong turmoil; however, it is growing thanks to numerous innovative endeavors and the search for more adequate solutions to health and social issues affecting the community, the patients, and the health carers themselves. Today we speak of PC not only for cancer and non-cancer patients but also for the simultaneous treatment and early and timely administering of PC. The various organizational models presented in the different regions and the changing approaches to welfare have echoed the guidelines suggested by the scientific and political institutions' choices, witnessed by the vast and courageous establishment of laws and documents. From the guidelines for palliative sedation to the suspension of treatments, from the Law on Early Treatment Provisions [18] to the heated cultural debate on euthanasia and assisted suicide, and from the training of healthcare providers to the supervision and staff support, there are many topics in which PC is reflected in Italy. Continued efforts to make further significant progress will ensure provision of the best service possible for those who need it.

References

1. Legge N. 38 del 15 marzo 2010 "Disposizioni per garantire l'accesso alle cure palliative e alla terapia del dolore".
2. Legge N. 39 del 26 febbraio 1999 "disposizioni per assicurare interventi urgenti di attuazione del Piano sanitario nazionale 1998-2000".
3. Decreto ministeriale del 28 settembre 1999 "Programma nazionale per la realizzazione di strutture per le cure palliative".
4. Piano Sanitario Nazionale per il triennio 1998/2000, "Un Patto di solidarietà per la salute".
5. Piano Sanitario Nazionale 2011/2013.
6. Decreto del Presidente del Consiglio dei Ministri DPCM 12 gennaio 2017: "Definizione e aggiornamento dei livelli essenziali di assistenza" – (LEA).
7. Conferenza permanente per i rapporti tra lo Stato, le Regioni e le Province autonome di Trento e di Bolzano, Accordo del 27 giugno 2007.
8. Intesa di Conferenza Permanente tra lo Stato, le Regioni e le Provincie autonome di Trento e di Bolzano del 25 luglio 2012.
9. Accordo del 10 luglio 2014 della Conferenza permanente per i rapporti tra lo Stato, le Regioni e le Province autonome di Trento e di Bolzano.
10. "Rapporto al Parlamento sullo stato di attuazione della Legge n. 38 del 15 marzo 2010 – triennio 2015/2017," Ministero della Salute.
11. Decreto Assessorato della Salute della Regione Sicilia N. 2167 del 2 dicembre 2015: "Organizzazione e sviluppo della rete locale di cure palliative".
12. Delibera della Regione Lombardia N. X 5918 del 29/11/2016 "Disposizioni in merito alla evoluzione del modello organizzativo della rete delle cure palliative in Lombardia: integrazione dei modelli organizzativi sanitario e sociosanitario".
13. DM n. 43 del 2007 "Regolamento recante: Definizione degli standard relativi all'assistenza ai malati terminali in trattamento palliativo".
14. Decreto Assessorato della Salute della Regione Sicilia del 1 settembre 2014: "Programma di sviluppo della Rete di cure palliative e terapia del dolore in età pediatrica nella Regione siciliana".
15. Elisabeth Kübler-Ross: "On death and dying," 1969.
16. S.I.C.P.: Documenti vari, sicp.it.
17. S.I.C.P.: "Core Curriculum" dei professionisti in Cure Palliative, sicp.it.
18. Legge n. 219 del 22 dicembre 2017: "Norme in materia di consenso informato e di disposizioni anticipate di trattamento".

Part V

Western Europe: Portugal

The Importance of the Interdisciplinary Team in Running Palliative Care Services in the Community

Bruna Burmeister, Sofia Amado Durão, Carla Marinho Teves, Rita Cunha Ferreira, Ana Sofia Simões, Tânia dos Santos Afonso, and Manuel Luís Vila Capelas

Concepts, Constitution, and Challenges of a Community-Based Palliative Care Team Approach

Nowadays, teamwork is thought to be the best way to manage various clinical disorders, trying to couple accuracy and scientific progress with a complete patient evaluation. A team's particular characteristics may either have beneficial effects or detrimental consequences on quality of care, team performance, and resource use [1, 2]. Teamwork has been inherent to palliative care philosophy since its origin. Admittedly, this "modus operandi" has been an example for other medical specialties [1].

B. Burmeister · C. M. Teves · M. L. V. Capelas (✉)
Universidade Católica Portuguesa, Institute of Health Sciences, Centre for Interdisciplinary Research in Health (CIIS), Portuguese Observatory for Palliative Care, Lisbon, Portugal
e-mail: luis.capelas@ucp.pt

S. A. Durão
Universidade Católica Portuguesa, Institute of Health Sciences, Centre for Interdisciplinary Research in Health (CIIS), Portuguese Observatory for Palliative Care, Lisbon, Portugal

Hematology and Marrow Transplantation Service – Centro Hospitalar Lisboa Norte, Lisbon, Portugal

R. C. Ferreira
Universidade Católica Portuguesa, Institute of Health Sciences, Centre for Interdisciplinary Research in Health (CIIS), Portuguese Observatory for Palliative Care, Lisbon, Portugal

Home Palliative Care Team of ACES Lisboa Ocidental/Oeiras, ARSLVT, Lisbon, Portugal
e-mail: ritafccferreira@netcabo.pt

A. S. Simões
Universidade Católica Portuguesa, Institute of Health Sciences, Centre for Interdisciplinary Research in Health (CIIS), Portuguese Observatory for Palliative Care, Lisbon, Portugal

Home Palliative Care Team & Hospital Palliative Care Support Team – Instituto Português de Oncologia de Lisboa, Francisco Gentil, Lisbon, Portugal

T. dos Santos Afonso
Universidade Católica Portuguesa, Institute of Health Sciences, Centre for Interdisciplinary Research in Health (CIIS), Portuguese Observatory for Palliative Care, Lisbon, Portugal

Hospital Palliative Care Support Team – Hospital Professor Doutor Fernando Fonseca, Lisbon, Portugal

M. Silbermann (ed.), *Palliative Care for Chronic Cancer Patients in the Community*,
https://doi.org/10.1007/978-3-030-54526-0_10

Models of Teamwork

There are three teamwork models, each distinguished from the other by the interaction among its members: (1) multidisciplinary, (2) interdisciplinary, and (3) transdisciplinary. These terms are often improperly used as synonyms [3].

In the multidisciplinary model, members have different professional backgrounds and specific responsibilities – instead of interacting with the other members, each professional provides an isolated care. The main limitation to this model is care fragmentation and consequent loss of a common aim [1, 2].

On the other hand, in the transdisciplinary model, roles and responsibilities are shared among members – they have the same duties in each shift. In this kind of approach, specific care needs can be neglected to the patient's detriment. Due to this major disadvantage, the transdisciplinary model is rarely used in healthcare services [3, 4].

Between these two models stands the interdisciplinary approach – members with different professional qualifications act together in a coordinated way. Some authors use the hand analogy: individual fingers with different abilities, function, and dexterity work together to achieve more than the sum of the individual fingers [1]. Jo Weis also said "an effective interdisciplinary team complements, expands, and enriches not only patient care but also the experience of providing that care" [5]. That is why the interdisciplinary team is generally the goal of specialized palliative care, especially in the community [3].

Interdisciplinary Model on the Community: Constitution, Advantages, and Challenges

A palliative care team should be built by adapting it to the patients' needs and, consequently, to the place where care is provided – community/home, hospice, or hospital. If the general practitioner with generalist palliative care knowledge plays a key role in the community setting, the hospice- and hospital-based care must have more qualified specialists [3], which includes not only doctors but also nurses, physiotherapists, social workers, and volunteers in the core team [6]. As the same patient (according to the disease trajectory) could benefit from any of these places of care, the collaboration among teams is crucial to ensure a continuity of adequate care [3].

The interdisciplinary palliative care team presents advantages and challenges for patients, families, and professionals, assuming that the final decision-maker is the patient. In order for a team to work effectively, the members must have a common purpose, an understanding of each other's role and an ability to integrate resources [3]. Role ambiguity and overload, interpersonal conflict, inadequate communication, and leadership management are some of the challenges faced by this kind of team. The teams should grow only when these problems are overcome, or when resolution techniques are implemented. As teams get larger, subgroups and alliances, lobby groups, and different agendas may distract the team from the main goal, creating a great pressure on the leadership [3].

Team Thinking: Interdisciplinarity and Leadership

Palliative care comprises, intrinsically, the construction of a care team. An interdisciplinary team is stronger, more robust, and more capable of dealing with complex interventions. Complementarity among all members guarantees the best capacity to respond to the needs of patients and families [7]. Care in the community should be reflected by the team that executes it, more than in any context, since it is this team who defines the image of community care at home [8].

Leaders have always been associated with a characteristic personality; considered as representatives of great acts and equipped with innate qualities, it is well known today that leadership can be learned and developed [9, 10]. Leadership is one of the team's pillars, which is supposed to be effective by managing the group in response to its needs, also assuming the role of problem-solvers [11]. The aspects associated with the act of leading come from an ability to share common goals and future projects, while also influencing others to follow the same ideals [9]. Leadership comprises a set of skills, such as intelligence, organization, and dexterity. However, these skills must be acquired and enhanced with programs for better training of the designated leaders [9, 11].

Bringing out the best of each member, leaders empower their teams for interventions. Additionally, it is the team that determines the success of the interventions made [7]. A community-based interdisciplinary team is, based on evidence, the best response to the needs of patients, families, and the community [8]. Acknowledging the diversity of these groups, we can understand the need for leaders to be just as diverse. Nevertheless, it is the leader's responsibility to mold its team and create better conditions for its development [1, 10]. A direct relationship between team satisfaction and its leadership is assumed, and better leaders potentialize its members, thus leading to better care for patients and families [8, 10].

Despite what has already been described, in a palliative context, leadership models are not specifically described in the literature. Leaders can be authoritarian, liberal, or democratic [9], and they may be more responsible for managing than leading, focusing mainly on aspects of system organization instead of the team itself [1]. It is known that smaller teams or teams with more experienced members can have a more democratic leadership. On the other hand, larger or younger teams might integrate more strict leadership. Some of the palliative care teams are led by members of greater seniority, considering hierarchical positions, and sometimes are coordinated externally. In these situations, there could be a lack of focus on palliative care. According to the literature, there is great diversity on this theme [9].

What can be expected from team leaders in palliative care, namely in the community? They should foster a high-performing team mentality, articulate with external resources, distribute tasks, and manage the information shared within the team. They should also enable retrospective moments and conflict resolution, promote trust, manage difficulties, and create opportunities for sharing and even moments of fun [1, 8–11]. This is understood as integrative leadership, that is, one in which individual competencies potentialize the group in the follow-up of patients and families. In the community, leadership assumes an even bigger responsibility, providing connected interventions, dealing with larger teams, and working in more complex social contexts [10].

Leaders should have the responsibility of creating moments of leisure and sharing moments of joy. In contrast, leaders should also manage moments of greater stress and provide space for mourning [11]. Enabling the team to share difficulties and successes helps them to manage emotions, which is something essential to the work done in palliative care [8].

Poor or unrecognized leadership and even an absence of it can create episodes of frustration and conflict among members, also risking failure to monitor patients and families [3].

An interdisciplinary team consists of the union of several health professionals, and this team should be built with a constructive leadership that recognizes the group's value. The team's strength should overcome that of the individuals and leaders should promote integrated actions among members. This is the recommended model in a specialized palliative care setting [1, 10].

The Patient, Family, and Society as Members of the Team in the Community

One of the main principles of person-centered care and the priority of palliative care professionals is the users' involvement. Patients and caregivers are people with unique identities, preferences, and characteristics, thus the need to recognize their potential contribution to the palliative care process and its outcomes [12].

Quality palliative care encourages users to be part of the assessment and intervention processes with professionals in the multidisciplinary team.

However, according to Iskander cited by Oliviere [12], this is not compatible with the reality of some settings. Despite a clear emphasis on patient autonomy, their empowerment, and respect for their opinion, there is actually a huge variety of operational philosophies [13].

Multiprofessional teams can also be very ambivalent about this issue. This is particularly true in palliative care, since it comprises dealing with a highly uncertain universe and having a great deal of pressure to be "the expert" in dying [12]. On the other hand, Iskander refers that a more informed population of patients and caregivers has recently emerged, questioning and requesting more complex care. This emphasizes the need for a partnership between a multidisciplinary team and its users, since they should be capable of orchestrating and ensuring care together.

For Tritter et al., as cited by Oliviere [12], user involvement represents "active and meaningful participation and consultation of users by the service to plan, execute, develop and evaluate this service. This should be done to a level the users feel comfortable with and considering their unique perspective. The level of involvement must be self-determined by users and cannot be expected to represent the user's community; it must be free to represent them." User involvement is a process composed of several elements and something that does not happen in a single event. Involvement can be experienced directly and indirectly at two levels: the individual and/or the collective. In order to establish a true partnership, there must be a commitment between health professionals and users at each level. Thus, for Tritter et al., the relationship between professionals and users is the core of this problem.

There is a series of prerequisites for the involvement of users in the multiprofessional team. Firstly, it stresses the need for a trustful relationship. Trust, empathy, and genuineness are fundamental elements in the relationship between patient/caregiver and professionals as team members [12]. The multiprofessional team must see the person as someone capable of understanding the treatment and care and offer explanations in a spirit of collaboration. Opinions must be taken seriously and users should feel safe to expose concerns, feelings, and thoughts. Additionally, the relationship between professionals allows users a space for refusal, expressing disappointment, and criticizing. The deliberation between professionals and patients/caregivers should allow them to express themselves from different points of view.

Payne cited by Oliviere [12] also refers to the systematic relationship between the elements, where the needs of the patient and the caregiver are considered as an ongoing process, emphasizing the bidirectional nature of the relationship between users and professionals. Contradiction, paradox, and ambiguity are commonly present in this relationship, given the constant changes in the disease trajectory, which is common in the palliative care setting. Moreover, the construction of a partnership between users and professionals where there is "an emphatic exploration of the issues in the hope that the final decision reached will be one where all parties can feel committed" should also be present [12].

Oliviere [12] states that the professional who respects the user as a unique and complete individual, even when very ill, recognizes the user as an "expert" and as better informed about their condition and body, allowing them to capture their individual voice in the process of involvement with the multiprofessional team. Patients and caregivers can contribute with their collective voice through their written testimonies, using creative art, and participating in consultations or even feedback groups.

Building a Team in the Community

Palliative care should be provided in teams. When there is no team, well-intentioned health professionals are caring for their patients, but they are not providing palliative care. Although there is a paucity of research relating to interdisciplinary palliative care teams, the available data demonstrates positive effects [14, 15].

Palliative care teams should be organized and respected. Nowadays, as shown in the literature, the development of interdisciplinary palliative care teams is primarily focused on delegating tasks and attributing roles to each member [16].

For these teams to work well, there should be a horizontal hierarchy where blended expertise creates a therapeutic synergy. Additionally, they should be led by a member of the team who can better influence a positive outcome.

Although there are a number of models for interdisciplinary teams in palliative care and this diversity should be encouraged, it is a complex specialty and requires compassionate expertise that cannot be delivered by one professional alone. These teams need resources such as adequate time, staff, communication, and a physical space to work in a community-based palliative care setting. Being able to maximize the quality of life for people challenged by serious illness requires many things, such as adequate training, high-level knowledge and skills, emotional maturity, and commitment [11]. Nevertheless, interdisciplinary teams are effective because they can rapidly adapt to different contexts.

Choosing staff is the most important part of developing a successful team. Jim Collins [17] says that the "who" should come before the "what." Picking the right people is much more important than defining the roles of each member. Members should support each other and effectively communicate difficulties to the leaders, such as insufficient staff. Members should also try to bring out the best in each other, maintaining a healthy equilibrium between mind and body. These individuals should be responsible for helping patients and families finding hope in challenging situations along the disease trajectory [11], and this requires several skills.

The community-based palliative care team also needs to learn how to address conflict within the group. Team members play a role in constructing and sustaining a high-functioning group, and each one must commit to the work's success. By this, we mean the whole is greater than the sum of the individual parts. Members should also commit to learn from new as well as senior members of the team. Moreover, individuals should know how to be a mentor and complement each other's knowledge. Table 1 lists outcomes of palliative care team functioning. Conflict should be expected but never avoided; it should be used as a vehicle for self-reflection, learning, and team growth [11]. Table 2 lists vulnerabilities and challenges that may result in conflict.

Table 1 Outcomes of palliative care team function

With colleagues – Builds trusting relationships with referring physician, nurses, and healthcare team through ongoing work together
Respect for their expertise
Comfort with what value the service has to offer
Rounding
Referrals
Ongoing communication
Verbally and in writing
Role-modeling effective management of conflict inherent in high-stress situations
For patient and families – Provides state-of-the-art clinical services
Open and honest communication
Symptom management

Table 2 Vulnerabilities/challenges of interdisciplinary team

Time consuming
More up-front costs and resources
Personality conflicts
Power struggles
Communication
Competitiveness
Splitting
Role confusion
Managing unrealistic expectations
Workload
Sharing of duties

Communication is the essential tool used to inform patient and family. It is the way the team can understand and address patients' needs and concerns [11]. If communication between health professionals and patients is to be improved, we need to understand why professionals use distancing strategies so frequently and find other approaches [14]. Learning communication strategies can reduce the risk of burnout, which has been linked to health professionals who feel they have insufficient skills in this area [18].

Ethical Issues

A palliative care team is not just a group of people gathered for a simple task. It is so much more than that. It encompasses joining people with different personalities and from different professional backgrounds to work based on deontological, legal, and ethical aspects.

When working in palliative care, the ethical issues are not just present in research and direct patient care but also within the team. The approach of these issues is not common [19]. However, if the team wants to achieve the best outcomes, it must work "all for one and one for all," similar to the Three Musketeers of Alexandre Dumas.

All team members, including the patient and their family, are unique individuals. Therefore, they have their own personal preferences, beliefs, and feelings. Their cultural background, projects, goals, and values should also be known and valued. If these characteristics are not adequately integrated, it can lead to internal conflicts.

Of the several ethical issues already reviewed in the literature [19], the autonomy principle, free expression, working together, and thinking outside of the box will be discussed here.

One of the most critical issues is autonomy and it is probably the most important one in a healthcare setting. The general concept of autonomy is self-government, a self-regulation that relies on both individual sovereignty and liberty, focused on the individual. It comprises an independence of others. In a healthcare setting, all individuals' autonomies must be taken into account and respected, from patient to family and healthcare professionals. When working as a team, there is a relational autonomy. In other words, the team must assume that the interdependence among members is vital and their own autonomy should be put aside and relational autonomy prioritized. In this model, choices should be made considering loyalty and friendship, which are essential in teamwork, and it is the only way to put the teams' interests above that of individuals.

Another ethical barrier is free expression. In modern society, people have the right to express their opinions freely. The team's goals and beliefs should be shared among members, always considering each individual as one of the team. Everyone should feel free to speak openly and discuss issues with other members. It is only by free expression that members can feel genuinely a part of the team and work together toward common goals, which should focus on improving the quality of life of patients and their families. When teams are able to accommodate different points of view, they are capable of achieving success.

Working together, another ethical challenge [19], implies accepting team rules when caring for the patient and family. Eventually, conflicts can arise between the individual's own beliefs and values and that of the team. This should be approached carefully, since the ultimate responsibility is of the professional, and it should be respected by others. The leader should work in order to promote the acceptance of different points of views and recognize that in some situations one individual's decisions and views prevail [19–21]. Put simply, expressing one's own views should be done freely and safely, providing acceptance within the team [22].

To promote and improve the quality of palliative care provided, it is necessary to achieve and respect the quality indicators developed within the team, usually based on national programs, and to provide evidence-based care. Therefore, it is essential to innovate and find new ways and strategies of caring to help patients have the best quality of life possible [23]. Ultimately, research is usually the standard action, which implies thinking outside of the box.

Teamwork in Palliative Care at Home: Challenges

Palliative care recognizes the value of working in interdisciplinary teams, where the outcomes are greater than the sum of the individual results. However, teamwork is difficult and challenging, and one must be aware of the internal and external threats so that they can be faced and overcome [24].

Informal and formal communication plays a central role in a team. It is one of the most important aspects when talking about challenges. Communication is supposed to be clear and easy. It is also expected that members develop trust and mutual respect, facilitating team growth [25–27].

As mentioned above, conflicts between team members are a potential challenge for an interdisciplinary team, but they can usually be solved by effective communication [1].

Formal communication must flow in a team so that every member shares and gets access to updated information about patients [25, 26], guaranteeing confidentiality. This is a challenge, especially with regard to healthcare in the community. As it is likely that different professionals are not at the patient's home at the same time, information must be shared, ideally electronically, and accessible to the whole team. However, electronic devices are not frequently available outside health institutions, and this requires professionals to leave information in writing for the other caregivers, potentially losing some of it.

In order to avoid losing information that would impact on the team's work, a systematic review stresses the importance of using electronic medical records and standardized patient assessments, communicating via secure e-messaging and having interdisciplinary team meetings [28]. The importance of these meetings is outlined in other studies [29, 30] not only for the process of delivering care but also for building and maintaining trust in a team. Finally, another challenge related to communication is the language used across different professional groups in an interdisciplinary team [24, 31].

It is known that limited resources impact negatively on professionals and this is also true in palliative care. Particularly, limited human resources may cause role conflicts and overload in an interdisciplinary team. In addition to that, working as a team consumes time and the absence of this resource results in frustration and a fragile team [24, 27]. Delivering care in the community has the feature of wasting time in commute, including dealing with traffic, driving long distances, and parking. This consumes resources, but it can also be an opportunity for team building and a chance for effective, frequent, and reciprocal informal communication [32].

The team's age may also present a challenge as, while it is being formed, there must be a supportive environment and time must be allocated. A relationship should be constructed; members should grow together, define their roles, and learn to communicate effectively with one another [27, 29]. On the other hand, in older teams the challenges may be due to self-sufficiency, stagnation, and the tendency for rejecting different opinions [1].

Additionally, team size is an important issue as it can be large enough to have separate alliances or subgroups, resulting in less contact among members and a lesser sense of responsibility for the quality of care being delivered by the whole team [1, 30]. This may also be present in teams that care for a dispersed community, such as in rural areas, where it may be necessary for professionals to be geographically distant from one another, resulting in less frequent contact and causing further challenges for successful teamwork [25, 26, 30].

Team organization is also a major problem. Roles and interprofessional boundaries must be clear, since role ambiguity may lead to conflicts and competitivity [1, 21, 24]. There ought to be interprofessional collaboration, responsibility, and compromise [1, 32], and this cannot occur without effort [24]. Moreover, leadership can also bring potential difficulties, and it is recognized that having a clearly defined leader can contribute to the success of an interdisciplinary team [1, 8].

Each member should contribute with their individual expertise and knowledge. They should not always rely on consensus of opinion or group-thinking, striving to promote creativity in solving problems [24, 33]. In contrast, they must be aware that this may potentially delay making decisions as there may be too many different inputs.

Supporting each other in a palliative care team, beyond patients and families, is not only an expected role but it is also a challenge. Members must be caring and provide mutual emotional support, especially in an emotionally charged environment, in order to prevent burnout syndrome [24, 29, 34].

Finally, specifically in the community, a team must also collaborate with other professionals, such as primary care providers, as they need support from palliative care specialists [25, 26].

Working as a team with unrelated members belonging to different organizations and dealing with different competencies and accepting others' abilities, qualities, and roles in the delivery of care is challenging [25, 26, 35]. Furthermore, it may also be necessary to collaborate with hospital professionals.

The Care Within the Team

Although less prevalent than in other healthcare sectors [34, 36, 37], burnout syndrome in palliative care is an issue that needs addressing. It is strongly related to workload, with a scarce number of professionals equipped with adequate knowledge and skills to deal with palliative care patients, and also to the strong impact that comes with helping patients in this critical moment of life. Fortunately, the interdisciplinary focus of community-based palliative care seems to carry a protective factor, facilitating communication between professionals and tightening their bond [34]. Job satisfaction has also been proven as another positive aspect, since it still presents high levels in this sector [38].

Burnout syndrome was initially described in the 1970s [39], and the current definition divides it into three categories: exhaustion and feelings of failure to give more, depersonalization and distancing from colleagues and patients, and reduced satisfaction in performance [40]. A related concept is compassion fatigue, which was first described by Jonison, relating symptoms such as decreased energy and depression to work-related stress [41]. Compassion fatigue is defined as the emotional exhaustion due to caring for patients [42], but differentiates from burnout because the former is focused specifically on the result of caring for patients and being empathetic, while the latter is influenced not only by the emotional load but also by the professional's own perspective on their work, the workplace environment, team management, and system dissatisfaction [43, 44].

Symptoms of burnout in a palliative care setting can be related to dealing with existential issues and delicate decisions, such as withdrawing treatment and discussing end of life with patients and families; constantly facing ethical problems might reinforce feeling burnt out [34]. Increasing time spent with patient and family can be a prevention and also a risk – intense relationships developed in a palliative care setting are usually marked by professional satisfaction due to the significance of the work done but also by patient suffering. Another area well documented as a risk factor is communication – lack of training and confidence in this area can lead to exhaustion and distancing oneself from work, as analyzed by Pereira et al. [34].

Several signs and symptoms can be present in workers from a palliative care team, thus the need to prevent it and treat it when necessary. Moreover, burnout is a long-term process and requires constant monitoring and care. Different strategies have been studied, and a recent investigation [45] shows that professionals working in community-based PC have significant differences in burnout categories compared to other sectors – they are less emotionally exhausted, but distance themselves more from work. Another interesting aspect is that levels of emotional exhaustion and depersonalization are similar among different professional categories in this specialty.

Ercolani et al. [45] also analyze different coping strategies in a community-based palliative care setting and conclude that acting positively, focusing on solving problems, and relying on religion are good ways to lessen the risk of burnout. In addition, it emphasizes the need for specific training programs based on the needs of professionals and levels of experience in home care. Another research suggests hope, resilience, and optimism are also ways of dealing with symptoms of burnout, while reinforcing the need for palliative care education for all professionals working in the area [46]. Finding time for self-care and being aware of its important are other crucial aspects of coping with burnout symptoms [38].

Thus, different validated questionnaires for assessing risk of burnout in palliative care teams can be used in the community setting [47–50], along with coping strategies already mentioned.

Specific strategies and programs should be created in each and every palliative care team to equip professionals with adequate knowledge in the area and prepare them to deal with the difficulties of working in a community-based team, which can differ from other settings. Focusing on education in palliative care, the gain of communication skills, and having a space to talk about the work challenges are paramount, and there is a need for further research in this area.

References

1. Crawford GB, Price SD. Team working: palliative care as a model of interdisciplinary practice. Med J Aust. 2003;179:S32.
2. Ciemins EL, Brant J, Kersten D, Mullette E, Dickerson D. Why the interdisciplinary team approach works: insights from complexity science. J Palliat Med [Internet]. 2016 [cited 2020 Jan 24];19(7):767–70. Available from: http://www.ncbi.nlm.nih.gov/pubmed/27104490.
3. Fernando GVMC, Hughes S. Team approaches in palliative care: a review of the literature. Int J Palliat Nurs MA Healthcare Ltd. 2019;25:444–51.
4. Mueller SK. Transdisciplinary coordination and delivery of care. Semin Oncol Nurs. 2016;32(2):154–63.
5. Weis J. Why interdisciplinary teams ten years later? J Palliat Med Mary Ann Liebert Inc. 2015;18:193–4.
6. Bartley C, Webb J-A, Bayly J. Multidisciplinary approaches to moving and handling for formal and informal carers in community palliative care. Int J Palliat Nurs [Internet]. 2015 [cited 2020 Jan 24];21(1):17–23. Available from: http://www.ncbi.nlm.nih.gov/pubmed/25615831.
7. Albers A, Bonsignore L, Webb M. A team-based approach to delivering person-centered care at the end of life. N C Med J [Internet]. 2018 [cited 2020 Jan 24];79(4):256–8. Available from: http://www.ncbi.nlm.nih.gov/pubmed/29991621.
8. Shaw J, Kearney C, Glenns B, McKay S. Interprofessional team building in the palliative home care setting: use of a conceptual framework to inform a pilot evaluation. J Interprof Care [Internet]. 2016 [cited 2020 Jan 24];30(2):262–4. Available from: http://www.ncbi.nlm.nih.gov/pubmed/27026192.
9. Aparicio M, Caldeira S. A Liderança de Enfermagem em Cuidados Paliativos. Tesela [Internet]. 2015;(17):1–8. Available from: http://www.index-f.com/tesela/ts17/ts10088.php.
10. Waldfogel JM, Battle DJ, Rosen M, Knight L, Saiki CB, Nesbit SA, et al. Team leadership and cancer end-of-life decision making. J Oncol Pract [Internet]. 2016 [cited 2020 Jan 24];12(11):1135–40. Available from: http://www.ncbi.nlm.nih.gov/pubmed/27601512.
11. Bernardo A, Rosado J, Salazar H. Trabalho em Equipa. In: Barbosa A, Pina PR, Tavares F, Neto IG, editors. Manual de Cuidados Paliativos. 3ª. Lisboa: Núcleo de Cuidados Paliativos do Instituto de Bioética da Faculdade de Medicina da Universidade de Lisboa; 2016. p. 907–14.
12. Oliviere D. User involvement – the patient and carer as team members? In: Speck P, editor. Teamwork in palliative care - fulfilling or frustrating? New York: Oxford University Press; 2006. p. 41–64.
13. Speck P. Power and autonomy in palliative care: a matter of balance. Palliat Med [Internet]. 1998 [cited 2020 Jan 22];12(3):145–6. Available from: http://www.ncbi.nlm.nih.gov/pubmed/9743832.
14. Wagner EH. The role of patient care teams in chronic disease management. Br Med J. 2000;320:569–72.
15. Higginson IJ, Finlay IG, Goodwin DM, Hood K, Edwards AGK, Cook A, et al. Is there evidence that palliative care teams alter end-of-life experiences of patients and their caregivers? J Pain Symptom Manage. 2003;25:150–68.
16. Lickiss JN, Turner KS, Pollock ML. The interdisciplinary team. In: Doyle D, Hanks G, Cherny N, Calmnan K, editors. Oxford textbook of palliative medicine. 3rd ed. New York: Oxford University Press; 2005. p. 42–6.
17. Collins J. Why some companies make the leap... and others don't. In: Good to great. Harperbusiness: New York; 2001. p. 1–320.
18. Ramirez AJ, Graham J, Richards MA, Cull A, Gregory WM. Mental health of hospital consultants: the effects of stress and satisfaction at work. Lancet. 1996;347(9003):724–8.
19. Farsides B. In: Speck P, editor. Teamwork in palliative care – fulfilling or frustrating Ethical issues in multidisciplinary teamwork within palliative care. New York: Oxford University Press; 2006. p. 167–82.
20. O'Connor M. Home-based palliative care and interdisciplinary teamwork. Aust Nurs Midwifery J [Internet]. 2014 [cited 2020 Jan 21];21(9):40–1. Available from: http://www.ncbi.nlm.nih.gov/pubmed/24812780.
21. Pype P, Symons L, Wens J, Van den Eynden B, Stess A, Cherry G, et al. Healthcare professionals' perceptions toward interprofessional collaboration in palliative home care: a view from Belgium. J Interprof Care [Internet]. 2013 [cited 2020 Jan 21];27(4):313–9. Available from: http://www.ncbi.nlm.nih.gov/pubmed/23181267.
22. Alderson P, Farsides B, Williams C. Examining ethics in practice: health service professionals' evaluations of in-hospital ethics seminars. Nurs Ethics. 2002;9(5):508–21.
23. National Quality Forum. A national framework and preferred practices for palliative and hospice care quality. Washington: National Quality Forum; 2006. p. 11–4.
24. Klarare A, Hagelin CL, Fürst CJ, Fossum B. Team interactions in specialized palliative care teams: a qualitative study. J Palliat Med. 2013;16(9):1062–9.

25. Macmillan K, Kashuba L, Emery B. Organization and support of the interdisciplinary team. In: Bruera E, Higginson I, von Gunten CF, Morita T, editors. Textbook of palliative medicine and supportive care. 2nd ed. Boca Raton: CRC press; 2015. p. 251–6.
26. Wenk R. Palliative home care. In: Bruera E, Higginson I, von Gunten CF, Morita T, editors. Textbook of palliative medicine and supportive care. 2nd ed. Boca Raton: CRC press; 2015. p. 287–92.
27. Mertens F, De Gendt A, Deveugele M, Van Hecke A, Pype P. Interprofessional collaboration within fluid teams: community nurses' experiences with palliative home care. J Clin Nurs. 2019;28(19–20):3680–90.
28. Fathi R, Sheehan OC, Garrigues SK, Saliba D, Leff B, Ritchie CS. Development of an interdisciplinary team communication framework and quality metrics for home-based medical care practices. J Am Med Dir Assoc. 2016;17(8):725–729.e10.
29. Shaw J, Kearney C, Glenns B, McKay S. Interprofessional team building in the palliative home care setting: use of a conceptual framework to inform a pilot evaluation. J Interprof Care. 2016;30(2):262–4.
30. Xyrichis A, Lowton K. What fosters or prevents interprofessional teamworking in primary and community care? A literature review. Int J Nurs Stud. 2008;45(1):140–53.
31. Jones M, Thistlethwaite J. Interprofessional practice in palliative care. In: MacLeod RD, Van den Block L, editors. Textbook of palliative care. Cham: Springer Nature Switzerland AG; 2019. p. 527–39.
32. Morgan S, Pullon S, McKinlay E. Observation of interprofessional collaborative practice in primary care teams: an integrative literature review. Int J Nurs Stud Elsevier Ltd. 2015;52:1217–30.
33. World Health Organization. Team building. Geneve: World Health Organization; 2007.
34. Martins Pereira S, Fonseca AM, Sofia Carvalho A. Burnout in palliative care: a systematic review. Nurs Ethics [Internet]. 2011;18(3):317–26. Available from: http://nej.sagepub.com/cgi/doi/10.1177/0969733011398092.
35. Groot MM, Vernooij-Dassen MJFJ, Crul BJP, Grol RPTM. General practitioners (GPs) and palliative care: perceived tasks and barriers in daily practice. Palliat Med. 2005;19(2):111–8.
36. Vachon ML. Staff stress in hospice/palliative care: a review. Palliat Med [Internet]. 1995 [cited 2020 Jan 22];9(2):91–122. Available from: http://www.ncbi.nlm.nih.gov/pubmed/7541687.
37. Rokach A. Caring for those who care for the dying: coping with the demands on palliative care workers. Palliat Support Care. 2005;3(4):325–32.
38. Sansó N, Galiana L, Oliver A, Pascual A, Sinclair S, Benito E. Palliative care professionals' inner life: exploring the relationships among awareness, self-care, and compassion satisfaction and fatigue, burnout, and coping with death. J Pain Symptom Manage. 2015;50(2):200–7.
39. Freudenberger HJ. Staff burn-out. J Soc Issues. 1974;30(1):159–65.
40. Maslach C, Jackson S. Burnout in health professions: a social psychological analysis. In: Sanders GS, Suls J, editors. Social psychology of health and illness. Hillsdale: Lawrence Erlbaum; 1982. p. 227–51.
41. Joinson C. Coping with compassion fatigue. Nursing (Lond). 1992;22(4):116–8.
42. Figley CR. Compassion fatigue: toward a new understanding of the costs of caring. In: Stamm BH, editor. Secondary traumatic stress: self-care issues for clinicians, researchers, and educators. Derwood: The Sidran Press; 1995. p. 3–28.
43. Mcholm F. Rx for compassion fatigue. J Christ Nurs [Internet]. 2006 [cited 2020 Jan 22];23(4):12–9. Available from: http://content.wkhealth.com/linkback/openurl?sid=WKPTLP:landingpage&an=00005217-200611000-00003.
44. Leiter MP, Maslach C. Six areas of worklife: a model of the organizational context of burnout. J Health Human Serv Adm. 1999;21:472–89.
45. Ercolani G, Varani S, Peghetti B, Franchini L, Malerba MB, Messana R, et al. Burnout in home palliative care: what is the role of coping strategies? J Palliat Care [Internet]. 2020 [cited 2020 Jan 22];35(1):46–52. Available from: http://www.ncbi.nlm.nih.gov/pubmed/30727827.
46. Frey R, Robinson J, Wong C, Gott M. Burnout, compassion fatigue and psychological capital: findings from a survey of nurses delivering palliative care. Appl Nurs Res [Internet]. 2018;43(May):1–9. Available from: https://doi.org/10.1016/j.apnr.2018.06.003.
47. Maslach C. The measurement of experienced burnout. J Organ Behav. 1981;2(2):99–113.
48. Endicott J, Nee J, Harrison W, Blumenthal R. Quality of life enjoyment and satisfaction questionnaire: a new measure. Psychopharmacol Bull. 1993;29:321–6.
49. Politi PL, Piccinelli M, Wilkinson G. Reliability, validity and factor structure of the 12-item General Health Questionnaire among young males in Italy. Acta Psychiatr Scand. 1994;90(6):432–7.
50. Carver CS, Scheier MF, Weintraub JK. Assessing coping strategies: a theoretically based approach. J Pers Soc Psychol [Internet]. 1989 [cited 2020 Jan 22];56(2):267–83. Available from: https://content.apa.org/record/1989-17570-001.

Part VI

Western Europe: Spain

Patients Suffering from a Chronic, Irreversible Illness: A Novel Study on the Psychological Intervention out of the Hospital

David Rudilla, Amparo Oliver, Laura Galiana, Claudia Valenzuela, and Julio Ancochea

Introduction

Since the 1980s, health psychology has been interested in identifying psychological aspects of patients suffering from rare, chronic, and advanced-stage diseases. This would be the case with chronic obstructive pulmonary disease (COPD), diffuse interstitial lung disease (DILD), and idiopathic pulmonary fibrosis (IPF). When compared with cancer patients, those suffering with IPF expressed similar or more severe symptoms and care needs [1]. However, the interventions in these patients were minor and limited to few variables, ignoring many other key issues in the perception of quality of life associated with the disease, and are presented in the Results section of this chapter.

The prevalence and incidence of idiopathic pulmonary fibrosis (IPF) varies in its definition and geographic location, with a prevalence of 1.25–63 cases and an annual incidence of 0.22–17.4 cases per every 100,000 inhabitants, with more cases in North America than in Europe [2]. It is the most frequent entity within the group of the National Institute of Immunology (NII), with an estimated prevalence in Spain of 13 cases per 100,000 women and 20 cases per 100,000 men, therefore affecting approximately 7000–12,000 patients, with a growing tendency [3, 4].

IPF is a chronic, irreversible, fibrosing lung disease with an unfavorable prognosis. The clinical course of patients with IPF varies from asymptomatic patients to those who have a progressive loss of lung function and on to others who may experience very rapid deterioration. Some patients may present episodes of sudden worsening, with acute respiratory failure, which we call acute exacerbations [5]. The combination of the poor prognosis, the uncertainty of the course of the disease, and the severe burden of the symptoms has a great impact on the quality of life both for patients and their relatives [6–8]. Although in recent years, with the appearance of two antifibrotic treatments, studies have been conducted, most of these trials focus on the modification of the disease measured by physiological parameters such as lung function. However, in many patients with IPF, there is no clear correlation between physiological parameters and outcome measures reported by patients regarding how they feel or cope with daily activities.

D. Rudilla
Pneumology, La Princesa University Hospital, Madrid, Spain

Air Liquide Healthcare, Madrid, Spain
e-mail: david.rudilla@airliquide.com

A. Oliver (✉) · L. Galiana
University of Valencia, Valencia, Spain
e-mail: amparo.oliver@uv.es; laura.galiana@uv.es

C. Valenzuela · J. Ancochea
Pneumology, La Princesa University Hospital, Madrid, Spain

Autonomous University of Madrid, Madrid, Spain
e-mail: j.ancochea@separ.es

M. Silbermann (ed.), *Palliative Care for Chronic Cancer Patients in the Community*,
https://doi.org/10.1007/978-3-030-54526-0_11

Table 1 Results for the basal line (n = 56)

	Min.	Max.	Mean	SD
Age	40	81	63.55	9.55
Anxiety	3	19	11.17	4.31
Depression	2	17	8.42	4.17
Demoralization	2	20	11.33	4.69
Quality of life	2	7	4.14	1.31
Spirituality intrapersonal	4	12	9.19	1.99
Spirituality interpersonal	2	12	10.42	2.03
Spirituality transpersonal	1	8	5.71	1.83
Threaten dignity	4	27	14.39	6.29
Preserved dignity	23	45	35.62	5.09
Dignity	35	72	50.01	9.31
Resilience	4	20	10.78	4.56
Confidential support	13	30	24.19	5.35
Affective support	12	25	19.82	3.84
Social support	25	55	44.01	8.95

More recent studies have examined the psychological needs of IPF patients and their families. Table 1 shows the studies that have explored the psychological aspects of the patient with IPF. Simultaneously, at the international level, IPF is becoming the leading indication for lung transplantation [9], and this could also introduce psychological symptoms associated with the uncertainty of this process. Anxiety and depression are known to frequently occur in patients with chronic respiratory diseases [8, 9]. In COPD, the intensity of dyspnea reported by patients is directly related to depression and the impairment of functional status [10].

Patients with diffuse interstitial lung disease (DILD) also report inadequate information regarding the disease process, an imprecise diagnosis, unsatisfactory treatment, and/or unacceptable side effects associated with therapy and poorly controlled symptoms of progressive illnesses. Ryerson et al. [6], in a study of patients suffering from DILD using the Center for Epidemiologic Studies Depression Scale (CESD), found that even a moderate degree of dyspnea experienced by patients with DILD resulted in a high incidence of depression. Therefore, depression and anxiety require special attention when assessing chronic lung diseases.

Pulmonologists have frequently emphasized their clinical impressions of the role that psychological components play in different respiratory pathologies. Holland et al. [11] corroborated the findings of Ryerson and his collaborators regarding the prevalence of anxiety and depression in DILD. They observed a growing presence of anxiety and depression across the spectrum of this disease without predilection for any particular sub-type.

Participating in a pulmonary rehabilitation program improves both mood and functional capacity, and enrolling in a local IPF support group may help reduce social isolation [12]. A palliative care program for patients and their caregivers focused in the home environment demonstrated significant improvements in health-related quality of life and respiratory symptoms [13]. However, studies that center on the relationship between psychological variables and the clinical manifestations of pulmonary diseases are still scarce [14–17]. Literature has established the presence of clinical symptoms of anxiety and depression in 21–50% of patients diagnosed with diffuse interstitial diseases, almost all with IPF. Recently, two papers have addressed the clinical impact of IPF on anxiety and depression. The first was exploratory in IPF patients and their relatives and found that a high incidence of anxiety was reported, and most considered psychological support essential [16].

The second study showed that the prevalence of anxiety and depression in patients with IPF was 25.9% and 21.4%, respectively [17]. However, most studies that address psychological variables are inconclusive, basically due to problems with sample size [18, 19], or because they focus solely on assessing the physical benefits of respiratory rehabilitation programs [20].

In the reviewed studies, patients with IPF were involved in almost all domains of life, but the areas most impacted were related to physical functioning, symptoms, and daily autonomy. The results significantly correlated with indicators used to assess the severity of IPF, with both physiological measurements and subjective indicators such as dyspnea. The degree of dyspnea was also associated with a depressive mood [21–24]. Duck et al. [25] identified three main themes in their interviews with patients with IPF: "fighting for a diagnosis," "loss of the life that they had previously led," and "living with idiopathic pulmonary fibrosis." Patients reported that they struggle to cope with a disease that limits their lives and progresses rapidly without sufficient treatment or support structures. These findings are in line with those reported by Sampson [26], in which patients diagnosed with IPF had a clear understanding of their prognosis, but little understanding of how their disease would progress or be managed.

There are few investigations of palliative care in advanced stages of IPF [18, 27–31], although problems related to symptom control and the deterioration of patients' quality of life are similar to those that occur, for example, in palliative cancer patients [32]. Thus, we have no information on the psychological profile of patients with IPF at the end of life: the presence of demoralization syndrome, spiritual needs, or perception of dignity. These three constructs, together with emotional distress, are most characteristic of patients at the end of life, having been the focus of oncological research but with less attention given to the importance of non-oncology issues.

The term "demoralization" is an alternative to the diagnosis of depression that seems to be more prevalent in patients with advanced chronic disease where discouragement, loss of meaning of life, helplessness, hopelessness, and feelings of failure characterize the mood of the patient [33]. Unlike the depressed patient, the patient with demoralization has no anhedonia and is able to enjoy some things. Mirjam and his collaborators [34] have recently described the ABCDE plan, which involves a comprehensive approach to the patient and which considers psychological intervention to be at the same level as the treatment of physical symptoms. This approach considers the participation of different professional profiles (pulmonologists, nurses, psychologists, etc.) a necessity.

Taking into account all these antecedents and needs of patients with IPF, this study presents the results obtained after a structured ambulatory psychological intervention.

Participants and Methods

Procedure and Design

After obtaining the permits from La Princesa University Hospital's Ethical Committee and patients' informed consents, patients diagnosed with IPF began psychological treatment at the Pulmonology Unit. For ethical reasons, as stipulated by the committee, a pre-test/post-test, non-randomized trial was carried out and no control group was set up, but everyone was offered to participate.

Pre-evaluations were carried out at the beginning of Session 1, and post-intervention evaluations were carried out at the end of the last session. The interventions took place between November 5, 2017, and June 7, 2018, in the consulting room of the psychology department of the DILD Unit, located in the Pulmonology Unit of the La Princesa University Hospital. The intervention consisted of three sessions of brief psychotherapy and focused on the essential dimensions of the person (dignity, demoralization, hopelessness, and spirituality), using counseling as a basic therapeutic methodology. The contents of the sessions were:

- 1st session: Who am I?
- 2nd session: Hope and demoralization
- 3rd session: Spirituality and dignity

Interventions were held every 2 weeks. A flowchart describing the study can be found in Fig. 1.

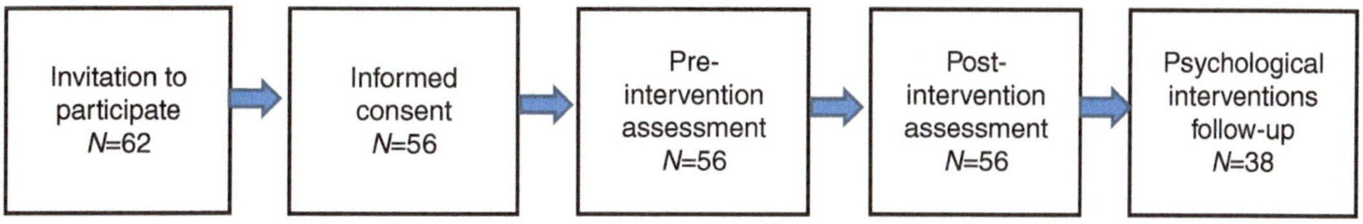

Fig. 1 Interventions

Sampling

The participants were patients diagnosed with IPF and were being followed-up by the Pulmonology Unit of La Princesa University Hospital.

The inclusion criteria were:

(a) Patients diagnosed with IPF being followed-up by the unit
(b) Adult patients (over 18 years old)
(c) Informed consent
(d) Survival expectancy greater than 6 months

The exclusion criteria were:

(a) Existence of a pact of silence (not knowing diagnosis or prognosis)
(b) Cognitive impairment (comprehension/expression problems)

Instruments

In addition to registering socio-demographic and clinical variables, the following instruments were administered:

(a) Hospital Anxiety and Depression Scale (HADS) [35, 36]. This instrument assesses affective disorders in the non-psychiatric hospital setting. It consists of 14 items with a four-point Likert response format (ranging from 0 to 3): seven for each subscale, anxiety and depression. The score for each subscale is 21 points, which is achieved with the sum of the items corresponding to each symptom. The reliability of the current application is 0.75 for anxiety and 0.71 for depression.
(b) Brief Demoralization Scale [37] that evaluates the demoralization syndrome by means of five brief elements with a Likert response that varies from none to a lot. Reliability measured by application is 0.85.
(c) Dignity Assessment Questionnaire (PPDS) [38]. Brief instrument to measure dignity in patients with and without palliative cancer, with an alpha in present application of 0.72. It consists of eight elements with a response scale of 0 (none) to 9 (a lot). It consists of two factors: preservation of dignity and threat of dignity.
(d) Spirituality (GES) [39]. Spirituality is associated with quality and meaning in life; it is a complex construct with more than 13 components [40] and is clearly different from religion or faith. The measurement tool consists of eight items that are answered with a five-point Likert scale ranging from 0 (nothing) to 4 (a lot). It includes three factors: intrapersonal, interpersonal, and transpersonal dimensions. The original Cronbach's alpha for this scale is 0.86
(e) Brief Resilience Scale [41]. This four-item scale was adapted and validated in Spain [42] with an internal consistency of 0.79 and in its current application has reached 0.92. Each item is scored on a five-point scale from 1 (strongly agree) to 5 (strongly disagree), and the highest scores reflect a greater resilience.
(f) Duke-UNC [43] Functional Social Support Questionnaire. Quantitative evaluation questionnaire of perceived social support relating to two aspects: people with whom intimate feelings can be communicated (confidential support) and people who express positive feelings of empathy (emotional or affective support). It collects values that refer to both confidential support and affective support. Each aspect is evaluated with a Likert scale with five options from 1 (much less than I want) to 5 (as much as I want). Overall reliability is 0.80.

Quality of life. Two elements of the EORTC-QLQ-C30 [38, 44] were used, which constitute the factor of the Global Health Scale. QLQ-C30 is currently used in several types of studies of people with cancer and other advanced chronic diseases. The use of the complete questionnaire was rejected and, as physical deterioration is inevitable in patients undergoing symptomatic treatment, it is recommended to use only the aforementioned indicators in studies. These studies also included patients with advanced respiratory diseases, and no comparative differences from cancer patients were found. Reliability of this measure in our patients was 0.75

Analysis

The equivalence of groups was tested according to whether the patients were following treatment with an antifibrotic. For the quantitative variables, *t* tests were performed for comparison of means of independent groups, with the appropriate correction to the diagnosis of compliance with the assumption of homogeneity of variances. Regarding categorical variables, χ^2 tests were used.

In order to view the clinical map of the essential dimensions, bivariate correlations were calculated. To know the differences between the results in variables of each of the types of intervention, *t* tests of repeated measures were carried out. In addition, the same tests were used to compare differences between interventions, except for independent samples. In all tests, the size of the associated effect was calculated. In the case of the effect size for the *t* tests, Cohen's d was calculated to determine the standardized difference between every two means under comparison. Cohen's d has values from 0 to infinity, with interpretation of small values at around 0.20, medium size around 0.50, and large size from 0.80 [45].

Results

The final sample consisted of 56 patients. 42% were women and 58% were men. 46% of the patients had been diagnosed more than 12 months ago, and 60% were on antifibrotic treatment. The rest of the characteristics can be consulted in Table 1.

When dividing the sample into two groups, depending on whether they were being treated with an antifibrotic, no significant baseline differences were found between both groups in gender ($\chi^2(2) = 1.373$; $p = 0.503$), marital status ($\chi^2(6) = 4.543$; $p = 0.604$), level of studies ($\chi^2(6) = 11.205$; $p = 0.082$), employment situation ($\chi^2(8) = 3.126$; $p = 0.926$), or diagnosis time ($\chi^2(8) = 14{,}494$; $p = 0.070$). Nor did Student's *t* test with independent samples correcting the error inflation find difference in age ($t(53) = 1.147$; $p = 0.256$).

Following, in Table 2, we appreciate the amount of significant correlations between key variables involved in the process of caring with dignity and also the intensity of these associations.

Regarding the changes after the interventions (Table 3), the *t* tests for paired samples showed statistically significant differences in all the variables ($p < 0.004$) except in depression ($p = 0.05$), transpersonal spirituality ($p = 0.075$), and confidential social support ($p = 0.465$). Bonferroni adjustment was applied to correct error inflation due to the simultaneous pairwise comparisons made.

Following these lines, Fig. 2 below more intuitively shows, in a visual display, the changes observed in the target variables after the intervention.

As shown in Fig. 2, as expected a priori, in some of the comparisons after the psychological intervention, the results are better except in depression, where there was an increase, although this is not significant. They also increase spirituality, quality of life, dignity, resilience, and social support. Regarding effect sizes, they were of great magnitude ($d > 0.8$) in quality of life and preserved dignity and of medium size ($0.8 > d > 0.5$) in intrapersonal spirituality and affective support.

Finally, several analyses of variance were carried out to test for the effect of using an antifibrotic. The results indicate that the changes already found are independent of the type of treatment being followed, with or without an antifibrotic (see Table 4).

Table 2 Relationships among the whole set of variables in basal line

	1	2	3	4	5	6	7	8	9	10	11	12	13
1. Anxiety	1												
2. Depression	0.629[a]	1											
	0.000												
3. Quality of life	−0.678[a]	−0.552[a]	1										
	0.000	0.000											
4. Demoralization	0.521[a]	0.469[a]	−0.332[b]	1									
	0.000	0.000	0.012										
5. Spirituality Intra	−0.270[b]	−0.189	0.284[b]	−0.223	1								
	0.044	0.163	0.034	0.099									
6. Spirituality Inter	−0.274[b]	−0.022	0.399[a]	−0.297[b]	0.561[a]	1							
	0.041	0.872	0.002	0.026	0.000								
7. Spirituality Trans	−0.338[b]	−0.425[a]	0.417[a]	−0.467[a]	0.343[a]	0.491[a]	1						
	0.011	0.001	0.001	0.000	0.010	0.000							
8. Preserved Dig.	−0.409[a]	−0.312[b]	0.454[a]	−0.329[b]	0.389[a]	0.321[b]	0.286[b]	1					
	0.002	0.019	0.000	0.013	0.003	0.016	0.033						
9. Resilience	−0.074	0.100	0.202	−0.114	0.196	0.339[b]	−0.103	−0.200	1				
	0.590	0.463	0.135	0.401	0.147	0.011	0.451	0.140					
10. Threatened Dig.	−0.387[a]	−0.467[a]	0.443[a]	−0.449[a]	0.160	−0.008	0.153	0.331[b]	0.131	1			
	0.003	0.000	0.001	0.001	0.238	0.955	0.260	0.013	0.335				
11. Dignity	−0.485[a]	−0.486[a]	0.547[a]	−0.483[a]	0.321[b]	0.170	0.260	0.770[a]	−0.020	0.857[a]	1		
	0.000	0.000	0.000	0.000	0.016	0.209	0.053	0.000	0.881	0.000			
12. Conf. Support	−0.386[a]	−0.062	0.295[b]	−0.089	0.112	0.479[a]	0.398[a]	0.144	0.235	−0.096	0.014	1	
	0.003	0.648	0.028	0.512	0.411	0.000	0.002	0.289	0.081	0.483	0.918		
13. Affective Sup.	−0.325[b]	−0.004	0.252	0.068	0.185	0.461[a]	0.371[a]	0.209	0.065	−0.181	−0.008	0.892[a]	1
	0.015	0.975	0.061	0.619	0.172	0.000	0.005	0.121	0.634	0.182	0.953	0.000	
14. Social Support	−0.370[a]	−0.039	0.284[b]	−0.024	0.146	0.485[a]	0.397[a]	0.176	0.169	−0.135	0.005	0.981[a]	0.963[a]
	0.005	0.775	0.034	0.859	0.282	0.000	0.002	0.194	0.214	0.322	0.971	0.000	0.000

Abbreviations: *Dig*. Dignity, *Conf*. Confidential, *Sup*. Support

[a]$p < 0.01$

[b]$p < 0.05$

Table 3 Results along the intervention

	Pre		Post					
	M	SD	M	SD	*t*	df	*p*	d
Anxiety	11.17	4.31	9.05	2.51	3.06	55	0.003	0.40
Depression	8.42	4.17	9.82	2.62	−2.00	55	0.050	0.27
Demoralization	11.33	4.69	9.82	2.62	−3.10	55	0.003	0.41
Quality of life	4.14	1.31	7.00	2.45	7.16	55	0.000	0.96
Spirituality intra	9.19	1.99	4.81	0.99	−5.33	53	0.000	0.72
Spirituality inter	10.42	2.03	11.27	1.91	−3.64	53	0.001	0.49
Spirituality trans	5.71	1.83	11.42	0.83	−1.81	53	0.075	0.25
Threaten dignity	14.39	6.29	11.33	4.09	3.28	55	0.002	0.44
Preserved dignity	35.62	5.09	42.41	1.86	−10.75	55	0.000	1.44
Dignity	50.01	9.31	53.75	5.40	−3.04	55	0.004	0.41
Resilience	10.78	4.56	12.92	4.27	−1.15	53	0.255	0.16
Social support	44.01	8.95	46.54	3.05	−2.04	49	0.046	0.29
Conf. support	24.19	5.35	23.62	1.39	0.73	55	0.465	0.10
Affective support	19.82	3.84	22.92	2.01	−5.19	49	0.000	0.73

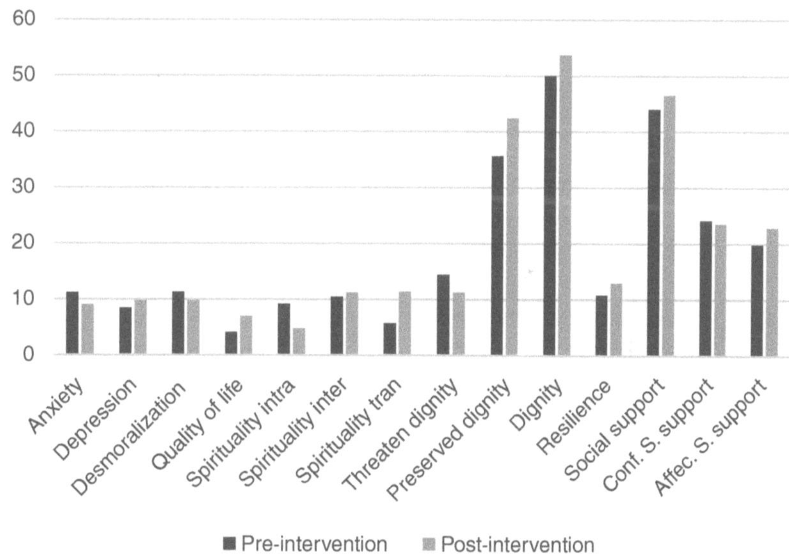

Fig. 2 Observed change in variables after the intervention

Table 4 Analysis of variance testing differences by type of treatment

Outcome	df	*F*	*p*	η^2
Anxiety	1	1.320	0.255	0.024
Depression	1	0.649	0.424	0.012
Demoralization	1	0.404	0.528	0.007
Quality of life	1	3.540	0.065	0.062
Spirituality intra	1	0.861	0.358	0.016
Spirituality inter	1	0.356	0.553	0.007
Spirituality trans	1	3.168	0.081	0.057
Dignity	1	0.179	0.674	0.003
Preserved dignity	1	0.036	0.851	0.001
Threatened dignity	1	0.175	0.678	0.003
Resilience	1	1.619	0.209	0.029
Confidential social support	1	0.668	0.417	0.012
Affective social support	1	0.275	0.602	0.006
Social support	1	0.000	0.995	0.000

Discussion

The objective was to evaluate the effectiveness of a structured psychological intervention to improve the quality of life of patients diagnosed with IPF. In general, the results showed that a brief psychotherapy intervention with content focused on the essential dimensions of the individual was beneficial for patients with IPF. As it happens in interventions of this style, anxiety levels were reduced in patients with early palliative profile [46–49]. The results of this study, however, do not show such improvement in terms of depression. The effects found in this work have not been statistically significant and with small sizes. These results are not far from those consulted in the depression literature that have been found when intervening in palliative patients [47, 48]. Possibly due to the same explanation: the depressive mood is explained by a demoralization and not by a depressive episode.

Along these lines, Houmann, Rydahl-Hansen, Chochinov, Kristjanson, and Groenvold [50] and Rudilla et al. [48] also found evidence that depression levels did not improve after interventions that address existential distress such as Dignity Therapy, but that they were even higher. These types of interventions in palliative patients do not seem to improve mood, although anxiety symptoms do.

Regarding the quality of life, psychotherapy showed positive and large effects on this variable. This result matches with what is proposed by Juliao et al. [47], Rudilla [48], and Chochinov et al. [51], among others. Finally, regarding the emotional distress caused by the lack of dignity, or the improvement of the spiritual dimension, results of this study also point to an improvement after the intervention, although only for some of the dimensions of spirituality (intrapersonal and interpersonal) and dignity and its dimensions. These results coincide with those found in different studies that use therapies of the essential dimension such as Dignity Therapy [47, 48, 52–54].

It is important to note that the results found that these benefits occurred both in patients treated with an antifibrotic and symptomatic treatment. There is a need for emotional support in patients with IPF.

In conclusion, it could be said that a brief psychotherapy session structured around the contents of existential anxiety has improved patients' quality of life, their dignity and spirituality, and also, to some extent, their emotional well-being. However, the fact that no previous studies aimed at patients with IPF have been carried out does not allow us to go in-depth in the elements for that success as there is no previous specific literature to compare it to. We can only provide some limited first or pilot evidence on the impact of this therapy in the medium term. It is still necessary to carry out follow-up measures to know if these changes are consolidated, as they suppose a personal resource in view of the progressive deterioration to which the patients with IPF are subjected, if maintenance is necessary, and, if so, what type. Nor have autonomy measures been taken that would allow us to know how psychotherapy impacts dependence.

For these reasons, it would be necessary for future research to address this problem with a larger sample size and clinical measures to study the possible replicability of the results found in this work. It is important to determine which interventions cover the needs of patients with IPF that have been neglected so far and, therefore, should be implemented by professionals. Another important aspect focuses on the quality of life of the palliative patient.

The evaluation carried out in this study of quality of life has been carried out with the global health status factor of the EORTC-QLQ-30, of simple application (thus avoiding the fierceness of evaluating with long and tedious questionnaires) and which has shown to be sensitive to studies with non-cancer palliative patients [48]. To include other questionnaires that determine quality of life through measuring symptoms in patients whose clinical deterioration implies a continuous loss supposes obtaining a negative result that may not reflect the true state of quality of life of the patient.

The evaluation of quality of life that focuses solely on the physical aspects neglects the possibility that patients can perceive a better quality of life in issues of a psycho-emotional nature and, therefore, can improve relationships with their relatives and others close to them [55]. The referred loss can result in worsening of mood (greater depression). It is important to emphasize these aspects when talking about "quality of life" in the patient with IPF.

Patients with serious illnesses tend to have great existential suffering, and in response to this need, specific interventions essentially focused on end of life (counseling, Kibo Therapeutic Interview [56]) have been developed. These types of interventions, in the context of the Spanish healthcare system, are not mandatory despite the recent commitment for increasing humanization of care. There are pathologies as adverse as lung cancer, such as IPF, in which protocoled treatments aimed at reducing existential suffering and emotional distress are being developed. These are rare or minor diseases; it is assumed from the start that they will conclude with a poor prognosis.

Advancements in the care of patients with serious illnesses must consider the entire person. The improvement of a treatment that increases survival rate implies that the set of treatments that affect the person, such as psychological and spiritual, be modified. In addition, each time the treatments are transferred to the patient's home environment, it is considered to be the best therapeutic space for the patient and his/her family. For this reason, the approach to the patient must have interventions that do not have the sole objective of admission or clinical worsening but should strengthen and provide coping strategies that allow the patient and his/her family to live day to day. It is necessary that health professionals' articulate mechanisms ensure that everyone (doctors, nurses, psychologists, patients, and caregivers) remembers that, before being patients, they are human beings.

By evidencing the usefulness of these interventions, we are attempting to stimulate a debate about a redesigning of end-of-life care protocols. Just as no one doubts the effectiveness of the case management nurse, approaches such as the intervention of the three psychotherapeutic sessions presented here are part of generic protocols for action. This has additional benefits such as avoiding treating groups of patients separately depending on their disease. By separating, it is inevitably labeled and sometimes even stigmatized, and with interventions like this, we are moving toward a more compassionate system of care, healthcare models that can be transformed into systems that honor the dignity of people, as was defended at the *International Conference on Improving the Spiritual Dimension of Whole Person Care: The Transformational Role of Compassion, Love, and Forgiveness in Health Care* in 2013 [57].

References

1. Callahan D. Death and the research imperative. N Engl J Med. 2000;324:654–6.
2. Nalysnyk L, Cid-Ruzafa J, Rotella P, Esser D. Incidence and prevalence of idiopathic pulmonary fibrosis: review of the literature. Eur Respir Rev. 2012;21:355–61.
3. Ancochea J, Xaubet A, Agüero R, editors. Fibrosis pulmonar idiopática. Madrid: Editorial Respira; 2015. p. 41–57.
4. Xaubet A, Ancochea J, Bollo E, Fernández-Fabrellas E, Franquet T, Molina-Molina M, et al. Normativa sobre el diagnóstico y tratamiento de la fibrosis pulmonar idiopática. Normativa SEPAR Arch Bronconeumol. 2013;49(8):343–53. https://doi.org/10.1016/j.arbres.2013.03.011.
5. Yount SE, Beaumont JL, Chen SY, Kaiser K, Wortman K, Van Brunt DL, et al. Health-related quality of life in patients with idiopathic pulmonary fibrosis. Lung. 2016;194(2):227–34. https://doi.org/10.1007/s00408-016-9850-y.
6. Ryerson CJ, Berkley J, Carrieri-Kohlman L, Pantilat SZ, Landefeld CS, Collard HR. Depression and functional status are strongly associated with dyspnoea in interstitial lung disease. Chest. 2011;139(3):609–16. https://doi.org/10.1378/chest.10-0608.
7. Overgaard D, Kaldan G, Marsaa K, Nielsen TL, Shaker SB, Egerod I. The lived experience with idiopathic pulmonary fibrosis: a qualitative study. Eur Respir J. 2016;47(5):1472–80. https://doi.org/10.1183/13993003.01566-2015.
8. Bausewein C, Farquhar M, Booth S, Gysels M, Higginson IJ. Measurement of breathlessness in advanced disease: a systematic review. Respir Med. 2007;101(3):399–410.
9. Bausewein C, Booth S, Gysels M, Kühnbach R, Haberland B, Higginson IJ. Understanding breathlessness: cross-sectional comparison of symptom burden and palliative care needs in chronic obstruc-

tive pulmonary disease and cancer. J Palliat Med. 2010;13(9):1109–18. https://doi.org/10.1089/jpm.2010.0068.
10. Funk GC, Kirchheinner K, Burghuber OC, Hartl S. BODE index versus GOLD classification for explaining anxious and depressive symptoms in patients with COPD—a cross sectional study. Res Rev. 2009;10(1):1. https://doi.org/10.1186/1465-9921-10-1.
11. Holland A, Fiore J Jr, Bell EC, Goh N, Westall G, Symons K, et al. Dyspnoea and comorbidity contribute to anxiety and depression in interstitial lung disease. Respirology. 2014;19(8):1215–21. https://doi.org/10.1111/resp.12360.
12. Ryerson CJ, Cayou C, Topp F, et al. Pulmonary rehabilitation improves long-term outcomes in interstitial lung disease: a prospective cohort study. Respir Med. 2014;108:203–10.
13. Bajwah S, Ross JR, Wells AU, et al. Palliative care for patients with advanced fibrotic lung disease: a randomised controlled phase II and feasibility trial of a community case conference intervention. Thorax. 2015;70:830–9.
14. Fulton BG, Ryerson CJ. Managing comorbidities in idiopathic pulmonary fibrosis. Int J Gen Med. 2015;8:309–18. https://doi.org/10.2147/IJGM.S74880.
15. Abu Youssefa HA, Sabryb Y, Sadekc M, Shabana M, Hafezd S. Study of the relationship of dyspnea with depression and functional status in patients with interstitial lung disease. Egypt J Chest Dis Tuberc. 2015;64(1):269–75. https://doi.org/10.1016/j.ejcdt.2014.11.019.
16. Van Manen M, Kreuter M, Van Den Blink B, Oltmanns U, Baroke E, Palmowski K, et al. What patients with pulmonary fibrosis and their partners think: a live, educative survey in the Netherlands and Germany. ERJ Open Res. 2017;3(1):00065-2016. https://doi.org/10.1183/23120541.00065-2016.
17. Lee YJ, Choi SM, Lee YJ, Cho Y-J, Yoon HI, Lee J-H, et al. Clinical impact of depression and anxiety in patients with idiopathic pulmonary fibrosis. PLoS One. 2017;12(9):e0184300. https://doi.org/10.1371/journal.pone.0184300.
18. Betancourt J, Torres del Castillo N, Hurtado H. Rehabilitación pulmonar en pacientes con enfermedad pulmonar intersticial difusa: estudio de casos. Rev Mov Cient. 2015;9(2):6–14.
19. Sgalla G, Cerri S, Ferrari R, Ricchieri M, Poletti S, Ori M, et al. Mindfulness-based stress reduction in patients with interstitial lung diseases: a pilot, single-centre observational study on safety and efficacy. BMJ Open Respir Res. 2015;2(1):e000065. https://doi.org/10.1136/bmjresp-2014-000065.
20. Swigris JJ, Brown KK, Make BJ, Wamboldt FS. Pulmonary rehabilitation in idiopathic pulmonary fibrosis: a call for continued investigation. Respir Med. 2008;102(12):1675–80.
21. The WHOQOL Group. Development of the World Health Organization WHOQOL-BREF quality of life assessment. Psychol Med. 1998;28:551–8.
22. Kaplan R, Bush J, Berry C. Health status: types of validity and the index of well-being. Health Serv Res. 1976;11(4):478–507.
23. Guyatt G, Berman L, Townsend M, Pugsley S, Chambers L. A measure of quality of life for clinical trials of chronic lung disease. Thorax. 1987;42(10):773–8.
24. Jones P, Quirk F, Baveystock C. The St. George's respiratory questionnaire. Respir Med. 1991;85:25–31.
25. Duck A, Spencer LG, Bailey S, Leonard C, Ormes J, Caress AL. Perceptions, experiences and needs of patients with idiopathic pulmonary fibrosis. J Adv Nurs. 2015;71(5):1055–65. https://doi.org/10.1111/jan.12587.
26. Sampson C, Gill BH, Harrison NK, Nelson AM, Byrne A. The care needs of patients with idiopathic pulmonary fibrosis and their carers (Canopy): results of a qualitative study. BMC Pulm Med. 2015;15:155. https://doi.org/10.1186/s12890-015-0145-5.
27. Molina J, Trigueros JA, Quintano JA, Mascarós E, Xaubet A, Ancochea J. Fibrosis pulmonar idiopática: un reto para la atención primaria. Idiopathic pulmonary fibrosis: a challenge for primary care. Semergen. 2014;40(3):134–42. https://doi.org/10.1016/j.semerg.2014.02.001.
28. Urrengoetxea LA, Solano CS, Barrenetxea MA, Moraza Cortés FJ, Quincoces AB, Sainz AC. Faseacelerada de la fibrosis pulmonar idiopática. Accelerated Phase of Idiopathic Pulmonary Fibrosis. Arch Bronconeumol. 2007;43(9):516–8.
29. Lindell KO, Liang Z, Hoffman LA, Rosenzweig MQ, Saul MI, Pilewski JM, et al. Palliative care and location of death in decedents with IPF. Chest. 2015;147(2):423–9. https://doi.org/10.1378/chest.14-1127.
30. Gainza D, Sanz EM, Alonso A, Varela M. Atención al final de la vida en los pacientes con fibrosis pulmonar idiopática. Med Paliat. 2017;24:21–5. https://doi.org/10.1016/j.medipa.2014.07.001.
31. Bajwah S, Higginson IJ, Ross JR, Wells AU, Birring SS, Riley J, et al. The palliative care needs for fibrotic interstitial lung disease: a qualitative study of patients, informal caregivers and health professionals. Palliat Med. 2013;27(9):869–76. https://doi.org/10.1177/0269216313497226.
32. Bradley B, Branley HM, Egan JJ, Greaves MS, Hansell DM, Harrison NK, et al. Interstitial lung disease guideline: the British Thoracic Society in collaboration with the Thoracic Society of Australia and New Zealand and the Irish Thoracic Society. Thorax. 2008;63 Suppl 5:v1–58. https://doi.org/10.1136/thx.2008.101691.
33. Kissane DW, Bobevski I, Gaitanis P, Brooker J, Michael N, Lethborg C, et al. Exploratory examination of the utility of demoralization as a diagnostic specifier for adjustment disorder and major depression. Gen Hosp Psychiatry. 2017;46:20–4. https://doi.org/10.1016/j.genhosppsych.2017.01.007.
34. van Manen MJ, Geelhoed JJ, Tak NC, Wijsenbeek MS. Optimizing quality of life in patients

with idiopathic pulmonary fibrosis. Ther Adv Respir Dis. 2017;11(3):157–69. https://doi.org/10.1177/1753465816686743.
35. Zigmond AS, Snaith RP. The hospital anxiety and depression scale. Acta Psychiatr Scand. 1983;67(6):361–70.
36. Quintana JM, Padierna A, Esteban C, Arostegui I, Bilbao A, Ruiz I. Evaluation of the psychometric characteristics of the Spanish version of the Hospital Anxiety and Depression Scale. Acta Psychiatr Scand. 2003;107(3):216–21.
37. Galiana L, Rudilla D, Oliver A, Barreto P. The Short Demoralization Scale (SDS): a new tool to appraise demoralization in palliative care patients. Palliat Support Care. 2017;9:1–8. https://doi.org/10.1017/S1478951516000973.
38. Rudilla D, Oliver A, Galiana L, Barreto P. A new measure of home care patients' dignity at the end of life: the Palliative Patients' Dignity Scale (PPDS). Palliat Support Care. 2016;14(2):99–108. https://doi.org/10.1017/S1478951515000747.
39. Benito E, Oliver A, Galiana L, et al. Development and validation of a new tool for the assessment and spiritual care of palliative care patients. J Pain Symptom Manage. 2014;47(6):1008–18.
40. Paul Victor CG, Treschuk JV. Critical literature review on the definition clarity of the concept of faith, religion, and spirituality. J Holist Nurs. 2019:898010119895368. https://doi.org/10.1177/0898010119895368.
41. Sinclair VG, Wallston KA. The development and psychometric evaluation of the Brief Resilient Coping Scale. Assessment. 2004;11:94–101.
42. Barreto P, Fombuena M, Diego R, Galiana L, Oliver A, Benito E. Bienestar emocional y espiritualidad al final de la vida. Med Paliat. 2015;22(1):25–32.
43. de la Revilla L, Bailón E, de Dios J, Delgado A, Prados M, Fleitas L. Validación de una escala de apoyo social funcional para su uso en la consulta del médico de familia. Atención Primaria. 1991;8(9):688–91.
44. Aaronson NK, Cull A, Kaasa S, Sprangers MAG. The EORTC modular approach to quality of life assessment in oncology. Int J Ment Health. 1994;23(2):75–96. https://doi.org/10.1016/0885-3924(95)94770-F.
45. Cohen J. Statistical power analysis for the behavioral sciences. Hillsdale: Lawrence Erlbaum; 1988.
46. Holland JC, Andersen B, Breitbart WS, et al. The NCCN distress management clinical practice guidelines in oncology. J Natl Compr Canc Netw. 2010;8:44884.
47. Julião M, Barbosa A, Oliveira F, Nunes B, Vaz Carneiro A. Efficacy of dignity therapy for depression and anxiety in terminally ill patients: early results of a randomized controlled trial. Palliat Support Care. 2013;11(6):481–9.
48. Rudilla D, Oliver A, Galiana L, Barreto P. Estudio comparativo de la eficacia del counselling y de la terapia de la dignidad en pacientes paliativos. Med Paliat. 2017;24:39–46. https://doi.org/10.1016/j.medipa.2014.09.005.
49. Levy MH, Back A, Benedetti C, Billings JA, Block S, Boston B, Bruera E, Dy S, Eberle C, Foley KM, Karver SB, Knight SJ, Misra S, Ritchie CS, Spiegel D, Sutton L, Urba S, Von Roenn JH, Weinstein SM. NCCN clinical practice guidelines in oncology: palliative care. J Natl Compr Canc Netw. 2009;7(4):436–73.
50. Houmann LJ, Rydahl-Hansen S, Chochinov HM, Kristjanson LJ, Groenvold M. Testing the feasibility of the Dignity Therapy interview: adaptation for the Danish culture. BMC Palliat Care. 2010;9:21.
51. Chochinov HM, Hassard T, McClement S, Hack T, Kristjanson LJ, Harlos M, et al. The patient dignity inventory: a novel way of measuring dignity-related distress in palliative care. J Pain Symptom Manage. 2008;36:559–71.
52. Chochinov HM, Hassard T, McClement S, et al. The landscape of distress in the terminally ill. J Pain Symptom Manage. 2009;38(5):641–9.
53. Chochinov HM, Kristjanson LJ, Breitbart W, et al. Effect of dignity therapy on distress and end-of-life experience in terminally ill patients: a randomised controlled trial. Lancet Oncol. 2011;12(8):753–62.
54. Albers G, Pasman HR, Rurup ML, de Vet HC, Onwuteaka-Philipsen BD. Analysis of the construct of dignity and content validity of the patient dignity inventory. Health Qual Life Outcomes. 2011;9:45.
55. Sanz A, Blancotoro L, Librada S, Julián-Caballero M, Del Valle M, Rocafort J. El concepto de calidad de vida en los profesionales de Cuidados Paliativos. Med Pal. 2008;15(3):165–70.
56. Rudilla D, Soto-Rubio A, Pérez MA, Galiana L, Fombuena M, Oliver A, et al. Psychological interventions in spirituality: a systematic review in palliative care. Med Paliativa (Internet). 2018;25(3):203–12. Available from: https://doi.org/10.1016/j.medipa.2016.10.004.
57. Puchalski CM, Vitillo R, Hull SK, Reller N. Improving the spiritual dimension of whole person care: reaching national and international consensus. J Palliat Med. 2014;17(6):642–56.

Community Palliative Care in Spain: The Critical Role of Nursing in Its Development

Maria Paz Fernández-Ortega and Julio César de la Torre-Montero

Introduction: Social and Cultural Considerations in Spain

Spain has had universal access to healthcare since the last century and palliative care has had a long history of nearly 30 years of evolution. Because of the idiosyncrasies of the nation and the existence of 17 autonomous regions governing their own competencies in health, there are a variety of programs and specialties that have been transferred to each autonomous government.

Palliative organizations were designed in the 1980s in accordance with the Social and Sanitary System (SSS) with a plan to interconnect the primary, secondary, and tertiary levels of health institutions. One priority was to address the insufficient continuity of care from hospital to home, the gap of time where patients are attended to at the end of life, usually at acute hospitals [1].

Palliative care was born together with the paradigm of oncology, which is currently undergoing a profound change; every scientific meeting that we attend shows that the use of social networks and digital information on the Internet as a means of communication is on the rise, echoing this new situation.

These new hopes are founded not only upon the personalization of the new therapies and initiatives that work in precise medicine [2] but also how professionals cope with all the new challenges.

Every type of cancer in this group of pathologies must be considered when we talk about the future. Beyond this point, oncology nursing is the art of caring for the "small details" regarding the patient's overall needs. And, in a large number of diagnoses, palliative care in cancer is a must when working in this field, from the very beginning of the diagnosis until the end of life.

Oncology and palliative nursing is one of the most important roles in caring for cancer patients, along with many other healthcare professionals who take part in this challenge.

Considering the existing demographic data, Spain could soon be among the countries with the oldest population in the world, with chronic conditions, multimorbidities, and disabilities that will continue to rise in number [3]. This will lead to a more complex social and health panorama requiring an urgent response from the government to ensure adequate health services.

Throughout the past 25 years, life expectancy from the time of diagnosis of virtually any type of cancer has evolved into survival rates hitherto

M. P. Fernández-Ortega (✉)
Institut Català d'Oncologia and University of Barcelona, Barcelona, Spain
e-mail: Paxfernandez2010@ub.edu

J. C. de la Torre-Montero
Oncology Nursing Care and Palliative Care, Comillas Pontifical University, Madrid, Spain
e-mail: juliodelatorre@comillas.edu

M. Silbermann (ed.), *Palliative Care for Chronic Cancer Patients in the Community*,
https://doi.org/10.1007/978-3-030-54526-0_12

unknown. This fact is paradigmatic in the case of breast cancer, where every year we update the former rate of survival by 5–10 years from the time of the first diagnosis. On the opposite side and still in a slow process of change, the diagnoses of diseases with a high mortality rate, such as pancreatic cancer or cerebral astrocytoma, are within the first year of the patient's evaluation.

With these figures, we manage the care of the cancer patient. The reflection on how we do our work can be seen by the looks of health professionals in hospital waiting rooms, which pass from a patient with little hope of survival to others who can practically be assured a cure.

The introduction of monoclonal antibodies in combination with classic chemotherapy at the beginning of the twentieth century later added to molecules that inhibit tumor growth processes (tyrosine kinase synthesis, EGFR inhibitors, VEGF, etc.); today, immunotherapy and treatments with CAR-T (chimeric antigen receptor T cell) provide new hope for combating most types of malignant tumors.

We have seen in our own personal experience that precision medicine is here to stay and has revolutionized the world of cancer treatment. The personalization of medicine, much broader than just in terms of treatment, has turned precision in nursing care into a daily occurrence, utilizing all our human potential [2].

If we go back to our peninsular past, we find the wonderful case of *Benjamina*, named after the paleontologist who discovered her at the excavations of Atapuerca (Burgos, Spain). Benjamina, about 530,000 years ago, was a girl with a great disability, born with craniosynostosis, where the bones of the skull merge prematurely and do not allow the brain to adequately develop. She was cared for until late in childhood; the fact is that, without special care, she would not have survived long: *Homo heidelbergensis* put the time from birth until the moment of the girl's death at about 10 or 12 years. The chronicle of care has been widely recorded in the literature, and at every historical time, doctors have recognized themselves as being the first to establish a specific way of caring for the patient. The care, and more specifically, special care, provided to Benjamina shows that the act of caring is the key to survival [4].

Florence Nightingale (1820–1910), nurse and former epidemiologist, was the first woman admitted into the British Royal Statistical Society. She was called "the lady of the lamp" for the night walks she took visiting the English soldiers that she attended to during the Crimean War. In her work, she highlighted two major and important points: the first, the quality of the care, based on the first epidemiological studies on hospital infections resulting from the poor conditions she observed in the field work – poor hygienic conditions and unscrupulous practices during the process of treating patients injured in war, who did not die from their wounds in battle, but rather from hospital infections. The second point is the explanation for the use of the lamp: the continuous attention to the patients as a novel method of care. This is one of the milestones in the so-called humanization of care in modern times and considered to be the cornerstone of palliative care [5].

If medicine has classically been considered as the art of healing, nursing, on the other hand, could be defined as the art of caring, with technique, with evidence, and, of course, with humanity. In the art of healthcare, the quality of care must be holistic, incorporating all the bio-psycho-social aspects of the patient, not forgetting any one of these areas. Three fundamental factors worth reiterating, with respect to patient care, are education, knowledge, and learning, followed by a continuous commitment to that care.

The United Nations' Sustainable Development Goals (SDGs) strategy guarantees equal access to healthcare, treatments, vaccinations, and food for all people of all ages, regardless of purchasing power [6].

This last statement, in reality, is subject to change, primarily due to not only economic reasons but also political reasons. The high cost of cancer treatments lowers the expectations of patients who must assume responsibility for part of or all of the expenses of their therapeutic procedures, so, in many cases, the only treatment that patients can afford is palliative treatment, many times in suboptimal conditions, especially in developing African or Latin American countries [7].

The Present-Day Palliative Care System in Spain

Many primary care professionals and specialists from hospitals were involved in and contributed to the development of the current palliative care system in Spain, with a lot of hard work and dedication. It was in 1984 that the first Spanish palliative unit was established, in Santander within a general hospital, followed by the *Canary Islands*, the Basque Country, and Catalonia in around 1986 [8].

Considering that all patients, as well as their relatives, have the right to be attended to during the dying process, various home care programs with different models and dependencies have been created in Spain since the 1980s. On December 18, 2000, the Foundation for the Development of the National Palliative Care Plan was approved at the plenary of the Inter-territorial Council of the National Health System in Spain, where palliative care was recognized as a health priority throughout the entire country, not distinguishing between the original diagnosis of the tumors, the type of cancer, and/or under what condition the cancer is to be treated [9].

In 1991, the Gregorio Marañón Hospital in Madrid created the biggest palliative care unit of any hospital, working jointly with community primary care teams under the umbrella of the national health service (INSALUD). They began with home care support teams called ESAD (Equipos de Soporte de Atención Domiciliaria).

However, primary care teams are not always the best trained and may not have the expertise, the necessary resources, or the means to attend to palliative patients who are treated by home hospitalization teams or home care support teams (ESAD) [10]. Their purpose is to support primary care professionals in the comprehensive and ongoing care of the following patients and their caregivers and families: (a) those who are in the advanced stages, (b) complex patients, or (c) those who have functional limitations [8].

Catalonia: The PADES Teams

The Catalonian network of social and sanitary services began in 1986 within the framework of the deployment of the program Vida al Anys ("Life in the Years"), contrasting the past focus which was adding "years to life." This program initiated the development of a range of services that integrated social and healthcare services in a single model for the benefit of advanced cancer patients. One of these services was the home care programs designed to support primary and community teams known as PADES (Programa d'Atenció Domiciliaria i Equips de Suport) [11].

In addition to giving individual attention, they are primarily there to control symptoms, to provide comfort, and to promote the well-being of the advanced patients, of their caregivers, and of the surrounding family, promoting the best care and death at home, when possible [12].

They play an important role in the management of complex cases, in the coordination of resources between healthcare levels, and also in training other professionals of the primary care network in the field of palliative and complexity care at the end of life [13].

The PADES' mission was to act as support for the other primary care professionals, mainly in the following circumstances: geriatric and/or chronic diseases that have been decompensated or are at an advanced stage, some conditions at the convalescence phase requiring specific care supervision such as endovenous treatment at home, advanced and palliative patients that express their desire to be at home instead of being hospitalized, and those patients with specific therapeutic or complex symptoms needing direct support at home from health professionals [14].

Types of Conditions and Support for Palliative Care

The PADES teams try to ensure that patients receive the best care, at any time or stage and in the right place or, at least, the most suitable one. The teams mainly focus on adult patients, but also there are some for onco-pediatric, in cities or rural areas. Multidisciplinary teams work on connecting the three different levels of health: primary, secondary, and tertiary.

In pediatric palliative cases, there is a multidisciplinary team (doctor, nurse, social worker, and psychologist) that treats the patient and his/her family as a whole. These teams move throughout the region so that the geographical dispersion increases the number of face-to-face visits, which are mitigated by telephone calls and telecommunication consultations [15, 16].

This provides the pediatric palliative services with data for unique research in the investigation into cultural and sociocultural aspects [17].

The Critical Role of Nursing Advocacy

Spain's regional reality is that access to treatments outside the community of residence is diminished by the administrative inconvenience that entails being able to receive the best treatment for a specific diagnosis in a hospital outside the autonomy of residence [13]. Sometimes it would be easier to go to an emergency room to get a cardiac monitor or, in some cases, to be admitted to an intensive care unit. Receiving the palliative care support in the community or at home can be very difficult.

Nursing care goes beyond physical or clinical needs and is often realized in the form of the emotional and supportive care that it brings to patients. The vital element is communication. The nurses' support is based on the communication skills of the professional nurse, who considers the patient as the center of the therapeutic dynamic. Communication is identified as the most positive and recognized element of palliative care and the most valued, both by patients and families.

In Spain, the main activities of the ESAD, PADES, and other team nurses are shown in Table 1.

The obstacles that the patients must face occur at multiple levels [18]. For instance, challenges at the bureaucratic level are often greater than those that can occur at the clinic or hospital. Another is related to the time of the medical referral and when to begin at the community level [19]. Another aspect is the cost, although it has been largely demonstrated that end-of-life home care is less expensive than hospital bills [20].

Table 1 Activities developed by palliative care community nurses

To work within a team with other medical and social work professionals with a patient-centered model and with a palliative philosophy
To work in a coordinated manner with other social services, primary care, and secondary or tertiary/acute health centers and hospitals in accordance with the patient's needs
To monitor the patient's condition with a therapeutic plan and establish a calendar of programmed visits according to the objectives established for each patient. To guide and advise patients and relatives, respecting their values and preferences and acting with ethics
To identify, assess, and address the patient's needs in a holistic and comprehensive manner and with a multidimensional vision
To train and teach caregivers and family members and to oversee techniques, such as subcutaneous administrations, to provide them with the most complete care guidelines to facilitate care at home by providing support and ensure safety
To provide individual and personalized medical, social, and emotional support
To resolve family and patient doubts that may arise with regard to their condition
To provide emotional support to patients, families, and friends pertaining to the environment at home
To prepare and facilitate the bereavement process at home or any other intervention required by the family. To follow-up grief and family after death

Bekelman et al. compared the costs at the end of life vs. place of death in seven different countries, for patients 65 years and older who died from cancer. They concluded that the costs in more hospital-centered countries – Canada, the USA, and Norway – were higher than the costs in Belgium, Germany, England, and the Netherlands and that intensive care admissions in the USA were more than double the cost of those in the other countries [21].

One explanation for the above statistics could be the fact that indirect costs are mainly assumed by the families, though, when hospitalization occurs, the costs are assumed by the National

Health System. In Spain, there are many examples of complementary therapies such as supportive care medications, physical rehabilitation, psychologists, and grief counselors to cope with end of life that are not included in the national health coverage, although their use is widely prescribed for cancer patients, especially at the advanced stage [22].

The guarantee of equity in access to treatments in our country is compromised in many communities due to budgetary imbalances and inequality in policies. These barriers are provoked more from political decisions than from the medical need of patients and the population.

Inequalities are clear, palpable, and demonstrable and we need to reverse the situation; scientific societies have already made statements denouncing the situation and calling for a reversal of the circumstances for many patients who live in our own country [23].

The Nurses' Role in Palliative Process

To "accompany," as an active verb, can be enumerated by the number of hours that health professionals, nurses, and doctors spend alongside the patient; this fervent accompaniment focuses on efforts to prevent a painful or distressing death, where the patient feels cared for and not abandoned to their fate. It has less to do with prescribing more medical interventions (which is easier for some professionals than listening to needs of the person at the end of life) and more to do with the effort required to order and provide compassionate care for patients and families.

Generally, all the professionals involved in the process – in the hospital and in the community context, from the people in charge of cleaning to the caregivers, auxiliaries, and technical staff to the rest of the experts – are proactive in their efforts to provide the best care. However, sometimes the lack of medication or technically sophisticated devices dedicated to managing symptoms and pain is supplemented in some way by accompanying the patient with genuine human care.

Finally, considering the patient as a whole and providing a comprehensive package of humane care should be the routine and not the exception.

Palliative Needs for Advanced Chronic Diseases Other than Cancer in the Community

Almost all National Care Plans of the 17 autonomous regions in Spain include palliative guidelines and have demanded that palliative care embraces all patients with life-limiting disease, irrespective of their diagnosis, in an equal manner [24].

Regarding access to palliative care, chronic patients should be referred as early as possible and not limit care to the last days or weeks of life. We know from previous research that palliative care, if integrated earlier than at the last moments in life, can offer better support and control of symptoms and has a more positive impact on the patient as well as on the family's grieving process after death [25, 26].

Among complex chronic patients, those who have advanced chronic conditions other than cancer may have multiple needs due to the life-limiting prognosis – on one hand, palliative care and, on the other hand, that they may also need curative and preventive measures from the health professionals [13].

These patients often have severe pain and a diversity of symptoms that necessitate supportive treatment and a palliative care approach. The physical and psychosocial needs of patients with chronic non-malignant lung disease are comparable to those with lung cancer.

Blay et al. found that 1% of the adult primary care population have advanced diseases. His study of advanced-disease patients was conducted in three primary care teams in Catalonia, with 251 patients mostly affected by dementia and chronic diseases; however, all presented with palliative needs, and the median age was 85 years old with an average survival rate of 23 months. For 47.3%, the place of death was their home, and 37.2% died in an intermediate care hospital and 15.5% in an acute care hospital; these findings coincided with the data reported in the literature in other regions of Spain and in other developed European countries [27].

Quality of Life and Future Challenges

Patient participation is the key issue in the palliative process, although it must be accompanied by the support and professional decisions of each of the disciplines that make up the team. Now, the patient is an active subject as far as the treatment is concerned. And above all, the patient must be asked what he/she wants to do and how far he/she wants to go.

Translating this last statement into the language of cancer patients, in the context of Spain and in general, means to facilitate the best and most appropriate treatments, as well as gaining access to the most advanced clinical trials. We try to provide the patient with the best supportive treatment when no therapy is indicated for the stage of the tumor, although we still have a long way to go.

It is well-worth considering the trend that has been booming in recent years – the idea of involving the patient in clinical decisions regarding medical and nursing care and techniques.

Another common issue concerning palliative care in oncology is the characterization of each of the diagnoses, molecular subtypes, and final classifications for treatment, which require a fine and precise differentiation so that, from the moment of diagnosis, the best and most appropriate therapeutic approaches to the disease are offered as options to each individual patient [5, 7, 26].

The relationship between human development, human rights, and bioethics can be debatable in the reality of an imperfect world, where bioethics must continue to respond to the different challenges of the evolution and development of technology [27].

It is important that professionalism includes the capacity for clinical judgment in decision-making, be it medical or nursing care, as we have the tendency to confuse patient autonomy and empowerment with decision-making. Some clinicians have defended a position to qualify the patient's empowerment, provided it is accompanied by clinical and critical judgment. That is, without the appropriate clinical perspective, the patient's critical view of his/her illness can be accompanied, among other things, by fear of pain, suffering from side effects, and, finally, death, whereby making an inadequate final decision perhaps causes harm to their health and well-being.

The classic example of the above lies in the treatment of lung cancer: treatments based on platinum salts in combination with radiotherapy, a traditional treatment in care procedures, have some harmful side effects including poor general condition and vomiting. Despite the unfortunate consequences, the short-term quality of life improves as the patient recovers ostensible respiratory capacity, pain levels decrease, and quality of life increases; with less pain, the patient moves better and his/her daily life activities (AVD) become more independent.

Greater initiatives regarding the training of professionals, in all areas of treatment and care, should be implemented. We need projects that help enforce better care [28].

References

1. Garralda E, Hasselaar J, Carrasco JM, Van Beek K, Siouta N, Csikos A, Menten J, Centeno C. Integrated palliative care in the Spanish context: a systematic review of the literature. BMC Palliat Care. 2016;15:49. https://doi.org/10.1186/s12904-016-0120-9. Review.
2. Goetz LH, Schork NJ. Personalized medicine: motivation, challenges, and progress. Fertil Steril. 2018;109(6):952–63. https://doi.org/10.1016/j.fertnstert.2018.05.006.
3. Instituto Nacional de Estadística. Proyecciones de población 2012–2052 [cited 21 Nov 2019]. Available at: http://www.ine.es/prensa/np744.pdf.
4. Gracia A, Martínez-Lage JF, Arsuaga JL, Martínez I, Lorenzo C, Pérez-Espejo MA. The earliest evidence of true lambdoid raniosynostosis: the case of "Benjamina," a *Homo heidelbergensis* child. Childs Nerv Syst. 2010;26(6):723–7. https://doi.org/10.1007/s00381-010-1133-y.
5. Attewell A. PROSPECTS: the quarterly review of comparative education. Paris, UNESCO: International Bureau of Education. 1998. xxviii(1):153–66.

6. United Nations. 2030 United Nations strategy and sustainable development. 2015. United Nations: New York. Accessed on 15 Jan 2020. Available at: https://www.un.org/sustainabledevelopment/sustainable-development-goals/.
7. de la Torre Montero JC, Gil Gómez N, Rives Bernal JL, Domenech Climent N, Ojer Perea A, Beorlegui Murillo P, et al. Cancer situation in Sub-Saharan countries: development of educational, diagnosis and treatment plans. Eur Soc Med Oncol Ann Oncol. 2018;29(suppl_8). https://doi.org/10.1093/annonc/mdy274.
8. Centeno C, Garralda E, Carrasco JM, den Herder-van der Eerden M, Aldridge M, Stevenson D, Meier DE, Hasselaar J. The palliative care challenge: analysis of barriers and opportunities to integrate palliative care in Europe in the view of national associations. J Palliat Med. 2017;20(11):1195–204. https://doi.org/10.1089/jpm.2017.0039.
9. Arrieta A, Hernández R, Meléndez A. Cuidados paliativos. Proceso asistencia integrado araba. Vitoria: Osakidetza-Servicio de salud vasco, Dirección Territorial de Álava-Departamento de Sanidad y Consumo. 2012. Spanish.
10. ESAD and Palliative Care Framework. Comunidad de Madrid (Spanish) Internet. Accessed on 20 Jan 2020. Available at: https://www.comunidad.madrid/servicios/salud/plan-integral-cuidados-paliativos.
11. Gómez-Batiste X, Martínez-Muñoz M, Blay C, Amblàs J, Vila L, Costa X, Espaulella J, Espinosa J, Constante C, Mitchell GK. Prevalence and characteristics of patients with advanced chronic conditions in need of palliative care in the general population: a cross-sectional study. Palliat Med. 2014;28(4):302–11. https://doi.org/10.1177/0269216313518266.
12. Generalitat de Catalunya. Programa d'atenció domiciliària, Equips de Suport PADES. Home care programme, Pades support teams [Catalan] Cited 4 Feb 2020. Available at: http://salutintegralbcn.gencat.cat/ca/ambits/Programa-datencio-domiciliaria-Equips-de-Suport-PADES/.
13. Limón E, Blay C, Ledesma A. Population needs, a call for changes in Primary Care. Aten Primaria. 2015;47(2):73–4. https://doi.org/10.1016/j.aprim.2014.08.001. Epub 2014 Nov 27. Spanish.
14. Generalitat de Catalunya. Institut d'Assistència Sanitaria. Atenció Palliativa al Malalt Terminal. (Palliative Care in the Terminal Patient). Web gencat.cat. Catalan. [Cited 11 Jan 2020]. Available at: http://www.ias.cat/ca/contingut/primaria/175.
15. Worster B, Swartz K. Telemedicine and palliative care: an increasing role in supportive oncology. Curr Oncol Rep. 2017;19(6):37. https://doi.org/10.1007/s11912-017-0600-y.
16. de Noriega Í, Barceló M, Pérez MÁ, Puertas V, García-Salido A, Martino R. Ingresos hospitalarios en cuidados paliativos pediátricos: estudio retrospectivo [Hospital admissions into paediatric palliative care: a retrospective study] [published online ahead of print, 2019 Mar 16]. An Pediatr (Barc). 2019;S1695-4033(19):30078–5. https://doi.org/10.1016/j.anpedi.2019.02.001.
17. Chocarro L, González P, Moreno A, Barceló M, Martino R. A grounded theory study of the perceptions and meanings associated with gastrostomies among parents of children with palliative needs. Int J Palliat Nurs. 2019;25(1):19–28. https://doi.org/10.12968/ijpn.2019.25.1.19.
18. Haun MW, Estel S, Rücker G, Friederich HC, Villalobos M, Thomas M, Hartmann M. Early palliative care for adults with advanced cancer. Cochrane Database Syst Rev. 2017;6:CD011129. https://doi.org/10.1002/14651858.CD011129.pub2. Review.
19. Brant JM, Fink RM, Thompson C, Li YH, Rassouli M, Majima T, Osuka T, et al. Global survey of the roles, satisfaction, and barriers of home health care nurses on the provision of palliative care. J Palliat Med. 2019;22(8):945–60. https://doi.org/10.1089/jpm.2018.0566.
20. Bekelman JE, Halpern SD, Blankart CR, Bynum JP, Cohen J, Fowler R, et al. International Consortium for End-of-Life Research (ICELR). Comparison of site of death, health care utilization, and hospital expenditures for patients dying with Cancer in 7 developed countries. JAMA. 2016;315(3):272–83. https://doi.org/10.1001/jama.2015.18603.
21. Molassiotis A, Fernández-Ortega P, Pud D, Ozden G, Scott JA, Panteli V, et al. Use of complementary and alternative medicine in cancer patients: a European survey. Ann Oncol. 2005;16(4):655–63.
22. Salvador J, Aparicio J, Baron FJ, Garcia-Campelo R, Garcia-Carbonero R, Lianes P, et al. Equity, barriers and cancer disparities: study of the Spanish Society of Medical Oncology on the access to oncologic drugs in the Spanish Regions. Clin Transl Oncol. 2017;19(3):341–56. https://doi.org/10.1007/s12094-016-1535-8. Epub 2016 Aug 25. Erratum in: Clin Transl Oncol. 2017 Apr;19(4):525.
23. Boland J, Martin J, Wells AU, Ross JR. Palliative care for people with non-malignant lung disease: summary of current evidence and future direction. Palliat Med. 2013;27(9):811–6. https://doi.org/10.1177/0269216313493467.
24. Wachterman MW, Pilver C, Smith D, Ersek M, Lipsitz SR, Keating NL. Quality of end-of-life care provided to patients with different serious illnesses. JAMA Intern Med. 2016;176(8):1095–102. https://doi.org/10.1001/jamainternmed.2016.1200.
25. Costa X, Gómez-Batiste X, Pla M, Martínez-Muñoz M, Blay C, Vila L. Living with advanced chronic obstructive pulmonary disease: the impact of dyspnoea on patients and caregivers. Aten Primaria. 2016;48(10):665–73. https://doi.org/10.1016/j.aprim.2016.02.008. Epub 2016 Jun 7. Spanish.
26. Blay C, Martori JC, Limón E, Oller R, Vila L, Gómez-Batiste X. Find your 1%: prevalence and mortality of a community cohort of people with advanced chronic disease and palliative needs. Aten Primaria. 2019;51(2):71–9. https://doi.org/10.1016/j.aprim.2017.07.004. Spanish.

27. Solbakk JH, Vidal SM. Clinical research in resource-poor settings. In: ten Have H, Gordijn B, editors. Handbook of global bioethics. London: Springer; 2014.
28. Drudge-Coates L, van Muilekom E, de la Torre-Montero JC, Leonard K, van Oostwaard M, Niepel D, Jensen BT. Management of bone health in patients with cancer: a survey of specialist nurses. Support Care Cancer. 2019. https://doi.org/10.1007/s00520-019-04858-2. [Epub ahead of print].

Collaborative Efforts in Developing Pediatric Oncology and Palliative Care Services in the Hispano-American and African Countries

Wilson Astudillo-Alarcón, J. Antonio Salinas-Martin, Jhon Comba Miranda, and Zemilson Bastos Brandão Souza

No child should die in the dawn of life– Danny Thomas, the founder of St. Jude

Introduction

Children's palliative care (CPC) is an interdisciplinary collaboration that seeks to improve the quality of life of all children and young adults with life-threatening conditions, as well as their families. It focuses on prevention and relief of various forms of suffering, regardless of the stage of disease, and comprehensively addresses the physical, psychosocial, and spiritual needs of the child and family. It is defined as "'active, total care' of a young person's body, mind, spirit, and family from life-limiting diagnosis until death." It is patient-centered and family-engaged, respecting and partnering with patients and families, pursuing care that is high quality and readily accessible integrated into the continuum of care, and equitable and improved care through research and quality improvement efforts. It is a human right and its integration into public healthcare systems is essential for achievement of the Sustainable Development Goal on universal health coverage [1–4].

CPC begins when illness is diagnosed and continues, regardless of whether or not a child receives treatment directed at the disease. It acknowledges that it helps to ensure an ongoing focus on quality of life with relief of symptoms so that the child's enjoyment of life can continue. It is optimally introduced when a life-threatening diagnosis is made or, for children with chronic diseases, when there is a decline in health status from baseline, growing in importance as part of the comprehensive treatment of end-of-life care and culminating with bereavement care. CPC

W. Astudillo-Alarcón (✉)
Paliativos Sin Fronteras / Palliative without Borders, San Sebastián Spain, Spain
e-mail: PSF@paliativossinfronteras.org

J. A. Salinas-Martin
Department of Radiation Oncology, CHUNSC – Hospital Universitario de la Candelaria, Santa Cruz de Tenerife, Spain

J. C. Miranda
Department of Pathology, Hospital Universitario Donosti, San Sebastián, Guipúzcoa, Spain

Z. B. B. Souza
Department of Oncology, Palliative Care and Pain Management, ACSC-HSJ/UNACON-Ministry of Health, Rio de Janeiro, Brazil
e-mail: zefma@zefma.com; zemilson@zefma.com

M. Silbermann (ed.), *Palliative Care for Chronic Cancer Patients in the Community*,
https://doi.org/10.1007/978-3-030-54526-0_13

facilitates informed decision-making by patients, families, and healthcare professionals and assists with ongoing coordination of care. CPC recognizes that there is always care to provide and something to do, such as attention to physical symptoms or emotional distress, regardless of the clinical situation. CPC responds to the ICPCN Declaration of Cape Town in 2009, stating "All children with life-threatening and life-limiting conditions have the right to quality palliative care provided by trained healthcare practitioners" [2, 4]. In this chapter we will review suffering in children, palliative care, cancer, and the importance of cooperation for improving oncologic and palliative care in low- and middle-income countries (LMICs).

Children and Suffering Related to Health (SHS)

CPC is a human response to serious health-related suffering (SHS) when it is associated with illness or injury of any kind. It is serious when it cannot be relieved without medical intervention and when it compromises physical, social, or emotional functioning [5]. CPC seeks to relieve the SHS associated with life-limiting, life-threatening conditions or the end of life for patients and their families [6] (see Table 1). Patients with serious illness experience a substantial burden of suffering with associated costs to society. Improving health through the prevention of suffering is an essential component of high-quality health systems and has the potential to generate economic benefits [5–7]. People younger than 20 years old represent 35% of the global population and 40% of the global population in least developed countries. Considering the distribution of SHS among adults and children in LMICs, children account for almost 70% of people affected by SHS associated with inflammatory disease of the CNS, about half of people with SHS associated with malnutrition and hemorrhagic fever, and about 10–20% with SHS associated with injury, leukemia, and HIV diseases [8]. The Lancet Commission of 2018 [5] goes on to state that in 2015 more than 5.3 million children aged 15 years or younger experience SHS worldwide and almost 2.5 million children die with SHS; more than 98% of these children are from developing countries. In high-income countries (HICs), children account for less than 1% of all deaths, whereas in LMICs, children account for more than 30% of all deaths associated with SHS.

Table 1 Type of suffering and palliative care needed [6]

Patient population	HICs palliative care need	LMICs palliative care need
Advanced chronic NCDs (non-communicable diseases)	High	High
HIV/AIDS	Moderate	Very high
Drug-resistant tuberculosis	Very low	High in some areas
Critical illness	High	High
Neonates with severe prematurity, birth trauma, or congenital anomaly	High	Very high
Severe non-progressive disabilities such as paraplegia and quadriplegia	Moderate	High
Severe social distress, such as extreme poverty or stigmatization	Low	High
Acute symptoms related to illness, injuries, or surgery	Not applicable	High
Health emergencies and crisis	Very low	High in some areas

Palliative Care

The number of children ranging from neonates to adolescents up to 19 years of age who need CPC each year may be as high as 21.6 million, with 8200 requiring specialist services and support for their families [8]. CPC provides treatments that aim to relieve suffering across multiple realms and to improve the child's quality and enjoyment of life. There is a great need for CPC services globally, but access to services is lacking in many parts of the world, particularly in resource-poor settings. The Global Atlas of Palliative Care at the End of Life estimates that more than seven million children need palliative care at the end of life [9]. Out of these seven million, nearly half of them (49%) are in Africa, with 97% needing palliative care and living in low-resourced settings. A review of CPC services in 2011 found that, despite the demand, 65.6% of countries have no known CPC activity, with only 5.7% having provision reaching mainstream providers, and these were in well-resourced countries [5]. While services do exist in low- and middle-income countries (LMICs), they are typically available in only one or a few institutions and are not integrated into healthcare systems. Countries' needs ranged from 21/10,000 in the UK to 120/10,000 in Zimbabwe, with the greatest need in low-resourced settings and those with high rates of HIV [8–10].

Approximately 400,000 children are diagnosed with HIV each year and are living in sub-Saharan Africa with greater incidence of malignancies and associated mortality. 3.4 million children are living with HIV/AIDS and almost 160,000 children younger than 15 years develop cancer each year. In South Africa it is estimated that between 600,000 and 800,000 children have palliative care needs [8–10]. Other conditions for CPC include severe prematurity; birth trauma; congenital anomalies; severe non-progressive disabilities such as paraplegia and quadriplegia; drug-resistant tuberculosis and injuries; endocrine, blood, and immune disorders; cancer; neurological conditions; kidney diseases; cirrhosis; and protein-energy malnutrition [11]. Hain et al. [12] identified from death certificates more than 376 conditions in the UK where CPC would have been useful, 32% of whom died from the 10 most common diagnoses. 67.7% of the seven million needing palliative care will die in perinatal conditions, 9.8% from congenital anomalies, 6.5% from HIV/AIDS, and only 3.2% from malignant neoplasms [11, 13]. The first 28 days of life – the neonatal period – is the most vulnerable time for a child's survival. Children face the highest risk of dying in their first month of life, with an average global rate of 18 deaths per 1000 live births in 2018. Comparatively, the probability of dying after the first month but before reaching age 1 was 11 and after age 1 but before turning age 5 was 10. Globally, 2.5 million children died in the first month of life in 2018 or approximately 7000 neonatal deaths every day, with one-third dying on the first day and the rest from 2 to 28 days [14]. Families benefit from the opportunity to prepare a plan prior to delivery. This planning involves supportive care for the mother during labor and delivery, involvement of the father when appropriate, and care plans that account for the various outcomes of the baby. Thus, despite external perceptions of CPC, the majority of children needing palliative care do not have cancer, but other life-limiting and life-threatening conditions. Children's palliative care is appropriate for the following conditions [1, 3, 4, 6]:

- Curative treatment is possible for critical illness or injury, severe malnutrition, or those awaiting solid organ transplantation, but may fail for children who have cancer or severe congenital heart disease.
- Intensive long-term treatment that maintains quality of life for chronic or potentially progressive conditions such as Duchenne muscular dystrophy, cystic fibrosis, severe immunodeficiencies including human immunodeficiency, virus infection, malignancies, multidrug-resistant tuberculosis, and HIV/AIDS.
- Progressive conditions without a curative option. These include infants with trisomy 13 or 18, type II osteogenesis imperfecta, and spinal muscular atrophy type I.
- Non-progressive irreversible conditions with extreme vulnerability to health complications, including children with severe developmental disabilities, such as those with severe cerebral palsy, hypoxic brain injury, or brain malformations.
- Neonates with limited life expectancy such as severe prematurity or congenital anomalies.
- Members of a family having unexpectedly lost a child from a disease or an external cause or during the perinatal period. These include fetal demise, encephalopathy, overwhelming sepsis in a previously healthy child, trauma from vehicle accidents, and burns.

Planning and implementing palliative care services should be based on the assessment of the type and extent of inadequately prevented or relieved suffering. The attention to local needs is necessary because palliative care services should be people-centered, tailored to the local needs of individual patients and families, with an interdisciplinary team that help ensure that emotional, spiritual, physical, and practical needs of children and families are identified and met [6]. Families' distress can be lessened by reviewing anticipated changes in appearance that occur as death approaches. CPC is crucial in acute cases such as those in Africa and in Latin America due to the poor conditions in which children reach hospitals. Thus, in Niger, 138 out of 461 children under the age of 2 die in the hospital within their first 2 months and 47% die within 24 hours of hospitalization [15]. In Mali, 345 out of 1644 children die during their admission and 40% within 24 hours of admission [16]. In Guinea-Bissau, 20% of all child deaths occur in the hospital or 12 months post-hospital [17]. High infant mortality from pneumonia, measles, and malaria requires that there be a good CPC from the time of the emergency and that they benefit from pain management and grief support. It is necessary that the child is without pain or distress. The philosophy of palliative care is the same with children as with adults, but the implementation of care is different because of the following [3, 4–6]:

- Children change continually as they grow from neonates to adolescents.
- Cognitive abilities and emotional maturity of children and adolescents make them more resilient.
- Good communication with patients and their families requires sensitivity to the child's developmental stage and to the language, culture, and illness and understanding of both the patient and family and their degree of trust in the healthcare system.
- Differences in the causes of life-threatening illnesses.
- Children require palliative care for longer periods than adults. They may need it for 1 day or a decade or more and, on average, the length of specialized CPC is about 40% longer than for adults.
- Children's dependence on others ranges from the total dependence of a neonate to the high degree of independence of some adolescents.
- Degree of difficulty of clinical decision-making. Authority for decision-making regarding care lies with the parents, not the child.
- Pediatric formulations and dosing of essential medicines. The pharmacokinetics of medicines is often different in children, but there is little or no evidence regarding the safety or effectiveness of some palliative medicines in children.

Pain is reported to occur, on average, in 67% for progressive nonmalignant conditions, 55% for HIV/AIDS, and 80% for cancer [8]. Alleviating the burden of pain, suffering, and severe distress associated with life-threatening or life-limiting health conditions and with end of life is a global health and equity imperative. Pain is much broader than just physical damage to tissues and causes distress for both the child and family [18]. Effective pain management includes identifying pain, assessing its severity, and performing preventive measures and treatment to either eliminate or reduce pain. There is a general agreement that pain in infants, children, and young people is often underestimated and undertreated. It is a multidimensional phenomenon with sensory, physiological, cognitive, affective, behavioral, and spiritual components, is subjective, and is experienced by children as well as adults.

The WHO two-step approach, which excludes codeine due to its severe side effects in children, is an effective strategy for the pharmacological management of persisting pain in children with medical illnesses. We recognize that codeine is more accessible in many hospitals and is inexpensive and widely available. It should be used in children older than 12 years for acute to moderate pain if paracetamol or ibuprofen alone is ineffective, but is not recommended for adolescents from 12 to 18 whose breathing might be compromised [19]. Tramadol is extensively used around the world, particularly where morphine is not available, and often with a good safety profile and analgesic efficacy. In clinical practice there is a large body of pediatric clinical experience regarding excellent safety and efficacy with the use of other mu-agonist opioids, namely, fentanyl, alfentanil, oxycodone, methadone, and buprenorphine. In neuropathic pain and visceral hyperalgesia, gabapentin and pregabalin are now used in most pediatric palliative specialist units. In the advanced management of pain in children with serious conditions, in order to provide excellent analgesics without oversedation, it may be necessary to combine nonopioids, opioids, adjuvant analgesics, and anesthetic or neurosurgical interventions with rehabilitative, and especially integrative, therapies [18].

Essential Package of Palliative Care and Pain Relief

Poor availability of essential palliative care medicines offers a formidable barrier to proper pain management with 89% of the world's population lacking adequate access. The 2017 WHO Essential Medicines List (EML) affirms the need for access to essential medicines, including opioids. There is an increasing crisis in accessibility, availability, quality, and affordability of WHO-recommended essential medicines for children. Member states are urged to ensure that they have "a medicines policy that will ensure the availability of essential medicines for the management of symptoms, including pain and psychological distress, in particular, opioid analgesics for relief of pain and respiratory distress." Access to essential palliative care medicines, such as oral morphine, in limited availability in LMICs has enormous but unrealized opportunities to improve the welfare of poor people at modest cost. Public financing and fully integrating an essential package of palliative care and pain relief interventions into national health systems can ameliorate a large part of the preventable burden of serious health-related suffering (SHS) [5] (see Table 2).

Table 2 Essential package of palliative care and pain relief health services [5, 6]

Medicines	Ibuprofen-naproxen, diclofenac
Amitriptyline	Lactulose
Bisacodyl (senna)	Loperamide
Dexamethasone, oral and injectable	Metoclopramide
Diazepam, oral and injectable	Metronidazole, oral and injectable
Diphenhydramine	Morphine, oral immediate-retard or injectable
Fluconazole, oral	Naloxone, injectable
Fluoxetine, sertraline, or citalopram, oral (> 8 years old)	Omeprazole, oral
Furosemide	Ondansetron, oral and injectable (>1 month)
Hyoscine, oral and injectable	Paracetamol
Haloperidol, oral and injectable	Petroleum jelly

The medicines included in this essential package for both adults and children meet three criteria: (1) they are necessary or essential to prevent or effectively relieve the specific symptoms or types of suffering most commonly associated with any of the 20 health conditions, (2) their safe prescription or administration requires a level of professional capacity that is typically available in a primary care setting if augmented by basic training in palliative care, and (3) in keeping with WHO guidelines, there must be medicines of their class that best balance accessibility on the world market, clinical effectiveness, safety, ease of use, and minimal cost [5].

It is very important that pediatric formulations are available, along with immediate-release liquid oral morphine. Pain in children is a public health concern of major significance in most parts of the world. The extremely limited availability in LMICs of morphine – the most essential of medicines to relieve SHS – is emblematic of the most extreme inequities in the world. The poorest 10% of countries have access to only 10 mg of morphine equivalent per patient in need of palliative care. This amount is sufficient to meet less than 2% of estimated palliative care needs for the relief of severe pain and dyspnea, and, according to INCB registries [20] from 2014, of the 298.5 metric tons of morphine available for medical use worldwide (average distribution in 2010–2013), only 0.1 metric ton

(100 kg) or less than 4% was distributed to LMICs. The cost to cover morphine equivalent pain treatment for all children over 15 years old would be one million US dollars per year. Pain control medication, including morphine, should be available in all environments as long as access can be controlled. It can be made universally accessible to remedy the abyss in access to care and offer a solution [5].

The health services of the essential package must be complemented with human resources: doctors and nurses with basic palliative care training, social workers, and other interventions for the relief of social and spiritual suffering to preserve the dignity of patients, to facilitate access to health interventions, and to prevent financial hardship and impoverishment. Opiophobia, the fear individuals have about prescribing/using opioids, exists in many parts of the world with beliefs such as there being a maximum dose of morphine that can be given safety; the fear of addiction, of tolerance, and of issues such as respiratory depression; the possibility of misuse; or the myth that children and babies do not experience pain.

Barriers and Challenges in Palliative Care

The integration of palliative care within health systems requires an understanding of population needs [7]. Palliation is needed not only for pain control in the final moments of life but should also be available at every part of the cancer pathway: at the time of surgery and radiotherapy and during chemotherapy. CPC has demonstrated that it improves not only the welfare of children and families but also the outcomes and reduces costs. There are many barriers associated with palliative care, such as a lack of policies supporting high-quality palliative care at regional and national levels, lack of medication availability, lack of integration into the health system, and lack of awareness of its need and available services [21]. It is time to recognize that children who need palliative care face tremendous barriers to accessing it, and there must be a priority to remove these barriers. The development of standardized programs and regional scorecards, incorporating qualitative and quantitative measures, could facilitate reporting and program development [22, 23].

As many children around the world are suffering needlessly due to pain and distress, there is a great need for training pediatricians, family physicians, pain specialists, and pediatric surgeons with basic skills in pain and symptom management [3] (including pharmacological and non-pharmacological methods), as well as the specific aspects of end-of-life care: communication skills, decision-making support, ethical issues, and psychological and spiritual dimensions of life and illness, including personal feelings about anxiety and grief. All physicians should be trained in basic approaches to prevent, assess, and manage symptoms and to communicate in a clear, caring, and collaborative manner with patients and families. Access to medications, in particular that of moderate-to-severe pain-relieving opioids, is essential to CPC development. While the majority of medications recommended for inclusion in the Essential Medical List (EML) for palliative care have been included, this does not always mean they are available. Fortunately, not all infants, children, and adolescents will need access to specialist palliative care; for many, an integrated approach by primary health providers should be adequate enough to meet their needs. Dedicated specialty CPC should be consulted for advanced clinical treatments and complicated decision-making regarding social and spiritual needs beyond what the primary care team can provide [21]. Many LMICs lack rehabilitation medicine specialists and services and long-term facilities to care for children with non-life-threatening but serious disabilities such as paraplegia or quadriplegia or those due to brain injuries or congenital anomalies. In addition, mental health services and social welfare programs may have limited capacity, are difficult to access, or are unavailable. In these countries, prevention for the relief of acute suffering and of suffering due to non-life-threatening conditions is often inadequate or unavailable.

Cancer in Children in Low- and Middle-Income Countries

Cancer is a leading cause of death for children, especially in LMICs where they are four times more likely to die of the disease than children in high-income countries (HICs). A child diagnosed with cancer in some low-income countries (LICs) has an 80% probability of dying, compared to less than 20% in HICs. An analysis of the Global Burden of Disease Study estimated a global incidence of 416,500 new cases of childhood cancer in 2017 that contributed to 11.5 million disability-adjusted life years (DALY) with 82% of this burden affecting low-, low-middle-, and middle-income countries [22–23]. Age can largely influence someone's ability to understand and communicate their early symptoms of cancer, making children particularly vulnerable to cancer. Early diagnosis can bring substantial reduction in mortality and long-term morbidity, but, to be fully realized worldwide, it must be accompanied by improved diagnostic and treatment facilities with universal access [24, 25]. Diagnostic delays necessitate more intensive therapy to control the malignancy, causing more economic burden to those paying and considerably more anxiety for patients and families. Inadequately treated illnesses create increased poverty, morbidity, loss of income, and impoverishment [26].

Nearly 40% of the world's children are expected to have undiagnosed cancer and are often neglected in cancer control planning efforts, despite the disproportionately high number of years of life lost due to missed opportunities to diagnose and treat cancer in LMICs. Other factors that influence this gap include high rates of co-morbidities (e.g., malaria, HIV, TB, diarrhea, and malnutrition); lack of diagnostic capability; insufficient resources and trained laboratory and radiological staff; paucity of trained nurses and doctors to treat patients, plus failure to retain those trained within LMICs; overall inadequate facilities and resources in hospitals; and lack of availability, accessibility, and affordability of good-quality essential medicines [27, 28] (all on the WHO list).

The most common worldwide childhood cancers are acute lymphoblastic leukemia (ALL) and tumors of the central nervous system, which make up 32% and 20.4% of childhood cancers, respectively. These are the most important cancers of childhood but frequently go underdiagnosed and under-reported in sub-Saharan Africa [27]. The "embryonal tumors" (neuroblastoma, renal tumors, and retinoblastoma) are confined largely to younger children, whereas cancers in adolescents include more epithelial tumors such as thyroid carcinoma and melanoma. The overall incidence of childhood cancer was more than five times higher in Africa compared with Europe and North America combined, due to the increased incidence of types of cancer other than ALL. In Western Africa, there was a significantly higher rate of lymphomas, retinoblastomas, and renal tumors, including 60% of the global incidence of Burkitt's lymphoma (BL). South Central Asia had the highest occurrence of ALL, Hodgkin's lymphoma, neuroblastoma, and central nervous system tumors [28]. BL arises in sub-Saharan Africa from a combination of the high prevalence of *Plasmodium falciparum* malaria [29] which produces a degree of T-cell immunosuppression resulting in B-cell proliferation within which the omnipresent Epstein-Barr virus also proliferates [26]. In 2018, de Martel et al. [30] found that an estimated 2.3 million infection-attributable cancer cases were diagnosed worldwide (13% of the global cancer incidence). GLOBOCAN 2012 showed that the four most important infectious pathogens for cancer incidence were *Helicobacter pylori*, high-risk human papillomavirus, and hepatitis B and C viruses which, together, caused more than 90% of infection-related cancers worldwide [30], *H. pylori* being the most important infectious cause.

For potential cure, three crucial factors are needed: (1) access to a timely and accurate diagnosis, (2) access to the most appropriate treatment, and (3) the efficacy of that therapy [31]. The initial, most worthwhile focus must be on the treatment of infection-related cancers as they all have a communicable disease connection and occur in places where considerable financial resources are needed in order to reduce infections.

For more than 80% of children, a cure for cancer is possible with treatments such as chemotherapy, surgery, and radiotherapy. Kaposi's sarcoma, retinoblastoma, and Wilms' tumor are potentially curable using standard therapies, provided they can be afforded by low-income communities [31]. In HICs, BL has a 90% survival rate and can be cured using intensive chemotherapy. An early diagnosis is very important because stage IV cancers have a survival rate of only 27%. Unlike for many adult cancers, it is not possible to improve the survival rate of childhood cancers through "prevention or early detection" – with a few notable exceptions, such as retinoblastoma, BL, Kaposi's sarcoma, liver tumors, and all HIV-associated tumors, where there is a hope of preventing them when formative measures (control of known infections, antiretroviral, and vaccinations) are applied rationally and persistently. Many carcinogenic infections have potentially modifiable risk factors for which prevention tools already exist.

Prescribing and delivering chemotherapy is frequently more complex. It needs the continual monitoring and assessment of patients receiving chemotherapy. There must also be adequate treatment facilities available, including surgery, radiotherapy, and a medical oncology team having the necessary palliative skills for delivering the chemotherapy. The delivery of cancer chemotherapy in Africa is further hindered by the widespread lack of healthcare professionals skilled in administering these agents, limited access to laboratories for blood count analyses, and insufficient effective antiemetic treatments. The manpower required to support the entire system must be trained and in place and adequate funding is needed to support these new developments [32]. The higher chance of curing children with cancer also requires the consistent availability, accessibility, affordability, and, above all, high quality of essential medicines. Sadly, the whole journey of medication – from production to the bedside – remains a big challenge [31].

To help staff respond quickly to infections and other causes of rapid clinical decline in children with cancer, an early warning system has been developed to facilitate identification, team communication, and management for children with cancer [31–35]. This early warning system was validated in Guatemala in collaboration with St. Jude Children's Research Hospital, where the system effectively reduced the number of children who deteriorated and decreased the need to transfer patients to an intensive care unit. In other LMICs, the so-called adapted treatment regimens have been helpful; for instance, the number of toxic deaths after initial treatments for BL may be reduced and managed by an additional few weeks of lower-intensity treatments. Other providers, in order to mitigate known chemotherapy toxicity in settings with less available supportive care, have studied the use of reduced chemotherapy doses, as well as low-cost modifications, to facilitate monitoring when measuring drug levels is not possible [25].

Toxic death is a leading cause of treatment failure for children with cancer in LMICs. The occurrence rate can be as high as 24–30% in higher-risk patients during the first month of therapy, with the risk depending on the type of cancer, the regimen used, and the supportive care available. Appropriate supportive care, especially at the beginning of treatment, is one of the biggest challenges of LMICs. Nutritional support, management of infections, and aggressive hydration (for hematologic cancers and bulky tumors) to prevent tumor lysis syndrome can effectively reduce the risk of early toxic death. In some areas of Africa, intestinal parasite therapy is routinely given before the start of chemotherapy to help protect children from common infections that can become overwhelming and potentially fatal when the child's immune system is weakened by malignancy as well as the treatment [25, 30, 34–36].

The reasons for abandonment of treatment, defined as four weeks or more of missed appointments during therapy, include poverty, the local cost of treatment, lower education of parents, distance from the cancer center, the type of cancer, and, in some cases, lack of patient care. In some settings, such as in rural Zambia, abandonment rates approached 50%. In Côte d'Ivoire (the Ivory Coast), nearly half of the children with Burkitt's lymphoma abandoned treatment shortly after the first administration, resulting in only a 6% cure rate. To address this problem, various strategies have been deployed. In Central America, only 6.5% of patients with anaplastic large-cell lymphoma abandoned therapy, perhaps because of its relatively short treatment duration. In El Salvador, in addition to free treatment, the implementation of a tracking protocol with community-based interventions for missed appointments successfully prevented abandonment in almost all patients; in Recife, Brazil, a comprehensive social support and educational program reduced abandonment from 16% to 0% [25]. When no oncologists are available, care can be provided by local physicians and nursing teams with the support of exterior staff trained at Harvard-based facilities. Some pilot programs in Malawi, Rwanda, and Haiti show that the absence of oncological specialists need not delay the implementation of mutually reinforcing efforts to prevent, screen, treat, and palliate cancer [25].

The 5-year survival rate of children with cancer has increased to 45% higher in HICs than in LMICs for ALL and up to 51% higher for children with brain tumors [25]. This progress partially reflects the optimized use of conventional therapies (cytotoxic drugs) through better risk stratification of patients, but these survival trends vary widely, and there are wide and persistent disparities between countries; for example, it is twice as high in Denmark and Sweden (around 80%) as in Mexico and Brazil (less than 40%) for children diagnosed as recently as 2014. In ALL, survival rates vary substantially worldwide, indicating major deficiencies in the diagnosis and treatment of a disease that is generally considered as curable. It is higher than 90% in several countries, including Canada, the USA, and nine European countries, but it remains below 60% in China, Mexico, and Ecuador. In September 2018, WHO established the 2018 Global Initiative for Childhood Cancer, which aims to achieve a global survival rate of at least 60% for all children diagnosed with cancer by 2030 thereby saving an additional one million lives [29]. This new target represents a doubling of the global cure rate for children with cancer. For diagnosed cases, the 5-year net global childhood cancer survival rate is currently 37.4% with large variation by region, ranging from 8.1% (4400–13,700) in Eastern Africa to 83% (81,600–84,400) in North America. Pediatric cancer survival rates in LMICs, however, range from 10% to 50% [31]. Investments that improve the quality of care, at both the health system and facility level, are needed to improve global childhood cancer outcomes [36]. From 2005 to 2006, cancer was among the top three causes of death in children aged 5–14 in Mexico, Brazil, and China.

In LMICs without specialized services, experience has shown that much can be done to prevent and treat cancer by the deployment of primary and secondary caregivers, using off-patent drugs, and applying regional and global mechanisms for financing and procurement. The management of cancer still poses enormous challenges [22]. There are a growing number of innovative programs that effectively address the challenge of treating childhood cancers in developing countries in spite of constrained resources. These can be and have been replicated around the world. For example, St. Jude Children's Research Hospital's international outreach program has partnerships with 15 countries that provide mentoring, consultation of clinical services, education, and research to strengthen children's cancer services in resource-poor countries. Several middle-income countries (MICs) have included cancer treatment in their national health insurance coverage with a focus on people living in poverty [33].

Barriers and Challenges in Cancer

Childhood cancers (CC) have higher cure rates than adult cancers, but programs tend to be concentrated in urban centers, and those in countries and capital cities publicizing multiple programs still may not be accessible to children in rural areas; therefore, best practice models may not reflect care elsewhere in the region. Despite improvements in awareness, services, and treatments, cancer still kills more than 100,000 children worldwide every year. Although provision of CPC can be challenging in LMICs, it is crucial precisely because 90% of children at risk for developing cancer live in LMICs where limited and curative therapy is less available. The governments must try to create essential supportive care resources and need to raise a global campaign to raise awareness of the signs and symptoms of cancer among the public and health workers to reduce missed or late diagnoses. There is a high rate of treatment refusal and subsequent abandonment, most frequently due to non-affordability and/or perception of incurability [31].

The Essential Medicines List proposed a list of 51 drugs – chemotherapeutics, antimicrobials, and supportive care medications – which are most critical to treat common pediatric cancers effectively [24]. Using the concept of graduated intensity treatment appropriate to their setting, healthcare systems can begin escalating treatment and using therapies which can offer a better chance of cure, where possible. This is how the successes in HIV were achieved over several decades [31]. There are low-cost drugs that, if made available, could greatly increase children's survival rates, but the drugs must be efficacious, free of contaminants, and not "false." For example, BL, which is the most common childhood cancer in Africa, is potentially curable at a cost of only US $50 per patient with a generic drug that has a 50% cure rate [36]. According to Eden et al. [31], most LMICs produce very few, if any, drugs within their country, especially anti-cancer medicines. All the drugs required are off-patent and generic but there are periodic episodes of lack of availability, accessibility, and affordability (in some countries) of these drugs and clinical anxiety about drug quality depending on where the drugs were procured.

Eden et al. [31] have shown in their survey that only a small number of LMICs, especially in India and China, buy from the USA or Europe due to the higher cost of drugs produced in these regions. An example of Brazil's experience with asparaginase is instructive; recently, several different brands of drugs especially those difficult to produce, like the enzyme L-asparaginase (a crucial drug for the treatment of ALL), have been shown to be contaminated and/or of low bioavailability. In 2017, anticipating a shortage of native asparaginase, the Ministry of Health in Brazil changed the national supplier to a foreign manufacturer that offered a new, lower-cost product, but this drug was less bioactive and contained contaminating proteins that increased the risk for immune-related side effects [25].This agent has been procured in at least five South and Latin American countries because it is much cheaper than proven products. Chemotherapy and other medications for the treatment and management of cancer are limited and, at times, not available. More worldwide attention to the adequate production of WHO essential medicines is required, especially cytotoxins, so that all children can access the appropriate medicines to enable potential cure. Collaboration across borders would help to develop consistency and facilitate "bulk buying" contracts with the potential for cost reduction and to improve availability and affordability.

Challenges for changing the situation of cancer in developing countries [5, 22, 32, 37–40]:

- Provide the urgently needed infrastructure to properly identify, register, and treat patients.
- Promote the training of oncologists and other cancer-related health professionals to develop regional guidelines specific to childhood cancer registration and treatment (abandonment, modalities, and palliation).
- Make drugs and equipment necessary to treat patients more available. It is necessary to deliver, install, and maintain adequate numbers of radiotherapy machines in each country, as well as linear accelerators, if possible.
- Improve access to healthcare and pathology services. The role of the pharmaceutical industry and others, such as device manufacturers, is critical.
- Opioids must be available for controlling the pain of patients with terminal cancers (and other diseases). It should be the right of cancer patients, no matter where they are, to have access to appropriate treatment of their disease.
- Establish informational campaigns to eradicate the stigma of cancer and put a stop to misinformation.
- Identification and evaluation of low-cost services through task and infrastructural shifts to

the benefit of health systems, even in wealthy countries.

- Coordinated financing and procurement to secure reduced prices and increased access to life-saving interventions.
- Improve everything that promotes greater survival rates, such as vaccinations and treatment against infections involved in cancer. As a third of cancers in Africa are currently caused by chronic infection, treatment and relevant vaccination programs must be funded and implemented worldwide.
- Place cancer as the primary concern for global health programs and renew their efforts to develop cancer drugs and other treatments that are accessible to all. Dedicate more funds to research and increase investments in diagnostic capacities.
- Effective diagnosis and treatment can be introduced, even in rural areas of LICs where specialized services are absent, as proven by successful examples.
- Effectively integrate prevention, early detection, treatment, and palliative care interventions for cancer into basic service packages covered by a combination of social insurance and tax-financed schemes.
- Increase and improve follow-up and registries of patients with cancer so that survival and its determinants, including treatment abandonment, can be measured.
- Provide universal coverage of cancer and palliative treatment, especially to the poorest, and implement universal health insurance that creates equity with respect to access to care.

The lack of specialists, surgeons, and hospitals equipped with diagnostic facilities and operating theaters and patients' inability to access and pay for surgical services in LMICs pose real problems and make it notoriously difficult to diagnose some of the more common malignancies in children (notably, leukemias and brain cancers) [27]. When healthcare professionals suspect cancer, weak referral systems can often prevent them from efficiently referring these patients on to pathology services for diagnostic testing, which inevitably leads to needless delays in treatment. It is essential for cancer advocacy groups, research funding organizations, and patient groups to stop advocating access to expensive (and often low-value) technologies, especially in LMICs, and to concentrate only on those interventions that have a meaningful impact on patients' lives. Governments must not insist on replicating those models established in HICs. It is possible that, for example, in place of medical oncologists, surgeons could be trained to deliver basic low-risk chemotherapy and nurses can be taught to deliver palliative care. The health planners' physicians/nurses need to carefully monitor and record every case, in addition to its outcome. They must try to create the essential supportive care resources and facilities before starting to treat patients and recognize that population-based cancer registries are key policy tools for all patients diagnosed with cancer and to monitor the impact of cancer prevention strategies and evaluate the effectiveness of the health system [35, 38]. Collaboration across country borders for the treatment of individual tumors has increased with the French-African Paediatric Oncology Group leading the way, linking 18 Francophone countries and 23 hospitals in specific tumor studies.

It would also helpful to expand the skill sets of general physicians and surgeons and to train more pathologists; more general and specialized surgeons and manpower are crucial. This includes concomitant enhancements in imaging and pathology [32]. Education and training of all professionals involved are cornerstones to improving the outcome of childhood cancers in a sustainable way. Access to educational materials and dedicating time for training are a challenge in LMICs. Websites such as www.cure4kids.org have transformed the ability to deliver and acquire educational information and are the core tool for communication. Additional training opportunities and materials for healthcare workers from LMICs working with CPC are found at https://sites.google.com/site/sioptrainingopportunities/home [24]. The lack of available chemotherapy and supportive care medications remains a challenge in LMICs. Reports with idealized solutions are very well but that time has passed. It is now necessary for coordinated and sustainable action.

Cost and effectiveness of treatment vary by type of childhood cancer. Although they are eminently treatable, the costs are relatively high for LMIC's health systems; Fung indicates that allocating resources to childhood cancer treatment is a cost-effective investment [29]. Alliances between public, private, and international agencies can improve the outcome of children with cancer in these countries [27, 29, 37]. In addition to medical treatments, over 90% of the population of low-income countries (LICs) lack access to radiation therapy, and it is very difficult for children in Africa needing radiotherapy to travel outside of their country to access this treatment. Radiotherapy, a key to improving survival for certain cancers, is scarce. In Afghanistan, Iraq, and sub-Saharan Africa, 25 countries do not have any radiation units; other countries have one unit per five million people (IEA 2013). It is worth emphasizing that the socioeconomic circumstance of the individual patient/parent is critical to the outcome, but so is the national context [24]. Prevention, early detection, and palliative care interventions for cancer can be effectively integrated into basic service packages covered by a combination of social insurance and tax-financed schemes [5, 38, 39].

Avoidable and Premature Deaths Associated with SHS

WHO defines death as premature if it occurs before the age of 70 as these are deaths that should not occur in the presence of effective and timely healthcare. The Lancet Commission of 2018 [5] showed that the proportion of child deaths in 2015 that can be considered avoidable is particularly high. Overall in LMICs, 4.3 million children died from 1 of 20 health conditions, and 3.8 million (88%) of these deaths are avoidable, compared with 1.1 million (93%) children in low-income countries, 2.2 million (89%) in lower-middle-income countries, and 0.4 million (73%) in high-income countries [5]. For low- and middle-income countries, more than 90% of child deaths associated with SHS are avoidable. Health systems can and should be strengthened through the incorporation of prevention, treatment, survivorship, and palliative care, especially in LMICs.

Children have their whole lives ahead of them, so saving their lives and those of active and young people has a far greater effect on countries' economic development than caring for older people. No longer can nations and people rely on hope; they must begin to act collectively to provide the required resources for CPC and to reduce the effects of cancer in children. In order to improve the palliative and oncological care of children, it is important to coordinate international cooperation among institutions. These efforts can improve patients' quality of life and reduce suffering by ensuring access to morphine for pain, as well as palliative care and psychosocial support. Our efforts to expand palliative care services must be focused on relieving the suffering of people with less resources. Energy and creativity must be summoned for furthering education regarding the integration of palliative care in the health systems of countries with short income. In an effort to surmount these challenges, a number of bilateral and regional collaborative childhood cancer initiatives have been developed in LMICs. These endeavors include forming partnerships with pediatric cancer centers in HICs, promoting capacity building, educating healthcare personnel, implementing treatment strategies, and establishing research programs adapted to local capacity and needs [29].

International collective action is necessary to ensure that all people, including poor people, have access to palliative care and pain relief. A well-functioning and balanced global system must both prevent non-medical use and misuse of medicines and ensure effective access to essential medicines for palliative care, including opioids for pain relief [5, 39–40]. Global institutions and those concerned with the health and welfare of children need to step up and contribute to closing this unacceptable gap in meeting the needs for CPC and healthcare for children with cancer [41]. The lack of staff in oncology research and palliative care requires a closer collaboration between researchers in HICs and LMICs, which must focus not only on the delivery of specific protocols but also on sharing skills to build an individual and organizational local capacity [41–42]. Cancer training and palliative care courses should integrate research methods for the entire team and present research as an essential and critical component to make them more effective; the African School of Pediatric Oncology Initiative is a model of subspeciality training in LMICs [43].

Many hospitals in emerging economies and most in low-income countries lack the basic infrastructure and personnel needed to treat diverse cancers. One of the greatest challenges is the paucity of trained pathologists in many LMICs. In sub-Saharan Africa, only 16 countries have access to basic pathology services – trained staff with the equipment needed to make a diagnosis of cancer. 35% of low-income countries reported that pathology services were generally available, compared to more than 95% in high-income countries. Throughout much of Africa, there is, on average, 1 pathologist for every 2.3 million people. In HICs, there is typically 1 pathologist for every 15,000–20,000 people. Many of the international twinning programs assist by providing modern-era remote telepathology review systems as interim measures until local services can be developed. It is necessary to call upon high-quality cancer institutions all over the world to establish collaborative ventures with African cancer institutes and public health services.

Conclusion

The death of a child in any culture or country, for whatever reason, is a tragedy for society. Therefore, the benefits of teaching and research collaborations among developed countries and low- and middle-income countries for better diagnostics, treatment of cancer, and palliative care services for children are manifold. This will help to improve health systems, reduce suffering, and make people live longer. Often in these countries, professionals in the general population are poorly educated, and hospitals do not have enough equipment or the essential medicines and structures to provide quality care, which leads to longer hospital stays, an increased risk of complications, and mortality. As Marie-Charlotte Bouesseau said in the SIOP in South Africa, "it is time to make things happen." It is a moral imperative/ethical duty of palliative care to transform the modalities of care, moving from the "umbrella strategy" to building the "house" of palliative care for patients and their families, the "house" being an analogy to describe an integrated, people-centered approach and the cultural transformation of health services [13]. We need to attend not just to the diseases but to the suffering of human beings.

World Bank income classifications, based on estimates of annual gross national income, are as follows: low-income countries (LICs), US$1045 or less; middle-income countries (MICs) that are subdivided into (a) lower-middle-income countries (LMIC), US $1046 to $4125, and (b) upper-middle-income countries (UMICs), US $4126 to $12,745; and high-income countries (HICs), US$12,746 or more.

Bibliography

1. ACT and the Royal College of Paediatrics and Child Health (RCPH). http://www.act.org.uk/content/view/77/127.
2. World Health Organization. WHO's definition of palliative care. http://www.whop.int/cancer/palliative/definition/.
3. Pediatric palliative care and hospice care commitments, guidelines and recommendations. Am Acad Pediatr Pediatr. 2019;132(5):966–72.
4. Hauer J. Pediatric palliative care. www.uptodate.com, Last visit, May 2019.
5. Knaul FM, Farmer PE, Krakauer EL, De Lima L, Bhadelia A, et al. Alleviating the access abyss in palliative care and pain relief- an imperative of universal health coverage: the Lancet Commission Report; 2018. www.thelancet.com, https://doi.org/10.1016/S0140-6736(17)32113-8.
6. Integrating palliative care and symptom relief into paediatrics. A WHO guide for health care planners, implementers and managers. WHO; 2018.
7. Sleeman K, de Brito M, Etkind S, Nkhoma K, Guo P, Higginson IJ, Gomes B, Harding R. The escalating global burden of serious health-related suffering: projections to 2060 by world regions, age groups, and health conditions. Lancet Glob Health. 2019;7:3883–92.

8. Connor SR, Downing J, Marston J. Estimating the global need for palliative care for children: a cross. Sectional analysis. J Pain Symptom Manage. 2017;53(2):171–7.
9. Connor SR, Sepulveda Bermedo MC. London: Worldwide Palliative Care Alliance; 2014.
10. UNAIDS FACT Sheet-World Day. 2017. Available online.: https://data.unicef.org/topic/child-survival/neonatal-mortality.
11. Downing J, Boucher S, Daniels A, Nkosi B. Paediatric palliative care in resource poor countries. Children. 2018;5:27. https://doi.org/10.3390/children5020037. www.mdpi.com/journal/children.
12. Hain R, Devins M, Hastings R, et al. Paediatric palliative care: development and pilot study of a "directory of life-limiting conditions". BMC Palliat Care. 2013;12:43.
13. Downing J. Boucher S, Ambler J. Brand T. et al. Inspiration, innovation and integration: highlights from the third ICPCN conference on children's palliative care; 20 May to 2 June 2018, Durban South Africa. e cancer. 2018:12_870. https://doi.org/10.3332/ecancer.2018.870.
14. UNICEF. Global.data.unicef.org/topic/child-survival/neonatal-mortality. https://data.unicef.org/topic/child-survival/neonatal-mortality.
15. Gamatie Y, Prual A, Wollo J, Huguet D. Are pediatric wards in developing countries only places to die? A study of prior to hospitalization risk-factors of death among 0–2 year old hospitalized children in Niamey-Niger. J Trop Pediatr. 1994;40:54–7.
16. Campbell JD, Sow SO, Levine MM, Kotloff KL. The causes of hospital admission and death among children in Bamako. Mali. J. Trop. Pediatr. 2004;50:158–63.
17. Veurum HE, Sodeman M, Biai S, Hedegard K, Aabi P. Increased mortality in the year following discharge from a paediatric ward in Bissau, Guinea- Bissau. Acta Paediatr. 2007;96:1832–8.
18. Downing J, Jassal SS, Mathews L, Brits H, Friedrichsdorf J. Pediatric pain management in palliative care. Pain Manag. 2015;5(1):23–5.
19. Palliative care formulary, PCG6. In: Twycross R, Wilcok A, Howard P, editors. 6th ed.; 2017. Haywarth House Study Centre. Palliative drugs.com.
20. International Narcotics Control Board. Availability of internationally controlled drugs: ensuring adequate access for medical and scientific purposes. New York, NY: United Nations; 2016.
21. Downing J, Powell R, Marston J, Huwa C. et al. Children's palliative care in low and middle income countries. Arch Dis Child. Published online. https://doi.org/10.1136/archdischild-2015-308307.
22. Farmer P, Frenk J, Knaul FM, Shulman N, et al. Expansion of cancer care and control in countries of low and middle income: a call to action. Lancet. Publish online. August 16 2010. https://doi.org/10.1016/S=140-67736(10)61152-X.
23. Caruso AE, Howard SC, Baker JN, Ribeiro R, Lam C. Reported availability and gaps of pediatric palliative care in low and middle income countries: a systematic review of published data. J Palliat Med. 2014;16:12. https://doi.org/10.1089/jpm.2014.0095.
24. Singh R, Challinor JM, Howard S, Israels T. Improving care for children with cancer in low-and middle income countries – a SIOP PODC initiative. Pediatr Blood Cancer. 2016;63:387–91.
25. Lam CH, Howard S, Bouffet E, Pritchard-Jones K. Science and health for all children with cancer. Science. 2019;363:1182–6.
26. Eden T. Childhood cancers in low and middle-income countries: prevention and potentially curable treatment? Cancer Control. 2017; ed69 cancercontrol.info/wp-content/uploads/2017/12/66-70-Eden.pdf.
27. Parkin DM, Stefan C. Editorial: childhood cancer in sub-Saharan Africa. e cancer. 2017;11:ed69. https://doi.org/10.3332/ecancer.2017.ed69.
28. Global improvement in cancer survival but international differences are still very wide. Lancet task force on Expanded Access to Cancer Care and Control in Developing countries. www.gtfccc.harvard.edu; 2011.
29. Fung A, Horton S, Zabih V, Denburg A, Gupta S. Cost and cost-effectiveness of childhood cancer treatment in low-income and middle-income countries: a systematic review. BMJ Glob Health. 2019:4e001825. https://doi.org/10.1136/bmjgh-2019-001825.
30. de Martel C, Georges D, Bray F, Ferlay J, Clifford GM. Global burden of cancer attributable to infections in 2018: a worldwide incidence analysis. Lancet Glob Health; 2019. https://doi.org/10.1016/S2214-109X(19)20488-7.
31. Eden T, Burns E, Freccero P, Renner L, et al. Are essential medicines available, reliable and affordable in low-middle income countries? J Cancer Policy. 2019;19:100180. https://doi.org/10.1916/j.Jcpo.2018.12.002.
32. Boyle P, Ngoma T, Sullivan R, Brawl O. Cancer in Africa: the way forward. ecancer. 2019;13:953.; www.ecancer.org. https://doi.org/10.3332/ecancer.2019.953.
33. About International Outreach. St. Jude Children's Research Hospital. Web 16 Feb 2011.
34. Global surveillance of trends in cancer survival 2000–14 (CONCORD-S): analysis of individual records for 37-513-025 patients diagnosed with one of 18 cancers from 322 population-based registries in 71 countries. Lancet. https://doi.org/10.1016/S0140-6736(17)3326-3.
35. Horton S, Gauvreau CL. Cancer in low and middle-income countries: an economic overview. In: Gelband H, Jha P, Sankaranarayanan R, editors. Cancer: disease control priorities. The International Bank for Reconstruction and Development/The World Bank. 2015;3:263–94.
36. Ward ZJ, Yeh JM, Bhakta N, Frazier AL, Girardi F, Atun R. Global childhood cancer survival estimates and priority setting: a simulation-based analysis. Lancet Oncol. 2019;20(7):972–83. https://doi.org/10.1016/S1470-20145(19)30273-6. E pub 2019, May 22.

37. Hesseling P, Israels T, Harif M, Chantada G, Molyneux E. Practical recommendations for the management of children with endemic lymphoma (BL) in a resource limited settings. Pediat Blood Cancer. 2013;60:357–62.
38. Knaul F, Horton S, Yerramilli P, et al. Financing cancer care in low-resource settings. In: Gelband H, Jha P, Sankaranarayanan R, editors. Cancer: disease control priorities. The international Bank for Reconstruction and Development/The World Bank. 2015;3:281–94.
39. Knaul FM Global task force on expanded access to cancer care and control in developing countries. 2011. www.gtfccc.harvard.edu.
40. Bhakta N, Force LM, Allemani C, Atun R, Bray F, Coleman MP, Steliarova-Fopucher E, Frazier L, Robison L, Rodriguez-Galindo C, Fitzmaurice V. Childhood cancer burden: a review of global estimates. Lancet Oncol. 2019;20:e42–53.
41. Astudillo W, Mendinueta C, De la Fuente C, Salinas A, Comba J, et al. La cooperación internacional en Oncología y Cuidados Paliativos. In: Astudillo W, Mendinueta C, Astudillo E, editors. Cuidados del enfermo en el final de la vida y atención a su familia. 6th ed. Pamplona, 2018. Eunsa, p. 1019–45.
42. Astudillo W, Mendinueta C, Astigarraga I, Salinas A. La necesidad de solidaridad oncológica y paliativa con los niños y adolescentes de países pobres y de recursos limitados. In: Astudillo W, Astigarraga I, Salinas A, Mendinueta C, Navajas A, De Souza C, Jassal S, editors. Medicina Paliativa en niños y adolescentes. San Sebastián: Paliativos sin Fronteras, 2015, San Sebastián, p 711–31.
43. Hessissen L, Patte C.,Martelli H, Coze C., Howards SC, Kili A., Gagnepain-Lacheteau A., Harif M. African School of Pediatric Oncology Initiative: implementation of a Pediatric oncology diploma program to address critical work force shortages in French speaking Africa. Journal of Global Oncology, 01 Oct 2010; 5:1–12. https://doi.org/10.1200/jgo.19.00161.

Part VII

United Kingdom

Transforming End-of-Life Care Through Advance Care Planning and Sharing of Information Digitally

Julia Riley and Joanne Droney

Introduction

Population ageing, frailty and the increased number of patients diagnosed with cancer make the management of dying patients an increasing global challenge [1, 2].

In England annual deaths are projected to increase from 501,424 in 2014 (38.8% aged 85 and over) to 635,814 in 2040 (53.5% aged 85 years and over). In the UK, care homes include residential homes for the elderly and nursing homes for patients requiring general nursing care. Hospices are units that provide specialist palliative care. Between 2004 and 2014, proportions of home and care home deaths increased (18.3%–22.9% and 16.7%–21.2%) whilst hospital deaths declined (57.9%–48.1%). If current trends continue, the number of deaths in care homes and homes will increase by 108.1% and 88.6%, with care home the most common place of death by 2040 [3].

J. Riley (✉)
Institute of Global Health Innovation, Imperial College, London, UK

The Royal Marsden and Royal Brompton Palliative Care Service, The Royal Marsden NHS Foundation Trust, London, UK
e-mail: Julia.Riley@rmh.nhs.uk

J. Droney
The Royal Marsden and Royal Brompton Palliative Care Service, The Royal Marsden NHS Foundation Trust, London, UK
e-mail: joanne.droney@rmh.nhs.uk

Hospital costs are the largest cost element of end-of-life care – in the final 3 months of life, the average cost is over £4500 per person who dies. The bulk of these costs are due to emergency hospital admissions [4].

An analysis of 9000 patients who had died in London and who had documented their preferred place of death revealed that 97.8% expressed a preference to die outside of hospital [5]. In 2018/2019 however, over half of patients in London died in hospitals. People in hospitals are at higher risk of unnecessary medical treatment. There is evidence that people receiving treatment in hospitals at the end of life are more likely to be encouraged towards additional medical treatments. This is the case particularly amongst cancer patients [6].

To sustain current trends, end-of-life care provision in care homes and the community needs to be doubled by 2040 [3]. This may be a conservative estimate given the increasing drive of health care providers to decrease unnecessary hospital admissions.

Modern medicine has become increasingly paternalistic and end-of-life care, particularly in Europe and the USA, has become more medicalised. Dying has become a medical event where in fact it should be a family, a social and a spiritual event. In modern medicine the family doctor is rarely available 24/7, 365 days a year. Services are progressively more fragmented and coordination of care is often poor [7, 8].

M. Silbermann (ed.), *Palliative Care for Chronic Cancer Patients in the Community*,
https://doi.org/10.1007/978-3-030-54526-0_14

Predictions indicate that more people will be dying, people will have a preference to die out of hospitals and the costs of hospital death at scale are prohibitive; alternative models of community care must be considered.

In order to provide a sustainable model of palliative care in the community setting, two key elements must be considered:

1. This model must be focused on the patient. Patients must be provided with sufficient and appropriate information about their diagnosis and prognosis to allow them to understand and make choices about how and where they die. How and where they die may be influenced by their families, friends and spiritual beliefs or lack thereof. In order to take these important factors into consideration, the patient must first be identified as having a limited prognosis and then be involved in a conversation to ascertain their bespoke needs. These conversations are often difficult for professionals to initiate. Training is thus required.
2. When considering new models of care, consideration must be given on how the urgent care services (e.g. the ambulance service) contribute to the care of dying patients and the interface and coordination between urgent care/community care/primary and secondary care health services.

Technology has the potential to revolutionise end-of-life care services if it addresses these two key areas: (a) technology in the form of advance care planning with the patient at the centre of end-of-life care decision-making and (b) where end-of-life decisions are kept up to date and communicated with all relevant health care providers.

In order to overcome the growing pressure on health care providers and to address the increasing costs, the use of technology has to be considered. Technology can help *share* the information that is captured once difficult conversations have been had with patients about their future care (e.g. cardiopulmonary resuscitation). Technology can enable the patients to have a care plan, *one single version* of the truth that is multidisciplinary, editable and accessible by all health and social care providers 24/7 across both acute and community sectors. Technology can improve *coordination* by sharing information in real time across acute and community health and care boundaries. Technology can *report outcomes* and help to identify best practice that can then be shared.

Redesigning end-of-life care models using technology is disruptive and represents a culture change. Success is dependent on the appropriate use and understanding of potential benefits. In terms of end-of-life care, for the technology to positively impact the pathway of end-of-life care patients, this cohort of patients who are in their last year of life should be identified. Once patients are identified, an advance care plan can be created.

Disrupting current ways of working and providing new models of care requires training of clinicians in the new pathway and feeding back to them how the new way of working has better outcomes for their patients.

End-of-Life Culture Change

If health services globally are to cope with the increasing demand for good end-of-life care, then a paradigm shift must occur: a shift from crisis end-of-life care that often requires unnecessary hospital admissions to planned end-of-life care. When end-of-life care is planned, a greater proportion of patients are enabled to die at home [9].

In order to plan care, clinicians need to be able to start difficult conversations with patients regarding their future, resuscitation and prognosis. In order to do this, they require training. Training is essential to the culture change.

Advance care planning is time consuming. Creating bespoke plans for individual patients requires time and thus should be remunerated. Policies need to be changed to show the emphasis on time taken to plan which results in decreased hospital admissions and decreased costs in the longer term. Upstream pain, for downstream gain.

In order to make planning part of routine work, patients who can benefit from having an advance care plan need to be identified proactively.

Historically, health care has been prescribed by doctors. Health care over time becomes medicalised. Creating the best model for end-of-life care for the future should involve joint decision-making with patients and clinicians. It does take time but it does give the patient the opportunity to include their cultural beliefs, their faith and their personal preferences in their future care.

End-of-Life Policy

Culture change requires system changes at all levels from patients to policy.

In England, there is a national policy to prioritise care for people at the end of their lives [10]. The information standard specifies the core content to be held in Electronic Palliative Care Coordination Systems (EPaCCS) and supports the national health care system's objective to increase the use of technology to help people manage their health and care. All EPaCCS must comply with this information standard. The dataset is known as the SCC11580 [11]. Embedding this objective in policy has driven advances in the quality of end-of-life care and incentivised innovation in this area.

Identification of Patients at End of Life

Algorithms

In order to improve end-of-life care, patients in their last 12 months of life need to be identified. Studies have shown that physicians over-estimate prognoses which results in a mismatch between patient wishes and actual care at the end of life [12, 13]. A number of studies have been undertaken to improve prognostication at end of life, but none has been consistently shown to be accurate or applicable in clinical practice. Although not routinely embedded into clinical practice, studies suggest that machine learning has potential to improve end-of-life care through better prognostication and identification of people who are approaching end of life. Several algorithms have been developed to predict those patients who have 6–12 months to live. One such example is the method used by Stanford University School of Medicine. Using deep learning and electronic health record (EHR) data in a pilot study, patients are automatically evaluated by algorithm, which brings patients who are likely to benefit from palliative care service to the attention of the palliative care team (PCT). This approach enables the PCT to reach out to patients [14]. Google AI has also developed predictive modelling regarding time of death [15].

Advance Care Planning

'Advance care planning' (ACP) is the term used to describe the conversation between people, their families and carers and those looking after them about their future wishes and priorities for care.

Advance care planning is a key part of improving care for people nearing the end of life and of enabling better planning and provision of care, to help them live well and die well in the place and the manner of their choosing. It enables people to discuss and record their future health and care wishes and also to appoint someone as an advocate or surrogate, thus making the likelihood of these wishes being known and respected at the end of life.

Preliminary evidence strongly supports the value of ACP in allowing patients to prepare for death, strengthen relationships with loved ones, achieve a sense of control, relieve burdens placed on others and through all these positively enhance hope. ACP has also been shown to strengthen patient-physician relationships, achieve higher congruence between surrogates and patients in their understanding of patients' end-of-life preferences and attain greater satisfaction with and less conflict about these end-of-life decisions. Data specific to end-of-life care practices are more limited but suggest ACP has positive outcomes such as increased hospice length of stay, less time spent in hospital and more deaths occurring at patients' place of choice [16–18].

Need for Control at End of Life

Advance care planning puts the patient in control. The patient makes their decisions and the clinician adds the clinical information. In a survey of 2649 Oregon physicians, Ganzini and colleagues studied the epidemiology of patient-assisted suicide (PAS) in Oregon as well as the characteristics of patients and physicians surrounding the request. The most common reasons for patients to request PAS were a loss of independence, a desire to control the circumstances of death, readiness to die and poor quality of life [19]. When patients make ACPs that are shared with all services who may care for them, they report feeling 'safe'. Many patients do not need round-the-clock carers if they know that, when they call for help, the right care will be delivered, in the right place, at the right time. This can only be done if the right information is shared.

Coordinate My Care: Description of an Innovative Model to Demonstrate the Positive Impact of Technology for Community-Based End-of-Life Care

An innovative, digital advance care planning service has been developed in London. The service is called Coordinate My Care (CMC). CMC is web-based, digital ACP. It aims to put the patients at the centre of their care and provide better coordinated services by improving communications between all health and social care professionals. The teams are joined together through the CMC record, which allows each professional involved in a patient's care to add and contribute to the clinical information.

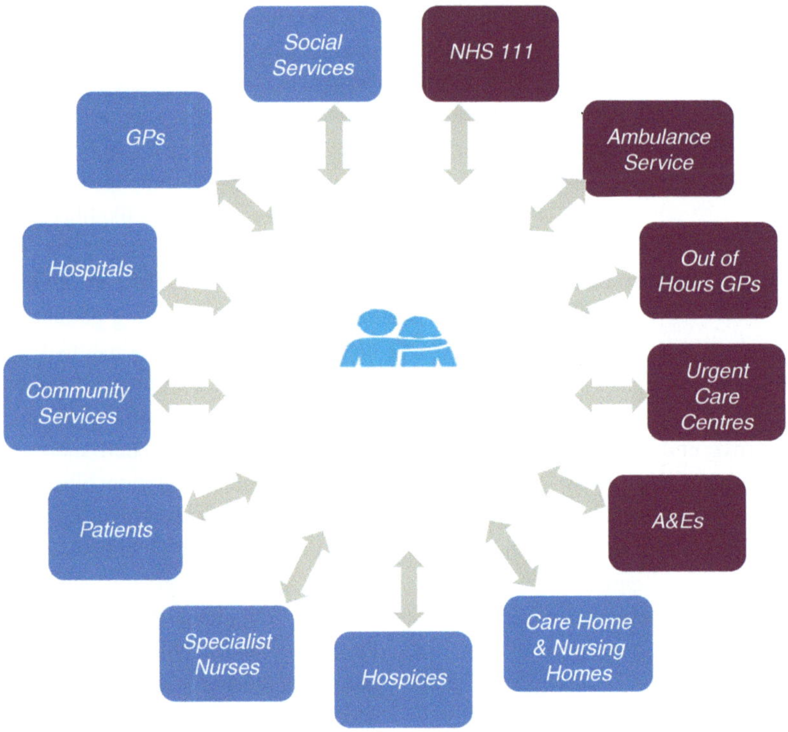

*CMC is a clinical service delivering **digital multidisciplinary urgent care planning** focused on coordinating urgent care around a patient's preferences and clinical needs. The service is underpinned by:*

- *A robust clinical and system training model*
- *A clinical and information governance framework*
- *A strong reporting offering*
- *An intuitive and highly interoperable IT platform*

CMC is 'one version of the truth' by a patient's multidisciplinary care team ensuring that urgent care services view live and accurate information.

Coordinate My Care (CMC) is a London-wide clinical service which facilitates the creation of advance care plans (ACPs), for all vulnerable patients such as patients with a life-threatening or life-limiting illness. Underpinned by a digital information care exchange, CMC allows patients to have their medical details, contacts, ACP, wishes about organ donation and goals of care recorded and shared with acute, primary and emergency health care providers, as well as hospices and care homes, in real time [20, 21].

The record care can be initiated by the patients (via myCMC online). If a patient initiates their CMC plan via myCMC online, they can do this at home with the support of their families and friends. They watch small videos that help them to understand the choices that they can make. Once myCMC is complete, patients can submit their plan to their chosen clinician or family doctor. The clinician then adds the medical details and an escalation treatment plan (i.e. what to do at 2 am in the morning). The clinician then approves the plan. Once approved, the plan is available to be viewed by all the urgent care services. The plan can be updated and edited at any time.

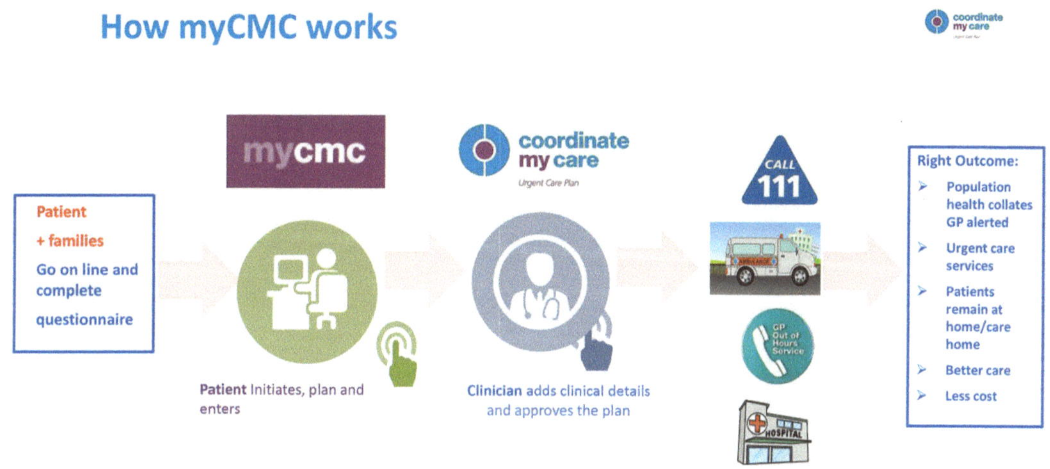

CMC acts as the Electronic Palliative Care Coordination System (EPaCCS) for London$_{11}$. Currently, 82,105 patients have CMC digital advance care plans, 35,322 of whom have died (data censored December 2019. Only 20.7% of patients with a CMC plan have died in hospital, as compared to the national average of 47%). 74% of patients with a CMC died in their preferred place. Analysis of 9027 CMC plans demonstrated that patients with a recorded preferred place of death (PPD) and a documented 'not for resuscitation' order had a 76% greater chance of achieving their PPD [20–23].

Additionally, CMC evaluation of 6854 plans showed patients are willing to engage in advance care and ceiling of care (CoC) planning. Benefits to patients of possessing a CoC include increased likelihood of dying in their PPD along with being more likely to die outside of a hospital setting. More patients with a CoC had a resuscitation decision made. Given this broader planning and decision-making process, patients are more likely to receive appropriate treatment and less likely to have interventions that are futile, inappropriate, distressing or contrary to patient wishes [24].

CMC evidence supports a broader, more comprehensive process to digital advance care planning giving patients the autonomy and ability to live and die the way they choose.

Sharing Patient Care Through Shared Multidisciplinary Care Plans

It is no longer realistic for an individual health care professional to be the sole carer for an individual patient. Care has in the future to be shared. Shared care requires the ability to share care plans. The care plans need to be multidisciplinary. These plans must have the ability to be edited in real time by multiple professionals in different organisations across the acute and the community sectors thus creating a digital, virtual care plan around the patient. This means that when the patient is in need of care, the generic services can respect the wishes and preferences of the patient and the care delivered is clinically the most appropriate way to manage the individual patient. For example, for over 12 months (December 2018 to December 2019), the urgent care services in London accessed the CMC care plans on average 2406 times per month[9]. Sharing information about a patient empowers the generic practitioners to deliver care that they may not otherwise be skilled to give.

Data

Data are shared routinely with the clinical service providers.

As the culture changes within the urgent care services, more CMC plans are viewed each month. The urgent care services include 111 (24/7 telephone advisory service for urgent medical care), out-of-hours GP service (family physicians who care for patients during the out-of-hours service) and the ambulance service.

Care Plan Views Per Month by Urgent Care Service

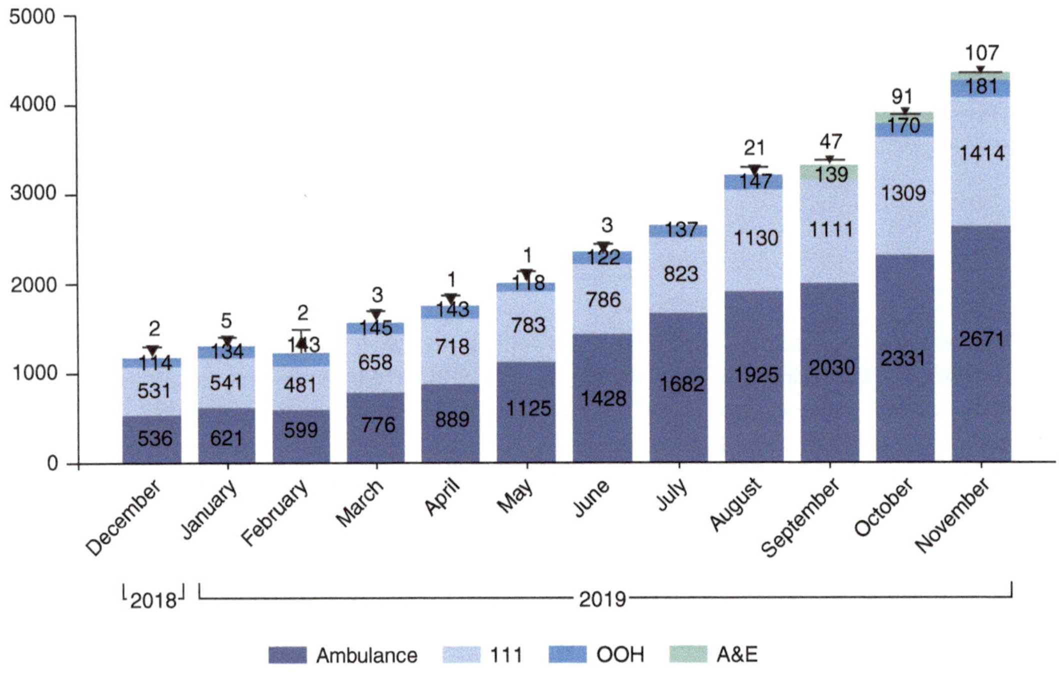

Place of Death

Place of death %	Year December 2018–2019			2010–3/01/2020
	National deaths 484,939	London deaths 48,342	Patients with Coordinate My Care plans deaths	Patients with Coordinate My Care plans deaths 35,631
Home	23.8	24		37.1
Care home	22.5	15.1		26
Hospice	5.9	6.0		15.4 (0.6 other)
Hospital	45.4	52.1		20.7

Case Study of Patient with Coordinate My Care Plan

A patient living in a nursing home has recurrent urinary tract infections. Each time she had an infection, she became confused and disoriented. On one occasion she fell out of bed and on another she had a seizure. Then she created a CMC care plan with her son and her key nurse in the nursing home. Some weeks later at 2 am, she became confused and disorientated and was walking in the corridor having lost her way to her room. The night nurse was new and did not know the patient and panicked. She called 999 (the ambulance service). On arrival the paramedics had already accessed the information about the patient on their mobile devices in the ambulance. The escalation treatment plan said to call the patient's son and start the antibiotics that were in the fridge. They called her son and gave her the medication. Her son arrived and calmed his mother. She stayed in the nursing home and responded well to the antibiotics. The patient was pleased not to go to the hospital and her son was relieved that his mother had not left the comfort of her nursing home.

Conclusions

When end-of-life care is well-planned, well-coordinated and centred around the individual patient, a greater number of patients die in their preferred place. Fewer patients have unnecessary admissions to hospital and costs of the last year of life are thus reduced.

Changing end-of-life care from crisis, reactive care to planned care requires a culture change. A culture change requires training: training to transform how the care is delivered. And the new transformed delivery of care requires technology to underpin it.

A combination of transformation and digitalisation of end-of-life care is a good model for sustainable care for terminally ill patients in the future.

Dying is a family, social, cultural and spiritual event. Modern medicine has medicalised death and increased hospitalisation of the dying. Future care of the dying requires training and technology to decrease medicalisation of death, making it a more personalised, social and spiritual event determined by the individual patient.

References

1. Etkind S, et al. How many people will need palliative care in 2040? Past trends, future projections and implications for services. BMC Medicine. 2017;15:102. https://doi.org/10.1186/s12916-017-0860-2.
2. Sleeman K, Brito M, Etkind S, et al. The escalating global burden of serious health-related suffering: projections to 2060 by world regions, age groups, and health conditions [published online May 22, 2019]. Lancet Glob Health. https://doi.org/10.1016/S2214-109X(19)30172-X.
3. Bone AE, Gomes B, Etkind SN. What is the impact of population ageing on the future provision of end-of-life care? Population-based projections of place of death. https://doi.org/10.1177/0269216317734435
4. Georghiou T, Bardsley M. Nuffield trust. Exploring the cost of care at the end of life. 2014.
5. Callender T, et al. The determinants of dying where we choose: an analysis of coordinate my care. Annals of Internal Medicine. 2017. https://doi.org/10.7326/M17-0695.
6. Davis C. Drugs, cancer and end-of-life care: a case study of pharmceuticalization. Soc Sci Med. 2015;131:207–14.
7. Mason B, et al. Coordination of care for individuals with advanced progressive conditions: a multi-site ethnographic and serial interview study. Br J Gen Pract. 2013;63(613):e580–8.
8. *The Way We Die Now* by Seamus O'Mahony (ISBN: 9781784974268).
9. Callender T, et al. The Determinants of dying where we choose: an analysis of coordinate my care. Annals; 2017.
10. http://endoflifecareambitions.org.uk/
11. Petrova M, Riley J, Abel J, et al. Crash course in EPaCCS (electronic palliative care coordination systems): 8 years of successes and failures in patient data sharing to learn from. BMJ Support Palliat Care. 2016; https://doi.org/10.1136/bmjspcare-2015-001059.
12. White N, et al. Survival in palliative care: how accurate are clinicians and who are the experts? PLOS One. 2016;11(8):e0161407.
13. James Downat et al. The 'surprise question' for predicting seriously ill patients; a systematic review meta-analysis. MSc CMAJ 2017.
14. https://ai.stanford.edu/~avati/bibm17.pdf
15. https://www.nature.com/articles/s41746-018-0029-1
16. Killackey T, Peter E, Maciver J, Mohammed S. Advance care planning with chronically ill

patients: a relational autonomy approach. Nurs Ethics. 2019:969733019848031
17. Bielinska A-M, Obanobi A, Riley J, Urch C. One year mortality: recognising the need for urgent or advance care planning in adults aged over 70 years old following emergency admission. BMJ Support Palliat Care. 2016;6(3):385.
18. Davison SN. Evidence base of Advance care Planning for patients with Advanced disease Research evidence leading to practical implementation. https://doi.org/10.1136/bmjspcare-2011-000053.18
19. Ganzini L, Nelson HD, Schmidt TA, et al. Physicians' experiences with the Oregon death with dignity act. N Engl J Med. 2000;24(342):557–63.
20. Smith C, Hough L, Cheung C, Millington-Sanders C, Sutton E, Ross J, Thick M, Riley J. Coordinate My Care: a clinical service that coordinates care, giving patients choice and improving quality of life. BMJ Support Palliat Care. 2012;2:301–7.
21. Riley J, Madill D. Coordinate My Care: a clinical approach underpinned by an electronic solution. Prog Palliat Care. 2013;2(4):214–9.
22. Callender T, Riley J, Broadhurst H, et al. The determinants of dying where we choose: an analysis of coordinate my care. Ann Intern Med. 2017; https://doi.org/10.7326/M17-0695.
23. Coordinate My Care data censored. 2019.
24. Broadhurst H, Droney J, Callender T, Shaw M, Riley J. Advanced care planning at end of life: The impact of anticipatory decision-making about ceiling of care in patients with a Coordinate My Care Urgent Care Plan. BMJ Support Palliat Care. 2018; In Press bmjspcare-2017-001414.R1

Routine Data and Minimum Datasets for Palliative Cancer Care in Sub-Saharan Africa: Their Role, Barriers and Facilitators

Matthew J. Allsop, Johnblack Kabukye, Richard A. Powell, and Eve Namisango

Background

In sub-Saharan Africa (SSA), 80% of cancers are incurable at the time of detection and diagnosis largely due to late-stage clinical presentation, limited funding and restricted access to curative therapies [1]. In 2018, there were over 770,000 new cancer cases and 514,000 cancer-related deaths across Eastern, Middle, Southern and Western Africa [2]. These figures are projected to continue to rise (up to 1.28 million new cases and 970,000 deaths) by 2030. Increasing incidence of cancer cases is attributed to factors that include ageing, the high residual burden of infectious agents (HIV/AIDS, human papillomavirus, hepatitis B virus) and lifestyle factors [3]. By 2060 an estimated 16 million people with cancer will die annually with serious health-related suffering; a 109% increase from 2016, with the fastest rise occurring in low-income countries (400% increase) [4].

Palliative care—the prevention and relief of physical, emotional, social or spiritual suffering associated with any chronic or life-threatening illness, from the point of diagnosis [5]—is a fundamental component of the essential services within universal health coverage [6]. It is also a realistic response to supporting equitable, accessible and cost-effective interventions for cancer care in SSA. Independent of cancer prevention and treatment efforts in the region, palliative care remains a critical and essential component of care, with proven effectiveness and cost-effectiveness in high-income countries (HICs) [7, 8]. Enormous strides have been made in the development of palliative care services in SSA [9, 10], but there remains a need for significant expansion of provision to meet demand. Across SSA, current provision of palliative care services is limited to 24 of 48 countries, up from only 5 in 2004, with fewer than 5% of people who need palliative care being able to access services in the region [10]. Moreover, whilst models of palliative care for adults in SSA is developing, models of service development, patient assessment and symptom management for paediatric palliative care are urgently needed [11].

A major challenge to developing palliative cancer care across Africa is the lack of local, reliable and valid data to ensure practice is evidence-based

M. J. Allsop (✉)
Leeds Institute of Health Sciences,
University of Leeds, Leeds, UK
e-mail: m.j.allsop@leeds.ac.uk

J. Kabukye
Uganda Cancer Institute, Kampala, Uganda

R. A. Powell
MWAPO Health Development Group, London, UK

E. Namisango
African Palliative Care Association,
Kampala, Uganda

Cicely Saunders Institute, King's College London,
London, UK
e-mail: eve.namisango@africanpalliativecare.org

M. Silbermann (ed.), *Palliative Care for Chronic Cancer Patients in the Community*,
https://doi.org/10.1007/978-3-030-54526-0_15

and replicable and reflects the needs of the population served [12]. Efforts are underway to explore how best to capture patient-level data and information to inform practice [13], this being part of a wider effort to improve the data and information underpinning provision of palliative cancer care in the region. This chapter outlines the role and potential value of routine data and a minimum dataset (MDS) in supporting palliative cancer care in SSA, highlighting barriers and facilitators to their collection and practical utilisation.

Routine Data Collection to Inform Palliative Cancer Care Delivery

'Routine data' describes datasets designed and developed primarily to support direct care provision, or for administrative and managerial purposes, rather than specifically for research. They can be generated at multiple points of interaction between patients, caregivers and health professionals. Routine data broadly exists across three levels: person, service and area (see Fig. 1) [14]. Person-level data may contain disaggregated data about individuals' demographic and clinical characteristics and the care they receive from facilities. Service-level data may focus on a service's capacity and provision (e.g. staff employed, case mix of diseases managed and number of patients seen). Area-level data may provide a regional overview, such as the number of health facilities in a region and number of overall cases of a particular disease.

To ensure that practice is informed by evidence and that any adjustments required to improve delivery and care quality can be implemented, data needs to be used effectively at all levels of a health system [15]. Individual-, service- and area-level data also have value to inform delivery of care for patients with cancer; collection of routine data has enabled the generation of datasets to provide valuable information regarding baseline patient demographics and characteristics, treatments, safety and toxicity and survival and recurrence rates.

Routine Data in HICs: United Kingdom

Across most HICs, recent decades have seen increasing developments in the technical infrastructure underpinning the collection, storage and processing of routine data. Supported by increasing and advancing infrastructure, the growth of electronic health records (EHRs) in HICs enables routine data to be collected about a person's communication and exchanged with health services across their life course. This practice of routine data collection across health services at all levels enables the generation of routine datasets with multiple uses, including for research and quality improvement [16] and supporting integration of services through data linkage (e.g. between primary and secondary care settings). With large, established datasets, EHRs and other routinely collected health data

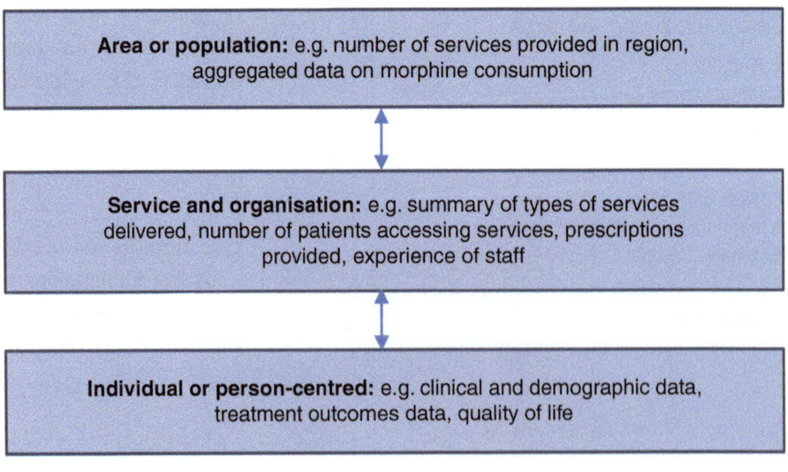

Fig. 1 Example of different levels of routine data for palliative cancer care services in SSA. (Based on Davies et al. [14])

are now enabling the exploration of approaches such as machine learning (i.e. identification of patterns and making predictions using large datasets) to improve clinical decision-making by palliative care professionals [17].

In the United Kingdom, the National Cancer Registration and Analysis Service (NCRAS) is responsible for the systematic collection, quality assurance and analysis of cancer registration data in England to support cancer epidemiology, public health, service monitoring and research [18]. Compiled datasets used by the NCRAS were designed for cancer outcome data, although their ability to support provision of clinical trial follow-up data is being explored [18]. NCRAS data are also used to provide data to the UK Office of National Statistics on new cancer cases and cancer survival, to monitor new cases of cancer in the population and to explore trends and geographic patterns to detect risk factors and cancer clusters. Data are additionally used by the UK National Health Service to assess the quality of care for individuals treated for cancer.

The example of NCRAS highlights the value of information technology (IT) infrastructure that enables data flow from the level of individual hospitals to create a national-level database. The creation of such a database has requisite criteria for sites from which data is drawn, including the use and adoption of certified EHRs, secure transfer platforms and sharing of health information and reporting of quality measures [19]. There have nevertheless been challenges, such as difficulties in the implementation of EHRs in secondary care settings, despite their universal adoption in primary care [20].

Routine Data in SSA

There is an increasing drive to develop approaches to the collection of data to inform care provision in low- and middle-income countries (LMICs). In SSA currently, large volumes of routine data are collected by healthcare staff (e.g. reporting for state and national government ministries of health, often completed through paper-based register ledgers) but the data are often unavailable to staff, including service managers, for meaningful use to inform quality improvement [21]. Receipt of timely data is necessary to inform efforts to improve quality of services, such as use of data when designing, testing and implementing changes using real-time measurement for improvement [22]. Routine data captured across services could be used in such ways to inform delivery and improvements in the provision of care. For example, through gathering clinical and demographic data at a health facility level, it is possible to explore the case mix of patients accessing care, when access occurs prior to an event (such as an onward referral or death) and the types of care they receive. There may also be scope to explore approaches to assessing the impact of health interventions for patients with cancer, with examples already existing for maternal and neonatal health [23].

In the context of palliative cancer care in SSA, advancements are being made in terms of policy supporting its development and the inclusion of palliative care in health budgets. This is increasing the reach and accessibility of care for patients with advanced cancer alongside efforts at the level of those providing care to patients with cancer (e.g. the use of volunteers who are trained as community home-based caregivers to provide palliative cancer care to those requiring support in community settings in Zimbabwe) [24]. However, despite developments in policy and provision, there remains a lack of local evidence to ensure practice is evidence-based and replicable and reflects the needs of the population served [12]. Developing the use and collection of routine data presents an opportunity to document existing provision to determine how and when services across settings are supporting patients with cancer and their families. This approach aligns with recommendations to develop cancer registries and health information systems that collect standardised data which is comprehensive and accurate so that decision-makers can make informed and evidence-based policy decisions [25]. Prior to the use of routine, standardised data being utilised to inform improvements in palliative cancer care in LMICs, there is a need to understand and address barriers to its access and use.

Barriers and Facilitators

Alongside availability and access to data, the situation is compounded broadly across LMICs by multiple additional generic barriers [26]. These include the following and are grouped as personnel, organisational and policy in nature:

Barriers

Personnel

- Demotivated staff involvement: Why should they get involved? What will they gain from their participation?
- Senior management under-appreciation of the potential value and role of data use at the service level.
- Low individual commitment and motivation (e.g. perceived attitudes, motivations and value and potential impact from the use of data).
- Insufficient skills in data collection, use and management core competencies (i.e. in the analysis, interpretation and presentation of data).

Organisational

- Structural barriers, including lack of Internet connectivity and lack of access to computers and power
- Not understanding the needs and preferences of those gathering and using data
- Data use culture (e.g. norms and values of leadership within organisations)
- Poor data quality (i.e. insufficiently timely or accurate)
- Inadequate availability of data (including both awareness of its location and how to combine data sources)
- System design (e.g. unable to respond to the changing needs of decision-makers, low usability)
- Relationships between actors who produce and use data
- Institutional factors influencing data use (e.g. authority figures influencing the role of information in decision-making and agenda setting)

Policy

- No expectations from national ministries of health for palliative care data
- No accountability expectations for data beyond donor agencies, many of whom have their individualised data reporting expectations and data needs

Despite these barriers, there are also known facilitators to the collection and use of data in LMICs [27], including:

Facilitators

Personnel

- Many staff will be responsive to additional skills acquisition.
- Annual performance reviews can embed routine data collection within their frameworks, tailoring expectations to grade level.
- Senior management can be the target of efforts to increase the appreciation of data—from its collection to management and decision-making—as they are the champions for ensuring change.

Organisational

- Many donor agencies are keen on health information management system (HMIS) strengthening, often supporting infrastructure developments (such as alternative power sources and uninterruptable power supply).
- Site-wide training opportunities could be initiated that explain the merits of effective quality data management and analysis, with a sensitised, tailored understanding of the needs and preferences of those gathering and using the data.

Policy

- There is a growing recognition and appreciation of palliative care amongst SSA policymakers. To effect positive palliative care legislation, those policymakers need data to ensure they are evidence-based.
- Rigorously gathered and presented data can be used as the underpinnings of effective advocacy to policymakers to effect positive palliative care legislation but also to ensure there is national budget provision to ensure its effective implementation.

This chapter discusses two examples where the application of routine data could support delivery and development of palliative cancer care services in the context of SSA and reflects further on the existence of barriers and facilitators to their development. More specifically, it focuses on the context of routine data use to guide palliative cancer care delivery in Uganda and the implementation of an MDS for palliative care across the region.

Routine Data Use for Palliative Cancer Care Provision in Uganda

Palliative Care in Uganda

Uganda's level of palliative care development is described as being at an advanced stage of integration in the health system (Group 4b) [28]. It was the highest-ranking African country and 35th country worldwide in the Quality of Death Index of 2015 that ranked 80 countries in terms of quality and availability of palliative care services for adult populations in the world [29]. At the recently concluded mapping of the development of palliative care in Africa, Uganda had the highest number of adult palliative care services amongst the 52 countries assessed [30].

Initially palliative care in Uganda was mainly provided for HIV/AIDS and cancer patients but is increasingly being extended to other life-limiting illnesses, such as persistent chronic respiratory conditions, advanced organ failure and chronic organ failure. Palliative care is currently provided across the various levels of service delivery, from primary to tertiary care settings, and also via hospices, home-based care programmes and non-governmental organisations [31].

The Uganda Cancer Institute—the major cancer care facility provider in Uganda—provides palliative care as an integral part of its cancer care. Primary palliative care is provided by the cancer care team, with the facility also using extended service provision (i.e. specialist palliative care service providers from Hospice Africa Uganda and Mulago Palliative Care Unit) to care for both patients that are referred and those in inpatient settings. Despite national guidance that palliative care should be provided from the point of diagnosis through to death and bereavement, most patients present at very late stages in the disease trajectory, resulting in poor prognoses and outcomes, limiting feasible work to end-of-life care. However, even in this unsatisfactory situation, the bereavement care component of palliative care is weak [32], despite the fact that the loss of a family member can generate grief and bereavement concerns which, if left unattended, can result in suffering and physical, spiritual and psychosocial morbidity [33].

Uganda is one of the few African countries that permits appropriately trained nurses to prescribe opioids for pain management and manufactures oral morphine locally [34]. In terms of policy frameworks, the country is in the final stages of developing a stand-alone palliative care policy, and palliative care is included in the *National Health Care Policy* and in the *Health Sector Strategic and Investment Plan II*, which are integral to the overall development of the Ugandan healthcare system. Additionally, palliative care is integrated into the education curriculum of medical and nursing schools and is monitored and evaluated nationally using indicators such as palliative care patients reporting pain.

Current Use of Routine Data in Palliative Cancer Care in Uganda

A health management information system (HMIS) has been implemented in Uganda to support the capture of routine data on healthcare delivery. All public and private health facilities in the country are mandated to report health data to the district through the HMIS [35]. For example, registers are in place to capture the diagnoses of all patients attending outpatient and inpatient services at public health facilities [36].

These registers were originally focused on issues considered important to public health and included multiple indictors relating to, for example, malaria, childhood diseases, maternal health, HIV/AIDS and tuberculosis. Consequently, there are minimal indicators on cancer and palliative care that are collected in the Ugandan HMIS. Whilst the burgeoning cancer epidemic demands changes in these priorities, there remains limited funding for cancer, amounting to only 2% of the current budget for HIV [37]. This has led to underinvestment in health IT for cancer; very few digital systems, or even comprehensive paper-based systems, have been developed. The current mandated HMIS utilises both the Open Medical Record System (OpenMRS) and District Health Information System (DHIS) platforms. OpenMRS is an electronic medical record solution used in resource-constrained environments [38]. The DHIS used is the DHIS2 platform, which enables ready-made reports to be generated that could cover reporting requirements for health services at all levels, enabling decisions to be made regarding services at health centres, as well as local, provincial and national health departments [39].

For cancer care in Uganda, limited data is currently available about people with cancer, the numbers of cancer cases and the services received by patients. Currently, data on cancer is recorded in the HMIS by health district headquarters. These data are gathered across government-run health facilities through routine, paper-based reporting to both the Municipal Council and health district headquarters. Data are then transformed into an electronic format when they are entered into the HMIS by staff at the health district headquarters. Data reported by government-run health facilities are captured across a range of reporting forms, which include items relating to cancer cases. For example, in the current 'Health Unit Daily Outpatient Diagnoses' reporting form, data is stratified by different age groups: 0–28 days, 29 days–4 years, 5–59 years and 60 years and above. Across age groups, cases of cervical, prostate, breast, lung, liver, colon, Kaposi's sarcoma and 'Cancer Others' are currently recorded. Alongside these data, data on cancer screening services accessed for both cervical and breast cancers are captured as part of the 'Integrated Family Planning Register'. This is the extent of current data recording specific to cancer. There is an absence of recording of contextual or detailed data, such as the staging of cancer at diagnosis or which treatments are accessed by people with cancer. Capturing such additional data, such as disease staging, could provide a coarse proxy measure to identify the point at which people with cancer are accessing services, alongside providing triggers for input from palliative cancer care teams.

Currently, in order to receive input from a palliative cancer care team, palliative care needs should be identified by an inpatient or outpatient facility, who should then count and record cases against the item, 'Need for palliative care'. Where pain management is identified as requiring palliative care involvement, this should be captured using the 'Pain requiring palliative care' item on a 'Health Unit Daily Outpatient Diagnoses' form. This is partly driven by the registration of oral morphine as a palliative treatment by the National Drug Authority, providing a route to strong opioids for pain management [40]. Cases where palliative care need or pain requiring palliative care has been identified should be reported via paper-based forms submitted to health district headquarters. A challenge with this process is the reliance on non-specialist teams across health facilities to identify the seriousness and stage of a progressive illness, with evidence that late referrals to palliative care are commonly occurring very close to death (i.e. a median of 5 days) [41]. Furthermore, recording a need for palliative care does not guarantee that those needs are addressed through a referral and subsequent access to a palliative service.

Existing routine data captured in Uganda may reflect objectives and priorities set by the Ministry of Health at a national level (e.g. capturing 'Pain requiring palliative care' to inform data on consumption of opioids and subsequent procurement). There may be scope to explore supplementation of existing datasets to create a valuable resource to guide decision-makers and managers at the service delivery level. Table 1 outlines the potential use of data currently captured when supplemented with demographic data, cancer staging information and recording of interactions with health services. Including such data could help to determine access to and processes of care for people with cancer across the different stages of the cancer trajectory.

Table 1 Overview of potential uses of routine data to inform delivery of care, including palliation, for patients with cancer in Uganda

Stage of cancer trajectory	Prevention	Diagnosis	Treatment	Palliation	Remission	Survivorship	Longer-term follow-up
Area or population	Determine cancer types with late presentation at a regional level to inform targeted cancer prevention strategies	Determine staging of disease at diagnosis	Determine time between diagnosis and onset of treatment	Determine timing of access to palliative care during cancer trajectory Understand extent of access to palliative care at regional and national level (e.g. number of patients with advanced cancer who access palliative care services)	Determine number of cases and service utilisation	Determine number of cases and service utilisation	Determine number of cases and service utilisation
Service and organisation	Identify number and characteristics of patients currently accessing available cancer screening programmes	Determine staging of disease at diagnosis, exploring variation by factors such as region, rurality, age, sexual orientation and cancer type	Understand pathways of care experienced by patients with different cancer types Identify treatment modalities used by specific cancer types Determine effectiveness of treatment regimens based on survival and person-centred outcome data	Determine palliative care need by those accessing the service Determine extent of pain management across different cancer types	Determine service utilisation by patients in remission	Determine service utilisation by survivors of cancer	Determine longer-term service utilisation, survival and subsequent health service utilisation

There are efforts currently to enhance the capture of routine data aligned to these data types for cancer care generally in Uganda. The Uganda Cancer Institute is working with the country's Ministry of Health to develop forms within the HMIS for routinely collecting detailed data on palliative care and cancer, including cancer stage and pain scores. Once developed, adapted forms may have value beyond the Uganda Cancer Institute to other facilities providing cancer care. Adaptation of forms to, for example, primary health facilities will create opportunities to understand wider access to, and use of, health services by patients beyond a specialised, tertiary care medical facility like the Uganda Cancer Institute.

Whilst there is scope to develop approaches to the capture and use of routine data to inform cancer care in Uganda, there exist multiple barriers and facilitators. Below we outline these across the health system, from the level of health facility personnel to organisation-level factors, and those relating to existing health and data policies in the country.

Use of Routine Data to Support Palliative Cancer Care Delivery in Uganda: Barriers and Facilitators

Whilst there may be potential value in utilising routine data in the context of palliative cancer care in Uganda, barriers and enablers similar to those for HMIS development more generally exist. The most pertinent ones are listed in Table 2, grouped into three categories: personnel, organisational and policy.

Minimum Dataset for Palliative Cancer Care in Sub-Saharan Africa

Whilst operational in a number of health fields, a MDS may not necessarily be as comprehensive as some HMIS datasets. Whilst comparably designed—composed of a standardised set of data items, with agreed definitions, across a number of domains that all participating agencies collect on a regular periodic basis—MDS can be more modest in ambition, focusing on the collection, storage, reporting and utilisation of a minimum or core set of data metrics.

In some countries, like in the United States, a palliative care MDS is embedded into federally mandated processes for clinical assessment of all residents in Medicare- or Medicaid-certified nursing homes and non-critical access hospitals [45]. It can also be less a regulatory requirement than a financially contingent one. Again, in the United States, reporting across various dataset metrics summarising utilisation data—i.e. who provides care, who receives care, where care is provided, the range and quality of hospice services, staffing levels and demographic, cost and payer data—is required by insurers and Medicare. For insurers, reporting links to direct billing to enable receipt of a daily per diem, with reporting to Medicare required on utilisation data. For the latter, sanctions for not reporting utilisation data include reductions in reimbursement.

In the vast majority of SSA countries, where there are no national or local regulatory obligations, or financial incentives, to collect routine data, information collected by palliative care services is at best inconsistent and at worst non-existent. Moreover, whilst aiming to integrate routine data for palliative cancer care into the HMIS of a country is the optimal goal, such a process can be protracted, with the need to negotiate existing stakeholders' demands and priorities, including those of any external funding agency with a pivotal role in supporting the HMIS. In this scenario, an MDS at the service level could be a useful interim development that in a shorter time-frame provides broadly comparable data to that which an HMIS would generate and which could be aggregated up across all providing sites to depict a national-level picture. The development of a core MDS therefore not only has potential utility in advancing palliative cancer care service provision but, given existing staffing limitations and data management challenges, may be the most feasible way forward in many SSA countries.

Table 2 Overview of barriers and facilitators to utilising routine data in the context of palliative cancer care in Uganda

Barriers to routine data use for palliative cancer care in Uganda	Facilitators to routine data use for palliative cancer care in Uganda
Personnel There is currently a low readiness for digital health across cancer services in Uganda, alongside users' low computer skills. There is no technical intervention set up to support and maintain the reporting of cancer data across health services.	**Personnel** Initiatives are available and training underway, for some individuals, in the management and analysis of data (such as in the development and implementation of new HMIS templates to align with cancer service provision).
Organisation Current IT infrastructure across health services remains a challenge. Furthermore, rural areas lack electricity and internet access so they require alternative approaches, such as local servers, which may be difficult to implement at scale. Paper-based HMIS are currently being used that are then entered into the digital HMIS by data clerks. This process risks transcription errors, reduces the near real-time potential of direct digital data entry and also creates duplication of data recording activities for facility staff. The private health sector in Uganda is large and informal and the governance surrounding data capture in such facilities is unclear, as is how their data is aggregated alongside public health facilities. Reporting of data creates opportunities to respond to highlighted needs, but with a limited health expenditure budget, the health system and its response to need can often be slow or not occur.	**Organisation** There are increasing examples of willingness to collaborate to understand the needs and preferences of those gathering and using data to inform optimal uses of routine data. A recent example is the collaboration between the Uganda Cancer Institute and Uganda Ministry of Health to develop the use of electronic medical records for patients with cancer. Open source systems are being developed to support secure data systems across health facilities in Uganda. Open source systems (such as DHIS II and OpenMRS) avoid commitment to expensive licences and enable collaborative reuse and development of software.
Policy Data to be collected by facilities has been determined by policymaker priorities around specific conditions, which has not historically included cancer. Limited indicator development has been carried out previously due to limited investment in cancer. Consequently, there are very few indicators relating to cancer and palliative care that are reported at the national level. Current information technology policy in Uganda makes it difficult to develop infrastructure to support routine electronic data capture across multiple sites. For example, there is no specific online privacy regulation within data protection laws for Uganda, and this may lead to concerns over the reliability or legality of electronic data. These are significant barriers as they may add to the inertia towards electronic data collection, despite the insecure, inaccessible and low-quality properties of some existing paper-based data collection processes.	**Policy** Strong political will and policy exists that mandates evidence-based decision-making, demonstrated through specific mention of cancer and palliative care data as a strategic priority area in the eHealth strategy for Uganda. The current eHealth strategy 2017–2021 [42] refers to cancer and palliative care where it is deemed a strategic objective. The granularity and ease of data collection may evolve in coming years with plans for the Ministry of Health to use information and communication tools, such as electronic clinical record systems and clinical information systems, to improve patient identification, support collection and management of patient data and inform clinical decision-making. The Government of Uganda records government support for the use of new approaches, for example, the use of mobile phones for data collection using the mTrac application, which uses the SMS (short message service) function of basic mobile phones to transmit data from paper forms to a central electronic database [43]. The Government of Uganda has a strong track record of working in partnership with development partners, including in the use of mobile platforms to bridge the gap in access to healthcare services and information, enabling faster and more effective coordination of healthcare and professionals, and digitisation of drug inventory and supply chains [44].

What Might a Palliative Cancer Care MDS Contain in SSA Settings?

Balancing the need for meaningful data with the practicality of a regularised exercise in low-resource environments, a palliative cancer care MDS could be characterised by metrics again across three operational domains: patient, service and area levels.

Individual or Person-Centred Level

- At this level, data could explore patients' socio-demographic (age, sex), clinical profiles (primary and secondary diagnoses, pathways to care, length of admission, medicine regimens and services received, onward referrals and mortality outcomes) and patient-reported outcome measures.

Service and Organisation Level

- At this level, data could explore the number of patients carried forward (monthly), number of new admissions, discharges, those lost to follow-up, deaths, the number of services provided (sites of care across home-based, outpatient, inpatient and day care), sources of referral and data on costs of care.
- Useful data could also be derived from exploring the number of staff at sites, their professional disaggregation, if they are full- or part-time (and if the latter, how much full-time is their equivalency) as well as the extent of duration in their profession, current job and the extent and nature of the palliative cancer care training they have received.
- Over time, and following strategic direction, such information could also help demonstrate the value of data, nurturing a culture at sites that appreciates data collection as more than a 'tick box' exercise but which can inform local decision-making and service development. Such a culture that attaches value to data could also act as a preliminary foundation block in attempts to encourage research at palliative care sites that actively includes local staff.

Area or Population Level

- At this level—and dependent upon the comparability of the MDS tools being used—data could be used to investigate variation across district, national and regional levels.
  - *District or provincial level:* Data could compare care provision with similar services (geographically or by size, capacity or case mix), identify potential service referral networks, determine best practices and lessons learnt that could be shared between not-for-profit providers operating at similar levels of service delivery and identify opportunities for linkages between services.
  - *National level:* Data could help define the reach and delivery of palliative care services across all aggregated palliative care providers, provide valuable insights into the nature and extent of current palliative cancer care need and those factors that can potentially impact upon patient outcomes, foster linkages between other front-line service providers, highlight inter-provider service differences and raise the profile of palliative care. These data can also be used for advocacy purposes, such as lobbying policymakers to include palliative care MDS in national HIMS for planning and budgetary purposes and ensure policy initiatives are embedded in evidence and attuned to actual needs.
  - *Regional level (SSA):* Data could facilitate intra-regional comparisons. Such data could again be used to provide benchmarking data that can supplement existing regional comparative work, supplementing these metrics with more clinically orientated metrics.

Such data usage could be derived from cross-sectional analyses but also from longitudinal analysis, using initial derived data as a benchmark against which to make service development comparisons over time. The proposed metrics provide a useful mix of data that can be used to understand quality within a complex system, including a mix of outcomes (what matters to patients), processes (the way work is being conducted) and structures (e.g. resources, equipment, governance [21]). Selection of outcome measures could then be used to inform improvement efforts with process measures used to assess how a service is operating.

Implications and Future Directions

Appropriate and effective health service development is partly premised on the availability and utilisation of useful, relevant and reliable data on current service provision and use. Some specialist health fields—especially those in LMICs that are significantly dependent upon external donor funding (e.g. HIV, malaria), where financial accountability for public expenditure is imperative—have access to large HMIS datasets. These data are collected on a routine basis by providers at the community level and are often aggregated up to the national level for reporting purposes. Such data can be rich in nature, providing information across multiple metrics.

Throughout this chapter we outlined a case for developing the use of such routine data in the context of services delivering palliative cancer care. There are multiple opportunities for using data to inform care delivery, with specific examples provided for existing provision of cancer care in Uganda and the role of an MDS across the SSA region. There is scope to gather and use data of differing levels of granularity, from the individual patient level through to service delivery and policymaker decision-making. Whilst multiple potential benefits exist from increased use and engagement with routine data, there are competing barriers and facilitators to achieving this in practice.

Common challenges across both personnel and organisation levels are the lack of readiness for digital health and the skills required to support the development, and maintenance of systems to capture and share routine data. There is scope to capitalise on wider developments across LMICs to address these barriers. Many LMICs are currently rolling out digital health approaches, presenting an opportunity to align efforts in palliative cancer care to increase electronic data capture and use. However, there is currently a lack of the requisite digital health workforce required to expand and sustain such approaches. Resources continue to be developed to target this gap in skills, such as work by MEASURE Evaluation. Together with the Global Evaluation and Monitoring Network for Health (GEMNet-Health), MEASURE Evaluation has developed an international health informatics curriculum to be used as in-service training for digital health staff [46]. This generic curriculum addresses key aspects of health informatics, including efforts to strengthen demand for and use of data, improving data quality and communicating the results of data demand and use interventions. There is scope to develop accompanying materials aligned specifically to cancer care at a country level, to determine specific uses and analyses of data that can be undertaken, understanding the content and availability of datasets for initiatives that involve centralisation and data linkage, and how these can be used to evaluate and improve existing provision of services for people with cancer. Examples of such programmes include advanced training courses for cancer registry staff by the African Cancer Registry Network and provision of data quality experts by the International Agency for Research on Cancer to provide training and technical assistance to registries globally.

Across SSA, development in the availability, quality and affordability of electronic mobile technology—such as telephones, personal digital assistants and electronic tablets—is creating an environment that is conducive to digital health approaches. This presents opportunities to collect data from healthcare facility registers and patients during health consultations and to transfer large quantities of data. An innovative solution utilising emerging technologies has been deemed an urgent health priority. However, this cannot be achieved without wider efforts to develop effective implementation of cancer care and control policies to improve pathways to care for people with, and at risk of, cancer [47].

These wider health systems strengthening efforts require policy-level advocacy for the importance and need for developing the extent of data capture on cancer, alongside strong leadership and clear policy direction coupled with the financial support to acquire essential technology, improvements in communication networks, and training for staff; all of which can help to promote implementation and use of routine data [48]. Furthermore, with the example of Uganda, there is scope to work in partnership with ministries of health to determine which mutually beneficial data could be captured on cancer that can inform both service delivery and policymaker decision-making. Such stakeholder engagement lends itself to user-centred design approaches to the development of health IT systems. Current data capture often involves paper-based systems conducted by healthcare workers, which is used by managers and ministries of health located some distance from the individual clinician collecting the data. There is a need to explore holistic perspectives in developing routine data collection approaches to explore whether the value and utility of data can be sought across all levels, alongside ensuring routine health information systems align with existing functioning health systems [49]. Efforts to move to routine data collection that may utilise digital health approaches need to ensure appropriate end user engagement to secure value and utility in collected data. It is hoped that by bringing about meaningful engagement with routine data, developments in the quality and scale of palliative cancer care delivery can be realised across countries in SSA.

References

1. Ferlay J, Soerjomataram I, Dikshit R, Eser S, Mathers C, Rebelo M, et al. Cancer incidence and mortality worldwide: sources, methods and major patterns in GLOBOCAN 2012. Int J Cancer. 2015;136(5):E359–86.
2. Globocan: All cancers [Internet]. International Agency for Research on Cancer. 2018. Available from: https://gco.iarc.fr/today/data/factsheets/cancers/39-All-cancers-fact-sheet.pdf.
3. Jemal A, Vineis P, Bray F, Torre L, Forman D. The Cancer atlas. American Cancer Society: Atlanta; 2016.
4. Sleeman K, Brito M, Etkind S, Nkhoma K, Guo P, Higginson I, et al. The escalating global burden of serious health-related suffering: projections to 2060 by world regions, age groups and health conditions. Lancet Glob Health. 2019;7:e883–92.
5. World Health Organization. WHO Definition of Palliative Care. https://www.who.int/cancer/palliative/definition/en/2020.
6. Knaul FM, Farmer PE, Krakauer EL, De Lima L, Bhadelia A, Jiang Kwete X, et al. Alleviating the access abyss in palliative care and pain relief-an imperative of universal health coverage: the Lancet Commission report. Lancet. 2018;391(10128):1391–454.
7. Gomes B, Calanzani N, Curiale V, McCrone P, Higginson IJ. Effectiveness and cost-effectiveness of home palliative care services for adults with advanced illness and their caregivers. Cochrane Database Syst Rev. 2013;6
8. Smith S, Brick A, O'Hara S, Normand C. Evidence on the cost and cost-effectiveness of palliative care: a literature review. Palliat Med. 2014;28(2):130–50.
9. Fraser BA, Powell RA, Mwangi-Powell FN, Namisango E, Hannon B, Zimmermann C, et al. Palliative care development in Africa: lessons from Uganda and Kenya. J Global Oncol. 2017;4:1–10.
10. Downing J, Grant L, Leng M, Namukwaya E. Understanding models of palliative care delivery in sub-Saharan Africa: learning from programs in Kenya and Malawi. J Pain Symptom Manag. 2015;50(3):362–70.
11. Harding R, Albertyn R, Sherr L, Gwyther L. Pediatric palliative care in sub-saharan Africa: a systematic review of the evidence for care models, interventions, and outcomes. J Pain Symptom Manag. 2014;47(3):642–51.
12. Harding R, Selman L, Powell RA, Namisango E, Downing J, Merriman A, et al. Research into palliative care in sub-Saharan Africa. Lancet Oncol. 2013;14(4):e183–8.
13. Okunade K, Bashan Nkhoma K, Salako O, Akeju D, Ebenso B, Namisango E, et al. Understanding data and information needs for palliative cancer care to inform digital health intervention development in Nigeria, Uganda and Zimbabwe: protocol for a multicountry qualitative study. BMJ Open. 2019;9(10):e032166.
14. Davies JM, Gao W, Sleeman KE, Lindsey K, Murtagh FE, Teno JM, et al. Using routine data to improve palliative and end of life care. BMJ Support Palliat Care. 2016;6(3):257.
15. Wagenaar BH, Hirschhorn LR, Henley C, Gremu A, Sindano N, Chilengi R, et al. Data-driven quality improvement in low-and middle-income country health systems: lessons from seven years of implementation experience across Mozambique, Rwanda, and Zambia. BMC Health Serv Res. 2017;17(Suppl 3):830.

16. Peltan ID, Beesley SJ, Brown SM. Can big data deliver on its promises?-leaps but not bounds. JAMA Netw Open. 2018;1(8):e185694.
17. Storick V, O'Herlihy A, Abdelhafeez S, Ahmed R, May P. Improving palliative and end-of-life care with machine learning and routine data: a rapid review. HRB Open Res. 2019;2:13.
18. Bhattacharya IS, Morden JP, Griffin C, Snowdon C, Brannan R, Bliss JM, et al. The application and feasibility of using routine data sources for long-term Cancer clinical trial follow-up. Clin Oncol (R Coll Radiol). 2017;29(12):796–8.
19. Bandopadhyay S, Murthy GVS, Prabhakaran D, Taylor P, Banerjee A. India and the United Kingdom—what big data health research can do for a country. Learn Health Syst. 2019;3(2):e10074.
20. Sheikh A, Cornford T, Barber N, Avery A, Takian A, Lichtner V, et al. Implementation and adoption of nationwide electronic health records in secondary care in England: final qualitative results from prospective national evaluation in 'early adopter' hospitals. BMJ. 2011;343:d6054.
21. Shah A. Using data for improvement. BMJ. 2019;364:189.
22. Perla RJ, Provost LP, Murray SK. The run chart: a simple analytical tool for learning from variation in healthcare processes. BMJ Qual Saf. 2011;20(1):46–51.
23. Dossa NI, Philibert A, Dumont A. Using routine health data and intermittent community surveys to assess the impact of maternal and neonatal health interventions in low-income countries: a systematic review. Int J Gynaecol Obstet. 2016;135(Suppl 1):S64–s71.
24. Khumalo T, Maasdorp V. The island hospice model of palliative care. Ecancermedicalscience. 2016;10:654.
25. Prager GW, Braga S, Bystricky B, Qvortrup C, Criscitiello C, Esin E, et al. Global cancer control: responding to the growing burden, rising costs and inequalities in access. ESMO Open. 2018;3(2):e000285.
26. Evaluation MEASURE. Data in Low- and middle-income countries: a review of the literature. North Carolina: MEASURE Evaluation; 2018.
27. Akhlaq A, McKinstry B, Muhammad KB, Sheikh A. Barriers and facilitators to health information exchange in low- and middle-income country settings: a systematic review. Health Policy Plan. 2016;31(9):1310–25.
28. Lynch T, Connor S, Clark D. Mapping levels of palliative care development: a global update. J Pain Symptom Manag. 2013;45(6):1094–105.
29. Economist Intelligence Unit. Quality of death index: ranking palliative care across the world. London: The Economist; 2015.
30. Rhee JY, Luyirika E, Namisango E, Powell RA, Garralda E, José Pons J, de Lima L, Centeno C. APCA atlas of palliative Care in Africa: IAHPC Press; 2017.
31. Rhee JY, Garralda E, Torrado C, Blanco S, Ayala I, Namisango E, et al. Palliative care in Africa: a scoping review from 2005-16. Lancet Oncol. 2017;18(9):e522–e31.
32. Gysels M, Pell C, Straus L, Pool R. End of life care in sub-Saharan Africa: a systematic review of the qualitative literature. BMC Palliat Care. 2011;10:6.
33. Mutedzi B, Langhaug L, Hunt J, Nkhoma K, Harding R. Improving bereavement outcomes in Zimbabwe: protocol for a feasibility cluster trial of the 9-cell bereavement tool. Pilot Feasibility Stud. 2019;5(1):66.
34. Jagwe J, Merriman A. Uganda: delivering analgesia in rural Africa: opioid availability and nurse prescribing. J Pain Symptom Manag. 2007;33(5):547–51.
35. Wandera SO, Kwagala B, Nankinga O, Ndugga P, Kabagenyi A, Adamou B, et al. Facilitators, best practices and barriers to integrating family planning data in Uganda's health management information system. BMC Health Serv Res. 2019;19(1):327.
36. Ministry of Health. The health management information system, vol. 1. Kampala: Republic of Uganda Ministry of Health; 2014.
37. Moten A, Schafer D, Farmer P, Kim J, Ferrari M. Redefining global health priorities: improving cancer care in developing settings. J Glob Health. 2014;4(1):010304.
38. Syzdykova A, Malta A, Zolfo M, Diro E, Oliveira JL. Open-source electronic health record systems for low-resource settings: systematic review. JMIR Med Inform. 2017;5(4):e44.
39. Dehnavieh R, Haghdoost A, Khosravi A, Hoseinabadi F, Rahimi H, Poursheikhali A, et al. The district health information system (DHIS2): a literature review and meta-synthesis of its strengths and operational challenges based on the experiences of 11 countries. Health Inf Manag J. 2018;48(2):62–75.
40. Nabudere H, Obuku E, Lamorde M. Advancing palliative care in the Uganda health system: an evidence-based policy brief. Int J Technol Assess Health Care. 2014;30(6):621–5.
41. Low D, Merkel EC, Menon M, Loggers E, Ddungu H, Leng M, et al. End-of-life palliative care practices and referrals in Uganda. J Palliat Med. 2018;21(3):328–34.
42. Ministry of Health. Uganda national eHealth strategy. Kampala: Republic of Uganda Ministry of Health; 2017.
43. World Health Organization. Strengthening accountability chains for maternal, newborn and child health in Uganda–mTrac. Geneva: World Health Organization; 2014.
44. GSMA. Uganda: Driving inclusive socio-economic progress through mobile-enabled digital transformation. London. 2018.
45. Thomas KS, Boyd E, Mariotto AB, Penn DC, Barrett MJ, Warren JL. New opportunities for Cancer health services research: linking the SEER-medicare data to the nursing home minimum data set. Med Care. 2018;56(12):e90–e6.
46. MEASURE Evaluation. Health informatics in low and middle-income countries: short course for health information system professionals course syllabus.

https://www.measureevaluation.org/resources/publications/ms-18-144/: MEASURE Evaluation; 2018.
47. Bhatt S, Evans J, Gupta S. Barriers to scale of digital health systems for cancer care and control in last-mile settings. J Global Oncol. 2017;4:1–3.
48. Kumar M, Gotz D, Nutley T, Smith JB. Research gaps in routine health information system design barriers to data quality and use in low- and middle-income countries: a literature review. Int J Health Plann Manag. 2018;33(1):e1–9.
49. Hotchkiss DR, Diana ML, Foreit KG. How can routine health information systems improve health systems functioning in low- and middle-income countries? Assessing the evidence base. Adv Health Care Manag. 2012;12:25–58.

Part VIII

Eastern Europe: Poland

Palliative Home Care in Poland: From Times of Political Turnovers to a Well-Structured Integrated System

Aleksandra Ciałkowska-Rysz
and Aleksandra Kotlińska-Lemieszek

Introduction

Palliative medicine in Poland is one of the youngest, dynamically changing disciplines of medicine. On the one hand, these changes result from the ageing of the population and the increase in incidences of lifestyle-related diseases and, on the other hand, from the progress made in the treatment of many illnesses, as well as the introduction of new, effective methods of symptomatic treatment. The funding system and legislative solutions have a significant impact on the situation in palliative care in Poland. Legislative changes introduced since the 1990s not only enabled the emergence of a new area in the Polish health-care system, but also ensured sources of funding and the necessary education of medical staff. However, a medical discipline which developed initially based on a civic movement required the definition of principles of functioning and standardisation, and earlier the assessment of the actual situation and available resources, as well as the precise definition of the target population of patients who are to be its beneficiaries. The first informal palliative care teams and the first voluntary teams at oncology hospitals have achieved a high degree of professionalism through coordinated organisation, education and the provision of the necessary financial resources.

Historical Background

Home-based care is the fundamental form of palliative care organisation in Poland, and its origins go back to the 1970s, when informal groups of volunteers started forming in order to look after terminally ill patients living at home. The next stage was the creation, since the 1980s, of non-profit organisations, often linked to churches and religious congregations, frequently associated with the Solidarity civic movement which was developing at that time in protest against the existing communist reality and which played a key role in social and political changes in Poland [1–3]. These groups consisted of clergymen and lay people, but medical assistance was the responsibility of professionals, doctors and nurses. The activities undertaken at that time were based entirely on voluntary work. The main objective of these organisations was to provide care to patients dying of cancer. The second important role of the organisations at that time was to educate medical personnel on pain management and to work towards changing the approach of the medical community and the general public to people who

A. Ciałkowska-Rysz
Clinical Department of Palliative Medicine, Medical University of Lodz, ŁódŹ, Poland
e-mail: olarysz@rmed.pl

A. Kotlińska-Lemieszek (✉)
Department of Palliative Medicine, Poznan University of Medical Sciences, Poznań, Poland
e-mail: alemieszek@ump.edu.pl

M. Silbermann (ed.), *Palliative Care for Chronic Cancer Patients in the Community*,
https://doi.org/10.1007/978-3-030-54526-0_16

were dying. At the end of the 1980s and the beginning of the 1990s, the first inpatient and home care units were established as components of the health-care system. In 1993, the National Council for Palliative and Hospice Care at the Ministry of Health was formed with the aim of developing the principles of palliative care organisation, drafting legal acts allowing free access to analgesics and educational programmes for physicians and nurses [2]. Professor Jacek Łuczak was the first President of the Council. In 1998, the Palliative Care Development Programme in Poland was approved. At the same time, the palliative medicine specialisation for physicians and specialisation in palliative care for nurses were also approved [4]. Thanks to the initiative of the National Council, the state budget allocated funds for palliative care. The reform of the health-care system in Poland in 1997 and the introduction of the Act on Universal Health Insurance also ensured access to public funds for entities operating outside the public health-care system [2]. Since the year 2000, there has been a rapid increase in the number of home care hospices operating in the public, non-profit and private sectors. All of them were treated equally by the health system and could obtain financing from health insurance for their activities for the benefit of patients. The vast majority of entities that initially based their activities on volunteering applied for public funding and employed medical staff. There are still several units that are fully based on voluntary work across the country, but they provide care to only a small number of patients. In other units, there are volunteers, who play an auxiliary role in the provision of medical care. In most of the units, campaign volunteering, mainly involving pupils and students, predominates. This type of volunteering organises civic campaigns on palliative care and raises funds for a given organisation.

Place of Palliative Care in the Polish Health-Care System

In Poland, palliative care is an integral part of the health-care system [2, 5]. Palliative medicine has been a medical specialty for physicians since 1999 [4]. The first diplomas for physicians were obtained in 2003. The diploma has since been awarded to 573 physicians [6]. The specialisation in palliative care nursing was approved by the Minister of Health in 1998 (first certificates for nurses—2006). These specialist diplomas have been awarded to 2142 nurses to date.

The most important legal acts constituting the basis for the functioning of palliative medicine units include the Act of 2004 on Healthcare Services Financed from Public Funds. This statute guarantees free access to palliative care and hospice care services. The legal act, defining in detail the list and conditions of guaranteed services in palliative and hospice care, is the Regulation of the Minister of Health on guaranteed services in the field of palliative and hospice care of 2009, and since then has been amended on numerous occasions (the last amendment took place in 2018) [5]. According to this regulation, palliative and hospice care services are provided free of charge under the following conditions:

- At home—in a home hospice for adults
- At home—in a home hospice for children under 18 years of age
- Inpatient—in an inpatient hospice or in a palliative medicine ward
- Outpatient—in a clinic for palliative medicine
- Perinatal palliative care

Access to these services is guaranteed by the state [7–9].

In Poland, so far, the state budget has not financed hospital support team services, and in recent years, the functioning of palliative day-care centres has not been financed, so these forms are few. The day-care centres that do operate are financed by local authorities or non-profit organisations.

The 2009 Regulation of the Minister of Health on guaranteed services in the field of palliative and hospice care lays down standards concerning the number of medical staff employed, professional qualifications and equipment of units, as well as the manner of providing care. Palliative care unit physicians should specialise in palliative medicine or complete a course organised by a unit authorised to train physicians according to a specialisation programme (with subjects including pain, somatic symptoms, psychological problems and communication).

In Poland since 2014, the Ministry of Health has been preparing maps of health needs in various fields of medicine; the last such map concerning palliative care was prepared for 2016. This document analyses the situation of palliative care and the resources as well as the needs for palliative care. It will serve to set the directions for the development of palliative care in the country in the years to come.

Home Palliative Care for Adults in Poland: Principles of Organisation and Integration with Other Forms of Professional Care

Home care is the most optimal form of help for a patient with an advanced incurable life-limiting disease and his or her family. The present chapter concerns home care for adults, excluding the activities of separate children's hospices managed by paediatricians. The basic principle of organising home care for sick adults in Poland is the 24-hour access to services, seven days a week. In accordance with the 2009 Regulation of the Minister of Health on guaranteed services in the field of palliative and hospice care, multidisciplinary home care teams are composed of doctors, nurses and psychologists; in most hospices additionally physiotherapists, chaplains, social workers and, in some hospices, also volunteers. According to the recommendations of the Regulation, one physician looks after a maximum of 30 patients in home care, and 1 nurse can take care of a maximum of 15 patients [5]. Visits of individual team members should take place depending on needs, but there should be no less than two visits per month by a doctor and at least two visits per week by a nurse [5]. Additional unscheduled visits are also possible in the event of an emergency. Patients requiring fewer visits should be redirected to outpatient care, while patients with symptoms that are difficult to control at home or with inefficient family support are redirected to inpatient care. Other members of the home care team visit patients with a frequency that depends on the individual needs of the patient and his/her family. The education of the staff involved should be in accordance with the services they provide. Volunteers working with patients should complete a palliative care volunteer course. In addition to specialist care, home care patients have free access to necessary specialist equipment such as pneumatic mattresses, infusion pumps, oxygen concentrators, rehabilitation equipment and more. Patients receiving home hospice care have the right to obtain services as part of basic health care (with the cooperation of palliative care teams with the family doctor and community nurse) and all specialist services offered within the framework of health insurance. They can also receive oncological treatment if there is an indication for such therapy.

In order to provide optimal care to the patient, home hospices are integrated into the inpatient and outpatient palliative care system. The healthcare system allows for the unlimited movement of patients between these forms of care in accordance with ongoing needs. Unfortunately, the number of beds in inpatient care is insufficient in some parts of the country, and the demand for this form of care is growing throughout Poland. Although the best place for patients to live in the last period of life and at the time of death is the home, an inpatient hospice may be the best option for a person living alone or with a family which, for various reasons, is unable to provide the patient with care in the last period of life. Home care patients are also admitted periodically to inpatient hospices or palliative care units in the event of developing symptoms which are difficult to alleviate at home, or the need for diagnostic and treatment procedures or family respite. Recently, in order to support families caring for patients at home, some home hospices have been implementing additional projects financed by the European Social Fund under Regional Operational Programmes for individual voivodeships. Within the framework of these programmes, professional carers are directed to the patient's home, and in some units, there are also physiotherapists, dieticians or psychologists who provide support to the patient's family to a greater extent than can be provided by the permanent hospice staff.

There are currently 476 home hospices for adult patients operating in Poland [6–9]. These are units meeting organisational standards, employing professional staff and receiving funding from the state budget. Patients receive free care there, but in many areas, the waiting time for care may constitute a limitation, since it may range from a few days to a few weeks. The latter situation absolutely needs to be improved and this is what the national consultant in palliative medicine at the Ministry of Health and the Board of the Polish Society of Palliative Medicine (PTMP) are expecting. In 2018, 56,820 patients benefited from home palliative care for adults in Poland (which is about 60% of over 95,000 patients who die from cancer in our country every year) [10]. Qualification to palliative care is made by a physician employed in a palliative care unit on the basis of an assessment and diagnosis in accordance with the International Classification of Diseases (ICD-10) [11]. Individuals with cancer diagnoses (ICD C and D) are eligible for palliative care in accordance with the Minister of Health's Regulation, regardless of the stage of disease progression and prognosis, if symptomatic treatment (e.g. pain treatment) is necessary. In addition, palliative care, including home care, may also be provided to patients with diseases classified under the ICD G code, with consequences of inflammatory diseases of the central nervous system, systemic CNS atrophies and sclerosis multiplex; the ICD B code, diseases caused by HIV; ICD L code, bedsore ulcers; ICD I code, cardiomyopathy; and ICD J code, with chronic respiratory failure. Among adult patients, approximately 80% of palliative care patients are cancer sufferers. Patients with other chronic diseases not included above are guaranteed long-term nursing care services in Poland.

Drugs Available at Patient Home

Patients in home care have access to all medications used for symptomatic treatment available in the country [12]. These drugs are prescribed by palliative care physicians or other physicians (e.g. family doctors), and the caregivers collect these prescriptions at the pharmacy. Most medicines are purchased for a low fee, as their cost is flat-rate and the patient bears a fixed fee of less than 4 Polish zlotys (the equivalent of about 1 US dollar). Some analgesics essential for cancer pain management, such as morphine in immediate release tablets or ampoules, are provided to the patients free of charge. The pain medications on the second step of the WHO analgesic ladder include tramadol, codeine and dihydrocodeine. If the pain is severe or very severe, patients may use strong oral opioids (morphine, oxycodone) or buprenorphine and fentanyl in transdermal formulations. Also methadone in syrup, tapentadol in controlled release tablets and a compound preparation of oxycodone with naloxone are available and reimbursed for patients with cancer pain. In case of breakthrough pain, patients can use morphine with a short duration of action (administered orally or parenterally) or transmucosal preparations of fentanyl (nasal, buccal or sublingual). For neuropathic pain, gabapentin and pregabalin are available and reimbursed. The amount of opioid medications prescribed is based on patients' needs and not limited [12]. Patients in home care can also benefit from enteral or parenteral nutrition if there are clinical indications for such procedures.

Challenges and Directions of Development

For many years now, there have been discussions in Poland concerning extending the indications for palliative care to other patient groups. As is well known, the current qualifications system based mainly on diagnosis favours cancer patients [11, 13]. It must be agreed that this patient population can benefit most from specialist palliative care, especially in view of the difficult situation of the health-care system in the country, the growing shortage of doctors and nurses, insufficient funding and the lack of effective reform to meet the changing needs of an ageing population. It should be added here that cancer patients, particularly those at advanced stages of the disease, may, in view of the many overlapping medical, psychosocial and spiritual needs, be difficult to handle by other physicians, such as family doctors or internists. These doctors are much more willing to continue the end-of-life care of patients suffering from other progressive chronic diseases such as cardiovascular or respiratory diseases. One should keep in mind, however, that according to the current definition of palliative care, the system of qualification for palliative care should not be based solely on diagnosis, but on the needs of the patient. This issue is the subject of an ongoing discussion among experts in our country, but it has not yet been possible to reach a consensus. It should be remembered that the actual needs for palliative care exceed the available resources by far, which can be allocated under the current financing of the health-care system in Poland [14]. Therefore, a separate direction of advancement is education in the basics of palliative care at the level of pre-graduate and postgraduate education [15]. Such education is provided within the framework of medical and nursing studies and during the specialisation of internal medicine physicians and oncologists. Improving the access to palliative care requires additional sources of funding. State resources are limited, and private insurance constitutes a negligible minority. Additional financing goes to hospices in Poland from non-profit organisations that raise funds from grants, civic collections and 1% of the income tax that each citizen can donate to a selected non-profit organisation. These resources are used to improve the quality of the offered palliative care services including, in particular, home care and often to provide financial support for the patient (e.g. by reimbursing expensive medicines or dressings) and for carers of the patient and the bereaved (e.g. children who have lost a loved one).

A large number of home hospices should ensure full access to this service, regardless of the place of residence. However, the distribution of home hospices is not even, and there are still places in some voivodeships where access to palliative care is very limited [7–9]. In recent years, attention has been drawn to inequalities in the access to care for patients living in urban and rural areas. Telemedicine may become a partial support for the care system in remote areas, providing 24-hour access, but currently these are just limited pilot schemes.

An important direction of activities carried out within the Polish Society of Palliative Medicine is pro-quality activity. Working groups are currently being set up to prepare guidelines and documentation for the quality certification of palliative care institutions.

Conclusion

Home-based palliative care is the primary care unit, recommended by choice, taking into account the wishes of the patients and their caregivers. This form allows for coordinated multidisciplinary teamwork and care of the patient in the familiar home environment. The success of these services, initiated in the 1970s and 1980s in the form of volunteer teams to the presently developed system integrated with the health-care system in Poland, was guaranteed by systematic and planned development based on the holistic palliative care approach.

References

1. Luczak J. Palliative/hospice care in Poland. Palliat Med. 1993;7(1):67–75.
2. Luczak J, Kotlińska-Lemieszek A, Kluziak M, Bozewicz A. Poland: cancer pain and palliative care. J Pain Symptom Manag. 2002;24(2):215–21.
3. Bogusz H, Pękacka-Falkowska K, Magowska A. Under the British roof: the British contribution to the development of hospice and palliative Care in Poland. J Palliat Care. 2018;33(2):115–9.
4. Bolognesi D, Centeno C, Biasco G. Specialisations in palliative medicine for physicians in Europe 2014-a supplement of the EAPC atlas of palliative care in Europe. Milan: EAPC Press; 2014.
5. Rozporządzenie Ministra Zdrowia z dnia 29 października 2013 r. w sprawie świadczeń gwarantowanych z zakresu opieki paliatywnej i hospicyjnej [Regulation of the Minister of Health on guaranteed palliative and hospice care services, 29 October, 2013] (Dz.U. z 2013 r. poz.1347).
6. Arias-Casais N, Garralda E, Rhee JY, de Lima L, Pons JJ, Clark D, Hasselaar J, Ling J, Mosoiu D, Centeno C. EAPC atlas of palliative care in Europe 2019. Vilvoorde: EAPC Press; 2019.
7. Ciałkowska-Rysz A, Dzierżanowski T. Stan opieki paliatywnej w Polsce w 2014 roku. [The condition

of palliative care in Poland in 2014]. Medycyna Paliatywna-Palliat Med. 2017;8(3):120–7.
8. Ciałkowska-Rysz A, Dzierżanowski T. Ocena sytuacji w opiece paliatywnej w Polsce w 2016 roku. [An appraisal of the situation of the palliative care in Poland in 2016]. Medycyna Paliatywna-Palliat Med. 2018;10(1):24–9.
9. Ciałkowska-Rysz A, Dzierżanowski T. Ocena sytuacji w opiece paliatywnej w Polsce w 2017 roku. [The appraisal of the situation of the palliative care in Poland in 2017]. Medycyna Paliatywna-Palliat Med. 2019;10(4):191–8.
10. Główny Urząd Statystyczny. Zdrowie i ochrona zdrowia w 2016 roku. [Central Statistical Office. Health and health care in 2016.] Warszawa 2017. http://www.stat.gov.pl (Last accessed 4 Oct 2019).
11. Ciałkowska-Rysz A. Wskazania do objęcia opieką paliatywną. [indications to extend palliative care]. Medycyna Paliatywna-Palliat Med. 2010;2(1):6–8.
12. Dzierżanowski T, Ciałkowska-Rysz A. Accessibility of opioid analgesics and barriers to optimal chronic pain treatment in Poland in 2000–2015. Support Care Cancer. 2017;25(3):775–81.
13. Ciałkowska-Rysz A, Dzierżanowski T, Łuczak J, Kotlińska-Lemieszek A, Krajnik M, Orońska A, Pakosz A, Pokropska W, Pyszkowska J, Stachowiak A, de Walden-Gałuszko K. Podsumowanie pracy Zespołu do spraw opieki paliatywnej i hospicyjnej (sierpień 2011 r. – czerwiec 2012 r.) [Summary of works of the expert task force on palliative and hospice care (August 2011 – June 2012)]. Medycyna Paliatywna-Palliat Med. 2014;6:177–89.
14. Ciałkowska-Rysz A, Pokropska W, Łuczak J, Kaptacz A, Stachowiak A, Hurich K, Koszela M. How much does care in palliative care wards cost in Poland? Arch Med Sci. 2016;12(2):457–68.
15. Luczak J, Okupny M, Wieczorek-Cuske L. The program of palliative medicine and care in the curriculum of sixth-year medical students in Poland. J Palliat Care. 1992;8(2):39–4.

Part IX

Southern Europe: Croatia

Palliative and Hospice Care in the Republic of Croatia: An Overview and Personal Experience

Renata Dobrila-Dintinjana and Marin Golčić

The Current State of Palliative and Hospice Care

The Republic of Croatia was established on June 25, 1991, when independence was declared from the Socialistic Federal Republic of Yugoslavia. Historically, from the very start of the Republic, there have been individual efforts pertaining to palliative care. However, only in 1994, those efforts resulted in the First Croatian Symposium on hospice and Palliative Care, which was organized in Zagreb by neurology professor Anica Jušić, who took a particular interest in the field of palliative care. Professor Jušić also helped to establish the Croatian Society for Hospice and Palliative Care within the Croatian Medical Association [1].

Unfortunately, there were no significant advances in palliative care for almost 20 years and palliative care relied on individual efforts. The Croatian Government finally formalized the "Strategic Plan for the Development of Palliative Care" on December 27, 2013. According to the National Program for the Development of Palliative Care, it was estimated that between 25,000 and 45,000 Croatian patients would require some form of palliative care per year, while 4000 to 5000 patients would require specialized palliative care [1, 2].

Based on previous European recommendations, the Croatian Health Insurance Fund (*Hrvatski zavod za zdravstveno osiguranje, HZZO*) estimated that up to 100 palliative care beds are required for each one million patients. As of 2019, HZZO operates a total of 20,468 beds in 63 hospitals in Croatia, five of which are Clinical Hospital Centers, three are Clinical Hospitals and five are Clinics, while the rest are specialized, general or county hospitals [3].

HZZO formally arranged for 6381 hospital beds for chronic disease patients, while out of that number, a total of 363 beds in 29 different hospitals are assigned for palliative care patients. The number of palliative care beds falls within the recommended estimate of 343–429 palliative care beds necessary for the Croatian needs. Out of 363 palliative care beds, 62 are available in specialized psychiatric hospitals, 61 in other specialized hospitals, 226 with the general hospitals and only 14 in the specialized establishment for palliative care "Hospice Marija Krucifiksa Kozulić." However, although 29 hospitals formally had palliative care beds, as of late 2017, only 22 hospitals actually had specialized teams for palliative care, and only 6 hospitals had a fast-track for palliative care patients. Due to an organizational decision, no Clinical Hospital Centers in Croatia have palliative care beds, requiring the transfer of palliative care patients to another

R. Dobrila-Dintinjana (✉) · M. Golčić
Department of Radiotherapy and Oncology, Clinical Hospital Center Rijeka, Rijeka, Croatia

M. Silbermann (ed.), *Palliative Care for Chronic Cancer Patients in the Community*,
https://doi.org/10.1007/978-3-030-54526-0_17

institution, the nearest of which could be located potentially hundreds of kilometers away. An additional issue is that only two institutions (specialized establishment for palliative care "Hospice Marija Krucifiksa Kozulić" in Rijeka and specialized hospital for lung diseases in Zagreb) predominantly treat palliative care patients with 50% or more of the beds in the establishment allocated for palliative care patients [3].

The specialized establishment for palliative care "Hospice Marija Krucifiksa Kozulić" (later referred to in this text as "the Hospice") is the only such establishment in Croatia and was founded by the Archdiocese of Rijeka in February 2013. The Hospice employs full-time nurses and carers, physiotherapists and other technical staff, while there is an agreement with the Clinical Hospital Center Rijeka to lend doctors to perform regular medical rounds. Historically, the majority of doctors working in the Hospice were oncologists, while there were also several anesthesiology and psychiatry specialists performing rounds. The Hospice has nine patient rooms, either one or two-bedded, along with all the other necessary contents. Other amenities include a small chapel and a quiet room for the visitors, while visits are allowed at any time of the day or night, and it is also possible to arrange for a family member to sleep in the Hospice. The Government covers patients' treatment and hospitalization, and no extra charges occur during the Hospice stay. In order to be admitted into the Hospice, patients need to have a medical confirmation from the specialist that all active treatment has been exhausted and that the patient is considered a candidate for palliative care treatment and is estimated to live less than three months. If these conditions are met, the family medicine physician signs referral papers which are then sent to the Hospice. Based on the available beds, the Hospice contacts and admits the patient [4].

Being a Catholic is not a prerequisite and the Hospice regularly cooperates with other Churches and their Ministers in order to offer its patients the maximum possible comfort and tend to their spiritual needs. Special care is taken when organizing funerals of the patients of other religions, and no rooms display any religious symbols unless the patient asks for it. The Hospice regularly interacts with other palliative care units and hospitals, both nationally and internationally, and while there are plans for several new hospices in Croatia, as of 2019, no similar institution has been established. There is also good interaction with the relatively new Department for Palliative Medicine in the Clinical Hospital Center Rijeka, which is led by Prof. Karmen Lončarek, whose individual efforts in developing palliative care have been crucial, especially for the Western region of Croatia [4].

During the first 4 years of its existence, the Hospice treated 902 patients, 768 of whom died in the Hospice in the same period, and is currently treating between 250 and 300 patients per year. Over 90% of the patients treated in the Hospice had malignant disease as a reason for admittance. The average time spent in the Hospice is 17 days, while the patients who died spent on average 13.7 days in the Hospice; the maximum stay permitted is 90 days. In the first 4 years, 15% of the patients died within 24 hours of admittance, and 23% of the patients died within 48 hours. Approximately 10–15% of the patients were discharged, either due to their wishes or if their medical condition did not necessitate an institutionalized palliative care treatment. Since 2016, the Hospice has also actively participated in scientific research. As of 2019, there have been six scientific publications (four of which are indexed in *current contents*) and one doctorate produced from the research conducted in the Hospice. The scientific focus of the research in the Hospice is predominantly analyzing factors that are associated with or affect the difference in the survival of the palliative care patients, although validation of the first Croatian quality-of-life questionnaire in palliative care (EORTC QLQ-C15-PAL) was also performed and published in 2018. Regarding survival analysis, it was shown that a physiotherapist evaluation of hospice patients might also be an independent biomarker of survival and could be used alongside previously known clinical biomarkers in the effort to analyze survival more precisely. Additionally, the data on 768 patients showed that the concomitant use of anxiolytics, antipsychotics and opioids, or using a large dose of opioids, was not associated with shorter survival of patients, highlighting the need for adequate treatment of the symptoms with the necessary doses of the medications. The research also showed that physicians underestimated pain in terminal cancer patients, highlighting the need for regular use of pain questionnaires in the hospice care, as well as suggesting the need for the development of specialized quality-of-life tools for the hospice patients [5–9].

The National Plan for the development of palliative care also recognized the need to establish 50–55 mobile palliative teams in Croatia. A mobile palliative team consists of a doctor and a nurse, while a county palliative care coordinator connects the palliative care professionals with the patient. The idea behind mobile palliative teams is the fact that many different patients might not require institutionalized care but require regular visits and follow-ups with the medical team. Mobile teams are especially crucial because Croatia is geographically very diverse, with over 40 islands with permanent settlements, resulting in the fact that many of the patients have limited access to health care. The first mobile team was set up in 2008 in Rijeka, which currently has five mobile palliative teams, the largest number in Croatia. As of 2017, there were only ten mobile palliative teams functioning in Croatia. Based on the data from the first 10 years of functioning mobile palliative teams in Rijeka, we know that the patient or family makes the majority of calls towards the teams, and only in 33% of the cases it is the family medical physician who contacts the team. The most common reasons for contacting the mobile palliative teams are: dehydration, pain, breathing difficulties and dyspepsia. On average, the team treats eight to ten patients per day and also offers psychological support to the family members; the total number of visits in the first 10 years was 26,401 [1, 10].

There are four Medical Schools in Croatia (Zagreb, Split, Rijeka and Osijek), with three of them offering mandatory palliative care education for undergraduate courses for medical doctors. Additionally, the Croatian Catholic University in Zagreb and the Faculty of Health Studies in Rijeka offer courses on palliative care. Also, the Croatian Institute for Emergency Medicine published National guidelines for the provision of hospital and ambulatory emergency care for palliative care patients, as the emergency medicine physicians treat a large number of palliative care patients. The limitations of providing palliative care are highlighted by the fact that there are no weekend services for mobile palliative teams, and there are no admittances to the Hospice over the weekend. Another issue applying to palliative care is the fact that there is no medical specialization in palliative care in Croatia, and only one doctor who, as of 2019, is specializing in geriatric medicine; additionally, there is no special formalized education for nurses, although there are several postgraduate courses available. Such discrepancies in the infrastructure and a relatively large number of beds allocated for palliative care patients and lack of education most likely lead to sub-optimal palliative care services in Croatia and resulting a substantial burden on families. Hence, although the government pays for the majority of medicines and medical services, there are many issues that families need to overcome when treating palliative care patients [1, 11].

A Personal Look from the Medical Perspective

Dr. Goran Golčić is a specialist in radiotherapy and oncology who works in Clinical Hospital Center Rijeka. Throughout most of his career, he worked in the Department for Radiotherapy and oncology, but currently works most of his time in the Department for Palliative medicine in Clinical Hospital Center Rijeka, as well as at the Hospice. "As a young doctor, my sole focus was to cure every cancer patient, however, during the years my attitude changed and I saw the quality-of-life as an equally important factor in oncology," says Dr. Golčić. There has been a considerable improvement in oncology recently, with many more diverse drugs with improved efficacy. "However, people are much more focused on quality control of the symptoms in recent years. I feel that dysthanasia is a huge issue in modern medicine, and we need to bring integrity and quality-of-life back to the patients, especially in the terminal phase." It is shown that countries that implemented palliative care also have a decrease in the total costs of the health care system as fewer resources are being spent, along with less burnout among physicians and nurses and higher quality of life among patients.

"Twenty years ago, there were no palliative beds, and patients would either be treated in acute hospitals or by loving family members if they had enough time, will and financial resources." Times have changed and there is a growing palliative care movement in Croatia, although not moving as fast as many would have liked. "Although entering the Hospice can be a daunting event, the staff really works as hard as they can in order to offer a comforting experience to both patients and their families. Once a month, family members of deceased patients gather in the common areas of the Hospice to socialize and communicate with each other and I feel this is helping with their grief"; he also mentions that the directors of the Hospice often organize trips and social events for the staff as burnout in palliative care is a recognized issue. Unsurprisingly, he adds, the future goal must be to invest in people and further education, along with a specialization in palliative care, which is considered a necessity both for doctors and nurses. "I think that we need to train to improve our communication skills towards the family, especially when delivering bad news to the patient and family. Being empathetic is something that patients recognize and value and is quite important for the grieving family. However, I do feel that medical professionals who work in palliative care also need psychological support and to focus on preventing burn-out syndrome." Compared to Western countries, Croatia also lacks a large volunteer base, which would immensely help, especially for at-home patients.

His wife, Dr. Lidija Gović-Golčić, is a family medicine specialist and a recipient of the St. Vitus Medal of Gratitude for her services in providing and developing palliative care in Rijeka, Croatia. Family medical practices in Croatia are generally location-based and usually have a base of 1200–2100 patients who can choose a different family medicine doctor every year. A large number of patients in the family practice base often leads to 100 or more visits per day, limiting time for palliative care patients who often require a much more significant proportion of the time. Several bureaucratic issues also limit the efficacy of family care physicians; for example, peroral nutrition supplements need to be recommended by a hospital specialist in order to be prescribed by a family medicine specialist.

Usually, when palliative care patients are discharged home, a family medicine physician visits the patient to determine the initial condition and needs, and then contacts community nurses. However, there are no real standards or algorithms in the treatment of such patients, and with many bureaucratic obstacles there is often a conflict between the emergency medical services, family practice and community nurses as to who will provide which service to the patient. Problems often escalate during the weekends when most medical services are unavailable to palliative care patients. Developing mobile palliative care teams has immensely helped family practice physicians as they provide services such as changing urinary catheters, giving parenteral medications, placing nasogastric tubes, etc. Similarly, having a specialized Pain Clinic in the nearby Clinical Hospital Center also helps patients as well as physicians. However, both of these services are weekday only and location-based, meaning there is a dramatic difference in palliative care depending on where patients live as well as the day of the week.

The need for radical changes is recognized, and this has led to the Team for the Development of Palliative Care being formed. However, advances are minimal due to many obstacles, such as education during working hours which is impractical for many physicians outside of the hospital, no proper definition and division of the work among different institutions and physicians, and the lack of connection between different institutions which should be included in the holistic approach towards palliative care patients.

There are some positive initiatives as well, such as the initiative of several professors of family medicine in Rijeka who have started to organize theme-based congresses in order to improve education, with the first congress theme being "Treating pain and oncology patients in everyday family medicine care." Additionally, although there are problems with the integration, a registry of palliative care patients was also formed recently. "In my opinion, palliative care patients should have a personal medical record which should combine all the data regarding the therapy, visits from family care, palliative care and emergency care physicians as well as community nurses. Currently, we have no such thing and with lack of algorithms in treating such patients and division of work, patients are reliant on the individual efforts from the family care physicians, which often result in a discrepancy of care amongst patients."

References

1. National program for the development of palliative care in Croatia, 2017–2020. Ministry of Health of the Republic of Croatia. 2017. https://zdravlje.gov.hr/nacionalni-program-razvoja-palijativne-skrbi-u-republici-hrvatskoj-2017-2020/3094. Accessed 24 Dec 2019.
2. Mid-Western Health Board. Report on the National Advisory Committee on Palliative Care. Department of Health and Children. 2001. http://hospicefoundation.ie. Accessed 24 Dec 2019.
3. Arranged health care providers in Croatia. Croatian Institute for health insurance. 2019. https://www.hzzo.hr/zdravstveni-sustav-rh/. Accessed 24 Dec 2019.
4. Marija K. Kozulić hospice web-site. The Archdiocese of Rijeka. 2015. http://hospicij-marijakozulic.hr. Accessed 24 Dec 2019.
5. Golčić M, Dobrila-Dintinjana R, Golčić G, Čubranić A. The impact of combined use of opioids, antipsychotics, and anxiolytics on survival in the hospice setting. J Pain Symptom Manag. 2018;55:22–30.
6. Golčić M, Dobrila-Dintinjana R, Golčić G, Petranovic D. How do hospice patients feel about hospice care – and is it important? Exploring the relationship between patient attitude to hospice care, survival and other patient characteristics in the setting of first Croatian hospice. Clin Soc Work Health Intervention. 2017;8:53–60.
7. Golčić M, Dobrila-Dintinjana R, Golčić G, Gović-Golčić L, Čubranić A. Physical exercise: an evaluation of a new clinical biomarker of survival in hospice patients. Am J Hosp Palliat Care. 2018;35:1377–83.
8. Golčić M, Dobrila-Dintinjana R, Golčić G, Pavlović-Ružić I, Stevanović A, Gović-Golčić L. Quality of life in a hospice: a validation of the Croatian version of the EORTC QLQ-C15-PAL. Am J Hosp Palliat Care. 2018;35:1085–90.
9. Golčić M, Dobrila-Dintinjana R, Golčić G, Pavlović-Ružić I, Gović-Golčić L. Do physicians underestimate pain in terminal Cancer patients? A prospective study in a hospice setting. Clin J Pain. 2018;34:1159–63.
10. Mozetič V. Ten years of mobile palliative care teams in Primorsko – Goranska county. 2018. http://domzdravlja-pgz.hr/. Accessed 24 Dec 2019.
11. National guidelines for the providing of hospital and ambulatory emergency care for palliative care patients. Croatian Institute for emergency medicine. 2015. https://www.hzhm.hr/source/smjernice/Nacionalne-smjernice-za-rad-izvanbolnicke-i-bolnicke.pdf. Accessed 24 Dec 2019.

Part X

Southern Europe: Montenegro

Palliative and Supportive Care in Oncology in Montenegro

Nada Cicmil-Sarić

Abbreviations

GDP General Domestic Product
GPs General Practitioners
IARC International Agency for Research on Cancer
IMRT Intensity-Modulated Radiotherapy
WHO World Health Organization

Introduction: General Considerations

In general, medicine can be divided into preventive, curative and palliative medicine. The need for palliative care in the world and in Montenegro is increasing significantly [1, 2]. According to the World Health Organization (WHO) definition of 2012, palliative care is comprehensive (health, psychological, social and spiritual) care with the aim of providing the necessary care to patients with inexhaustible illness that significantly shortens life expectancy [3]. Although there are many medical conditions in the areas of geriatrics, neurology, psychiatry, polytrauma, chronic cardiology states, autoimmune and other diseases, the term palliative care is primarily associated with malignant diseases. For a long time, the most important parameter for successful oncological treatment was the length of life of the patient. Modern times have brought about a different concept: the relationship between significance of length of life and quality of life is equally balanced: 50% vs. 50%. Recent studies have shown that palliative care reduces symptoms and improves quality of life for both the patient and their family caregivers. This reduces unnecessary emergency department visits, hospitalizations and time spent in the intensive care unit [4–7]. Studies have found that some patient groups receiving palliative care live longer than those treated with traditional medical methods alone [8]. Recent studies on the degree of clinical symptom severity in cancer patients have found not only a reduction in visceral crisis, but also an improved quality of life and better survival rates of palliative-treated patients relative to the control group [9–11]. Considering the contemporary need for palliative care and its application, one could also discuss the most appropriate name for this area of medicine. Namely, in addition to care, it includes various forms of treatment, interventions, psychological, spiritual and social support for the patient and his family members. Palliative care of an oncology patient by current definition begins when the measures and possibilities of active-specific oncological treatments are exhausted. A holistic approach to palliative care actually begins from the moment of diagnosis of

N. Cicmil-Sarić (✉)
Clinical Center for Oncology and Radiotherapy,
Clinical Center of Montenegro,
Podgorica, Montenegro

M. Silbermann (ed.), *Palliative Care for Chronic Cancer Patients in the Community*,
https://doi.org/10.1007/978-3-030-54526-0_18

malignancy and the communication of this fact to the patient and his family. Palliative treatment, on the other hand, is appropriate at every age and stage of cancer. Finally, when the disease progresses so much that the patient can no longer bear its consequences, palliative medicine assists the patient with a dignified acceptance of inevitability and helps the relatives in their grief. Care should be carried out in a multidisciplinary environment in a polite, open and sensitive way. Teamwork, communication and the highest level of trust are the "holy trinity" of palliative care. Good communication skills are a prerequisite for quality interaction between the patient and the health professionals, but also between the patient and his/her family and among the various health care professionals and the care-related services.

World population has reached 7.5 billion [12]. Each individual human community in the world has its own history, culture, tradition, religion, customs, geography and climate. All these factors have the greatest influence on the organization of the state, the social system, the law and the social and economic status of the population. Viewed in this framework, each community has its own specificities for the organization of public health care as well as palliative care.

Montenegro: Health System in Montenegro, Malignant Diseases in Montenegro and Oncology Facilities in Montenegro

Montenegro is a multi-ethnic, multi-religious and multi-cultural country in Southeast Europe on the Adriatic Sea. Montenegro has an area of 13,812 square kilometers. According to the last population census taken in 2011, Montenegro had 620,079 inhabitants [13]. The Montenegrin health system encompasses both the public and private health sectors. In addition to the Montenegrin Clinical Center located in the capital city of Podgorica, public health has 7 general hospitals, 18 health centers, 3 special hospitals, 3 smaller health centers, the Public Health Institute, the Emergency Medical Service, the Blood Transfusion Institute and the association of the Montenegrin pharmacies, Montefarm. The Institute for Physical Medicine, named the Rehabilitation Center Simo Milošević and the Rudo Institution are providers of medical and technical aids and also belong to the public health sector. The private health sector has 786 units, including medical, dental and pharmaceutical, which are not networked between them. As of a few years ago, part of the private sector facility (361 medical facilities and 27 providers for medical and technical tools) has been networked with public health [14]. The Clinical Center and Institute for Public Health are institutions at the tertiary level of health care (including educational and scientific research activities, independently or in cooperation with Medical and other faculties). The Faculty of Medicine of the University of Montenegro was established in 1997.

The health care system of Montenegro is a work in progress, and there are currently 2061 physicians. The number of physicians per 1000 inhabitants increased to 3.3 (2018), which is approaching the European standard (3.4) [15].

The Montenegrin Health Insurance Fund is the main (and could be said to be the only) bearer of the costs of health services to Montenegrin people who are insured. In Montenegro, various forms of private and supplementary health insurance are not yet available or are only sporadically available in everyday practice. The health care system accounts for 4.64% of General Domestic Product (GDP) (as of 2017). The annual State Health Expenditure per capita is 329 EUR (2018) [16].

According to data released by the IARC (The International Agency for Research on Cancer), Global Cancer Observatory, published in Geneva in September of 2018, the global cancer burden is estimated to have risen to 18.1 million new cases and 9.6 million deaths in 2018. The data from Montenegro fits into this gloomy statistic [16]. Montenegro has a National Cancer Registry established in 2013. The most recent valid statistical data from this field originates from this paper, published by the Institute for Public Health of Montenegro. The National Cancer Registry of the National Institute for Public Health recorded 2784 new cases of malignant neoplasm registered in Montenegro (out of which 325 cases were non-melanoma malignant tumors of the skin). In Montenegro, 1549 people in the affected area died all of those neoplasms which are subject to mandatory reporting [17]. The oncology and radiotherapy clinic in Podgorica, the capital, is a tertiary health care institution. Presentation and treatment of the vast majority of malignant diseases in Montenegro are gravitated to the Oncology and Radiotherapy Clinic in Podgorica. Oncological diagnosis and treatment are performed by two other institutions: The Center for Hematology in Podgorica and the Brezovik Special Hospital in Nikšić, which is designated for the treatment of malignant lung tumors. The oncology and radiotherapy clinic in Podgorica have a capacity of 25 beds in the radiotherapy unit and 25 beds in the medical oncology department. One unit in each department is intended for intensive care. The Department of Medical Oncology has a daily hospital for outpatients. Conformal radiotherapy, intensity-modulated radiation therapy and brachytherapy are all performed at the radiotherapy unit.

Palliative Medicine and Palliative Care in Montenegro

The National Palliative Care Plan in Montenegro is not defined. National Programs for the Prevention of Malignant Diseases as well as contemporary curative treatment for malignant patients have had priority so far. In 2011, the Ministry of Health of Montenegro issued a document entitled: *The Project for Improvement of Good Governance in Montenegrin Healthcare System. Admission of Good Management in the Health System in Montenegro.* The document states the following: "The prerequisite for work in this area is the development of palliative care standards, development of guidelines, training of personnel in terms of acquiring knowledge, skills and attitudes and formation of dedicated capacities. At least 3 to 5% of the bedding division should be chosen for the purpose of providing palliative care. Palliative care mainly requires the engagement of nurses and technicians in 24 hours. It is necessary to find a model and stimulation for nurses and doctors for this and for this type of work. It is necessary to provide adequate equipment, materials and medicines for the disposal of palliative patients at home." [18]. Montenegro Health Development Master Plan 2015–2020 states the following: "Palliative care: Demographic and epidemiological trends are increasing the number of elderly and chronic patients, changing the image of the traditional family, which has led to a different approach to the problem of death. The obligation to care for elderly, chronic and dying patients is transferred from the family to society and, to a large extent, to the public health system. Palliative care for patients with advanced and incurable disease and their environment means integral care for the consequences of illness (pain, nausea, shortness of breath, exhaustion and delirium) and psychosocial needs for a better quality of life until death. This includes patients with malignancies, organ failure, neurological diseases, psychiatric illnesses, HIV, etc. Palliative care is now being carried out partly on the primary level, through the services of a nursing home and home treatment by an elected doctor, which does not satisfy the real needs. In the forthcoming period, it is necessary to pay special attention in the field of palliative care, to the development of educational programs and to organizing multidisciplinary teams for palliative care (physician, nurse, social worker, physical therapist, occupational therapist, dietician and psychologist). Palliative care must become an integral part of integrated healthcare through palliative teams, palliative wards or hospices" [19].

Herein, we will consider how the significance, definition and understanding of palliative care, together with the objective conditions, affect the way of treatment of patients in Montenegro with malignant illness in the terminal stage of the disease.

All decisions about the treatment of patients with malignant diseases in Montenegro are made within a multidisciplinary oncology team: both when it comes to specific oncological treatment and when it comes to the use of symptomatic therapy and palliative care in the terminal stage of the disease. The obligation of palliative care in oncology in Montenegro is shared by the family of the patient and hospital specialist medical treatment institutions, that is, all existing primary, secondary and tertiary levels. To date, options for creating hospices have been considered on several occasions, but the idea has not yet been realized. When it comes to hospital palliative care, it is mostly performed at the specialist departments of internal medicine of seven regional medical centers and at the Oncology and Radiotherapy Clinic of the Clinical Center of Montenegro. Patient care is conducted utilizing the available resources, health care staff: nurses, technicians and physicians. The staff caring for the terminal oncology patient has no additional education, training or stimulation for this type of work. This organization of work creates the risk of lack of adequate accommodation for potentially curable oncology patients who need to receive specific oncology drugs and/or radiation. The long stay of terminal patients in oncology wards also causes high costs of hospital days. In practice, in part, we seek to address this problem by directing patients to outpatient radiation and treatment within a daily hospital. In order to best solve the complex condition of the terminal oncological patient being treated in hospital, specialists from all branches of medicine are involved. The importance of the presence of two psychologists at the Oncology and Radiotherapy Clinic should be emphasized.

In Montenegrin society, there is still a strong sense of the importance of family and a sense of duty and care that family members should provide to their ill relative. The loved ones and their feelings translated into a word of compassion and comfort are certainly of the most importance when it comes to palliative care. When it comes to professional help, it can be said that family doctors and oncologists are involved in palliative care of Montenegrin patients with malignant diseases to the greatest extent and in a wide variety of ways. However, most palliative cancer patients are cared for at home. The family physician is the best expert in the disease, comorbidity, cultural, social and economic circumstances of his or her patient. The Faculty of Medicine in Podgorica, within the curriculum of general medicine studies and training of family medicine specialists, has modules of lectures and practical classes in oncology. The Center for Science of the Clinical Center of Montenegro has been conducting continuous medical education for many years, the content of which includes oncology and especially the part related to palliative care of patients. There are no specific mobile palliative care units in Montenegro.

The family physician and the home health services are the main providers of the services needed by these patients. The modern age and the temptations of a new consumer society, a hectic life, large commitments and over-employment, and enormous efforts to secure material benefits for the family present a great burden for the whole world, and especially for the inhabitants of developing countries, including Montenegro. These circumstances leave less time for family members to devote themselves to their sick relative sufficiently and in the desired manner. Volunteer work was once very prevalent in Montenegro. More recent, modern times have brought about changes: volunteerism as a category is no longer present in many areas of life or in health. In the field of palliative care in general, as well as in the field of oncological palliative care, volunteerism is minimal in Montenegro at the moment.

The most important areas related to the content and quality of human life in the terminal phase of the disease are pain therapy, nutrition, treatment of anemia syndrome, psychological support and physical rehabilitation.

Palliative measures and resources are generally applied at the primary level of health care. The exception is radiation and surgical interventions.

According to the World Health Organization (WHO), two-thirds of patients with malignancies have pain during their illness; that is, approximately 12 million people worldwide are currently suffering from chronic cancer pain [20, 21]. In Montenegro, the treatment of pain by oncological patients is prescribed by the oncologist and is carried out by family and general practitioners (GPs). We work with anesthetists to perform blockages and neurolysis. We do not have a specialized pain clinic. The range of drugs ranges from non-steroidal antirheumatics, spasmolytics, light opioids and heavy opioids: long-acting and short-acting.

We do not have strong mid-length opioids. We also have coanalgesics, primarily from the group of anesthetics and psycho pharmaceuticals.

When it comes to the nutrition of a terminal oncology patient, in addition to standard infusion solutions, saline, Ringer's, Hartman's, glucosaline and glucose, dietary supplements such as Fresubin and Supportan drinks are available. The Health Fund is reimbursing the costs of these preparations. We also often use Megace syrup, which has a very good effect, but health insurance does not offset the cost of this preparation. Kabiven emulsion is used for partial or total parenteral nutrition. Nutritional advice can be obtained from the specialist at the Institute of Public Health of Montenegro.

In addition to standard anemia medications, the use of erythropoietin alpha is of great importance.

Palliative interventional radiological and surgical procedures such as palliative irradiation, biliary stent, vena cava stents, nutritional and protective gastrostomy, irrigator application, vaginal douching, cannula maintenance, catheter changes and oxygen for home use are available to the patient. We pay great attention to the success of decubitus prevention, infection and treatment of infection. Regular sterile patient dressing, decubital mattresses, adult diapers, numerous orthopedics as well as toiletries are available for the sick.

Conclusion

In conclusion, it should be repeated and emphasized that the material resources (facilities, bedding, medicines and supplies) and human resources (professional knowledge and skills) available in Montenegro for the care of palliative oncology patients are much better than the way or models of their implementation.

In order to implement palliative oncology care in daily practice and life in Montenegro, we propose the following recommendations:

- By law, to define the name, model of organization, financing, activities and activists for the implementation of palliative care as a vital and integral part of health care and to draw conclusions within the framework of the Master Plan of Health Development in Montenegro.
- To work on the continuing education of medical students, family physicians and GPs in primary health care, breaking the fear of opiates and preparing the patient and family for the inevitable outcome.
- Improve cooperation and communication with specialists in regional medical centers in their field of knowledge and implementation of palliative medicine, thus strengthening the patients' confidence and improving the rational use of bedding in hospital settings.
- The preservation of the family tradition and the assistance of family members in the palliative care of a sick relative should be encouraged.
- Work should be done to organize the outpatient clinic for pain therapy, to provide nutritional advice and psychological and spiritual support.
- Improve the existing mix of competences of health palliative and social care, clearly define their competences and strengthen their cooperation.
- Consider introducing palliative medicine specialization into the regular system of specialist medical studies.
- Complete the work of the palliative care team with the presence of a priest.
- Form patient support associations and include volunteers in the work of the palliative team.
- Work to establish a hospice.

Acknowledgment and Dedication As the saying goes, "To realize the meaning of its existence, the human being has to do three things: to leave offspring, to build a house and write a book." I'm not writing a book, but I have the opportunity to participate in creating a joint masterpiece. I owe thanks to Professor Michael Silbermann, who gave me the honor and the opportunity to take part in the writing of this book. This text is in remembrance of and is dedicated to all of my patients and their families: those who are with us and those who, unfortunately, are not.

References

1. Murtagh FEM, Bausewein C, Verne J, Iris Groeneveld E, Kaloki YE, Higginson IJ. How many people need palliative care? A study developing and comparing methods for population-based estimates. Palliat Med. 2014;28(1):49–58.
2. Wilson BE, Jacob S, Yap ML, Ferlay J, Bray F, Barton MB. Estimates of global chemotherapy demands and corresponding physician workforce requirements for 2018 and 2040: a population-based study. Lancet Oncol. 2019;20:769.
3. Available from: https://www.who.int/cancer/palliative/definition/en.
4. Available from: https://www.capc.org, documents America's Care of Serious Illness 2019.
5. Kavalieratos D, Corbelli J, Zhang D, et al. Association between palliative care and patient and caregiver outcomes: a systematic review and meta-analysis. JAMA. 2016;316(20):2104–14.
6. Cassel JB, Garrido M, May P, Del Fabbro E, Noreika D. Impact of specialist palliative care on re-admissions: a "competing risks" analysis to take mortality into account. J Pain Symptom Manag. 2018;55(2):581.
7. Khandelwal N, Kross EK, Engelberg RA, Coe NB, Long AC, Curtis JR. Estimating the effect of palliative care interventions and advance care planning on ICU utilisation: a systematic review. Crit Care Med. 2015;43(5):1102–11.
8. Temel JS, Greer JA, El-Jawahri A, et al. Effects of early integrated palliative care in patients with lung and GI cancer: a randomized clinical trial. J Clin Oncol. 2017;35(8):834–41.
9. Basch E, Deal AM, Kris MG, et al. Symptom monitoring with patient-reported outcomes during routine cancer treatment: a randomized controlled trial. J Clin Oncol. 2016;34(6):557–65.
10. Denis F, Basch E, Septans AL, Bennouna J, Urban T, Dueck AC, Letellier C. Two-year survival comparing web-based symptom monitoring vs routine surveillance following treatment for lung cancer. JAMA. 2019;321(3):306–7.
11. Basch E, Deal AM, Dueck AC, et al. Overall survival results of a trial assessing patient-reported outcomes for symptom monitoring. JAMA. 2017;318(2):197–8.
12. Available from: https://www.worldometers.info/world-population/.
13. Available from: https://en.wikipedia.org/wiki/Montenegro.
14. Available from: www.mzdravlja.gov.me › rubrike › pzu.
15. Zdravstveni sistem 2017-2018 pdf. Available from: www.mzdravlja.gov.me.
16. Available from: https://gco.iarc.fr.
17. Malignant neoplasms in Montenegro 2013. Podgorica: Institute of Public Health of Montenegro, Center for Control and Prevention of Non-communicable Diseases, Registry of Malignant Neoplasms of Montenegro, 2018.
18. Strategy for optimization of secondary and tertiary health care levels with implementation action plan. 2011. pdf. Available from: www.un.org.me › Library › Health › 3a.
19. Master plan razvoja zdravstva Crne Gore 2015-2020.pdf. Available from: www.mzdravlja.gov.me › strategije.
20. World Health Organization. National cancer control programmes, policies and managerial guidelines. 2nd ed. Geneva; 2002.
21. Atasoy A, Bogdanovic G, Aladashvili A, Cvijetic Z, Dediu M, Cicmil-Saric N, Nersesyan A, Athanasiou A, Serdar Turhal N. An international survey of practice patterns and difficulties in cancer pain management in Southeastern Europe: a Turkish & Balkan Oncology Group common initiative. J BUON. 2013;18(4):1082–7.

Part XI

North Africa: Egypt

The Critical Contribution of an NGO to the Development of Palliative Care Services in the Community – Encouraging Outcome of the Tanta Project in Egypt

Mohamed Ahmed Hablas

Introduction

Egypt is located in the northeastern corner of Africa. Egypt's heartland, the Nile River valley and delta, was the home of one of the principal civilizations of the ancient Middle East.

Gharbia is one of the governorates of Egypt. It is located in the north of the country. Its capital is Tanta, which is 90 km north of Cairo, and 120 km south east of Alexandria. The total area of Gharbia governorate is 1942 km^2, making it the tenth largest governorate of Egypt, with a population of 5 million people (Fig. 1). There are three main hospitals that serve cancer patients in the governorate: Tanta Cancer Center, Tanta University Hospital, and Gharbia Cancer Society Hospital.

In many countries, palliative care is still not recognized as a medical discipline. Palliative care teams and programs are difficult to finance because most of the health systems do not pay or underpay for their services. Most palliative care programs begin by nongovernmental organizations as government policies can obstruct, permit, or promote palliative care programs in most countries.

The Gharbiah Cancer Society is a charity, nonprofit, and nongovernmental organization, located in Tanta city, the capital of Gharbiah governorate. The society was announced in 1966. The main target at that time was to give social and financial support to cancer patients and their families. For example, artificial limbs and stoma care. It was a leading step in the area.

Members of the society are oncologists from Gharbiah, community representatives, and local social leaders. The activities of the society are run through an executive committee composed of five oncologists, a social worker, two business men, and a politician who are interested in cancer control and social activities.

On 1985, the necessity for introducing a modern radiation therapy services in the area was behind the effort for starting a campaign for charity support to finance radiation therapy department. The government at that time had provided an area of 418 m^2 to start a new building for the society, and it was exclusively built by public fund raising. Although this available land is a limited area, we designed the building to contain all the necessary equipment for the cancer patient care in the area. With time, other services were introduced like chemotherapy and surgery. These services are free of charge and state funded. In 2011, the Gharbia Cancer Society has started its palliative care services.

M. A. Hablas (✉)
Palliative Care, Gharbiah Cancer Society, Tanta, Egypt

M. Silbermann (ed.), *Palliative Care for Chronic Cancer Patients in the Community*,
https://doi.org/10.1007/978-3-030-54526-0_19

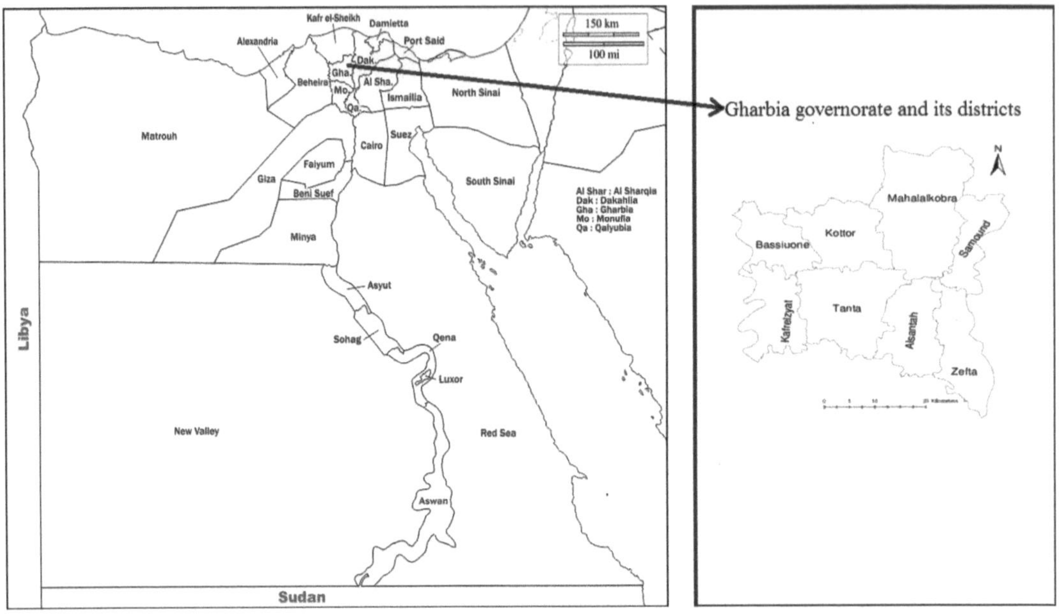

Fig. 1 Map of Egypt showing the location of Gharbia governorate and its eight districts

Obstacles to Palliative Care Program

In the Western health-care system, palliative care is provided mostly in hospices. However, there is a shortage of available hospices. Inability to fulfill enrollment requirements for hospice admission and lack of integration of palliative care in most health-care systems are challenges that face those who care for terminally ill patients in developed countries. The main discipline involved in the palliative circle of care in developed countries is shown in Fig. 2.

Developing countries face different spectra of obstacles. Lack of resources directed to palliative care, administrators' unawareness of the role of hospice care in health-care system, poor physicians' understanding and training on medical care in the final stages of diseases, and the unreasonable expectations of patient and families are some additional challenges as shown in Fig. 3.

In the Egyptian palliative care circle, we need to improve the knowledge and palliative care principles of health workers, enhance the education of nurses, doctors and pharmacists, work on policies of narcotics and pain killers' dispensing, and ensure its availability to the terminally ill patients.

Egypt is a country where religion plays a pivotal role in daily life. Charity "Al-Zakah" is one of the five pillars of Islam. During the entire month of Ramadan when donations are at their peak, we run a campaign to collect money for expensive equipment. We purchase linear accelerators, imaging machines, and lab equipment depending on the amount of donations received annually. We believe that hospice care can only be financed using the same approach. It is unrealistic to request financing for hospice care in countries struggling to provide the basic services for infectious disease control and sanitation [1].

Approaches developed in the USA and Western countries can be tailored to our culture taking into consideration that there are some advantages in Egyptian culture. Family ties are strong, and most patients are surrounded by their beloved ones during the difficult phases of their illnesses.

Family members usually request their involvement in the daily care of the patients. Their presence assures the patient and raises his/

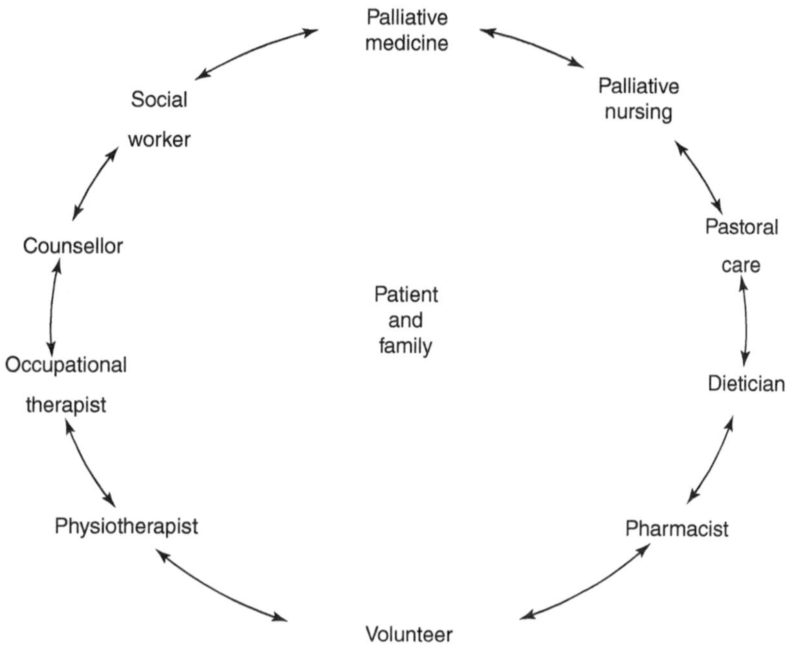

Fig. 2 The palliative circle of care in developed countries

her morale. Although it's difficult to provide accurate information to families in societies in which issues such as informed consent, living will, or health-care proxy are unknown, the same rules governing the Western medicine cannot be applied.

When Muslims are sick, their friends and relatives tend to visit and sometimes in rather large numbers for rather extended visits. Western trained health-care workers may find this somewhat unusual, but consideration should be given to the point where the visitors are in some way impeding the delivery of care. Near the end of the patient's life, the family may wish to read passages from the Qur'an or recite *Shahadah* that bears witness to Allah being the only God and Muhammad (pbuh) being the messenger of Allah. The Shahadah is one of the five pillars of Islam, and it is generally desired that these be the last words heard by and on the lips of the patient in this life.

One concern regarding the use of opioid analgesics may be that morphine-induced sedation might interfere with the ability of the patient to recite the *Shahadah* or hear the Qur'an being read. Some families may not wish their dying relative to be fully informed regarding his/her illness. While this is certainly not unique to Islam, it is perhaps somewhat more common in Muslim families than in Western families today. In some instances, the patients and relatives may be engaged in what has been termed "mutual pretense" (Bluebond-Langer, 1978), that is, both the patient and his/her family know that the patient is dying, but the topic is avoided with each pretending that the other doesn't know the real situation [2].

Illiteracy remains a major problem hindering development of palliative care program in many countries around the world. Spreading the word about our mission of relieving suffering rather than cure requires extra effort; therefore, we make sure to educate patients and families about our role in helping patients. Paying attention to the unique structure and limitations of our society will help establish a successful relationship with the patients and their families.

There are many other barriers to palliative care programs in Egypt; for example, the patients prefer to be linked to one doctor; surgical oncologist, medical oncologist, and so on, and there are also no protocols for palliative care, and families prefer home care rather than hospice care. There

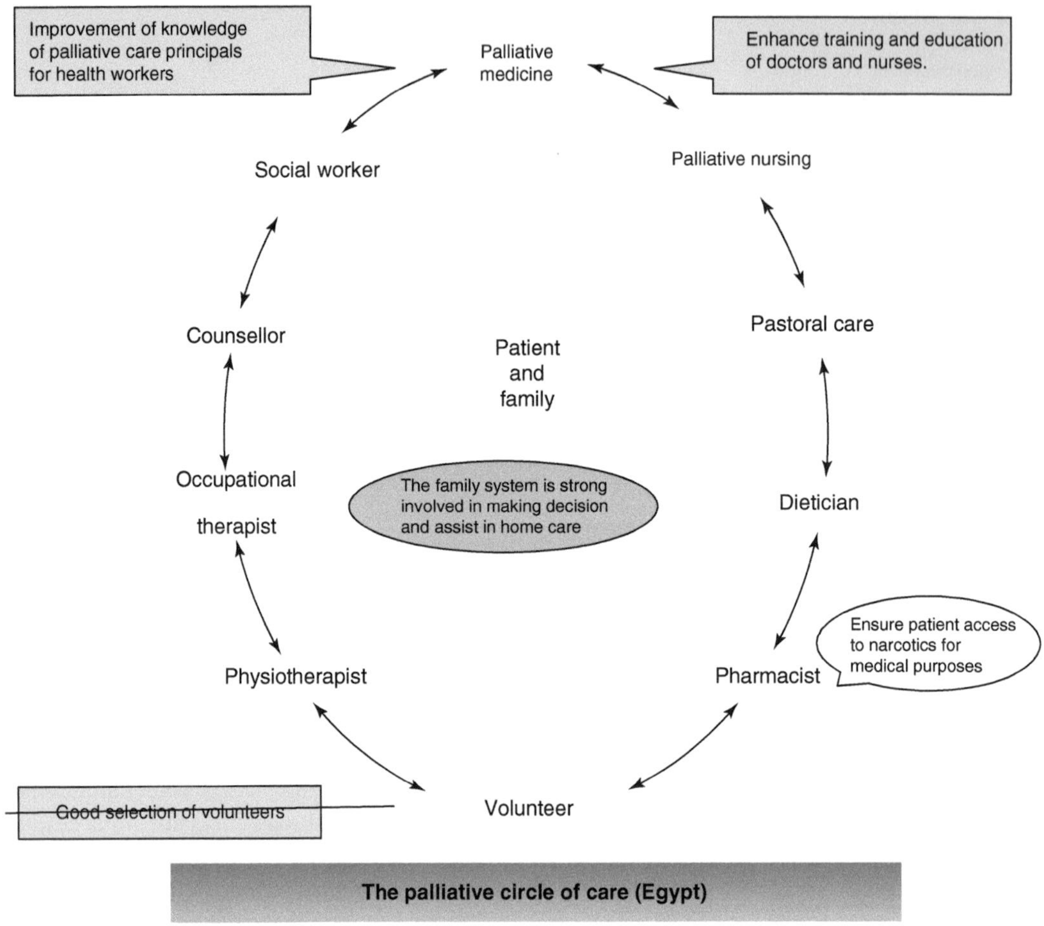

Fig. 3 Palliative care circle in Egypt and what needs to be improved

is no carrier attraction for doctors, psychologically and financially, and the doctors can be an obstacle to improving palliative care due to their lack of basic training. Beside there's limited availability of and access to narcotics, as well as busy unaware health authorities of palliative care.

The Status of Cancer in Egypt

The status of cancer in Egypt is showing that most patients are diagnosed at advanced stage. There will be an expected increase in cases over the next decades due to increasing number of cancer hospitals and diagnostic facilities, aging of the population and limited cancer control interventions (Fig. 4).

Review of 9-year-data of Gharbiah population-based cancer registry (Middle East Cancer Consortium, MECC) from 1999 to 2007 revealed 3480 cancer cases/year, with age-standardized rate (ASR) of 161.7/100,000 for males and 120.8/100,000 for females. Liver cancer is the most frequent cancer in male, and breast cancer is the most frequent cancer in females as shown in Fig. 5. About 70% of cases present in advanced stages (III and IV) as shown in Fig. 6. According to Alsarafy et al., 73% of Egyptian patients with advanced cancer referred to palliative care died at home with poor control of pain and other symptoms, while 27% died at hospital [3]. Pain was the most common symptoms among Egyptian.

Opioid consumption in Egypt is among the lowest worldwide, indicating largely inadequate

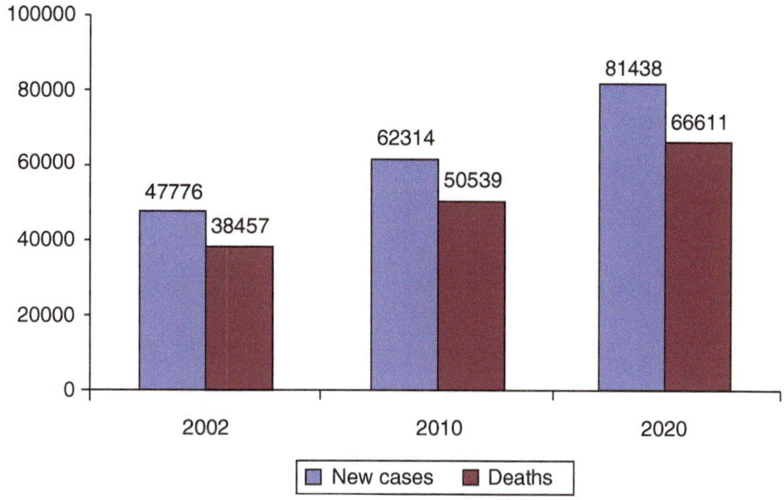

Fig. 4 Cancer burden in Egypt according to Globocan 2002

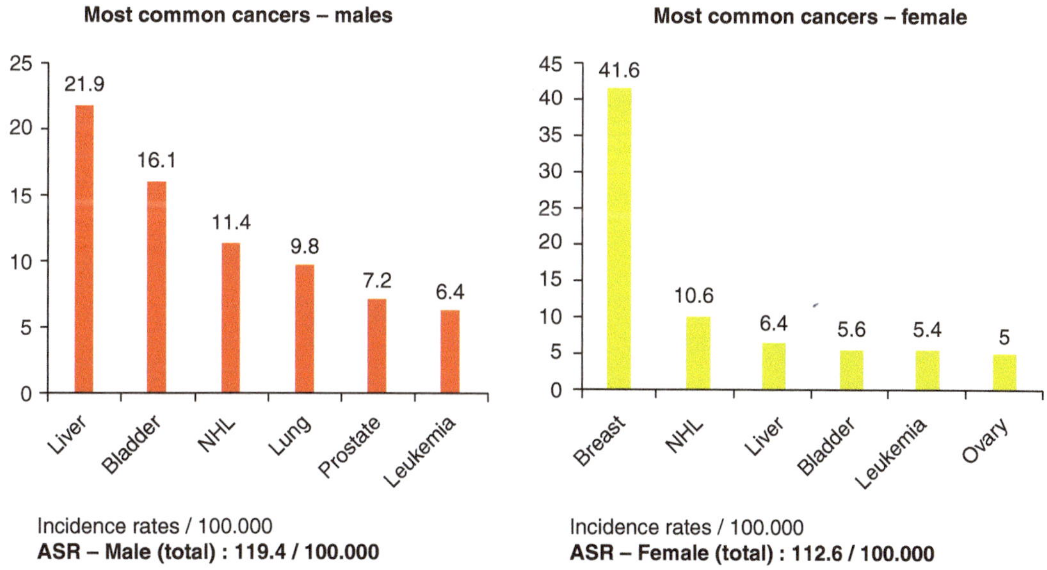

Fig. 5 Most common cancers in Egypt according to Gharbia Population-Based Cancer Registry

cancer pain control [4]. Based on the data published in the annual report of the International Narcotics Control Board, the average opioid consumption in Egypt during 2008–2010 was 62 defined daily dosed for statistical purposes (S-DDD) per million inhabitants per day, and with this, Egypt was ranked 115th among 184 countries [5].

According to the Pain and Policy Studies Group (PPSG) at the University of Wisconsin, morphine consumption in Egypt in 2010 was 0.1818 mg morphine equivalents/capita (Fig. 7).

Strategy of Our Palliative Care Program

There are many reasons why cancer pain is not adequately treated at present in Egypt including absence of national policies on cancer pain relief and palliative care; lack of awareness on the part of health-care program workers, policy makers, administrators, and the public that most cancer pain can be relieved; shortage of financial resources and limitation of health-care delivery systems and personnel; concerns that the medical use of opi-

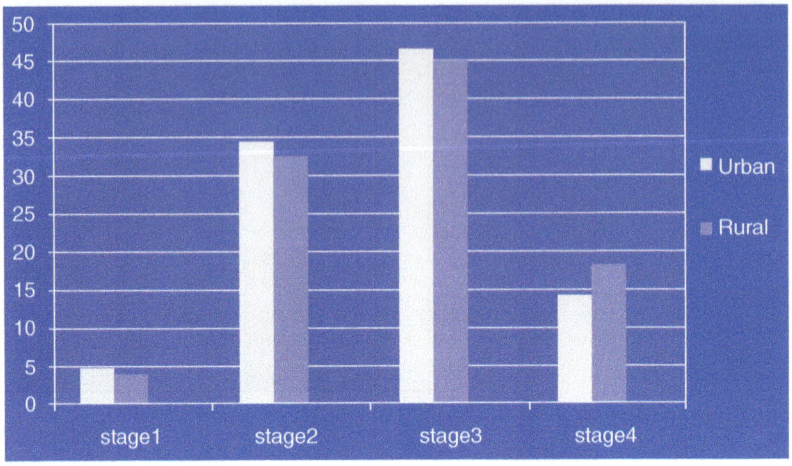

Fig. 6 Breast cancer staging in Gharbia, 1999–2006

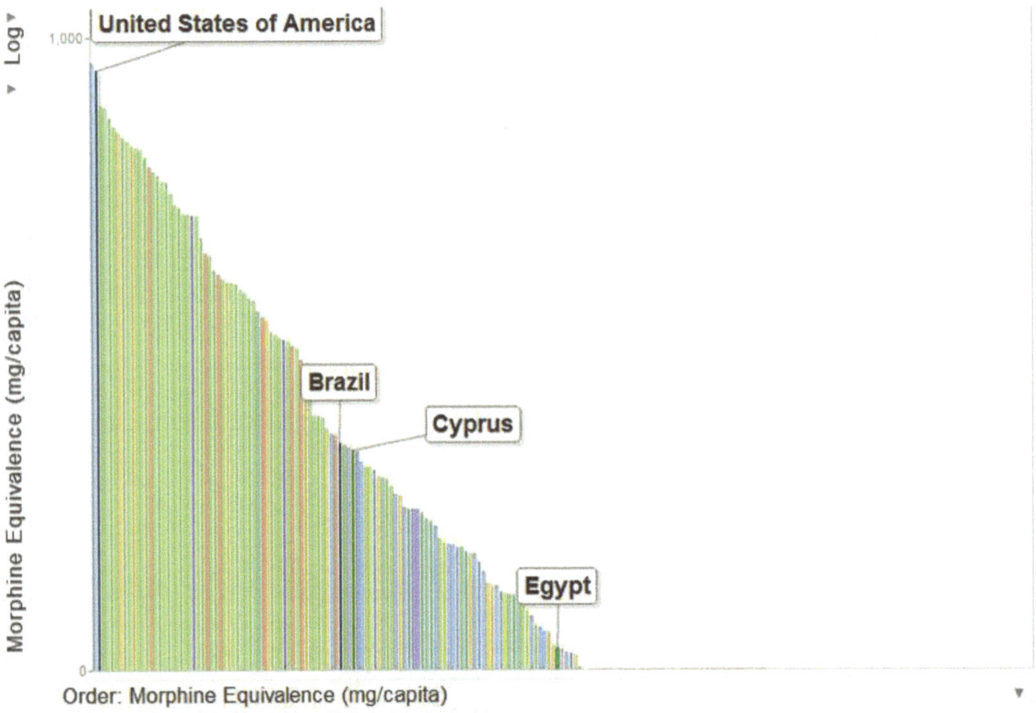

Fig. 7 Morphine consumption per capita pain and policy studies group

oids will produce psychological dependence and drug abuse as well as legal restriction on the use and availability of opioid analgesics [6].

To respond to these issues, the World Health Organization (WHO) advocates a strategy with the following key components: national or state policies that support cancer pain relief through government endorsement of education and drug availability; educational programs for the public, health-care personnel, regulators, and so on; and modification of laws and regulations to improve the availability of drugs, especially the opioid analgesics [6] (Fig. 8).

On April 2011, the Gharbia Cancer Society started a comprehensive palliative care services with ten-bed inpatient unit, 6-day/week outpatient clinic, and home care activity including nurse visits, phone consultation, and family education. All palliative care equipment were provided by public donations (Fig. 9). The palliative

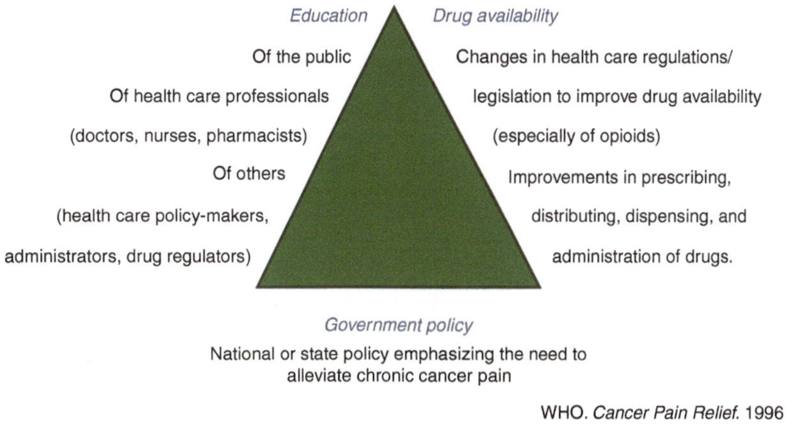

Fig. 8 WHO Foundation measures for implementing cancer pain relief programs

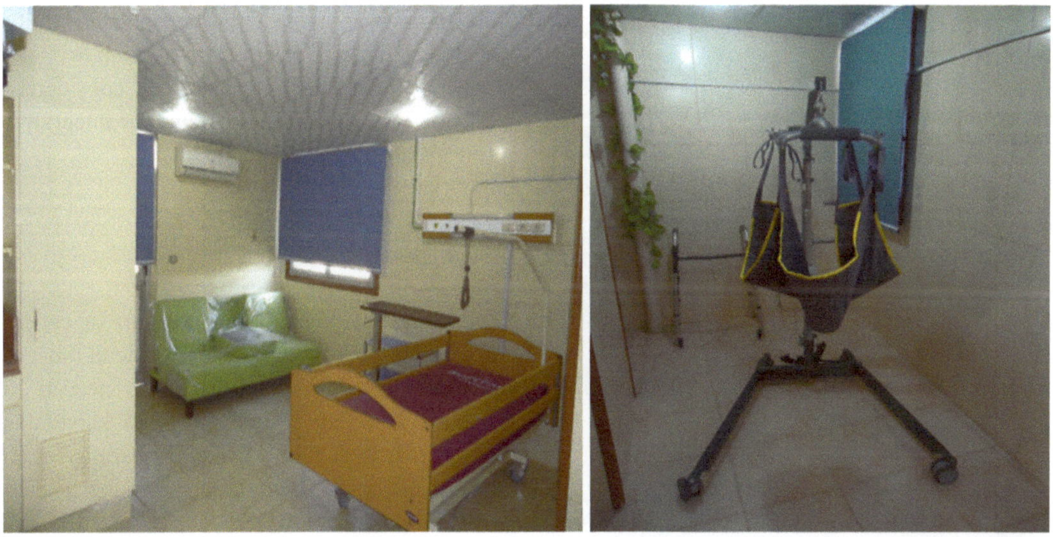

Fig. 9 Palliative care unit and room equipment

care team included one consultant, one fellow, two residents, one social worker, and six nurses.

Education

We believe that education was probably the most important thing to start with. Through collaboration with National Cancer Institute, Bethesda, Maryland, and the San Diego Hospice and the Institute for Palliative Medicine and Middle East Cancer Consortium, a fellowship training program was developed for a medical oncologist in palliative medicine and End-of-Life Care training course for nurses.

A physician from the Gharbia Cancer Society has received a specialist-level training in palliative care in San Diego Hospice and the Institute for Palliative Care. The trainee visited San Diego Hospice six times as International visiting fellow for 5 weeks each visit over a period of 30–48 months. The training focused on symptom management, care for terminally ill patients, prescription and doses of pain medications, and principles of home care. The training also included integrative medicine approaches, spirituality and end-of-life care, communication, examples of other successful international palliative care programs, career development, and planning.

The Gharbia Cancer Society started a nursing education program with emphasis on communication skills, pain recognition and control, and comfort care, and we sought physicians willing to care for terminally ill patients. Doctors treating

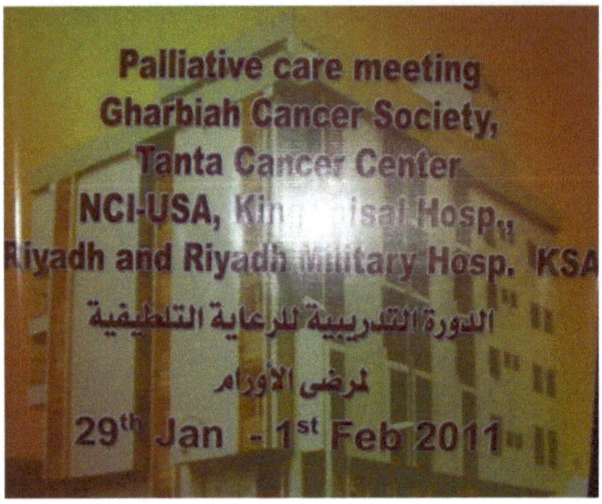
Palliative care meeting
Gharbiah Cancer Society,
Tanta Cancer Center
الدورة التدريبية للرعاية التلطيفية
لمرضى الأورام
29th Jan - 1st Feb 2011

Fig. 10 Training course for nurses in collaboration with National Cancer Institute, USA, and King Faisal Hospital, Saudi Arabia

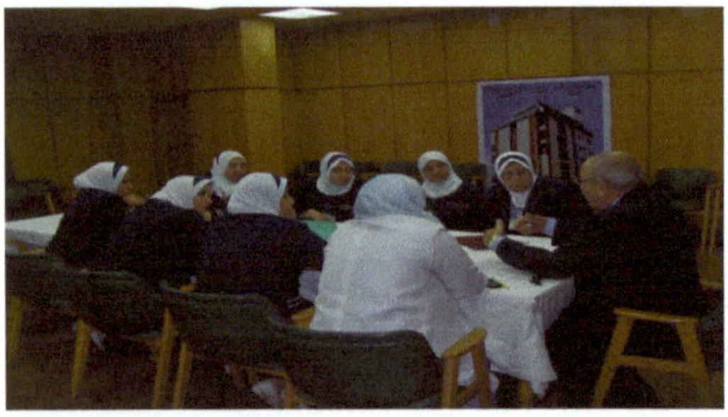

Fig. 11 Nurses' education program

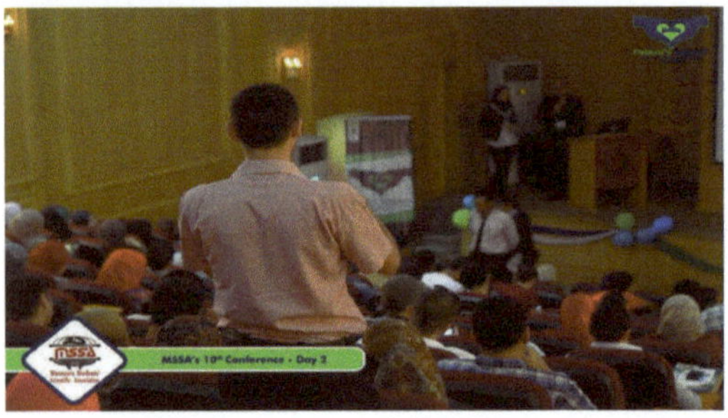

Fig. 12 Presentation of our work at the national conference

patients with cancer are aware of the medical problems that their patients face. Most of the physicians do not get formal training in hospice care in developing countries. We believe that training of doctors working in the field of cancer will be more beneficial to the patients. Through formal lecture series and in-service training of our staff, we provide the staff to start the hospice unit rather than hiring a new crew [1].

Individual discussions were important to educate other members of staff, such as pharmacists and administrators. Participation in national scientific meetings to present our work was essential to spread the knowledge about palliative care (Figs. 10, 11, and 12).

In 2019, through collaboration with Middle East Cancer Consortium (MECC) and the Medical section/International Coordination of Anthroposophic Medicine and the International Federation of Anthroposophic Medical Associations (IVAA), we were invited to a workshop aiming to provide anthroposophic and traditional medicine training to nurses and practitioners in oncology centers considering inclusion of palliative-oriented integrative interventions.

Drug Availability

Pain management is an integral part of cancer care. Proving opioid medicine is difficult most of the time. Extensive paper work is needed to receive pain control medicines. To solve this problem, we dedicated a separate pharmacy with proper staffing and secretarial personnel to dispense pain medication.

In Egypt, the only strong opioids registered for use are sustained-release morphine 30 mg, injectable and transdermal fentanyl patches, and injectable morphine, which are available only in small amounts, mainly for treating acute pain. The oral form of immediate-release morphine is not registered for use. The Egyptian Narcotics Control Law limits to 420 mg the amount of oral morphine that can be given in a single prescription. Local authorities in Gharbiah accepted our request that any patient in need of pain medication can have the recommended dose of opioids. To some extent, the problem of availability was solved and now we are getting enough supply of opioids.

In a period of 8 years, symptom management and palliative care were provided to more than 900 patients with advanced malignancies.

The opioid consumption was increased by several folds.

We also succeded in importing other types of opioids which are not registered in Egypt as the immediate-release morphine and sustained-release and immediate-release oxycodone.

Government Policy

Government policy in Egypt is still not greatly supporting pain relief and palliative care. We are in need of national governmental home-based palliative care program and organization of a national master or diploma degree in palliative care with reasonable training hours.

Conclusion

The major challenges for the program were inadequate public and health professionals' awareness of palliative care services and lack of vehicles and finances to cover home visits. The initial results of the program warrant allocating more resources for coverage of a large number of trainees and instituting a home visits program.

The future directions include instituting a home care services, continuing educational activities, expanding the palliative care teams, and disseminating our experience to other developing countries in Africa and the Middle East.

References

1. Hablas A. Palliative care in Egypt: challenges and opportunities. J Pediatr Hematol Oncol. 2011;33:S52–3.
2. Aljawi DM, Harford JB. Palliative care in the muslim-majority countries: the need for more and better care, contemporary and innovative practice in palliative care, Prof. Esther Chang (Ed.), InTech, https://doi.org/10.5772/32452. 2012. Available from: http://www.intechopen.com/books/contemporary-and-innovative-practice-in-palliative-care/palliative-care-in-muslim-majority-countries-the-need-for-more-and-better-care.
3. Alsirafy Samy A, Elmesidy Salah M, Abou-Elela Enas N. Where do Egyptian palliative care patients with cancer die? J Hosp Palliat Med. 2010;27:313–5.
4. Alsirafy S. Opioid consumption in Egypt, (Kasr El-aini). J Clin Oncol Nucl Med. 2012;8(1–2):1–3.
5. International Narcotics Control Board. Narcotic drugs: estimated world requirementsfor 2012; statistics for 2010. New York: United Nations; 2012.
6. World Health Organization WHO cancer pain relief: with a guide to opioid availability 1996, pp. 42–43.

Part XII

North Africa: Sudan

Republic of Sudan - Palliative Care - Hope for the Future

Geraldine Damanhuri and Mohja Marhoom

Introduction

The year 2019 has been significant in the modern history of the Republic of Sudan – a year of political unrest and turbulence with peaceful demonstrations and protests by the population, asking for positive political change to take place.

July 17, 2019, demonstrated a change in the governing ruling political structure within Sudan with the signing of an agreement for a new transitional Government. This gave hope to the Sudanese people for constructive change to take place especially in health care, education and economic affairs.

Dr Akram Ali Al-Tom has been appointed Minister of Health (MOH), a highly experienced health care professional (HCP) within local and global health care. He is committed to advancing sustainable development and universal health coverage for marginalised and dispossessed groups in society. The MOH is considered well placed to start the enormous process of improving and developing an effective health care system, giving hope to the population of Sudan, for better health care including palliative care.

In December 2019, a meeting between delegations of Sudanese Palliative Care Health Care Professionals with representation from the World Health Organisation took place with the new MOH. Special reference was given to the need for the urgent provision and availability of palliative care symptom control medications. There was a call for integration of palliative care in all health care settings in Sudan [1]. This was deemed a positive meeting by the Palliative Care delegation.

History

Dr Anne Merriman, the Founder and Director of Policy and International Programmes Hospice Africa, introduced palliative care to Uganda in 1993, a neighbouring state to Sudan. She continues to be involved in the hospice movement promoting holistic care for the palliative, end-of-life care patient [2].

> "Every pain that is relieved and every symptom that is improved is a little resurrection for our patients"

Due to Dr Anne Merriman and other inspirational leaders such as Dame Cecily Saunders, Professor Irene Higginson and Professor Marie Fallon in the field of palliative care, freedom from pain is now recognised worldwide as a human right.

Due to the coronavirus pandemic there has been postponement of some of the proposed projects. However, the intention is that in the future they will be realised.

G. Damanhuri (✉)
Comboni College of Science and Technology, Khartoum, Sudan

M. Marhoom
Sudan Medical Specialization Board, Khartoum, Sudan

M. Silbermann (ed.), *Palliative Care for Chronic Cancer Patients in the Community*,
https://doi.org/10.1007/978-3-030-54526-0_20

However, this right is still denied, for many reasons to people throughout the world [2] including Sudan and Khartoum.

A small number of health care professionals (HCPs) over the years have travelled to the Hospice in Uganda having recognised the absence of palliative care education within Sudan. These HCPs also recognised the importance of personal and professional development. They were initially supported by the Principle of Comboni College of Science and Technology (CCST) in Khartoum and the African Palliative Care Association (APCA). Hospice Africa Uganda was responsible for the teaching, education and training of a group of Sudanese health care professionals which included doctors, nurses and psychologists.

Palliative care training in Africa has been a hospice function since the opening of Island Hospice and Bereavement Services in Harare, Zimbabwe, in 1979 [3], St Luke's Hospice, Cape Town, and Highway Hospice, Durban, in 1980. The initial palliative care training was for 'volunteers' as caregivers and bereavement carers [4]. Historically, importance has been given to the volunteer within the hospice movement.

Background

Those Sudanese health care professionals educated in Hospice Africa Uganda included a senior nurse, Sr Halima Ali, recently completing her PhD and currently practicing at the National Cancer Institute (NCI), Medani, outside Khartoum. Sr Ali has been responsible for the development of the NCI hospital specialist palliative care (SPC) team and is promoting innovative structures between hospital palliative care and community/home care. She has developed a volunteer team that is involved in visiting patients in their homes, wound care, stoma care and lymphedema drainage.

Successive Deans of the NCI have been supportive to Sr Ali in the promotion of the 'continuity of patient care in the community' and 'holistic care' concepts. Sr Ali also promotes the concept of 'patient centred care' and works closely with Dr Rana Samir, a family physician based in Medani organising and educating family doctors.

Clinical Nurse Specialist (CNS) in Palliative Care, Alfaki Adam is in clinical practice at Soba University Hospital, an educationalist, educator/lecturer in Khartoum University and Comboni College, nearing completion of his PhD and collaborates with Sr Ali.

Dr Mutasim Mursi, Clinical Oncologist and General Director of East Oncology Centre in Al Gedarif, outside Khartoum is in contact with the NCI in Medani.

Dr Nahla Gafer, Oncologist and Palliative Care Clinical Practitioner in Khartoum Oncology Hospital (KOH), is responsible for the palliative care unit. Dr Gafer is also responsible at Comboni College Khartoum for the short courses, including the 'Introduction to Palliative Care' course aimed at health care professionals. Sr Ali, CNS Alfaki Adam, Senior Nurse Sarah Abdelrahman, Dr Marhoom and Dr Mohammed Mahgoub (Clinical Oncologist) have supported in the past and contribute to this course when possible.

Dr Mohja Marhoom, Family Physician and specialist in palliative care, supports the palliative care unit in KOH. Dr Marhoom is an educationalist and clinical practitioner with innovative ideas regarding extending palliative care within the family doctor's role in primary care. She currently has an innovative proposal under review by the Sudanese Medical Specialization Board (SMSB). Dr Marhoom along with CNS Alfaki Adam is part of the team involved in the development of a four-year BSc Honours Degree Specialist Nursing Course for Palliative, Cancer, Critical and Maternity Care.

Senior Nurse Sara Abdelrahman has a specialist interest in paediatric palliative care. She is collaborating with senior management nurses in developing nurse practice within Sudan and developing palliative care education for health care professionals. Senior Nurse Abdelrahman is assisting in the development of structures and processes including good 'evidence based' practice, management and clinical guidelines within the hospital environment. These are early days.

Management, administration and clinical structures of patient care, both medical and nursing, are being reviewed by the Ministry of

Health and Ministry of Higher Education and Scientific Research within the new Sudanese Government.

Dr Jackline Edwards, palliative care practitioner and public health specialist, is involved with promotion of community palliative care and is a member of the team in the development of the new Comboni Palliative Care Volunteers' (CPCVs) lecturing and training.

These pioneers promote education, research and clinical practice in palliative care in Sudan contributing to the 'Hope' of a nation. The population will potentially experience palliative, holistic care benefiting in the future from effective bereavement, pain and symptom control management [5].

Hospice—A Multi-Professional Team

For many years there have been discussions and meetings among palliative care educationalists and clinical practitioners regarding the development of palliative and end-of-life care in hospital and community care services, leading now to the most recent intense call from Palliative Care Clinical Nurse Specialist Alfaki Adam and others:

"We need a hospice"

This intense call in recent times is now loud. Hospice service provision is now seen as the way forward to promote and achieve good pain and symptom control, end-of-life care, a 'good death' and a role model for best practice. There is currently no effective home care and community palliative care in Khartoum.

In Sudan, there is a shortage or non-availability of important analgesic pain and symptom control medication, including morphine sulphate, in the hospitals and in the community. This is an enormous challenging issue [6].

It is recognised within 'specialist palliative care' that the family members watching a loved one coming to the end of his/her life with symptoms not controlled, including pain, can lead to feelings of guilt and failure, 'failing the loved one' in time of need [7] contributing to bereavement and mental health issues including depression [8]. There is little or no bereavement support in Sudan [9].

The vision and hope for the future is the recognition of the need for the development in teaching of health care professions, including social workers, in the skills to attend to the issues surrounding loss, grief and bereavement [10, 11]. A badly managed death has consequences and has an impact on the living [12].

The following case study demonstrates challenges faced by the palliative care patient and HCPs in Sudan with regard to access to morphine sulphate in addressing a cancer patient's symptom of pain.

Case Study: Lack of Access to Appropriate Analgesia

Mona (name protected), 27 years of age, lives in White Nile State, 4-hour journey from Khartoum, married with two young children and abandoned by her husband when diagnosed with cancer of the cervix in 2014. She has no income and is supported sometimes by her mother. She received chemotherapy and radiotherapy free of charge with an initial good response. However, progressive disease has reoccurred.

Not suitable for further treatment, Mona was referred to the palliative unit as an out-patient, presenting with abdominal pain, somatic and neuropathic. Symptom control assessment was made, and titration of morphine sulphate immediate release (IR) commenced. Only 5 mg and 15 mg morphine sulphate (IR) tablets are available, and sometimes only 5 mg IR tablets are available.

There are no morphine sulphate slow release (SR) tablets, transdermal analgesia patches or higher dosage morphine IR tablets available.

Mona is currently requiring 105 mg Morphine Sulphate (IR) 4 hourly, that is, 630 mg morphine sulphate (IR) in 24 hours.

Therefore, taking 21 × 5 mg Morphine Sulphate IR tablets every 4 hours = 126 tablets in 24 hours (if only 5 mg IR tablets are available).

Mona is also required to take adjuvant medication for pain and symptoms control including diclofenac sodium 50 mg BD and pregabalin 150 mg BD. For her extensive cervix wound, she is prescribed antibiotic powder and local analgesia gel, and she attends to her wound herself. Constipation prevention requires Mona to take local herbal laxatives, and dietary advice is given by the Palliative Care Unit.

Mona comes monthly to Khartoum to collect the morphine and adjuvant medication. The morphine is free; however, adjuvant medication is not. She cannot afford the adjuvant medication. In front of this suffering, when asked how she was coping, she said:

> "I am OK but taking 21 pills every four hours to swallow, which I barely can do, is making me suffer more than the physical pain. Taking 21 pills and more, makes me depressed."

As can be seen in this short case study, we are looking at one aspect of care, pain control, which demonstrates the enormous challenges being faced by HCPs and patients in addressing effective pain control. Attention is required from the new Ministry of Health (MOH). The hope for the future is that the new MOH will listen, recognise and address this urgent need by ensuring all patients have access to appropriate and timely analgesia.

Hospice Feasibility Study/Proposal

In January 2019, there was a call for a Hospice as a centre of excellence by 'Palliative Care for the Future Team' (PCFT), a group of health care professionals. A feasibility study was requested by the Principal of Comboni College of Science and Technology (CCST). This serious progressive work has reached the current position, which is, meeting with and surveying community leaders, health care professionals and local population within a specific geographical area. This work continues, and the target area has a population of approximately 2 million people or more. The aim of this feasibility study is the consideration of the development of the first Modern Hospice to service a specific geographical area in Khartoum owned by the people and supported by the Government.

Comboni Palliative Care Volunteers' (CPCVs) First-Year Celebrations, 2020

The first palliative care course for CPCVs, which began on Saturday, 26th January 2019, was recognised and supported by CCST, and it took place over four Saturdays. CPCVs was founded by Dr Mohja Marhoom, and co-founded by Geraldine Damanhuri. After they recognised a desire from students, teachers, educationalists, community workers and HCPs to assist in the care of the palliative care patient and their families, the CPCVs was born [13].

Batch two of the palliative care course was completed in December 2019. A third course is planned for June 2020. There are currently 48 names on the waiting list to attend the course. Some volunteers teach on the course, including Dr Jackline Edwards, Senior Nurse Sara Abddelrahman, CNS Mahasin Ibrahim and CNS Alfaki Adam, and Dr Martina Lowisebra is involved in effective coordination.

The CPCV's first-year celebration of working volunteers was well attended, 600 people on the night, with lecturers, HCP's, students, spiritual, diplomatic, community and business leaders and of course the wonderful happy, joyful volunteers who made the evening happen.

Events included provision of food; African dancers; north Sudanese, south Sudanese, Ethiopian and Yemini dancers; and great fun. Other acts included poetry and comedy which made everyone laugh. Volunteers' personal experiences and stories from clients were expressed. The message given was:

> "Palliative care is about life and living"

In 2019, hands-on practical care, education and research were carried out giving a common purpose bringing unity and hope to the volunteers and clients.

In 2019, the Comboni Palliative Care Volunteers carried out practical tasks including translation in clinics, hand massage for both patients and co-carers, patient storytelling, listening, recording and documentation. Over 200 persons received hand massages between July and

November. Research projects took place and service evaluation for service improvement continues. The following are comments from the evaluation form using client's own words:

> "hand massage reduced the stress in my body and gave me the good idea for life"
> "Please spread the importance of therapy so that people will get knowledge about it"

Volunteers are currently working over three sites including a charity guest house for cancer patients, a palliative care unit within a state cancer hospital and a TB unit. At the TB unit, there were many young patients, this meant, adapting the service to meet their needs. Hand massage and storytelling will continue. With the introduction of 'English language', 'how to look after your health', singing and art-therapy courses, ongoing evaluation of the service will take place.

A volunteer overheard two young patients speaking: When one said

> "they only want to make us happy,"

the other young patient responded

> "we deserve to be happy."

CNS Damanhuri and Dr Marhoom introduced teaching on the 'pain assessment tool' to nurses in the Khartoum Oncology Hospital in the wards and in the chemotherapy treatment areas. This resulted in a request by the nurses for further training in 'palliative care'. There were many difficulties in carrying out this service due to the lack of practical resources, long nurse working hours and political unrest at the time in Khartoum.

A small group of nurses persevered in attending a short 'introduction to palliative care course' in-house, which included pain and symptom control, communication skills, breaking bad news and ethics [14]. The course was completed by teaching 'hand massage' to the nurses, which they appreciated.

Palliative Care Audit and Research

Three small audit/research projects [15] were completed. Written permission was given by the General Director of the Oncology Hospital which made it possible with the support of the Matrons and the collaboration of oncology registrars, nurses, patients, co-patients and volunteers to complete the projects. The following are summaries of the three projects.

Project One

A conversation with nurses employed within an oncology hospital in Khartoum on cancer and palliative care nurse education and training issues. The aim was to get a baseline to quantify if there was a need for education in both theory and clinical practice for nurses working within oncology (please refer to Fig. 1). The population sample had 30 nurses. Ninety per cent of the nursing sample had not received any training in palliative or oncology care. Forty-three per cent did not know what 'palliative care' meant, and 23% did not know if their patients were under curative or palliative care.

One nurse wrote:

> "we have not received any training, but we are in desperate need to have the proper training and knowledge to be capable enough to look after the patients"

Project Two

Listening to the cancer patients. Results of a completed patient satisfactory survey on the Gastro-Intestinal (GI) wards in a cancer hospital.

The aim of this project was to give the patient and their carers a voice in cancer service development, to engage in the positive transformation of the quality of the patient's experience, to promote audit and research development on the frontline for health care professionals, and to recognise and promote education and training needs for health care professionals, administrators and managers. The population sample was 20 females and 16 males, all receiving chemotherapy treatment.

The results of the audit clearly showed a need for a conversation to take place within the hospital management team regarding patient–doctor diagnosis disclosure (refer to Fig. 2).

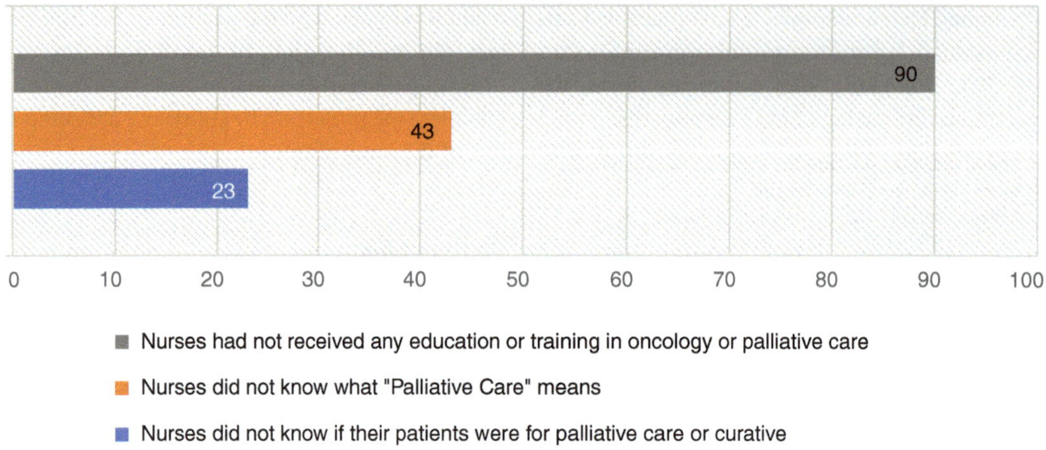

Fig. 1 Reasons for education and training requested by nursing staff

Fig. 2 The need for doctor/patient discussion on patient diagnosis disclosure

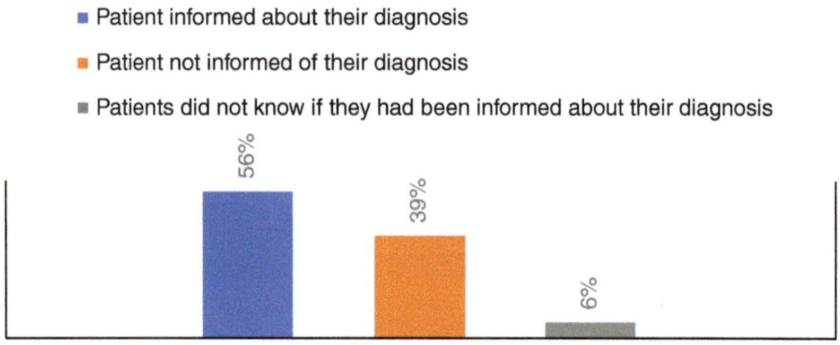

Figure 3 demonstrates the need for a conversation to take place within the hospital management team with special reference to consent for treatment. Fifty-eight per cent of patients were not informed of the side effects of chemotherapy before treatment, and 3% did not know if they had been informed.

Referring to Fig. 4, there was a clear message from patients and co-carers regarding the need for housekeeping/hygiene/infection control improvement.

Project Three

Oncology registrars within a cancer hospital respond to a questionnaire on palliative/symptom control recognition, education, management and cancer service development. The aim of this 'snap' audit was to begin to access the experiences of the oncology registrars over one day, concentrating on pain and symptom control and associated issues which they observe in their everyday practice. The sample population was 15 oncology registrars.

Eighty per cent of oncology registrars recognised that they had palliative care patients on their caseload, and 20% did not; however, this could be explained as to the specific patient caseload and area of work of the oncology registrar on the day the audit took place (refer to Fig. 5).

The four leading symptoms recognised by the oncology registrars were pain, nausea, vomiting and shortness of breath. Attention to psychological symptoms such as anxiety and depression was also recorded.

Oncology registrars were clear in their request for service improvement (please refer to Fig. 6). Service improvement requests included

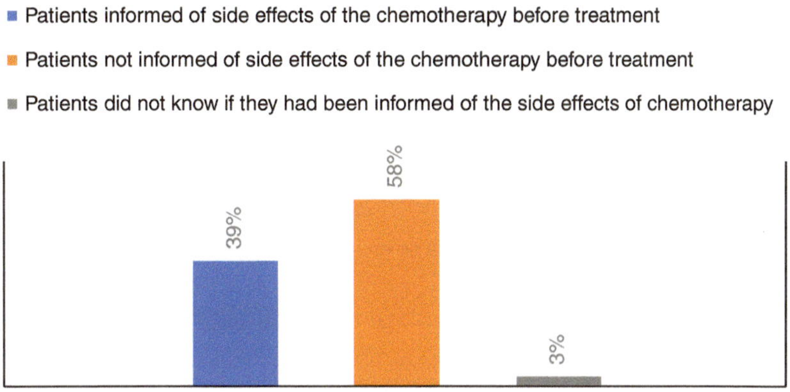

Fig. 3 The need for ethical issues regarding consent for treatment to be addressed

Lack of cleanliness, poor ventilation, poor air condition, dirty bathroom facilities and bedding, lack of access to clean sheets and water, concerns regarding insects on the ward. Would like better availability of staff and access to nutritionists, social and financial support. Patients would like privacy and better access to medication

Fig. 4 Patients' concerns on the gastro-intestinal cancer chemotherapy ward

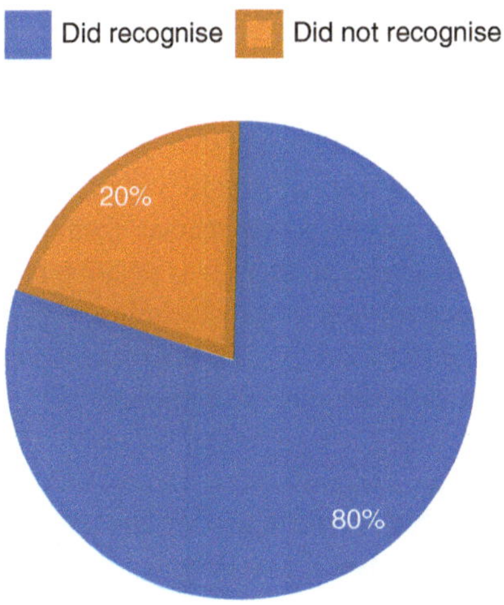

Fig. 5 Oncology registrars requests for service improvement

waiting times for patients, organisation of clinics, privacy for patients, ratio of number of patients to available registrars, cost of and access to medication for patients and the referral process to be improved. More than 90% of the oncology registrars requested palliative care teaching/training both in theory and clinical practice.

Oncology registrars also requested improved availability of investigations for patients, better filing systems and an isolation room for neutropenic patients.

Summary of Recommendations

Recommendations for the above three projects include the opening of a conversation between the hospital management team, the medical, nursing, pharmacy and university HCP's curriculum planners, on pain and symptom control. Recognising that patients are in pain and acknowledging that the nurses and registrars recognise that their patients are in pain and are requesting the resources to carry out effective care.

Further recommendations include the need for attention to housekeeping, infection control issues, medical ethics recognition, provision and availability of effective pain relief and symptom control medications, and education both in clinical practice and theory. There is an urgent need to review clinical, management, ethical and administration guidelines. Further audit and research are required for development of best international practice [16].

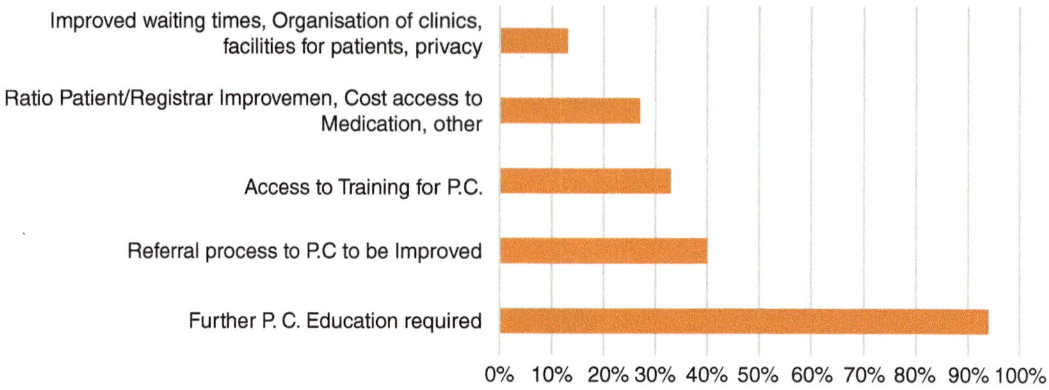

Fig. 6 Oncology registrars requests for service improvement

Palliative Care and Higher Education Hope for the Future

A Bachelor of Science Honours degree course for Special Nursing in Palliative Care, Cancer Care, Critical Care and Maternity is awaiting approval by the Ministry of Higher Education. A new nursing faculty building and library for nursing has been approved by Comboni College of Science and Technology. December 2020 is the provisional starting date for the nursing degree course.

A Post Graduate Diploma in Palliative Care is being discussed and is awaiting approval by the Ministry of Higher Education. Currently, Comboni College of Science and Technology has a short six-day course over 6 weeks including clinical teaching during the six-week 'Introduction to Palliative Care' aimed at HCPs which is approved by the Ministry of Higher Education.

October – Breast Cancer Awareness Month, Sudan, 2019

A health care initiative by the DOH in Sudan took place in October 2019 promoting awareness of breast cancer. The Sudan Medical Specialisation Board (SMSB) family doctors requested part of the final celebration time to include a presentation, titled

"Breast Cancer – How Can Palliative Care Help?"

The family doctors and volunteers responded to the following questions with a show of hands

(a) *How many people here present know a family member who has/had breast cancer?*
(b) *How many of these persons experienced pain?*
(c) *How many of these persons died from the disease?*

There was a show of hands, the taboo of cancer was publicly challenged, this was an effective demonstration that patients in Sudan have cancer and pain and some do not recover from cancer.

In the discussion, there was positive feedback on the need to look at the discipline of palliative care in the community. The conversation on palliative care 'home care' was opened.

Medani, National Cancer Institute (NCI) Palliative Care Week Celebration

Multi-professional palliative care was celebrated officially in Medani in October 2019 for the first time. The aim of the celebration was to create awareness to the public and local HCPs of palliative care issues, current service provision, recreation for patients and co-patients and training for health professionals and volunteers.

Activities included home care visits, screening symptoms of patients presented on the day, information leaflets, posters produced and disseminated, exhibitions and videos, rest areas for adults and paediatric cancer patients, wound dressing and lymphedema training, and distribution of food and juice. The event was documented by the local university and the mass media. It was a very successful palliative care awareness campaign week. Congratulations.

Conclusion

Palliative care in Sudan has seen an extraordinary year of energy within both education and health domains. Future plans include meetings between Medani and Comboni Khartoum volunteer groups to share skills. There is potentially a new higher education palliative/cancer care BSc honours four-year degree course in nursing, awaiting approval by the Department of Higher Education. At a multi-professional level, a potential diploma in palliative care is being planned. A hope for a hospice in Khartoum in the future is gaining ground. There is now an awareness and participation of family physicians in palliative care. There is an energetic push for access to effective analgesia especially morphine sulphate. Collaboration is happening between palliative care specialists. Palliative care in Sudan is looking forward to a hopeful future. An African proverb says:

> "If you want to go fast, go alone. If you want to go far go together"

References

1. Grant L, Downing J, Luyirika, Murphy M, Namukwaya L, Kiyange F, Atieno M, Kemigisha E, Hunt J, Snell K, Murray SA, Leng M. Integrating palliative care into national health systems in Africa: a multi-country intervention study. J Glob Health. 2017;7(1):010419.
2. Merriman A. Audacity to love. Bringing hope and peace for the dying. The story of Hospice Africa. 2010. Irish Hospice Foundation Morrison Chambers, 32 Nassau Street, Dublin 2 http://www.hospice-foundation.ie.
3. Mkwananzi S. Focus on training in palliative care at Island Hospice , Zimbabwe. African Palliative Care Association. J Palliat Care. 2005;1(2):205–13.
4. Gwyther L. Intergrating palliative medicine into medical curricula. Family Practice Conference, Mtata, 2005.
5. Randal F, Downie RS. The philosophy of palliative care – critique and reconstruction. Oxford, UK: Oxford University Press; 2006.
6. Chaplin D. Developing an end-of-life pathway to improve nurses' bereavement care. Nurs Times. 2009;105(1):20–1.
7. Parkes CM. The dying patient. BMJ. 1998;316(7140):1313–5.
8. Shear MK. Complicated grief. N Engl J Med. 2015;372:153–60.
9. Bereavement Care Services Standards. Bereavement Services Association and Cruse Bereavement Care, 2013.
10. Parkes CM, Weiss RS. Recovery from bereavement. New York: Basic Books; 1983.
11. Sealey M, Breen LJ, Connor M, Aoun SM. A scoping review of bereavement risk assessment measures: implication for palliative care. Palliat Med. 2015;29(7):577–89.
12. Stroebe W, Stroebe MS. Bereavement and health. Cambridge: Cambridge University Press; 1987.
13. Scott R, Howlett S. Volunteers in hospice and palliative care – a resource for voluntary services managers. 2nd ed. Oxford: Oxford University Press; 2009.
14. Walshe C, Preston N, Johnson B. Palliative care nursing. Principles and evidence for practice. 3rd ed. London, UK: Open University Press; 2018.
15. Addington-Hall JM, Bruera E, Higginson IR, Payne S. Research methods in palliative care. Oxford: Oxford University Press; 2007.
16. Wee B, Hughes N. Education in palliative care – building a culture of learning. Oxford: Oxford University Press; 2007.

Part XIII

North Africa: Morocco

Cancer and Palliative Care in Morocco

Asmaa El Azhari

Introduction

Cancer is the second leading cause of death in Morocco and the number of cancer patients has increased significantly in recent years.

The mission of epidemiological surveillance of cancer in Morocco is assumed by the Registre du Cancer du Grand Casablanca (Cancer Registry of Greater Casablanca Region, or RCRC) which indeed provides essential data on the descriptive epidemiology of cancers in the Greater Casablanca region.

The population of this region is 11% of the total population of the country and one-fifth of the total urban population in Morocco—this is a representative sample, allowing an extrapolation to the entire population of the country [1].

According to the RCRC, the evolution of cancer between 2004 and 2012 has increased in terms of the both number of cases recorded and the overall incidence (Fig. 1) [2]. In addition to the normal course of cancer and the epidemiological transition, this increase can be explained by the many changes that took place in Morocco during this period.

Since its creation in November 2005, the Lalla Salma Foundation for Cancer Prevention and Treatment (FLSC) has worked to improve the management of cancers in Morocco, as evidenced by the impact of actions such as the organization of media awareness campaigns, the implementation of an early detection program for breast and cervical cancer, the improved accessibility and supply of care, and the strengthening of the capacity of care in oncology centers [2].

In the same context, the National Cancer Prevention and Control Plan (PNPCC) 2010–2019 was implemented, not only to reduce the morbidity and mortality rates attributable to cancer, but also to improve the quality of life of patients and their relatives within a comprehensive and integrated care system; this plan is based on impartiality, human service and equity to guarantee the rights of the patient.

Indeed, for the first time in Morocco, palliative care appears to be a strategic axis within the national health plan, in this case regarding cancer, on the same level with prevention, early detection and diagnosis, and treatment (Fig. 2).

The palliative care axis is the fourth strategic axis of the PNPCC 2010–2019; it includes four actions broken down into 13 measures oriented toward the promotion of pain management and covers the needs of patients with cancer in palliative situations (Chart 1).

There are two types of medical coverage in Morocco: (a) Compulsory Health Insurance or AMO for employees, the self-employed and students and (b) the Medical Assistance Plan or RAMED for the most deprived, which allows free access to healthcare without prior social security contributions.

A. El Azhari (✉)
Palliative Care Department, Mohammed VI Center for the Treatment of Cancers, UHC Ibn Rochd Casablanca, Casablanca, Morocco

M. Silbermann (ed.), *Palliative Care for Chronic Cancer Patients in the Community*,
https://doi.org/10.1007/978-3-030-54526-0_21

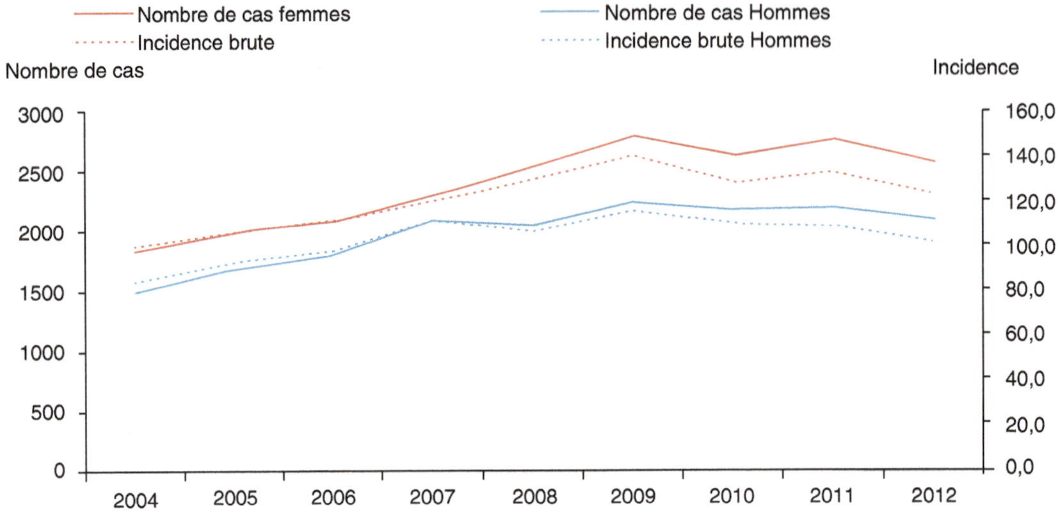

Fig. 1 Evolution of the number of cases and gross incidence in all type of cancer according to gender between 2004 and 2012, RCRC

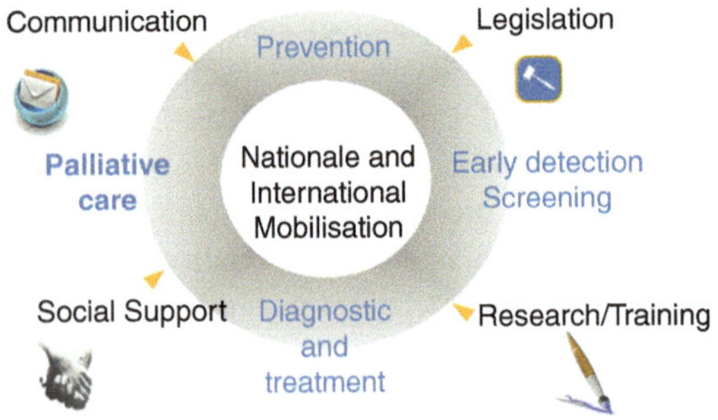

Fig. 2 Conceptual Frame of the PNPCC 2010–2019

Palliative care programs for cancer patients are largely free and provide outpatient care and home visits for patients with AMO and RAMED, including hospitalization for patients with RAMED. This allows cancer patients to access care regardless of their financial condition.

Chart 1 Actions of the Palliative Care Axis of the PNPCC 2010–2019

1. Developing pain management (5 measures: 62–66)
2. Ensuring family and social support (3 measures: 67–69)
3. Ensuring the development and extension of networked palliative care (4 measures: 70–73)
4. Developing research in palliative care (one measure: 74)

Evolution of Palliative Care in Morocco

The year 1995 is considered to be the year that witnessed the birth of palliative care in Morocco and is marked by the introduction of absorbable morphine (oral route); for the first time, the pain of cancer patients was treated with a strong opioid.

Since then, several steps have been taken by the Moroccan government and medical community for the development of palliative care.

Since the year 2000, a university degree in pain management can be attained in three cities in Morocco: Rabat, Casablanca and Oujda.

In 2002, a home-care program called AMAD—Assistance Medicale a Domicile—was launched by Professor Abdelatif Benider, the Head of Oncology at the University Hospital in Casablanca; this program lasted for 10 years.

With the creation of the FLSC in 2005, the first pain unit was established at the National Oncology Center in Rabat. The establishment of the 2010–2019 PNPCC played a critical role in developing and extending palliative care.

From 2012 to 2019, palliative care units were set up in different regions of Morocco; in addition to outpatient care, almost all of them were strengthened by teams who paid home visits.

The cities of Casablanca, Rabat, Marrakech, Meknes, Oujda and Fez all have palliative care units at oncology centers located at university or tertiary hospitals.

During the same period—on the political level—in addition to the development of the PNPCC 2010–2019, the Ministry of Health adopted a sectoral health strategy (SSS) 2012–2016 that included actions to develop palliative care to address the burden of pain. However, both the body responsible for carrying out these actions and the budget allocated are not mentioned in this 2012–2016 SSS. The project to institutionalize and decentralize palliative care to regional and provincial hospitals and to primary healthcare was established through a ministerial circular issued in 2015; its application did not take place.

A national guide to palliative care was published in 2018 by the Ministry of Health in partnership with the FLSC.

The goal of the PNPCC was to ensure the total coverage of cancer patients in need of palliative care by the year 2019.

So, how is palliative care perceived by the community? Are health professionals prepared to adopt a perspective of care and support rather than a curative approach at any given time in the development of incurable cancer? What political, legal and organizational obstacles hinder the expansion of, and then the access to, palliative care? Can we talk about community palliative care in Morocco?

To better understand the current situation of palliative care in Morocco, we must first understand the attitude toward palliative care in Moroccan culture.

The Culture of Palliative Care in Morocco

The failure to cure cancer remains a taboo for the majority of oncologists in Morocco today, especially as the approach toward the care of the patient is (most of the time) paternalistic and not patient-centered.

Therefore, the doctor takes full responsibility for the process, from start to finish—a start that will most likely be marked by the omission of prognostic information. A relentless therapy is the logical continuation of this conspiracy of silence, making it difficult for patients to access palliative care; some will access it very late, during the last days of their lives, when the majority will not stand a chance.

When the oncologists realize that their goal—healing—is no longer attainable, they withdraw as they consider that their mission is over. They hand the patient over to the community, which is not prepared to provide this type of support; the patient then lacks the human, material or emotional resources to cope with the end of life.

The unsupported chronic phase implies a sudden interruption of care, or continuity of care, except through various institutions that are unrelated to palliative care [3], and the transition from hospital to community is not done properly.

Yet, according to reports from palliative care teams in Morocco, patients and their families do seek palliative care—they accept dying but refuse to suffer. Few of the patients or their families refuse opioid therapy due to cultural connotations or a complete misunderstanding about morphine. On the other hand, the majority of health professionals in Morocco are morphinophobic.

Since the creation of palliative care teams, the number of patients treated by these units has increased over the years. On the one hand, despite the paternalistic mentality that dominates the medical sector and the thanatophobia (fear of dying) that pervades it, several oncologists have become aware of the importance of integrating palliative care into the overall care of the patient and, when treatments become ineffective, that much of the process can be delegated to the community. On the other hand, according to the palliative care teams, almost all the patient-family units in care adhere to palliative care programs; for them, it is a new way of experiencing death; it no longer represents suffering and is no longer synonymous with heartbreak. They now experience it as it once was, before medicalization invaded the moment of death, as a natural process where new emotional opportunities are to be explored.

Community acceptance of palliative care has also led to an increase in the demand for palliative care in the community. This transition has been a positive factor in facilitating the inclusion of more and more cancer patients into each unit's palliative care program. However, this development has not been accompanied by a proportional increase in either human or material resources. The decentralization of the prescription of opioids and the minimal provision of palliative care at different levels of health (regional, provincial, primary healthcare) have not evolved proportionnally either.

Apart from the organizational obstacles which slow down this decentralization as well as the philosophical beliefs regarding palliative care in the medical environment, there is also a certain reluctance among health professionals to accept or practice palliative care because of morphinophobia and fear of being confronted with the suffering of the patient at the end of life, not out of lack of compassion, but due to a great lack of training.

Palliative Care Education

As mentioned earlier, since 2000, programs for university degrees in pain management exist in three Moroccan universities. This diploma program includes modules that treat the management of different types of pain (post-surgical, trauma, rheumatology, emergency room, etc.) allocating a single module for cancer pain and palliative care. Continous training, the content of which is exlusively dedicated to palliative care, has been provided at the Casablanca University Hospital by the team from the palliative care unit of the Mohammed VI Center for the Treatment of Cancers since 2015. It is the personal initiative of the members of this team and the director of aforementioned center. Admittance to this six-module training is free of charge in order to facilitate access, and thus raises awareness among the greatest number of health professionals. However, this certificate is not recognized by the medical school of casablanca and has no academic value.

From 2015 to 2019, the FLSC has focused on training all palliative care teams, providing theoretical and practical training by facilitating mobility and the teams taking up residence at the palliative care unit in Casablanca to carry out internships.

In fact, this unit is currently considered as the reference center for palliative care training as its palliative care program serves the largest number of cancer patients in palliative care, almost 1000 patients annually.

In 2015, a reform in medical studies required medical students to attend basic palliative care training in 20-hour compulsory segments during their fifth year of medical studies.

The application of this reform will take place during the 2019–2020 academic year in some medical schools in Morocco. In the dispensation of this theoretical segment, health professionals dedicated to palliative care do not intervene—it is entirely entrusted to the anesthesiologists.

However, palliative care is not only the treatment of pain, but a whole philosophy that should be passed down and taught not only by educators but also by health professionals who are exclusively dedicated to palliative care and are faced every day with the challenges of managing biopsychosocial and spiritual suffering and grief, not only at hospitals but also at the home of patients and their families.

There is no palliative care specialty in Morocco. Doctors who specialize in palliative care and practice in Morocco received their academic training abroad. Currently, to our knowledge, there is no government project that recognizes palliative care as a specialty.

In summary, currently, the quantity as well as the quality of training in palliative care remains poor in Morocco and is not supported by any definitive government measures.

Access to Opioids

As the majority of palliative cancer patients reside in the community, an oral immediate-release opioid should not only be available for hospital patients but should also be supplied by community pharmacies [4]. In addition, morphine is on the World Health Organization (WHO) list of essential medicines for palliative care [5].

Three opioids are available in Morocco: morphine, fentanyl and methadone; the use of the latter is not authorized for the treatment of pain, except for when weaning from narcotic drugs. It can therefore be said that the two opioids most used are, first, morphine and, then, fentanyl.

Morphine is available in either quick and prolonged-release oral tablets or as a solution for injection. The oral form is dispensed at the oncology centers free of charge for patients with RAMED-type medical coverage. For the rest, it must be purchased at a city pharmacy. The price of oral morphine remains expensive compared to the purchasing power of the Moroccan population.

Fentanyl is available as a patch and oral tablets as well as a solution for injection. The transdermal and oral forms are rarely dispensed at the hospital and most of the time must be purchased by patients. Their costs are often unaffordable.

According to Moroccan law, any community pharmacy has the right to store and dispense opioids in accordance with certain regulatory requirements. However, only a few community pharmacies located in the cities where the regional oncology centers are sell morphine or fentanyl.

The reluctance of pharmacies to dispense opioids can be explained by the cumbersome administrative hassles associated with Moroccan regulations regarding the storage and dispensing of opioids. Patients needing opioid therapy who do not live in the cities that provide it will need to travel, sometimes long distances. A prescription for oral morphine or fentanyl, according to Moroccan law, is valid for 28 days, and a prescription for injectable morphine is valid for only 10 days.

Only one laboratory in Morocco supplies oral morphine to the market and runs out of stock frequently, leaving no alternatives. The possibility for the rotation of opioids is obviously limited given the availability of only two types of opioids.

Pediatric forms of opioids do not exist. Morphine in oral solution or in powder form to prepare the solution is not marketed in Morocco.

Any specialist or general practitioner has the right to prescribe opioids, but currently only palliative care doctors and anesthesiologists prescribe them.

Palliative Care Programs

The palliative care units in Morocco today are specialized units and offer a model of mixed care; that is to say, the same palliative care unit with its corresponding team provides palliative care at home, at hospital and as outpatient consultations. They care for patients with various levels of complexity, and each team is trained by doctors and nurses.

There are two types of cancer patients in palliative care programs: patients referred by their oncologist from the public or private sector and patients whose cancer is diagnosed late and are referred by their treating physician, followed by a multidisciplinary consultation meeting with the palliative care team. The latter constitutes most of the patients in palliative care programs.

Only patients residing in urban areas of those cities that have a palliative care unit can benefit from home care.

There are no palliative care support teams at provincial hospitals or at primary health centers to take over once access to the specialized palliative care unit becomes impossible or when the patient presents a minimal level of complexity not specified in specialized palliative care.

This leads to two extremely complex situations: one, the distress of patients who cannot access specialized palliative care units due to geographic, economic or physical obstacles, and the other, the saturation of palliative care units as only cancer patients in palliative situations can be admitted.

Healthcare professionals are reluctant to take care of these patients, even when they show minimal complexity, due to a lack of training in basic palliative care. In addition, today there is no palliative care network to coordinate between the different levels of care, nor any budget allocated to the palliative care program; there is no national palliative care program per se in Morocco. Palliative care, therefore, remains at the tertiary level, and the participation of the community is limited to the patient's family, who takes responsibility for all of their biopsychosocial needs.

We can represent this model as a chain of rings which, in fact, only has two rings, one at either end of the two extremes: tertiary level and community, and all the intermediate rings which should contribute to the decentralization of palliative care and proper integration into the community do not exist: link nurses, support teams at the primary healthcare level, teams of volunteers, respite hospitalizations in provincial hospitals and so on.

There is no pediatric palliative care unit, only a palliative care team that takes care of children as well as adults.

Conclusion

Cancer and its treatments are a source of weakness, not only for patients but also for the people who surround them, who undergo and bear the entire burden of care—the communication with health professionals in addition to psychological and spiritual support [6].

The biggest challenge for health systems is how to integrate palliative care in an efficient, sustainable manner while adapting to community parameters [7].

The vulnerabilities of our healthcare system are essentially centered around either the moment of integration of palliative care or the transition of the patient from the hospital back to the community; in addition, many health professionals have morphinophobia and/or thanatophobia. The first points can be remedied through a project to decentralize palliative care by means of a network that involves all parties concerned for the proper community care of the patient and the latter by strengthening education in palliative care.

From our point of view, tangible political commitment through advocacy and the designation of budgets allocated particularly to palliative care are necessary to take a step forward in the care of cancer patients in palliative situations.

References

1. Registre des Cancers de la région du Grand Casablanca pour la période 2008-2012, edition 2016: 8.
2. Plan national de prévention et de contrôle du cancer 2010-2019 Synthèse: 22.
3. Saunders S, Killackey T, Kurahashi A, et al. Palliative care transitions from acute care to community-based care - a systematic review. J Pain Symptom Manag. 2019;53(4):721–34.
4. Sharkey L, Loring B, Cowan M, et al. National palliative care capacities around the word: results from the Word Health Organization noncommunicable disease country capacity survey. Palliat Med. 2018;32(1):106–13.
5. World Health Organization. WHO model list of essential medicines, https://apps.who.int/iris/bitstream/handle/10665/325771/WHO-MVP-EMP-IAU-2019.06-eng.pdf?ua=1. 2019, Access Jan 2020.
6. Hendricks BA, Lofton C, Azuero A, et al. The project ENABLE Cornerstone randomized pilot trial: protocol for lay navigator-led early palliative care for African,-American and rural cancer family caregivers. Contemp Clin Trials Commun. 2019;16:100485.
7. Nguyen HQ, Ruel N, Macias M, et al. Translation and evaluation of a lung cancer intervention for community practice. J Pain Symptom Manag. 2018;56(5):709–18.

Psycho-oncological Support for Children with Cancer and Their Parents: The Soleterre Foundation Experience With the PIOP's Program

Imane Benlekbir and Damiano Rizzi

Soleterre and Its Intervention Method

The international pediatric oncology program (Programme International d'Oncologie Pédiatrique, PIOP) was created to protect the right to health and life for children and adolescents with cancer. Launched in 2005 in Ukraine, the program is now operational in five countries: Italy (starting in 2012), Ivory Coast (2010), Morocco (2010), and Ukraine and Uganda (2014). The program has also been launched in India.

It is a complex organization designed to act on the various factors that determine access to and quality of care. The complex nature of oncological diseases, which includes emotional, financial, and social factors, requires simultaneous actions in several areas: medico-scientific, psychological, social, and community-based. To increase survival rates, Soleterre first decided to act on healthcare systems, improving them by targeting infrastructures, availability of medication and equipment, and medical and paramedical training. Upgrading these areas is the only way to impact the timeliness and quality of diagnoses and the treatments availability and efficiency. However, an integral part of treatment is the management of children and families, psychological and social needs, based on a therapeutic alliance with all subjects of care.

Since childhood cancer is a global health issue, it is easy to understand why this program should be multidisciplinary and involve many other actors in the community. The international pediatric oncology program addresses each country's specific weaknesses in order to meet their needs. With this in mind, the Soleterre Foundation works on seven themes according to each specific environment:

Health Education

The primary prevention, defined as health education, aims to prevent objectionable behaviors and promote those that are recommended to raise children in healthy environments while minimizing risk factors. Critical actions in this regard are educating mothers and children on lifestyle, nutrition, and hygiene, and awareness of and research on the protection of the health environment.

Early Diagnosis

Early diagnosis and treatment can increase survival rates and limit the temporary or permanent debilitating consequences of the illness. Early

I. Benlekbir
Psychology, Education Science,
Rabat, Rabat Salé Zamour Zeir, Morocco
e-mail: imane.benlekbir@soleterre.org

D. Rizzi (✉)
Department of Psychology, Soleterre
Foundation – Policlinico San Matteo, Pavia, Italy
e-mail: damiano.rizzi@soleterre.org

M. Silbermann (ed.), *Palliative Care for Chronic Cancer Patients in the Community*,
https://doi.org/10.1007/978-3-030-54526-0_22

diagnosis is determined by the quality of, and access to, the basic pediatric healthcare system and by the level of awareness of parents and communities. Critical actions in this regard are awareness, information, and education for general physicians, pediatricians, parents, and communities (particularly in peripheral areas), training and linking peripheral, non-specialized medical staff with relevant pediatric oncology units, and provision of powerful diagnostic tools.

Medical Care

To improve survival rates, treatments must be effective and fast, and initiated immediately after a diagnosis. Drugs (chemotherapy as well as painkillers and anti-inflammatories), medical supplies, and equipment (in case surgery is necessary) must be readily available. Critical actions in this regard are structural improvement of relevant services through the provision of surgical, diagnostic, and rehabilitation instruments and modernization (hospital wards, operating rooms, dormitories, and playgrounds), provision of medication and hygienic and sanitary equipment, and national and international transport and care for highly severe cases.

Psycho-social Educational Support

Pharmacological and surgical treatments should be combined with psychological, social, and educational support. Some of the actions focus directly on children, along with support for parents and the department's medical and paramedical staff. Critical actions in this area are continuing training and meetings for physicians (pediatricians, general practitioners, psycho-oncologists, etc.), psychological monitoring for sick and cured children and their parents and for the medical and paramedical staff, art therapy and therapeutic clown activities, leisure and play activities at the hospital, and awareness sessions in schools.

Temporary Residences

A facility outside of the ward where families and children with cancer who are receiving outpatient care can be housed has three advantages. First, it helps families who can't afford to move to health centers where care is dispensed; second, it frees up space for new patients; third, the relationships created within this space significantly reduce the drop-out rates. Therefore, temporary family housing is a safe place where families can deal with the trauma of illness and cope with difficult treatments in a familiar and peaceful environment; they also facilitate health activities. Critical actions in this area are opening and managing temporary residences, training local staff in welcoming visitors, contracting and connecting with healthcare institutions, and promoting participation and collaboration of the multidisciplinary team (physicians, psychologists, paramedics, educators, and volunteers).

Networking

Networking between international oncology departments and civil society organizations is necessary to share experiences and best practices and develop new joint project strategies. In some cases, civil society organizations that help children with cancer are small entities that need specific training to better manage a non-profit and reach institutional and private donors and stakeholders in the most impactful way possible. It is crucial to support local organizations to ensure project sustainability and heighten awareness among local communities and the civil society. Critical actions in this area are developing twinning arrangements with Italian centers of excellence or between south–south hospitals, creating and strengthening parent and hospital volunteer associations, and creating networks of national organizations.

Awareness and Advocacy

Awareness-raising and advocacy aim to protect the rights of children with cancer and break the stigmatization of the pediatric oncologic pathology. On the one hand, there is a need to raise community awareness on the rights of children and adolescents with cancer; on the other hand, policy makers must be encouraged to ensure these rights by complying with international agreements, formulating relevant national and supranational laws, and combatting corruption in healthcare systems. The key actions in this area are communication, raising awareness and advocacy for the various stakeholders, including policy makers, and local sharing of service costs.

The Program in the Various Hosting Countries

The program is active in several countries, as follows:

In *Italy*, with 2160 new diagnoses per year for 60 million inhabitants, Soleterre helps 350 patients who come to the pediatric oncology center of the Policlinico San Matteo Foundation, located in Pavia (north of the country), and in the pediatric oncology department of the SS Ospedale Annunziata de Taranto (south of the country) with psychological support for patients, parents, and medical staff, and with scientific research activities. Survival rates in Italy are 82%; the most frequent childhood cancers are leukemia (32%), tumors in the central nervous system (13%), lymphomas (16%), neuroblastomas (8%), and other cancers (31%). Italy has a national pediatric oncology plan and a national cancer registry.

In the *Ivory Coast*, of 570 new childhood cancer diagnoses per year for a total population of 23 million, Soleterre helps 260 children per year and approximately 90 family members who receive psychological support and treatment in the pediatric oncology department of the Treichville University Hospital in Abidjan. They take part in recreational and educational activities. An emergency fund has been created in the country for the purchase of medications for families who cannot afford to buy them and provides for 105 children every year. Approximately 90 minors and their families are hosted every year in temporary residences built by Soleterre. Educational sessions pertaining to early diagnosis for local physicians are organized every year in collaboration with the hospital teams. Activities are organized throughout the country with the Lalla Salma Foundation and the Franco-African pediatric oncology group (Groupe Franco-Africain d'Oncologie Pédiatrique, GFAOP). The survival rate is 22%, and the most frequent cancers are Burkitt non-Hodgkin's lymphomas (38%), kidney tumors and nephroblastomas (42%), leukemia (6%), and other types of cancers (14%). The country has set up a national pediatric oncology plan but no national cancer registry.

India counts 670 children diagnosed with cancer every year for a population of approximately 33 million (just for the state of Kerala, the location of the program). On average, Soleterre has helped 1500 children per year; approximately 110 families were hosted in a temporary residence created in collaboration with the "KanKids" organization and the Trivandrum Regional Cancer Center. Subsequent to this initiative, signatories are preparing the implementation of a psychological, nutritional, and educational support system and a palliative care program. Within the country, survival rates were 67% in 2017; most frequent tumors were leukemia (30%), central nervous system (18%), lymphomas (10%), and other cancers (42%). India applies a pediatric oncology plan and has a national cancer registry.

In Morocco, approximately 1200 new cases of childhood cancers are recorded every year in a population of about 35 million. Soleterre provides psychological support to 400 children and to 270 family members treated every year in the oncology department of the Rabat hospital, the Mohammed VI Hospital in Marrakech, and the Hassan II Hospital in Fez. The project also includes continuing training in information sharing and best practices in pediatric oncology to approximately 70 physicians per year. In Marrakech, the project benefits from the collaboration of AMAL (Association des Malades Atteints de la Leucémie, Leukemia Patients' Association). An informative web portal was created in 2015 (www.chop.ma). It is managed in collaboration with the Rabat Hospital and has counted approximately 400,000 visits and 40,000 visitors since its inception. Official survival rates are not published. The most frequent cancers are kidney tumors and nephroblastoma (41%), leukemia (18%), Burkitt non-Hodgkin's lymphomas (15%), and other cancers (26%). The country applies a national pediatric cancer plan and has a national cancer registry.

Ukraine reports 1018 new diagnoses for a population of 45 million. Soleterre provides psychological support and treatment to 800 children and 350 family members hospitalized each year at the Cancer Institute in Kiev and pediatric neurosurgery wards in Kiev and Lviv. A total of 370 children and their families have been hosted in the temporary residence during treatment, 240 families have benefitted from an emergency fund, and 46 general practitioners and pediatricians were trained in the factors and issues specific to pediatric oncology (early diagnosis, emotional support, etc.). The primary partner of Soleterre in Ukraine is the Zaporuka Foundation. The most frequent types of childhood cancers are leukemia (30%), brain tumor (13%), lymphoma (10%), kidney cancer (6%), and other cancers (41%). There is no pediatric oncology plan; there is a national cancer registry.

In *Uganda*, with 2093 new childhood cancers diagnosed every year for a population of 41 million, Soleterre provides care and psychological support to 100 children and as many families admitted to Mary's Lacor Gulu Hospital in northern Uganda, hosted in a Soleterre residence. They receive socio-sanitary care and psychological support in group or individual sessions. There is no official data on survival rates. The most frequent pediatric cancers are kidney tumors and nephroblastoma (47%), leukemia (9%), Burkitt non-Hodgkin's lymphomas (34%), and other cancers (10%). The country applies a national pediatric oncology plan and has a national cancer register.

Temporary Residences

In 2013, the Soleterre Foundation conducted a survey to understand how the etymological meaning of the word "welcome" is perceived in the various cultures of the temporary residences that are directly managed (or managed by partners). The word seems to have a common root in "gathering" and "receiving expressions of love." We wanted to analyze the semantics from a psychological point of view in the area of pediatric oncology. This forced us to begin studying existing literature and topics of the hosting relationship, not only with the child but also with the family.

Talking about hosting in pediatric oncology brings us into a world of "recent discovery." Hospitality in oncology is a fairly new area of psychology called psycho-oncology. It didn't exist as a clinical support activity for cancer patients until the 1980s, although there are traces of it as early as the 1950s in the United States. The International Psycho-oncology Society (IPOS) was created in 1984, and the European Society for Psycho-social Oncology was created 2 years later. In Italy, the first psychology department focusing on the cancer patient was created in Genoa in 1980, at the national cancer research institute and at SIPO, the Italian psycho-oncology society, founded in 1985.

This shows that from a psychological point of view, cancer in young patients is universally recognized as a source of great emotional distress for the child, for their family, and for the healthcare team. Here, we are adding another essential element to our discussion: the healthcare team. Although, in some respects, it appears "easy" to identify the patient in the care relationship, it should be noted that, for the purpose of this study, we are including the members of the medical and paramedical teams, the parents, and the organizations into a therapeutic alliance that should be considered as a wide-spectrum entity that is not solely targeting the hospital environment and patient care. This approach is based on the assumption that a tumor in a child is a critical event causing serious suffering and anxiety. In addition to the essential and inevitable need for physical care, being sick also requires psychosocial support.

Therefore, we want to understand the psychological impact of tumor diseases on children and their families. Moreover, we seek to study how the hosting relationship is part of the care relationship and identify the strengths and areas for improvement.

A review of the literature we used for this study (in particular, the weight of a stressful event in Ljungman et al. 2003; Hockenberry et al., 1997; Kazak et al., 1997) led us to examine the best way to investigate the care–hosting relationship.

To this end, a group of psychologists and psychotherapists conducted face-to-face and virtual meetings in 2013, with a starting point of data collection on the meaning of the term "WELCOME" for the sick child in pediatric oncology departments in five countries: Italy, Ukraine, India, Morocco, and the Ivory Coast. The international dimension is due to the strong interdependence of the situation.

The idea was to grasp the lexical semantic aspect and the psycho-social connotations, both imaginary and real, in the various cultures involved in the study, using the existing literature in pediatric oncology (studies on children and parents) that included 11 specific papers, 64 scientific articles, 2 studies by AIEOP (Italian pediatric hematology oncology association), 4 studies by IPOS (International Psycho-oncology Society), and 4 studies by AIRTUM (Italian cancer registry association). In addition to these studies, research was conducted in five pediatric oncology departments in Italy (in collaboration with the Institute of Hospitalization and Scientific Care (IRCCS) Foundation - Policlinico San Matteo di Pavia and the pediatric clinical and surgical sciences department), in Ukraine (in collaboration with the Kiev Cancer Institute and Pediatric Oncology Sciences Academy), in India (with the Trivandrum Cancer Institute and the Indian Cancer Society), in Morocco (with the Mohammed VI University Hospital in Marrakech), and in the Ivory Coast (in collaboration with the Treichville University Hospital in Abidjan).

The target group was the parents of children admitted to pediatric onco-hematology departments with a diagnosis of onco-hematological pathology: the sample included 150 parents (30 parents per country). The study consisted of a 17-question questionnaire (translated and administered by expert investigators).

Here are the answers to the main questions:

(a) Do you find differences between life in your country and life in the hospital's city?

	Yes (%)	No (%)
Ukraine	66.70	33.30
Ivory Coast	93.30	6.70
India	70.00	30.00
Morocco	93.90	6.10
Italy	50.00	50.00

(b) What are they?

Ukraine	75%	Treatment is better, but cost of living is too high
Ivory Coast	66%	Costs too high (food, accommodation, treatment, transport)
India	53%	Better equipment, treatments, and physicians
Morocco	71%	Cost of living is higher, the city is busier, travel is too expensive and difficult, and the family is far away
Italy	64%	A busier, more chaotic city but better services and better organization

(c) Did you have any problems at the hospital?

	Yes (%)	No (%)
Ukraine	73.3	26.7
Ivory Coast	83.3	16.7
India	53.3	46.7
Morocco	53.3	46.7
Italy	39.3	60.7

(d) What were they?

Ukraine	%
Not enough blood donors	17.1
Cost of treatment	17.1
Proper nutrition for the children	14.3
Erroneous or incomplete diagnoses	11.4
Long wait time for lab tests	11.4
Overcrowded department	11.4
Addressing psychological needs	8.6
Hostile attitude of the staff	2.9
Finding accommodation prior to hospitalization	2.9
Poor health conditions for the child	2.9
Ivory Coast	**%**
Financial issues: many tests required and excessive costs	92.0

Ivory Coast	%
Cost of medication	4.0
Shortage of medication and staff for nights and holidays	4.0
India	%
Lack of information on the hospital and amenities	24.1
Financial problems	20.7
Too long wait time	20.7
Lack of understanding with the staff (language and other issues)	10.3
Overcrowding	6.9
Hostile environment/people	6.9
Irrelevant response	3.4
Lack of information on patients and treatments	3.4
Poor hygiene conditions	3.4
Morocco	%
Problem with department orientation, lack of information, and too many forms to fill every day	50.0
Cost of tests and drugs too high	18.8
Need to come and go several times per day in an unknown city since there is no accommodation at the hospital for the companion	18.8
Too many tests prior to treatment	6.3
No answer	6.3
Italy	%
A busier, more chaotic city but better services and better organization	64.3
Less traffic	7.1
Physicians are more caring and the environment is more patient-friendly	7.1
Cost of living	7.1
Higher cost of living but better services	7.1
No answer	7.1

In line with the review of literature on creating pictures of mental illnesses (Illness Representation Model, IRM) and of Leventhal's self-regulation model, the primary psychological need expressed by respondents pertained to the knowledge and expectations of the disease. This need was directly expressed as a "request for additional information" (30.9% in India, 50% in Morocco, 14.7% in Ukraine, and 32.1% in Italy). This resulted in representation models more relevant to the possibility of personal adjustments. The IRM could also be indirectly facilitated by the request for a "more empathic attitude of physicians and staff" (60% in the Ivory Coast, 10.3% in India, 63.3% in Morocco, 41.2% in Ukraine, and 42.8% in Italy). This second IRM component would be created based on information from people the patient identified as authorities (i.e., physicians, psychologists, and staff).

In general, this type of expressed need would be part of a psycho-educational (cognitive component) and socio-affective (emotional component) dimension that, if appropriately addressed, could improve the parents' and children's emotional confinement capacity and upgrade therapeutic compliance.

Regarding the social aspect, the main requests revolved around the complex socio-economic conditions and the difficulty of access to health systems and care (in the Ivory Coast: "financial issues and excessive costs" (92%); in India: "a better place to undergo treatment" (67.6%); in Morocco: "cost of tests and drugs too high" (18.8%); in Ukraine: "treatments too costly and transfusions charged to patient" (17.1%). In Italy, although the situation is totally different in terms of access to treatment, 14.1% of the subjects express "a desire for better financial availability" when facing illness.

The results of the social aspects of the study confirm the principle of health being an element of social justice. Unfortunately, it is still far from effective for every human being, which inspires us to confirm our mission to implement the right to treatment everywhere in the world.

Psychological Support

Research and clinical practice data on pediatric oncology show how the disease has been defined as a biographical rupture, a sudden event that patients and their families struggle to accept and explain since it is always a unique experience.

Implementing psychological support in pediatric oncology departments and in Soleterre residences creates a relationship, opening a space for physical sensations and disturbing thoughts often expressed in a state of extreme suffering. One of the primary activities is to create an environment that facilitates recognition, sharing, and partial new representation of the "disturbance" so that it can evolve into a possible transformation. This is done with the help of a functional approach to absorb and metabolize the disturbance by progressively transforming it into an element that can be integrated into their autobiography.

If we try to understand illness as an event that triggers a series of biographical interruptions, we must also consider that the human spirit is capable of accessing and representing in a new, more explicit, and cognitive form, the available information that seems to conflict with unconscious and automatic procedural routine.[1] The life event that we represent as an illness, including all the correlates of pain, fatigue, and physical and mental symptoms, is often internalized as an unadjusted experience. It would be more accurate to say that an "other," "foreign" experience is internalized. A true, foreign self that in some cases becomes intolerable to the point that one runs the risk of feeling a break in identity continuity and consistency.

If accepted, the provision of psychological support offers the possibility of a conscious and participatory approach in which patients and family members can try, with the help of the psychologist, to put into words the traumatic experience of the illness and give it meaning. A story is not only a message from a sender to a receiver: it is also a path that they must create together. It is a mentalizing process, creating a narrative "me" that gives the illusion of identity consistency that progressively integrates some episodes that otherwise would be separated and lost. The mentalization process generates evaluation and reorganization of the mental content.

This illustrates the need to help patients and families to emerge from the silence in which they often lock themselves to give voice and content to the numerous and conflicting emotions that freeze when facing a diagnosis, particularly if it is serious or debilitating. Consequently, patients must recover the dignity of a name, the space, and a time for words.

The psychologist embodies the spirit of those who make this transformation with the patients and family members to create meaning together. Through a continuous reiteration of this process, the method is adequately adopted. This creates a process allowing one to transform the indescribable into images by placing it in a context that makes it less frightening (A. Ferro).

The child is an active subject in the story, and by identifying with characters, they are able to get in touch with their emotions and enter a plane of perspective where everything has a place.

[1] *Regolazione affettiva, mentalizzazione e sviluppo del Sé*, P. Fonagy, G. Gergely, E. Jurist e M. Target, Edizioni Raffello Cortina, 2005

Bibliography

1. Regolazione affettiva, mentalizzazione e sviluppo del Sé, P. Fonagy, G. Gergely, E. Jurist e M. Target, Edizioni Raffello Cortina, 2005.
2. Associazione Italiana di Ematologia e Oncologia Pediatrica AIEOP. Tutti bravi. Milano, Raffaello Cortina Editore, 1998.
3. Società Italiana di Psico-OncologiaStandard, opzioni e raccomandazioni per una buona pratica psico-oncologica, SIPO Società Italiana di Psico-OncologiaGiornale Italiano di Psico-OncologiaVol. 13 - N. 2/2011.
4. La psicologia clinica in ospedale. Consulenza e modelli di intervento, Carlo Alfredo ClericiLauraVeneroni, edizioni Il Mulino, 2014.
5. Bertolotti M, Peirolo C, Geuna T, Cappelli P, I pazienti stranieri e le loro famiglie: il doppio trauma. XI Congresso Nazionale SIPO Società Italiana di Psico-Oncologia. Bologna, Atti del congresso Nazionale SIPO, 2009.
6. Dell'Antonio A, Ponzo E. Bambini che vivono in ospedale. Roma: EdizioniBorla; 1982.
7. Ekman P. Biological and cultural contributions to body and facial movment in the espression of emotions, in Explaining Emotions, a cura di A. O. Rorty. Berkeley, University of California, 1980.
8. Harris PL. Il bambino e le emozioni. Milano: Raffaello Cortina Editore; 1989.
9. Lüscher M. Il Test clinico di Lüscher. Abano Terme: Piovan Editore; 1993.
10. Massaglia P, Bertolotti M. Psicologia e gestione del bambino portatore di tumore e della sua famiglia. Milano: Raffaello Cortina Editore; 1998.
11. Scarponi D, Trombini E, Rizzardi M. Il risalto delle emozioni del volto dell'adulto in oncologia pediatrica: un'indagine sperimentale. Scienze dell'Interazione. 1998;5(1):19–27.
12. Scarponi D. Tutto il tempo che conta. Bologna: CLUEB; 2003.
13. Scarponi D, Mazza S, Puglisi I, Trombini G, Pession A. Bambini oncologici in ospedale. Gruppi terapeutici ad orientamento analitico. Cagliari: Atti del congresso Nazionale AIP; 2005.
14. Trombini E, Scarponi D, Rizzardi M, Weiss H, Paolucci G, Trombini G. Sofferenza psicologica e differente contenimento psicosomatico nella coppia genitoriale del bambino oncologico. Parma: Tipografia Benedettina; 1998.

15. G. Ljungman, P.J. Mc Grath, E. Cooper, K. Widger, J.Ceccolini, C.V. Fernendez, G. Frager, K. Wilkins. "Psychosocial needs of families with a child with cancer". Journal of Pediatric Hematology/Oncology 2003;25:223–31.
16. M. Hockenberry-Eaton, B. Manteuffel, S. Bottomley. "Development of two instruments examining stress and adjustment in children with cancer". Journal of Pediatric Oncology Nursing 1997;14:178–85.
17. A. E. Kazak, L. Barakat, K. Meesske, D. Christakis, A. T. Meadows, R. Casey, B. Penati, M.L. Stuber. "Posttraumatic stress, family functioning and social support in survivors of childhood leukaemia and their mothers and fathers". Journal of Consulting and Clinical Psychology 1997;65:120–9.

Part XIV

East Africa: Kenya

Provision of Palliative Care Services for Cancer Patients in the Community in Africa

John K. Weru and Esther W. Nafula

Introduction

The World Health Organization (WHO) defines palliative care as an approach which improves quality of life of patients and families facing the problem of life-threatening illness, through the prevention and relief of suffering by means of early identification and impeccable assessment and treatment of pain and other problems—physical, psychological and spiritual [35]. The primary goal of palliative care is therefore achievement of the best quality of life for patients and their families [9].

The number of mortalities due to non-communicable diseases (NCDs) has been rising globally, and these diseases are currently among the leading causes of death in many countries. WHO [36] predicts that by 2030, NCDs will be the biggest cause of death in the Sub-Saharan region. Cancer is also a significant public health problem in the region [24]. In 2012, there were 645,000 new cancer cases and 456,000 cancer-related deaths in Africa.

Cancer rates in Africa are expected to grow by over 400% over the next 50 years with the WHO estimating 70% of new cases will be in the developing world by 2020 [6]. It was estimated that 24.7 million people were living with HIV/AIDs in 2013 accounting for 70% of the global disease burden with 1.4 million new infections in 2013 alone [13, 32].

Non-communicable diseases (NCDs) are non-infectious, non-transmissible and of long duration with generally slow progression (APCA 2016). They are divided into four categories, namely, cardiovascular diseases (heart attacks and stroke), cancers, chronic respiratory diseases (chronic obstructive pulmonary disease) and diabetes (20 APCA 2016). The global burden of NCDs is projected to approach epidemic levels in developing countries [1, 19]. In 1999, NCDs were responsible for 60% of deaths in the world and 43% of the global burden of the disease [33]. It is estimated that by 2020, NCDs will cause up to 73% of deaths and 60% of the disease burden [33].

Due to high rates of poverty, it is still common for patients in Africa with incurable illnesses to die in pain and without appropriate care [20]. Approximately 80% of patients with malignancies are diagnosed at later stages where cure is not possible and most end up needing palliative care [26]. Access to treatment is largely controlled by the patient's or family's ability to pay and their geographical location with specialized care often being far away from many communities [26]. Palliative care is only available to less than 5% of those who need it despite various

J. K. Weru (✉)
Department of Medicine, Aga Khan University Hospital, Nairobi, Kenya
e-mail: John.weru@aku.edu

E. W. Nafula
HCG-CCK Cancer Centre, Nairobi, Kenya

M. Silbermann (ed.), *Palliative Care for Chronic Cancer Patients in the Community*,
https://doi.org/10.1007/978-3-030-54526-0_23

programs and national palliative care associations emerging in Africa [7]. End-of-life care is given lower priority by governments compared to preventive and curative services which are often more expensive [26].

Despite many governments investing in preventive and curative medicine, disease burden is still rising with many Africans not being able to access or afford life-prolonging treatments [26]. With increasing awareness creation among various populations, diseases such as HIV and cancer that previously led to premature deaths are now chronic conditions that confer an increase in burden of symptoms and functional decline in patients [23, 30]. Many patients are suffering for extended periods of time with life-limiting conditions which are often treated in the acute care settings with multiple hospital visits rather than being adequately supported within the community. Many patients even at the end of life have multiple emergency room visits due to inadequate symptom control or lack of adequate or trained caregivers at home [2].

Background

Palliative care is a relatively new field in Africa, and its development is hampered by lack of integration into healthcare systems or policies [22]. Out of 53 countries, 4 countries, namely, Kenya, Uganda, South Africa and Tanzania, have integrated palliative care into their healthcare policies or used it as part of a strategic plan focusing on cancer treatment [21]. Two countries namely Rwanda and Swaziland have stand-alone national palliative care policies [22]. Uganda has made palliative care for HIV and cancer patients a priority in their National Health Plan with Hospice Uganda and two other hospices in Mbarara and Hoima focusing on home-based care (HBC) [26]. Other African countries have also developed community-based palliative care services such as Botswana, Ethiopia, Tanzania and Zimbabwe [26], with Botswana having home-based care programs integrated into their national health system. There are minimal resources with huge shortages of healthcare providers trained in palliative care [7]. Due to these challenges, a community-based approach of providing palliative care has been found to be cost effective in Africa [8].

The WHO defines community-based palliative care as those services offered at a community health center or those run with community participation [37]. Such services involve the community in trying to solve their own problems and are usually initiated by help of the local authorities [37]. Palliative care services are offered by trained healthcare providers, trained volunteers, community health workers or untrained sensitized volunteers [37]. Palliative care in Sub-Saharan Africa is mostly provided through home-based care [8].

A home-based care approach is where patients stay in their own homes and are cared for by their families or community volunteers together with hospice teams [24]. Patients are visited at home by palliative care providers who provide medical care, nursing advice and psychosocial support [37]. In a study exploring home-based palliative care, Grant et al. [7] carried out a survey in three countries namely Kenya, Uganda and Malawi. Their study found that most patients were poor and had been made poorer by the financial burden of treating cancers. Most patients were referred to palliative care after exhausting their financial resources. Most of these patients were not able to travel far to access healthcare. The palliative care teams sometimes had to look for ways of providing food, necessities and sometimes even school fees to patients and their families. The patients were therefore visited in their homes by community volunteers who worked with the palliative care teams. In this study, the provision of services was similar in the three countries. Palliative care teams brought knowledge to the communities changing their attitudes toward death and dying. Many relatives who took care of their loved ones had greater satisfaction with being in the comfort of their own homes.

Community-based palliative care has been shown to improve quality of care and patient outcomes while also minimizing costs of treatment [4]. This approach is also associated with decreased acute care health service use as most symptom control can be done at home [27]. Community-based palliative care aims to avoid futile treatment while providing holistic care and support for the patients and their families [16].

Current Burden of Disease

The enormous burden of cancer associated with the myriad of physical and psychosocial suffering demands quality, timely provision of palliative care in developing countries. Despite this, the access to this service is significantly limited. Moreover, there are poor or no policies that recognize palliative care as an essential component of healthcare, and there is inadequate training for both healthcare professionals and the public about palliative care. Nevertheless, based on these issues, could there be any approaches that best suited provision of Palliative care (PC) services to cancer patients and their families in the continent?

Palliative Care Approaches Suitable in Africa

A number of approaches are applicable in the African context, but there is minimal data to form a solid evidence base. However, the WHO has recommended a public health strategy (PHS) as the best approach for establishing and/ or integrating palliative care into a country. The public health approach comprises of preventing measures, prolonging life where possible with the eventual aim of promoting the health of entire populations through the organized efforts of society [10]. In 1990, the WHO described the first strategy for the establishment of a palliative care program—the three pillars of palliative care: (i) government policy, (ii) education and (iii) availability of medicines (opioids) (World Health Organization, 1990a). Public health strategies must therefore be incorporated into all levels of healthcare systems and be community based with specific contextualization. The African Palliative Care Association (APCA) advocates for patients' access and safe management of controlled medicines. For this to be feasible, palliative care services must be integrated at all levels of healthcare throughout the society [29].

Policies

To effectively integrate palliative care for cancer patients into developing countries' healthcare systems, appropriate national policies, education of healthcare workers and the general public, and culturally appropriate implementation of palliative care services at all levels of society must be assured. Governments in developing countries have been encouraged to include palliative care in the National Health Plan, policies and related regulations as well as to devise a mechanism for funding and/or service delivery models that support palliative care service delivery [29]. Unfortunately, most countries in Africa have not yet included palliative care in their national policies or regulations.

Service Delivery Models

Palliative care services in developing countries need to be delivered in a way that meets the cultural, spiritual and economic needs of the people (Merriman 1999). Therefore, there is need to identify organizations that have the potential to become bench marks, the patient population they are caring for and to engage with community, clinical and administrative leaders to help them to identify the need for palliative care for their patients and families [28, 29]. In order to provide palliative care for all, it needs to be integrated in the existing health infrastructure into all levels of society—from community level upward to the tertiary level and downward to the community so a down up; up down approach into all levels of health care system, from health centers to tertiary care fcilities. The community thus becomes the epicenter of care, improvement of the same, data production and policy formulation. For this to happen, funding is an unavoidable necessity [3]. This is evident from a study conducted to determine the place of death and its predictors among palliative care patients with cancer with the findings that the place of death is influenced by the socio-demographic characteristics of patients, the characteristics of their caregivers and health service factors [15, 17]. Several models of providing PC to cancer patients have been proposed:

(a) Home-based care (HBC) has been the most common service model in Africa, because it is cheap and, most of the time, acceptable to the patient and family, as well as respecting their cultural practices [12] (Merriman 2002). Various models are included within the HBC system; Community HBC (CHBC); Integrated community-based home care (ICHC); Hospice care with HBC services; Hospital-supported HBC services; Outreach services that include HBC; Government District Level HBC services and Home Visiting. CHBC and ICHC are the two models with greatest opportunity for palliative care integration [31]. The best practice model was judged to be ICHC followed by CHBC with volunteers being very crucial in community-based palliative care [5]. The volunteers are indispensable as they are aware of community needs and norms something most skilled caregivers are lacking. In the African setting, the volunteers are trained through hospice programs and often work as part of the interdisciplinary team [14].

    They are able to offer support to patients in their own homes and coordinate with skilled healthcare providers trained in palliative care to review the patients when needed [7].
(b) In-patient service model—where patients are admitted at a hospice—is practiced in some countries. The cost effectiveness of this model is questionable.
(c) Outpatient clinics and day care where patients visit a palliative care facility for services
(d) Hospital-based palliative care programs are another way of extending palliative care services to those in need. This is an affordable model as it takes advantage of sharing the resources within the hospital. The hospital team then liaises with a HBC team to ensure continuity of care for patients [25].
(e) Hospital outreach services: this model has the potential to avert hospital admissions in generally overcrowded services in low-resource settings and may improve the quality of life of patients in their home environments [11]. The down side of this is that it is hospital led and there could be conflict of interest in its implementation.

Whatever model is envisaged, it is important that the standard of care is ensured across.

Challenges for community PC in Africa include the following:
The evidence above details the fact that home-based PC service is the model best suited for Africa and has been advocated as being cost-effective and culturally appropriate [18]. The major challenge faced by all PC services is reaching those with the greatest need, often the rural poor. Challenges include:

1. Poor or lack of Governments on opioids availability, accessibility, prescribing, storage and dispensing [34].
2. Misunderstanding the definition of palliative care by patients, communities, policy makers, donors and support organizations.
3. Penetrating and changing long-held myths and beliefs taught to clinicians regarding use of morphine and other opioids.
4. Providing PC for the poor requires provision of basic support such as food as well as facilitating access to PC services.
5. The changing palliative care needs in the wake of increased non-communicable diseases in Africa.

Meeting these challenges may entail:

- Morphine powder reconstitution in the health facilities

- Enabling nurses and Clinical Officer trained in PC to prescribe opioids
- Introducing well-structured home-based PC services in the continent
- Advocacy and education in palliative care to all healthcare providers
- Clear PC definition—support care without pain and symptom control up to the end of life—is supportive care and not PC. Pain control without supportive and holistic care is anesthesiology and not PC. Both holistic support and pain and symptom control are essential for PC, anything less will lower standards and renew suffering.

Conclusion

The incidence of non-communicable diseases has been rising globally and currently accounts for many deaths. Cancer being one of the NCDs is expected to rise exponentially in Africa. Eighty percent of cancer patients are diagnosed in later stages of disease where cure is not possible, making the need for palliative care to be great. African governments however are still focused on investing in curative and preventative measures instead of addressing the growing need for palliative care. Very few countries have integrated palliative care into their policies or created stand-alone policies.

The WHO (1990) recommends a public health strategy as the best approach in provision of palliative care in Africa. It is useful for establishing or integrating care into health systems. Community-based care involves participation of the communities in creating working palliative care models. Currently home-based care models are used widely in Africa because they are cheap and readily acceptable to patients and their families. Care is provided in the patient's home by trained healthcare providers working with volunteers. Many challenges are still encountered such as inaccessibility of palliative care services to many rural populations and opioid shortages. As the practice of palliative care continues to improve in Africa, many patients needing the services will be reached as governments accept to create and implement policies.

References

1. Airhihenbuwa CO, Ogedegbe G. Noncommunicable diseases in Africa and the global south, 2016.
2. Agarwal S, Banerjee J, Baker R, Conroy S, Hsu R, Rashid A, Camosso-Stefinovic J, Sinfield P, Habiba M. Potentially avoidable emergency department attendance: interview study of patients' reasons for attendance. Emerg Med J. 2012;29(12):e3.
3. Barbera L, Taylor C, Dudgeon D. Why do patients with cancer visit the emergency department near the end of life? CMAJ. 2010;182(6):563–8.
4. Brumley R, Enguidanos S, Jamison P, Seitz R, Morgenstern N, Saito S, McIlwane J, Hillary K, Gonzalez J. Increased satisfaction with care and lower costs: results of a randomized trial of in-home palliative care. J Am Geriatr Soc. 2007;55(7):993–1000.
5. Claxton-Oldfield S, Claxton-Oldfield J. Should I stay or should I go: a study of hospice palliative care volunteer satisfaction and retention. Am J Hosp Palliat Med®. 2012;29(7):525–30.
6. Costa A. Will our planet be able to cope with the cancer burden in the next decade? Semin Oncol. 2001;28(2):140–2. WB Saunders
7. Grant L, Downing J, Namukwaya E, Leng M, Murray SA. Palliative care in Africa since 2005: good progress, but much further to go. BMJ Support Palliat Care. 2011;1(2):118–22.
8. Harding R, Higginson IJ. Palliative care in sub-Saharan Africa: an appraisal 2004. London: Department of Palliative Care and Policy, Kings College; 2004. p. 1–106.
9. Harding R, Stewart K, Marconi K, O'Neill JF, Higginson IJ. Current HIV/AIDS end-of-life care in sub-Saharan Africa: a survey of models, services, challenges and priorities. BMC Public Health. 2003;3(1):33.
10. Higginson IJ, Koffman J. Public health and palliative care. Clin Geriatr Med. 2005;21(1):45–55.
11. Hongoro C, Dinat N. A cost analysis of a hospital-based palliative care outreach program: implications for expanding public sector palliative care in South Africa. J Pain Symptom Manag. 2011;8:1–10.
12. Jagwe JG, Barnard D. The introduction of palliative care in Uganda. J Palliat Med. 2002;5(1):159–63.
13. Joint United Nations Programme on HIV/AIDS (UNAIDS), UNAIDS global report 2013.
14. Kelley AS, Morrison RS. Palliative care for the seriously ill. N Engl J Med. 2015;373(8):747–55.
15. Kikule E. A good death in Uganda: survey of the needs for palliative care for terminally ill people in urban areas. BMJ. 2003;327:192–4.
16. Luckett T, Phillips J, Agar M, Virdun C, Green A, Davidson PM. Elements of effective palliative care models: a rapid review. BMC Health Serv Res. 2014;14(1):136.
17. Masucci L, Guerriere DN, Cheng R, Coyte PC. Determinants of place of death for recipi-

ents of home-based palliative care. J Palliat Care. 2010;26:279–86.
18. Merriman A, Kaur M. Palliative Care an Appraisal Editorial. Lancet. 2005;365:1909–10.
19. Murray CJ, Lopez AD. Mortality by cause for eight regions of the world: Global Burden of Disease Study. Lancet. 1997;349(9061):1269–76.
20. Murray SA, Grant E, et al. Dying from cancer in developed and developing countries: lessons from 2 qualitative interview studies of patients and their carers. BMJ. 2003;326:368–72.
21. Mwangi-Powell F, Dix O. Palliative care in Africa: an overview. Afr Health. 2011;33(5):19–21.
22. Ntizimira CR, Nkurikiyimfura JL, Mukeshimana O, Ngizwenayo S, Mukasahaha D, Clancy C. Palliative care in Africa: a global challenge. Ecancermedicalscience. 2014;8:493.
23. Phillips JL, Currow DC. Cancer as a chronic disease. Collegian. 2010;17(2):47–50.
24. Rhee JY, Luyirika E, Namisango E, Powell RA, Garralda E, Pons-Izquierdo JJ, Lima L, Centeno-Cortes C. 2017. APCA atlas of palliative care in Africa.
25. Sepulveda C, Habiyambere V, et al. Quality care at end of life in Africa. BMJ. 2003;327:209–13.
26. Spence D, Merriman A, Binagwaho A. Palliative care in Africa and the Caribbean. PLoS Med. 2004;1(1):5.
27. Spilsbury K, Rosenwax L, Arendts G, Semmens JB. The impact of community-based palliative care on acute hospital use in the last year of life is modified by time to death, age and underlying cause of death. A population-based retrospective cohort study. PLoS One. 2017;12(9):e0185275.
28. Stjernswa¨rd J, Foley KM, Ferris FD. The public health strategy for palliative care. J Pain Symptom Manag. 2007;33:486–93.
29. Stjernswa¨rd J, Foley KM, Ferris FD. Integrating palliative care into national policies, 2007.
30. Tanko MN, Vento S. The challenge of lymphomas in sub-Saharan Africa. Lancet Oncol. 2010;11:610–2.
31. Ugandan Census 2002 Ugandan Bureau of Statistics www.ubos.org. Accessed 29.8.05.
32. UNAIDS, W. Global report 2013. Joint united nations Programme on HIV/aIDS (unaIDS) Joint united nations Programme on HIV/aIDS (unaIDS), 2013.
33. Unwin N, Mugusi F, Aspray T, Whiting D, Edwards R, Mbanya JC, Sobgnwi E, Rashid S, Alberti KGMM. Tackling the emerging pandemic of non-communicable diseases in sub-Saharan Africa: the essential NCD health intervention project. Public Health. 1999;113(3):141–6.
34. WHO. Cancer pain control. 2nd ed. Geneva: WHO; 1996.
35. WHO Palliative Care WHO 2002. http://www.who.int/hiv/topics/palliative/palliativecare/en accessed 29.8.05.
36. World Health Organization. The protocol for the WHO study on the effectiveness of community-based programmes for NCD prevention and control (No. NMH/NPH/NCP/03.09). Geneva: World Health Organization; 2003.
37. World Health Organization. Planning and implementing palliative care services: a guide for programme managers, 2016.

Part XV

East Africa: Uganda

Current State of Palliative Care in Uganda

Elizabeth Namukwaya, Amos Deogratius Mwaka, Eve Namisango, Mark Donald Mwesiga, and Julia Downing

Introduction

The Need for Palliative Care in Uganda

Each year an estimated 20 million people worldwide are in need of palliative care during the last year of their lives. Many more require palliative care (PC) prior to the last year of their lives. It is also estimated that 40–60% of all people that die need PC [1]. Palliative care is aimed at relieving severe health-related suffering associated with life-limiting or life-threatening conditions [2]. It is estimated that 45% of the 56.2 million deaths that occurred globally in 2015 endured severe health-related suffering [2]. Of the 56.9 million global deaths in 2016, 40.5 million (71%) were due to non-communicable diseases (NCDs). The leading causes of NCD deaths in the same year were cardiovascular diseases (17.9 million deaths), cancers (9.0 million) and respiratory diseases including asthma and chronic obstructive pulmonary disease (3.8 million) and diabetes (1.6 million deaths) [3]. Therefore, most adults in need of palliative care have chronic, non-communicable diseases. On the other hand, patients with communicable diseases including drug-resistant tuberculosis and the Acquired Immune Deficiency Syndrome (AIDS) also need palliative care; AIDS represents 5.7% of the global need for palliative care [1].

The majority of people with severe health-related suffering (80%) are from low- and middle-

E. Namukwaya
Palliative Care Education and Research Consortium, Kampala, Uganda

Department of Medicine, School of Medicine, College of Health Sciences, Makerere University, Kampala, Uganda

A. D. Mwaka (✉)
Department of Medicine, School of Medicine, College of Health Sciences, Makerere University, Kampala, Uganda

E. Namisango
African Palliative Care Association, Kampala, Uganda

Cicely Saunders Institute, King's College London, London, UK
e-mail: eve.namisango@africanpalliativecare.org

M. D. Mwesiga
Palliative Care Association of Uganda, Kampala, Uganda
e-mail: mark.mwesiga@pcau.org.ug

J. Downing
Palliative Care Education and Research Consortium, Kampala, Uganda

Department of Medicine, School of Medicine, College of Health Sciences, Makerere University, Kampala, Uganda

International Children's Palliative Care Network, Assagay, South Africa

M. Silbermann (ed.), *Palliative Care for Chronic Cancer Patients in the Community*,
https://doi.org/10.1007/978-3-030-54526-0_24

income countries (LMICs). Therefore, most people in need of palliative care live in low- and middle-income countries (LMICs) [1, 2]. Almost 98% of the children who need palliative care live in LMICs, and almost half of them live in Africa [2]. In 2016, over three quarters of NCD deaths (31.5 million) occurred in the low- and middle-income countries [3]. In Uganda, the need for palliative care has been estimated mainly through morbidity and mortality data. The World Health Organisation estimates that 1% of the population needs palliative care [4]; therefore, as the current population of Uganda is 40,308,000 [5], an estimated 403,080 Ugandans need palliative care. The need for palliative care in Uganda is increasing due to an increasingly ageing population, the increase in the number of non-communicable diseases and the relatively high prevalence of HIV/AIDS [2, 6]. In 2016, there were an estimated 297,000 deaths in Uganda; 33% of these were due to NCDs: 9% were cancer related, 10% cardiovascular, 2% chronic respiratory diseases, 2% were due to diabetes and 10% other NCDs [7, 8]. HIV/AIDS continues to be a major health concern in Uganda. In 2016, the Uganda Population-based HIV Impact Assessment (UPHIA) estimated that there were 1.2 million adults and 95,000 children living with HIV in Uganda; 23,000 died from AIDS-related illnesses [9, 10].

Most patients with NCDs in Uganda, especially those with cancer, present with advanced stages of the disease and need palliative care [11–13]. Those who are diagnosed early may not be able to sustain treatments as most care must be paid for out-of-pocket [14]. Without regular treatments, these conditions progress to advanced, irreversible states. In addition, most patients with advanced chronic diseases that have progressed to organ failure, such as advanced heart failure, renal failure and liver failure, and may need transplants cannot access these options because of financial constraints. Their best accessible and affordable options are usually palliative care [15, 16].

Development of Palliative Care in Uganda

It is now just over a quarter century since all components of PC, as defined by the WHO, were introduced in Uganda [17]. The pioneers of PC in Uganda built on the foundations laid by the then-existing HIV/AIDS services, such as The AIDS Support Organization (TASO), that were already providing some elements of palliative care for HIV/AIDS patients [17]. The pre-antiretroviral therapy HIV era played a pivotal role in the development of palliative care in Uganda because most treatments at that time were mainly for symptom control and, therefore, most funding for HIV/AIDS also funded palliative care development and provisions [17]. Uganda employed the WHO's four-pillar approach to the integration of palliative care into healthcare services [18]. These four pillars include:

1. Implementing palliative care services that are integrated into all healthcare systems at all levels, including palliative home care as part of primary care [18, 19];
2. Initiating required training in palliative care for all clinicians who treat people with palliative care needs, including training in basic palliative care for all primary care workers;
3. Assuring safe accessibility of essential palliative medicines, including oral fast-acting morphine;
4. Updating existing policies on palliative care and creating new ones where there are none.

A fifth pillar (research) was later added in recognition of the role of research in the development of palliative care service delivery [20]. This chapter reviews the current state of palliative care in Uganda based on these five pillars.

(i) *Implementing Palliative Care Services Integrated in Healthcare Systems at all Levels*

Uganda has made significant progress in providing palliative care services that are integrated into the health system. By 2006, Uganda was one of the 20 countries in the world ranked amongst those in the advanced integration category in palliative care [21]. The 2011 mapping of global palliative care developments undertaken by the Worldwide Palliative Care Alliance reported that in Africa, only Uganda had achieved advanced integration of palliative care into its health system (Group 4b) [22]. Uganda was the highest-ranking African country and 35th country worldwide in the Quality of Death Index of 2015 that ranked 80 countries in terms of quality and availability of palliative care services for adult populations in the world [23]. In addition, Uganda had the largest number of palliative care services among the countries surveyed in Africa for the recent African Palliative Care Association (APCA) Atlas of 2017 [24]. It is estimated that there are 5.87 PC services per million people in Uganda, and this is second only to Swaziland in Africa which has the largest number of PC services per population [24]. By 2016, 90 out of the 112 districts (80%) in Uganda have at least one palliative care service centre (Fig. 1). Palliative care is provided at the national referral, regional referral, district and health centre (HC) IV level, HC III, private health facilities, in standalone hospice centres and non-governmental organisations. The majority of palliative care is integrated into the healthcare system and is provided by 216 hospital-based palliative care services [24]. Most home-based palliative care is provided by 13 of the 229 palliative care services in Uganda [24]. Among all these services, there are two specialised services specific for children's palliative care [24]. Palliative care is also extended to other special populations including the elderly, prisoners, armed forces and those with disabilities [25, 26]. Palliative care is provided for both cancer and non-cancer conditions including HIV, chronic organ failure and chronic progressive neurological conditions. Palliative care clinical guidelines are included in the national clinical guidelines,

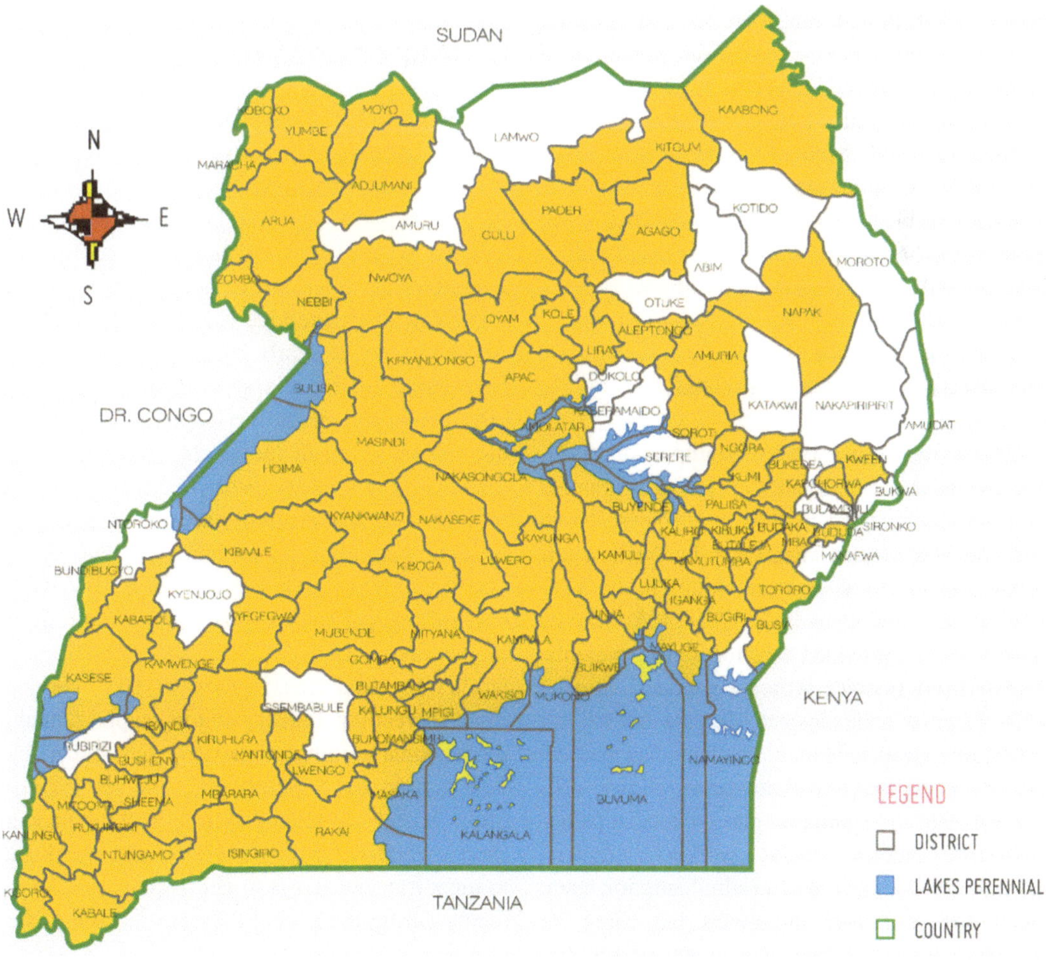

Fig. 1 Map of palliative care service coverage in Uganda. (Permission to use this map was obtained from the Palliative Care Association of Uganda)

and these are useful in guiding clinicians in patient care [27]. Baseline research done in Uganda when palliative care services were starting revealed that patients with terminal illness prefer to die at home [28]. This finding, coupled with the fact that most Ugandans live in rural areas with limited access to healthcare facilities, shows the importance of home- and community-based models of service provision, especially at the end of life. The next section will describe the services which provide home-based and community-based palliative care in Uganda.

Home-Based and Community-Based Palliative Care

Thirteen services offer most of the home-based and community-based palliative care services in Uganda [24]. In addition, there are also hospital palliative care services that offer home-based palliative care. These include, but are not limited to, Gombe Hospital, Mildmay Uganda Hospital, Lubaga Hospital, Mengo Hospital, The AIDS Support Organisation and Kabale Hospital palliative care services. These 13 services that offer most of the home- and community-based palliative care will be described briefly below.

Hospice Africa Uganda (HAU)

HAU was founded in 1993 in Kampala and initiated palliative care in Uganda [17]. HAU expanded in 1998 and founded two other hospices at two sites: Mobile Hospice Mbarara in the Western part of Uganda and Little Hospice Hoima in the Mid-Western region of Uganda. By 2018, HAU and its other sites had provided care for 32,918 patients: 15,564 from Hospice Africa Uganda, Kampala, 12,142 from Mobile Hospice Mbarara and the rest from Little Hospice Hoima. The team has medical doctors specialised in palliative care, clinical officers specialised in palliative care, specialist palliative care nurses, social workers, trainers, community volunteers and an administration team. HAU does not have in-patients but cares for patients at the above three sites in out-patient clinics at the HAU health facilities, outreach sites and at home; their coverage for home-based care is limited to a radius of 20 km from their offices. They also offer paediatric palliative care services at the Uganda Cancer Institute. HAU's service matrix includes, but is not limited to, pain and symptom management, psychosocial and spiritual care, bereavement support and day care services for patients and their families enrolled in their care program. Patients are referred to HAU by trained community volunteers from their home communities or by healthcare workers from hospitals, while some are self-referred. The majority of patients seen by HAU are cancer patients. Other activities carried out by HAU include training of healthcare workers in palliative care within Uganda and the rest of Africa, research and morphine reconstitution [29].

Kawempe Home Care

Kawempe Home Care was started in 2007 and provides palliative care services for the Kawempe division of Kampala and Nangabo sub-county in the central part of Uganda. The team consists of a medical doctor, nurses, counsellors, community volunteers, a driver and an administration team. The focus of this service is PC mainly for HIV/AIDS patients. By early 2019, 4800 patients had been cared for by this service, and there were 1998 active patients in service: 91.4% adults and the rest children, including 24 with cancers. A total of 291 home care visits were made from the time of its inception until early 2019, and most patients were seen as out-patients. Other activities run by the organisation include HIV/AIDS counselling and testing, provision of antiretroviral therapy for HIV/AIDS patients, prevention of mother to child transmission of HIV, cervical cancer screening, family planning support, health professional training in palliative care and education support for orphans [30]. The service also offers hostel accommodations for children with cancer who live far from Kampala and are unable to meet transport costs to get to scheduled treatments during the period they are receiving chemotherapy or radiotherapy.

Joy Hospice Mbale

Joy Hospice was established in 1998 in Mbale in the Eastern part of Uganda. The service provides palliative care for people in Eastern Uganda including the Bugisu sub-region, parts of Teso, Bukedi and Karamoja. This hospice service also receives referrals from Western Kenya. The service offers out-patient services, in-patient palliative care, and home-based palliative care. The team consists of clinical officers trained in palliative care, palliative care nurses and doctors and an administration team. Additional services include pain and symptom management, psychosocial support and end-of-life counselling [31].

Rays of Hope Hospice Jinja

Rays of Hope Hospice was founded in 2005 and provides palliative care for patients with life-limiting illnesses in the Busoga sub-region and Buikwe District in the Eastern part of Uganda, an area of about 10,000 km^2 with a population of 3.5 million people. Activities at this centre include clinical palliative care services. In 2019, the centre had 456 active patients in care: 52% with cancers, 26% with advanced HIV/AIDS, 9% with HIV/AIDS and cancer, and 13% with other severe diseases and injuries. The service offers poor patients transport refunds, meets costs for diagnostic tests, food and upkeep, counselling, day care clinics, bereavement support, school fees, housing support, training of volunteers and the community and capacity development for the staff [32].

Hospice Ngora (FADO-T)

Faith Action Development Organisation-Teso is a Christian private healthcare initiative established in 2005 in the Teso region in Eastern Uganda. FADO-T provides home-based palliative care services and the provision of food and water purification agents, bedding and clothing [33].

Hospice Tororo

Hospice Tororo is a non-governmental organisation that was established in 2011 and provides home-based, community- and outpatient-based palliative care for patients with cancer, HIV/AIDS and other chronic diseases in the Eastern region of Uganda, including the districts of Mbale, Manafwa, Busia, Malaba and Butaleja. The service also offers palliative care services to patients admitted to the three hospitals in Tororo. The care team is comprised of nurses, a social worker, a driver, managers, advocacy personnel and community volunteers. Activities carried out by the service include pain and symptom control, psychosocial support, spiritual care, end-of-life counselling, bereavement support, cancer screening and community sensitisation on palliative care to reduce stigma. The service is also involved in training healthcare workers and community workers in palliative care [34].

Kitovu Mobile Home Care

Kitovu Mobile Home Care was established in 1987 by the Medical Missionaries of Mary in response to the needs of patients with HIV/AIDS who preferred to be cared for in their homes. The program started as an outreach program for Kitovu Hospital. The program offers mobile (outreach) and home-based clinical services for patients with HIV/AIDS, tuberculosis and cancer living in the rural areas around Lake Victoria in Uganda and in-patient care for patients admitted to Kitovu Hospital. The program team is made up of medical workers, social workers, counsellors and community facilitators and volunteers. Their service matrix includes offering antiretroviral therapy to HIV/AIDS patients, spiritual support, grief and bereavement care, and psychosocial support, especially to vulnerable children and widows, as well as building resilience of caregivers. The catchment area of Kitovu is one where the HIV epidemic led to the loss of many parents, leaving grandparents to care for young children. The Kitovu Mobile Home care has programs to empower grandmothers, orphans and vulnerable children, with education for the latter. The program has youth and adolescent empowerment activities to help reduce the risk of HIV transmission and also builds resilience among grandmothers who have orphans to care for [35].

New Life Hospice Arua

New Life Hospice Arua (NELIHA) serves palliative care patients in the greater West Nile region, nearby communities of the Democratic Republic of Congo and parts of South Sudan. It currently operates within the premises of Arua Regional Referral Hospital. On average, the hospice attends to over 200 patients monthly. It has a team of Palliative Care Nurses and volunteers who reach communities and homes to care for those with palliative care needs. They care for patients within a 5-km radius from the hospital. They also conduct community sensitisation on cancer [36].

Peace Hospice Adjumani

Peace Hospice Adjumani was started as a community-based organisation in 2014 and was registered as a non-government organisation in 2015. Since its inception, 4150 patients have been cared for. The program offers home-based care, trains caregivers of patients and Village Health Teams (VHTs), and is involved in awareness campaigns for palliative care. Patients seen include those with cancer, HIV/AIDS and organ failure including patients with chronic renal and heart failure. The program also offers home-based care for the refugee population from South Sudan [37].

St. Francis Hospital, Naggalama

The palliative care services at St. Francis Hospital, Naggalama, was established in 2013 with the support of the Palliative Care Association of Uganda and APCA. The care team consists of a palliative care nurse, a nursing assistant and a pastoral caregiver. The palliative care team cares for geriatric patients as well as patients suffering from other chronic illnesses such as cancer, diabetics and HIV/AIDS. Patients are cared for at the out-patient department, the in-patient wards and in the community. They are also involved in the training of staff, caregivers and healthcare teams. The team collaborates with, and receives external support from, palliative care specialists from the USA who are also involved in training the staff in palliative care [38].

St. Francis Hospital, Nsambya Home Care Program

The Nsambya Home Care program was founded in 1987 to continue care for the increasing number of HIV/AIDS patients after their discharge from hospital, as they could not all be accommodated on the wards. It is one of the departments of Nsambya Hospital, and it started with a staff of three, but currently has 67 established staff members and 50 community volunteers [39]. The program targets HIV-infected and affected families, and serves communities living within a radius of 21 km from the hospital. Their target population is about 200,000 people with HIV living in the districts of Kampala, Wakiso, Mukono and Mpigi. The program also operates a clinic at Ggaba landing site [40]. By 2017, the program was established and had cared for 17,183 patients, 7366 of whom are in active care and are on antiretroviral treatment (ART). Services are offered through home-based care, out-patient clinics and outreaches. Services offered include HIV counselling and testing, diagnosis and treatment of opportunistic infections, for example, tuberculosis, provision of ART, social support to orphans and vulnerable children, a paediatric and adolescent clinic, and legal, psychosocial and nutrition support for patients. The program also provides community mobilisation on issues pertinent to HIV care including, but not limited to, counselling and testing, safe male circumcision, hygiene and sanitation [40].

Palliative Care Volunteers in Community Palliative Care

Community volunteers are a key component to the provision of palliative care in communities in Uganda. Community volunteers have been essential for increasing advocacy, awareness and acceptance for palliative care in the community. They also supplement the work of the palliative care teams and identify patients in need of palliative care, particularly in rural settings where the hospice teams may not easily be reached. In addition, they help to provide physical, emotional and spiritual care for patients while in their own homes [41]. Being part of the community, and because they are fully aware of the values and norms of their communities, these volunteers give culturally acceptable care and, therefore, patients and their families are willing to participate in the palliative care activities. Community volunteers are trained by the various palliative care services to empower them to provide adequate and appropriate information to the communities regarding cancers and HIV and to advise on family planning, health promotion, preparing wills and using herbal medicines. Some volunteers support patients in day care activities. Volunteers are often recruited through churches, and they call on their church networks for support [42, 43]. Hospital and community volunteers are important for supporting patients, especially with their psychosocial and spiritual needs, as well as linking them to palliative care services [43, 44].

Palliative Care Service Coordination and Governance

One of the factors that has enabled the integration of palliative care into Uganda's healthcare system has been the presence of a system that coordinates and governs palliative care services and activities. Palliative care is currently coordinated by the Department of Clinical Services in the Ministry of Health, where there is a palliative care desk. In addition, a new post of Assistant Commissioner, Palliative Care and Hospice Services has been established in the Ministry of Health, and the occupant of the post will oversee palliative care activities throughout the country. Palliative Care Association of Uganda (PCAU) was founded in 1999 and was registered as a non-government organisation in 2003. PCAU was founded mainly to support and promote the development of palliative care and palliative care professionals in Uganda. In this regard, PCAU provides leadership and coordinates civil society efforts for integrating palliative care into patients' care. Palliative care providers and those interested in palliative care are members of this organisation. The key activities of PCAU include supporting integration of palliative care services in every district of Uganda through training and mentorship, advocacy for palliative care and increasing awareness for palliative care. PCAU acts as the centre for data and information on palliative care service provision in Uganda and provides governance for palliative care. PCAU organises quarterly updates for all its members to improve and update knowledge on palliative care and palliative care services [45]. PCAU works in partnership with the Ministry of Health (MoH) to accredit palliative care facilities and has led several projects including the development of a palliative care policy for Uganda. On a broader scale, PCAU works with APCA, which oversees palliative care activities on the African continent [46]. APCA was founded in 2004 and works across the continent to promote palliative care for all in need, providing information to improve awareness of palliative care, strengthening systems by integrating palliative care at all levels of the healthcare system and building a sound evidence base for palliative care in Africa.

(ii) *Training for Clinicians Who Treat People with Palliative Care Needs*

Education has been a key factor in the development of palliative care in Uganda; for several years, Uganda has been a centre for palliative care training of health professionals from all over Africa. Education in PC has targeted clinical officers, medical doctors and nurses in service, medical and nursing students, allied health professionals (including counsellors, social workers, occupational therapists, physiotherapists, pharmacists, teachers, lawyers and spiritual leaders), volunteers, traditional healers, and patients and their families. Education among healthcare providers has improved attitudes toward palliative care, reduced opiophobia and increased general practitioners' provision of palliative care and referrals to palliative care specialists [47]. The main institutions in charge of PC training include: the Institute of Hospices and Palliative Care in Africa /Hospice Africa Uganda (IHPCA/HAU), APCA, the Makerere Mulago Palliative Care Unit in Makerere University, Mildmay Uganda and PCAU. By 2017, 60% of medical and 27% of nursing schools had PC as a mandatory component of their undergraduate curriculum, and 20% offered PC as an optional course [24]. Medical and nursing students undergo both summative and progressive assessments in palliative care. Palliative care assessments are included in the written and clinical examinations of medical, nursing and postgraduate specialist training. Palliative care has also been integrated with social work and social science schools at the university level.

At the start of palliative care in Uganda, champions for palliative care were identified in medical and nursing schools and were central in integrating palliative care into these schools as well as into postgraduate specialist training for doctors. Palliative care courses offered by training institutions in Uganda include short certificate courses, diploma courses, a Bachelor of Science degree in palliative care, a postgraduate diploma in general palliative care and a postgraduate diploma in paediatric palliative care. A masters' program in palliative care is at advanced stages of being approved and will begin in the near future. The program will be accredited through Makerere University. Training will teach healthcare workers generalist, intermediate and specialist PC skills. By 2017, over 10,000 health and healthcare-related professionals had been trained by the IHPCA/HAU. These included 3260 medical students, 3461 health professionals and managers, 83 volunteers, 92 health tutors, 347 palliative care initiators from other African countries, 80 rapid prescribers, 195 graduates with a diploma in palliative care and 86 graduates with Bachelor of Science degrees in palliative care. The Makerere Palliative care unit had trained 4630 individuals by 2018; these included medical and nursing students from within and outside of Uganda, clinical officers, nurses and doctors in service, and doctors that are undergoing postgraduate training in internal medicine, family medicine, Ear, Nose and Throat and the gynae-oncology fellowship programs [48]. A new palliative care diploma program has been introduced in the Mulago School of Nursing and Midwifery. Palliative care training programs employ different methods of training including didactic lectures, experiential learning and clinical placements during which clinical modelling is done.

The key to good service provision is having the right and competent leadership. Most palliative care in Uganda is provided and led by specialist palliative care nurses. For this, a leadership fellowship program was established for palliative care nurses in Uganda in 2015 by the Makerere Mulago Palliative Care Unit in collaboration with the University of Edinburgh with the aim of developing and enlarging the capability of nurses from all over Uganda to be leaders in palliative care. These nurses are mentored by nurse leaders from the United Kingdom. The program has equipped palliative care leaders with leadership, governance, research and advocacy skills [49].

(iii) *Safe Accessibility to Essential Palliative Medicines*

Pain and other symptom control are a key goal in palliative care. Therefore, essential palliative care medicines should be available to achieve this goal. Safe accessibility to essential palliative care medicines has been crucial in the development of palliative care in Uganda. Essential medicines for palliative care, including oral morphine, are now part of the Essential Medicines and Health Supplies List for Uganda, supported by the Ministry of Health. This implies that these medicines are available at all government health institutions in Uganda at no cost to the patients. Uganda has also gone a step further to ensure that the available palliative care medicines can be readily accessed, especially in the rural areas, by being the first country to amend statutory instruments to allow people who are not doctors to prescribe oral morphine. This was to supplement the efforts of the few medical doctors who, by law, were the only health workers allowed to prescribe narcotic medications. The Narcotic Drugs and Psychotropic Substances (Control) Act was reviewed in 2004 to legally allow nurses and clinical officers with appropriate training to prescribe morphine. Most of these trained nurses and clinical officers are based in the rural districts of Uganda. An evaluation of prescribing nurses across Uganda found that the nurses were competent to assess and manage pain and to prescribe morphine and other medications appropriately [50].

The control of morphine use is multi-sectoral involving the Ministry of Internal Affairs, Ministry of Justice and the National Drug Authority, among others, according to the regulations for narcotic use in Uganda and the International Narcotics Control Board (INCB). Through a public–private partnership between the Government of Uganda and Hospice Africa Uganda, oral morphine is locally reconstituted and distributed through the existing national medicines distribution system. The National Medical Stores (NMS) and Joint Medical Stores (JMS) are central to the distribution process of essential palliative care medications, including oral morphine for public and private health institutions. These stakeholders work in collaboration with the PCAU to support and monitor the use of morphine in order to limit stock-outs and potential abuse. The Ministry of Health and PCAU support the accreditation of sites for the use of opioids and delivery of palliative care services based on standard criteria. All these efforts have led to the increase in Uganda's consumption of opioids over the years. In 2002, national guidelines for the use of Class A medicines were developed and have guided the use of morphine in the country. The Uganda Clinical Guidelines also gives guidance to the use of other essential palliative care medicines for various symptoms under the palliative care section [27].

(iv) *Policy Development*

A draft policy for palliative care in Uganda has been developed and is in the advanced stages of acquiring approval. Although there is no standalone palliative care policy yet in Uganda, palliative care is recognised and promoted in several official documents of the government and the Ministry of Health, and these have laid the foundation for developing a palliative care policy and streamlined the provision of palliative care services. For example, palliative care is included as one of the priorities in Uganda's National Development Plan II as well as in the National Health Policy II and is well-elaborated in the Health Sector Strategic and Investment Plan II as an essential integral component of current healthcare in Uganda. Palliative care is also included in the National HIV/AIDS Framework.

(v) *Research*

Research has been critical in guiding the planning and development of clinical services. Notably, a community assessment/survey of needs at the beginning of palliative care services in Uganda was crucial to understanding patients' preference for home-based care at the end of life [28]. This survey confirmed the necessity of the home-based model for the provision of palliative care. Research has also highlighted the urgent need for palliative care in health facilities [51–53] and identified palliative care service models to ensure accessibility to all in need based on this demonstrated demand. For example, Mulago National Referral Hospital has employed a model of care that provides PC at three levels including generalist, intermediate and specialist levels, as recommended by the WHO [47].

A biennial palliative care conference is held to disseminate best practices and research to palliative care specialists. There are both national and international palliative care research collaborations among researchers in Uganda and researchers at the University of Edinburgh, Kings College London, Cardiff University, Indian Association of Palliative Care, International Children's Palliative Care Network and University of Leeds. Research training is done by all the palliative care training institutions. There are several palliative care providers who are undertaking a PhD in palliative care training and research. In addition, there is an honorary professor of palliative care in Makerere University who engages in rigorous research activities in Uganda.

Challenges Facing Palliative Care in Uganda

Despite the many successes in implementing, training and establishing strategies to ensure essential palliative care drug availability, palliative care in Uganda still faces challenges. Only about 10% of patients who need PC in Uganda access it [54]. In 2010, 80% of the 16,526 patients who died of cancers in Uganda had moderate to severe pain, and 50% of the 112,065 people who died from HIV-related illnesses had moderate to severe pain [55]. According to Treat the Pain Report in 2010, only 2.6% of patients who needed pain relief in Uganda received it [55]. In those districts with palliative care, not everyone has access to it, largely due to the lack of home-based care teams and the inadequate number of trained healthcare providers in palliative care; another challenge is the high patient to health professional ratio that hinders the provision of quality services. In many facilities, there are frequent shortages of essential medications, which is a barrier to adequate symptom control.

Regarding training and education, not all health education institutions have teaching programs on palliative care; this is mainly due to the shortage of trained tutors and lecturers. In addition, there is still limited knowledge and skills for palliative care across all levels of the health system, including policy and service providers at the community and patient levels. This has led to palliative care services being perceived as only end-of-life support for the dying, resulting in late referrals and poor integration [56]. Also, palliative care services mainly offer care to cancer and HIV/AIDS patients with very few services offering palliative care for other chronic health conditions due to limited funding for palliative care. Therefore, there is still inadequate access to essential palliative care services by patients in need.

There is also a lack of recognition of PC practitioners in the national health scheme and their appropriate deployment in the public service. Much research in palliative care has been done in the country, but there are few clinical trials; this has constrained its use in clinical practice and policy. There has been limited funding for creating palliative care activities. Most of Uganda's centres of PC rely on external donor funding. The unpredictable nature of such financing, particularly in the current global economic crisis, raises issues of sustainability and highlights the need for a national policy and implementation framework. The absence of a national policy on palliative care constitutes a major challenge with serious implication to the country's level of financial investment in palliative care and scale-up.

Conclusion

There has been significant progress made in furthering palliative care in Uganda over the past 25 years. Most notably, there has been an increase in the number and quality of services in the country; palliative care services are now available and accessible in most districts in Uganda. Significant progress has also been made by training health professionals and non-health professionals in palliative care. In addition, research in palliative care has increased, and some of it has influenced practice and local policy. With regard to drug availability, most of the essential medicines for palliative care are now on the Essential Medicines and Health Supplies List for Uganda and are provided free of charge in public healthcare facilities. However, there is still an enormous need to further develop and improve home-based and community-based palliative care services, making the programs sustainable and less dependent on donations. There is also a need to sustain consistent medicine supplies as well as funding for research and to establish palliative care policy. The national policy on palliative care would, in turn, guide the development and improvement of palliative care services through strategies that include increasing financial investments in palliative care, training and promoting research to inform service.

References

1. Connor SR, Bermedo MCS. Global atlas of palliative care at the end-of- life. London: Worldwide Palliative Care Alliance; 2014.
2. Knaul FM, Farmer PE, Krakauer EL, De Lima L, Bhadelia A, Kwete XJ, Connor SR. Alleviating the access abyss in palliative care and pain relief - an imperative of universal health coverage: the Lancet Commission report. Lancet. 2018;391(10128):1391–454.
3. World Health Organization. Global Health Observatory (GHO): NCD mortality and morbidity. [Cited on 12th February 2020]. Available from http://www.who.int/gho/ncd/mortality_morbidity/en/.
4. Palliative care -World Health Organisation. [Cited on 12th February 2020] available from: https://www.who.int/news-room/fact-sheets/detail/palliative-care.
5. Uganda bureau of statistics - UBOs 2019. [Cited on 30th September 2019] available from: https://www.ubos.org/.
6. Merriman A, Mwebesa E, Zirimenya L. Improving access to palliative care for patients with cancer in Africa: 25 years of Hospice Africa. e-cancer Med Sci. 2019;13:946.
7. Non- communicable diseases country profiles 2018 -Uganda. [cited on 10th February 2020] Available from: https://www.who.int/nmh/countries/uga_en.pdf.
8. Uganda-Global cancer observatory. [cited on 2nd October 2019] available from: http://gco.iarc.fr/today/data/factsheets/populations/800-uganda-fact-sheets.pdf.
9. Uganda Population HIV-based HIV Impact Assessment. Uganda fact sheet –WHO - Afro-World Health Organisation. [Cited on 8th October 2019] available from: https://www.afro.who.int/sites/default/files/2017-08/UPHIA%20Uganda%20fact-sheet.pdf.
10. Uganda-UNAIDS [cited on 10th February 2020.] available from: https://www.unaids.org/en/regionscountries/countries/uganda.
11. Mwaka AD, Garimoi CO, Were EM, Roland M, Wabinga H, Lyratzopoulos G. Social, demographic and healthcare factors associated with stage at diagnosis of cervical cancer: cross-sectional study in a tertiary hospital in Northern Uganda. BMJ Open. 2016;6:e007690.
12. Galukande M, Mirembe F, Wabinga H. Patient delay in accessing breast cancer care in a sub-Saharan African Country: Uganda. Br J Med Med Res. 2014;4(13):2599–610.
13. Ministry of Health Uganda report on NCD survey 2014. [Cited on 10th October 2019] available from.: https://health.go.ug/community-health-departments/non-communicable-diseases.
14. Medicine prices in Uganda –World Health Organisation. [cited on 10th February 2020] available from: https://www.who.int/medicines/areas/technical_cooperation/MedicinePricesUganda.pdf.
15. Lunyera J, Stanifer JW, Ingabire P, Etolu W, Bagasha P, Egger JR, et al. Prevalence and correlates of proteinuria in Kampala, Uganda: a cross-sectional pilot study. BMC Res Notes. 2016;9:97.
16. Naicker S, Ashuntantang G. End stage renal disease in sub-Saharan Africa. In: Chronic kidney disease in disadvantaged populations. Elsevier; 2017. p. 125–37.
17. Merriman A. Uganda: current status of palliative care. J Pain Symptom Manag. 2002;24(2):252–6.
18. Stjernaward J, Foley KM, Ferris FD. The public health strategy for palliative care. J Pain Symptom Manag. 2007;33:486–93.
19. Care, WHO Integrating Palliative. Symptom relief into primary health care: a WHO guide for planners, implementers and managers: World Health Organization; 2018.
20. Harding R, Selman L, Powell RA, Namisango E, Downing J, Merriman A, et al. Research into palliative care in sub-Saharan Africa. Lancet Oncol. 2013;14(4):e183–8.
21. Lynch T, Connor S, Clark D. Mapping levels of palliative care development: a global update. J Pain Symptom Manag. 2013;45:1094–106.
22. Alliance, Worldwide Palliative Care. Mapping levels of palliative care development: a global update. London: Worldwide Palliative Care Alliance; 2011.
23. Economics Intelligence Unit. The 2015 quality of death index. Ranking palliative care across the world. London: EIU; 2015. [Cited on 12th February 2020] Available from: https://eiuperspectives.economist.com/sites/default/files/2015%20EIU%20Quality%20of%20Death%20Index%20Oct%2029%20FINAL.pdf.
24. Rhee JY, Luyirika E, Namisango E, Powell RA, Garralda E, Pons JJ, et al. APCA atlas of palliative care in Africa. Houston, TX: IAHPC Press; 2017.
25. Kiwanuka, R. Palliative care for the deaf community in Uganda. ehospice 2015. [Cited on 13 February 2020] available from: https://ehospice.com/international_posts/palliative-care-for-the-deaf-community-in-uganda/.
26. Compassionate cell-mates-improving access to palliative care and HIV services in Masaka prison in Uganda. e-hospice 2016. [Cited on 13th February 2020] Available from https://ehospice.com/africa_posts/compassionate-cell-mates-improving-access-to-palliative-care-and-hiv-services-in-masaka-prison-uganda/.
27. Uganda Clinical guidelines 2016.Ministry of Health. [cited on 14th February 2020] Available from https://www.health.go.ug/content/uganda-clinical-guidelines-2016.

28. Kikule E. A good death in Uganda: survey of needs for palliative care for terminally ill people in urban areas. BMJ. 2003;327(7408):192–4.
29. Hospice Africa Uganda. [Cited on 13th February 2020] Available from: http://uganda.hospiceafrica.or.ug/.
30. Kawempe Home care. [Cited on 13th February 2020] Available from: https://kawempehomecare.org/who-we-are/.
31. Email communication from Joy hospice team member received on 12th February 2020.
32. Rays of Hope Hospice. [Cited on 13th February 2020] Available from: https://www.raysofhopehospicejinja.org/about-us-vision-and-mission.
33. Global directory for palliative care services and organisations. [Cited on 10th October 2019] Available from: https://hospicecare.com/global-directory-of-providers-organizations/listings/details/1886/.
34. Hospice Tororo. [Cited on 13th February 2020] Available from: http://www.hospicetororo.com/about-us.
35. Kitovu mobile. [Cited on 13 February 2020] Available from: http://www.kitovumobile.com/about-us.
36. New life Hospice Arua. [Cited on 13th February 2020] Available from: https://pcauganda.org/fund-raising-for-the-construction-of-the-first-hospice-in-west-nile/.
37. Bringing Palliative care to Southern Sudan refugees. [Cited on 13th February 2020] Available from: https://eapcnet.wordpress.com/2019/10/07/winning-posters-from-berlin-bringing-palliative-care-education-to-south-sudanese-refugees-in-uganda/.
38. Nakafeero. A rural hospital initiates a successful palliative care service-St. Francis Nagalama hospital, Uganda. E hospice 2015. [Cited on 13th February 2020]. Available from: https://ehospice.com/africa_posts/a-rural-hospital-initiates-a-successful-palliative-care-service-st-francis-naggalama-hospital-uganda/.
39. Massavon W, Nsubuga M, Lundin R, Penazzato M, Nannyonga N, Namisi C, et al. Nsambya community Home-Based Care complements national HIV and TB management efforts and contributes to health systems strengthening in Uganda: an observational study. ISRN Public Health. 2014;2014:623690.
40. Nsambya home care. [Cited on 13th February 2020] Available from: http://www.nsambyahospital.or.ug/department/home-care/.
41. Jack BA, Kirton JA, Birakurataki J, Merriman A. The personal value of being a palliative care community volunteer worker in Uganda: a qualitative study. Palliat Med. 2012;26(5):753–9.
42. Grant L, Brown J, Leng M, Bettega N, Murray SA. Palliative care making a difference in rural Uganda, Kenya and Malawi: three rapid evaluation field studies. BMC Palliat Care. 2011;10:8.
43. Volunteering –Hospice Africa Uganda. [Cited on 13th February 2020] available from: http://uganda.hospiceafrica.or.ug/index.php/careers/volunteering.
44. Jack BA, Kirton J, Birakurataki J, Merriman A. A bridge to the hospice: the impact of a community volunteer programme in Uganda. Palliat Med. 2011;25:706–15.
45. Palliative Care Association of Uganda. [cited on 13th february 2020]. Available from https://pcauganda.org/.
46. About APCA –African Palliative Care Association. [Cited on 13th February 2020] Available from: https://www.africanpalliativecare.org/about/about-apca/.
47. Downing J, Batuli M, Kivumbi G, Kabahweza J, Grant L, Murray SA, et al. A palliative care link nurse programme in Mulago Hospital, Uganda: an evaluation using mixed methods. BMC Palliat Care. 2016;15(1):40.
48. Leng M. Building momentum for palliative care, transforming lives, changing systems, bringing hope. 10th anniversary conference for Makerere Mulago Palliative care Unit . Makerere College of Health Sciences 9th–10th August 2018. [Cited on 27th may 2020 Available from: https://cairdeas.org.uk/resources/conference-lecture-posters-and-presentations.
49. Downing J, Leng M, Grant L. Implementing a palliative care nurse leadership fellowship program in Uganda. Oncol Nurs Forum. 2016;43(3):395–8.
50. Downing J, Kivumbi G, Nabirye E, Ojera A, Namwaga R, Katusabe R, et al. An evaluation of palliative care nurse prescribing: a mixed methods study in Uganda. BMJ Support Palliat Care. 2018;8:A6.
51. Leng M, Okongo F, Knights D, Downing J, Batuli M. Who needs palliative care; assessment of needs in two regional referral hospitals in northern Uganda. Proceeding of Makerere University Annual Scientific Conference September 2014. At: Imperial Royal Hotel Kampala-Uganda [cited on 13th February 2020] Available from: https://www.researchgate.net/publication/280830291_WHO_NEEDS_PALLIATIVE_CARE_ASSESSMENT_OF_NEEDS_IN_TWO_REGIONAL_REFERRAL_HOSPITALS_IN_NORTHERN_UGANDA.
52. Jacinto A, Masembe V, Tumwesigye NM, Harding R. The prevalence of life-limiting illness at a Ugandan National Referral Hospital: a 1-day census of all admitted patients. BMJ Support Palliat Care. 2015;5:196–9.
53. Lewington J, Namukwaya E, Limoges J, Leng M, Harding R. Provision of palliative care for life-limiting disease in a low income country national hospital setting: how much is needed? BMJ Support Palliat Care. 2012;2:140–4.
54. Nabudere H, Obuku E, Lamorde M. Advancing palliative care in the Uganda health system: an evidence-based policy brief. Int J Technol Assess Health Care. 2014;30(6):621–5.
55. Access to Palliative care 216 Uganda fact UPR sheet [cited on 13th February 2020] available from.: https://pcauganda.org/wp-content/uploads/2017/02/PC-FACTSHEET_Final-1.pdf.
56. Powell RA, Mwangi-Powell, Kiyange F, Radbruch L, Harding R. Palliative care development in Africa: how can we provide enough quality care? BMJ Support Palliat Care. 2011;1(2):113–4.

Part XVI

East Africa: Rwanda

Palliative Care: Challenges and Opportunities – A Comparison of the Fee-for-Service System of the United States with Rwanda's Public Health Approach

Christian R. Ntizimira, Blaise Uhagaze, Olive Mukeshimana, Eric Kabisa, Scholastique Ngizwenayo, Sandra Urusaro, and Mary L. Dunne

Palliative Care in the United States

Dame Cicely Saunders, founder of the innovative St. Christopher's Hospice in London, visited the United States and inspired the development of the American hospice movement. In 1972, psychiatrist Elizabeth Kübler-Ross, author of *On Death and Dying* [1], testified before the US Senate on the subject of death with dignity, expressing her support for home care and hospice [2]. Florence Wald, a former Dean of the Yale School of Nursing, led the founding of Connecticut Hospice in 1971, and Declan Walsh, MD, founded the first inpatient palliative care program at the Cleveland Clinic in 1987 [3].

The US Medicare Hospice Benefit, introduced in 1982, defined hospice as end-of-life care that excluded curative treatment. The 1995 SUPPORT Study painted a grim picture of death in U.S. hospitals: poor communication, overuse of intensive care, and appalling levels of patient and family suffering [4]. These findings helped increase national engagement in both quality-of-life and end-of-life issues, including grant funding to palliative care to benefit all patients living with serious illness, applying the patient-centered philosophy and interdisciplinary team approach of hospice to patients of any age, at any stage of serious illness.

Clinical palliative care is practiced at three levels: primary (basic skills for all providers), secondary (specialist care), and tertiary (academic practice, teaching, and research) [5]. Hospice and Palliative Medicine was recognized as a medical subspecialty in 2006. In 2020, there are an estimated 7600 board-certified palliative care physicians in the United States [6], which represents an estimated shortage of 18,000 based on optimal need for specialists [7]. This increases the importance of primary palliative care services delivered by non-palliative care clinicians.

C. R. Ntizimira (✉)
City Cancer Challenge Foundation, Kigali, Rwanda
e-mail: ntizimira@citycancerchallenge.org

B. Uhagaze · E. Kabisa
Rwanda Palliative Care and Hospice Organization, Kigali, Rwanda

O. Mukeshimana · S. Ngizwenayo
Kibagabaga District Hospital, Kigali, Rwanda

S. Urusaro
Partners in Health/Inshuti Mu Buzima, Kigali, Rwanda

M. L. Dunne
Supportive Care Medicine, Nuvance Health, Poughkeepsie, NY, USA

Distinguished Careers Institute, Stanford University, Stanford, CA, USA
e-mail: mdunne@nuvance.org

M. Silbermann (ed.), *Palliative Care for Chronic Cancer Patients in the Community*,
https://doi.org/10.1007/978-3-030-54526-0_25

In 2019, the Center to Advance Palliative Care (CAPC) reported that 72% of US hospitals with 50 or more beds had a palliative care team, compared with 7% in 2001 [8] as shown in Fig. 1. The Joint Commission, a US accrediting organization, launched an Advanced Certification for Palliative Care Program in 2011, and over 1900 hospital-based programs have been certified [9].

Palliative care in the community setting is most often provided through established delivery systems, such as office- or clinic-based visits, home care, hospice, and skilled nursing facilities. The goal is to support a person's life at home or place of residence by maximizing quality of life and providing care based on patient preferences and goals. At present, there is no nationwide data on US community-based palliative care. In a 3-year CAPC survey of community-based palliative care providers, 890 programs responded, representing 3162 sites of care. Programs by operator are shown in Table 1. The majority (70%) treat adult patients only;

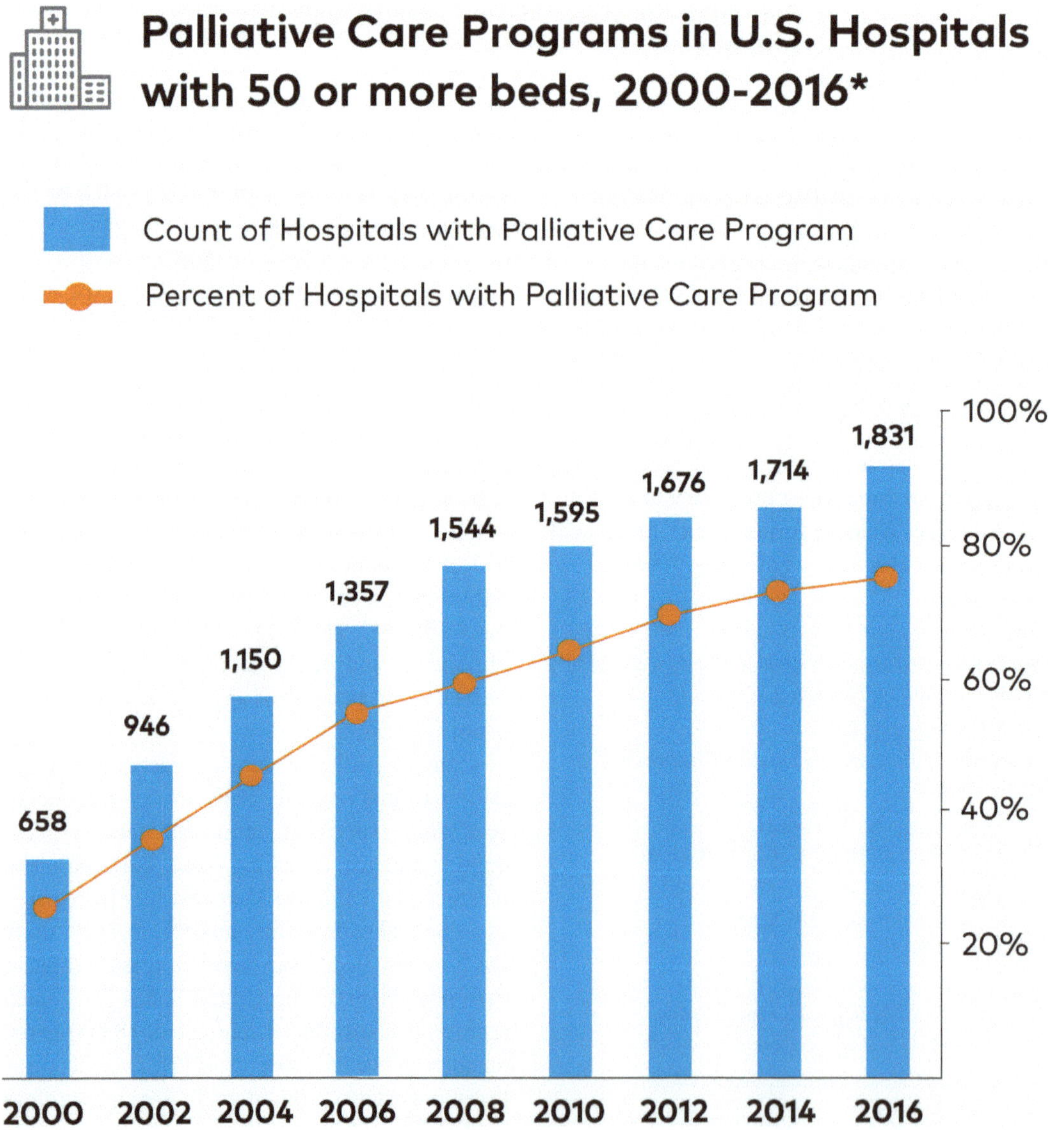

Fig. 1 Palliative care in US hospitals with 50 or more beds, 2000–2016 [9]. (Source: Center to Advance Palliative Care)

Table 1 Community-based palliative care programs by operator [10]

Total	Hospice	Hospital	Office	Long-term care	Home Health Agency
3162	33%	32%	14%	11%	10%

Table 2 US hospices. Report to the Congress: Medicare Payment Policy. Hospice services [13]

Year	Number	$ CMS spending	Non-profit (%)	For profit (%)	Government (%)
2000	2255	2.9 billion	59	31	11
2015	4199	16.8 billion	23	65	4

Table 3 Who pays for end-of-life care? [14]

Payer	Medicare	Medicaid	Private insurance	Self-pay, charity
% total	85.4	5	6.9	2.7

24% treat both children and adults; 6% focus solely on children [10].

In 2016, the Joint Commission developed a certification program for community-based palliative care [11]. By the end of 2017, 91 programs had been certified (personal communication January15, 2020).

Hospice services are available in every state. To be eligible to receive care under the Medicare or Medicaid hospice benefit, an adult patient must be certified as having a prognosis of 6 months or less, endorse care focused on comfort, and give up disease-modifying treatment. Pediatric patients are an exception, as the 2010 Affordable Care Act mandated that children enrolled in state Medicaid or Children's Health Insurance Programs must be allowed to receive hospice care along with cancer treatment [12]. Tables 2 and 3 show US hospice characteristics.

Home is the most common place of death in hospice. Eighty percent of Americans say they wish to die at home, but less than 40% do so [15]. For the first time since the early twentieth century, home surpassed the hospital as the most common place of death in 2017, although hospital deaths remain common [16].

Palliative care growth has paralleled improvements in cancer diagnosis and treatment, as well as the articulation of the "cancer control continuum," from prevention, screening, and diagnosis through treatment, survivorship, and end-of-life care [17]. There is a robust literature on the value of palliative care integration in oncology services. In 2010, Temel and colleagues published a landmark clinical trial randomizing 151 advanced lung cancer patients to usual oncology care with or without specialist palliative care. The palliative care group demonstrated better quality of life, fewer depressive symptoms, improved end-of-life care, and lived almost 3 months longer [18]. These findings galvanized national momentum to implement and study palliative care in oncology services. Temel continues to investigate palliative care integration in oncology to elucidate the elements that confer benefits [19]. Hui recently concluded that interdisciplinary specialist palliative care in stand-alone clinics is the gold standard for integration in oncology due to the impact on multiple patient and caregiver outcomes [20]. However, such a resource-intense system is not accessible to many patients. Research is needed to evaluate optimal models for a variety of care settings.

It is pertinent to briefly review the US health care system, as it affects the entire cancer control continuum. In 2017, the United States spent about $3.5 trillion, or 18% of Gross Domestic Product, on health care, more than twice that of other countries [21]. This is due to many factors, including the speed with which the U.S adopts new technologies and treatments; the lack of cost transparency and limits on price negotiation; the higher costs the United States pays for materials, devices, drugs, and providers; and a decentralized and fragmented system of insurances, both public and private. With no universal health insurance, the US system has many gaps.

The types of coverage are shown in Table 4. (They are not mutually exclusive as people can be covered by more than one type of health insurance during the year.)

The 2010 Affordable Care Act (ACA), or Obamacare, was the biggest change in US health care since the 1965 establishment of Medicare

Table 4 2018 Sources of US health insurance plans [22]

Plan type	Private	Medicare	Medicaid	Veterans
% covered	66	18	17	1

(for persons 65 and older) and Medicaid (for low-income persons) [23]. As a result of the ACA, the number of uninsured non-elderly Americans decreased from over 46.5 million in 2010 to just below 27 million in 2016.

Most people in the US obtain private health insurance through an employer. However, not all workers are offered coverage or, if offered, can afford their share of the premiums. Employers are increasingly shifting costs to employees via high premiums, high deductibles, co-payments, and co-insurance. Such escalating cost-sharing means that an increasing proportion of the population is underinsured, delaying or not accessing care because of cost [24]. Greater cost-sharing is associated with worse adherence to treatment, which disproportionately affects the poor [25].

The US cancer mortality decreased by 26% from 1991 to 2015 [26]. More Americans receive a cancer diagnosis each year and more patients survive [27], reflecting the aging of the population as well as advances in screening, detection, and treatment. The number of US cancer survivors is expected to increase to 20.3 million by 2026 [28].

The National Cancer Institute (NCI) is the principal US agency for cancer research and training. Part of the National Institutes of Health, an agency in the US Department of Health and Human Services, the NCI coordinates the United States National Cancer Program. There are 71 NCI-designated cancer centers, located in 36 states and the District of Columbia, funded by the NCI to deliver groundbreaking cancer treatment [29]. More than 1500 cancer centers, found in every state, are accredited by the Commission on Cancer of the American College of Surgeons, which made palliative care a condition of accreditation in 2014 [30].

The dramatic improvements in cancer therapy, especially novel immunotherapies and genome-guided treatments, confound clinicians' ability to determine and communicate prognostic information to patients and families [30]. While palliative drugs can ease symptoms and may prolong life in some settings, patients often have a poor understanding of their prognosis and believe their treatment will be curative [32]. Such misunderstanding may delay palliative care and hospice referral.

The median monthly price of many cancer treatments is approximately double the median monthly US household income. Newly approved cancer drugs have list prices of $100,000 per year or more, and the cost of older drugs continues to rise rapidly [33]. Insured patients' share of some treatments ranges from 20% to 30%, and uninsured persons may be responsible for the entire cost. Health care costs and income losses are a leading cause of bankruptcy, especially among cancer survivors [34]. Financial hardship is associated with poor compliance [35], poorer quality of life, and worse survival [34]. Physicians' failure to disclose the cost of treatments has been called "financial toxicity," impairing patients' well-being [36].

For many Americans, cancer survival means living with a complex chronic condition. They need long-term support in survivorship: prevention, surveillance, ongoing management of the multidimensional consequences of cancer and treatment, and coordination of generalist and specialist providers [37].

In 2019, there were 43.5 million unpaid US caregivers, whose numbers will not keep pace with the rising numbers of senior citizens [38]. Family or informal caregivers (unpaid friends, neighbors, community members) are critical to a patient's well-being and compliance, from diagnosis through treatment and survivorship [39]. Caregivers are expected to execute clinical tasks that would previously have been performed by trained health care staff [40], and they receive little support from the health care system [41]. Only about 30% of caregivers report being asked about their experience or their need for assistance by health care professionals [42], though caregiving increases mortality risk [43]. According to the Partnership for Solutions, the number of hours spent caregiving increases with caregiver age, as shown in Fig. 2 [44].

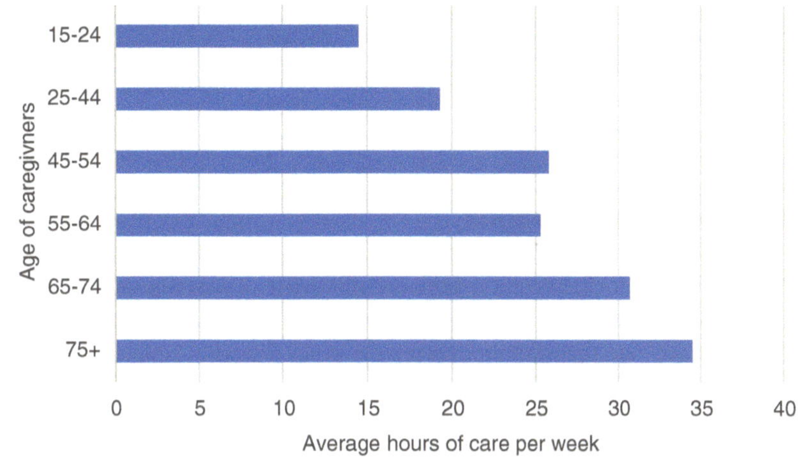

Fig. 2 Number of hours dedicated to caregiving by age of family caregiver [44]

There is a scarcity of formal or paid caregivers in the United States. Low wages, few or no benefits, low job satisfaction, lack of career development, and immigration restrictions all contribute to this shortage [45].

Future Trends in the United States

The US health care delivery and financing system, while complex and politically charged, is in a period of transformation. The ACA accelerated change by creating the Center for Medicare and Medicaid Innovation (CMMI) to implement and scale innovative models to address the "triple aim" of better quality, better health, and lower cost [46]. As of 2019, the percentage of Medicare payments with alternative payment models had increased to 38% [47].

The US model of hospice care is increasingly outdated as the line between curative and palliative treatments is blurred by new treatments and best practice data. At present, Medicare beneficiaries must make the "terrible choice" between cancer treatment and hospice care [48]. CMMI is piloting new models that expand access to palliative care specialists, including the Oncology Care Model, which aims to provide higher quality, more highly coordinated oncology care at the same or lower cost, and the Medicare Care Choices Model, which allows Medicare beneficiaries to receive disease-modifying care while enrolled in hospice [49]. A number of Medicare Advantage models, such as Aspire Health, focus on multidisciplinary home-based palliative care [50]. The Veterans Administration Medical Centers offers expanded-access hospice, including concurrent cancer therapy [51]. There are also value-based programs in the private sector, such as Aetna's Compassionate Care Program, which allows the seriously ill to enroll in hospice while still receiving curative treatment [52]. Understanding the effects of various value-based payment models is a critical area of research to develop public policy.

The Palliative Care and Hospice Education and Training Act, pending in Congress in 2020 [53], would amend the Public Health Service Act to increase palliative care training in medicine, pharmacy, nursing, social work, chaplaincy, and allied health disciplines, as well as create national educational and advocacy programs.

The promise of interoperable electronic health records, so critical in oncology care, has not yet been realized. Clinical medicine is on the threshold of "learning health care systems" that can analyze data, generate evidence, and provide new insights into care and research [54], including prioritizing patients for palliative care services [55].

The current US health care system is not structured to meet the needs of the growing number of people with cancer and other chronic conditions. This crisis presents an opportunity to transform serious illness care to be more patient-centered, accessible, culturally inclusive, coordinated, and team-based. The US policymakers must work to overcome persistent gaps and challenges, expanding coverage, improving quality, and reducing the level and growth of health care costs.

Palliative Care in Rwanda

The World Health Organization defines palliative care as an approach that improves the quality of life of patients and their families facing the problems associated with life-threatening illness through the prevention and relief of suffering by means of early identification and impeccable assessment and treatment of pain and other problems, physical, psychosocial, and spiritual [56]. Hippocrates (c. 460 BC–c. 370 BC), the father of the modern medicine, stipulated in the Hippocratic Corpus that "It is far more important to know what sort of person has the disease than what sort of the disease the person has." By treating the disease, we can miss treating the patient, but by treating the patient, we cannot miss treating the disease. Caring for patients and their families involves more than treatment of disease itself, but must consider the environment, feelings, emotions, cultures, context, and perception of care as defined by the patient. End-of-life care, as part of palliative care services, proves difficult to manage across societies due to various challenges: inadequate support systems for the process of dying, death as a difficult topic to discuss, and the impact of community-oriented versus individualistic sociocultural values on the dying process [17].

In the past 25 years, Rwanda has made remarkable steps toward recovery, both in terms of psychological healing as a society and in key global health indicators such as in maternal and child mortality and access to anti retro-viral medication [57, 58]. An important indicator of progress in Rwanda is life expectancy, which was 28 years in 1994 compared with 62 years in 2015. The country has been able to rebuild national security and stability, reinvigorate the economy, and rebuild the health sector.

In 2011, Rwanda became the first African country to adopt a stand-alone national policy on palliative care, as well as palliative care strategic and implementation plans. A platform for the continuum of care has been set up with a focus on vulnerable populations. In particular, Rwanda has a community-based health insurance scheme that provides access to treatment for the poorest members of the population. However, there are still many issues which threaten the improvement of developing countries like Rwanda, such as inadequate health infrastructure, lack of access to health education, high population growth, and devastating diseases such as cancer, HIV-AIDS, and tuberculosis.

The Rwandan government uses a public heath approach to address health issues [59], from infectious disease to non-communicable disease, as a principle of equity. Access to health care services is not considered a luxury but a necessity for all Rwandan citizens. The same approach has been used with the national policy in palliative care. A program to train physician, nurses, and social workers from various health care settings began in 2012 with the aim to integrate palliative care services throughout the system, following the HIV/AIDS model started by the United States' President's Emergency Plan for AIDS Relief (PEPFAR) supported by Intrahealth and Mildmay. This introduced the training of trainers at district hospitals in partnership with the Rwanda Ministry of Health.

Another indicator of progress is opioid availability in Rwanda. Physical pain is a symptom common to cancer patients and others who need palliative care. Over the last century, research has demonstrated the efficiency and effectiveness of morphine to relieve pain and reduce suffering. Today, morphine is the gold-standard medication in palliative care, especially among cancer patients. Through effective pain management, a patient's comfort and dignity is preserved.

In the preamble of the Single Convention on Narcotics Drugs, 1961, as amended by the 1972 Protocol Amending the Single Convention on Narcotics Drugs, 1961, it is specified that: "*...Desiring to conclude a generally acceptable international convention replacing existing treaties on narcotic drugs, limiting such drugs to medical and scientific use...*" [59]. The accessibility and availability of opioids is a core palliative care principle. Unfortunately, there is profound inequality of access to medication: the richest 10% of the world's population live in countries that receive nearly 90% of the opioid pain relief medications [60]. The top four consuming countries are the United States, Canada, Australia, and New Zealand, with the rest of world sharing the remaining 15% [61]. Today the Rwanda Ministry of Health produces its own morphine syrup, which is on the List of Essential Medicines in Rwanda, and the supply chain has improved so that patients at the village level can access morphine through district pharmacies. According to the Rwanda Biomedical Center, the implementor institution from the Ministry of Health, morphine consumption grew from 0.2 kgs per year in 2007 to almost 10 kgs in 2019. The Government of Rwanda also revised the law governing narcotics drugs, psychotropics, and precursors in Rwanda (Official Gazette n*15 of 09/04/2012, Law n* 03 of 15/02/2012) to allow nurses and other allied health professionals to be trained to prescribe morphine in their practice. Figure 3 shows the supply chain of morphine syrup in Rwanda, from the central Medical Procurement and Production Division (MPPD), overseen by the Non-communicable Disease (NCD) Division of the Ministry of Health, through the health system to the local level via Community Health Workers (CHW) and Health Posts.

CHWs, who are elected by their villages and trained and supervised by national guidelines, play an important role in primary health care delivery. Rwanda has leveraged the strength of its people, using CHWs to reduce the burden of major diseases (HIV/AIDS, tuberculosis, malaria, and cancer) and improve the health care system [62]. This has demonstrated the potential of human resources to deliver services, collect data, and bring change [63]. More than 210 Home-Based Care Practitioners (HBCPs), lay persons who provide longitudinal care to chronic patients after receiving a six-month training in NCD and palliative care services, work at the village level to support patients and their families and report to the health center.

According to GLOBOCAN, an estimated 10,704 new cancer cases and 7662 cancer-related deaths occurred in Rwanda in 2018. The survival rate of cancer patients is appallingly low in the developing world, including Rwanda. The main gaps for cancer control in Rwanda include ignorance, poor awareness, and myths about cancer in the general population; limited screening and

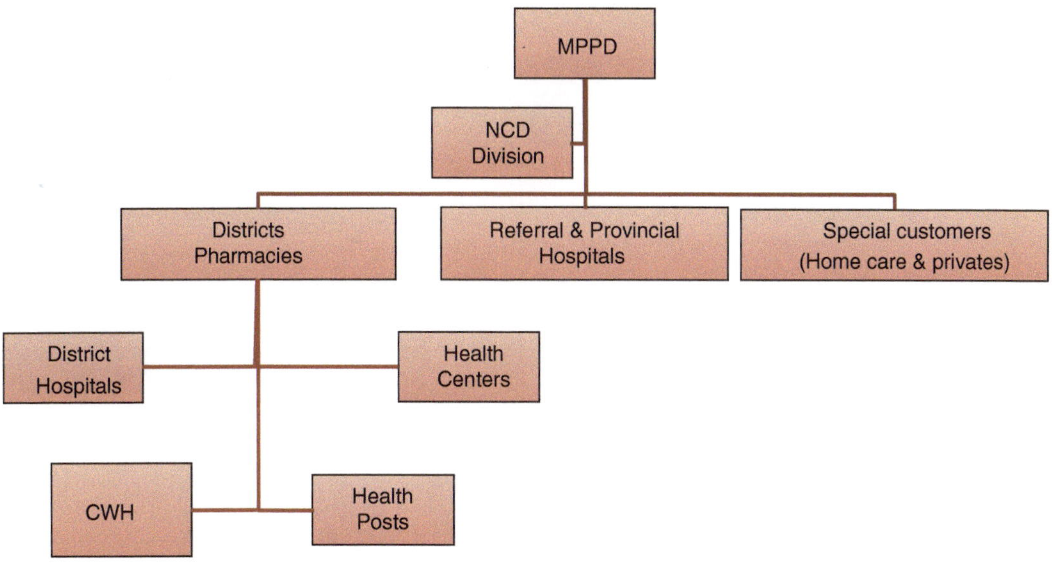

Fig. 3 The supply chain of morphine in Rwanda

early detection; and inadequate diagnostic and treatment facilities.

Cancer diagnosis is carried out at the level of tertiary and teaching hospitals, including the Butaro Cancer Centre of Excellence (BCCOE) in rural Northern province, which has pathology laboratories and advanced medical imaging equipment. BCCOE is supported by Partners in Health, a non-profit American organization with a philosophy of social justice and equity for poor and vulnerable populations [64]. Cancer treatment is provided at the same facilities, where patients benefit from surgery, chemotherapy, and palliative care.

Palliative care is a critical component of cancer care in Rwanda, as most cases are identified at advanced stages. Palliative care services are integrated throughout the Rwanda health system, including teaching, referral, provincial and district hospitals, and community health centers, with community services provided through HBCPs [65].

The public–private partnership developed by the Rwandan Ministry of Health with non-governmental organizations and local civil society has validated a multisectoral approach to solutions. In that context, the Ministry of Health signed a Memorandum of Understanding with the Rwanda Palliative Care and Hospice Organization, a local non-profit organization providing palliative care services in patient homes, to support HBCPs in the development of services at the village level. Figure 4 illustrates the comprehensive model of palliative care in Rwanda, using a multisector collaborative approach.

Patients diagnosed with advanced cancer, whether in BCCOE or in Kigali, are referred to the district hospital near their villages to receive supportive care. Depending on the general condition of the patient, the district hospital will refer to the Health Center or the community level, where HBCPs or CHWs are trained to be the "eyes and ears" of physicians. A nurse trained in palliative care visits patients at home with HBCPs and reports to the district level. The local organization provides important psychological support for patients and family caregivers, including after the death of the patient. These partnerships have created a strong synergy between the public and the private sectors.

The Rwanda Ministry of Health has developed an NCD model of care, encompassing all

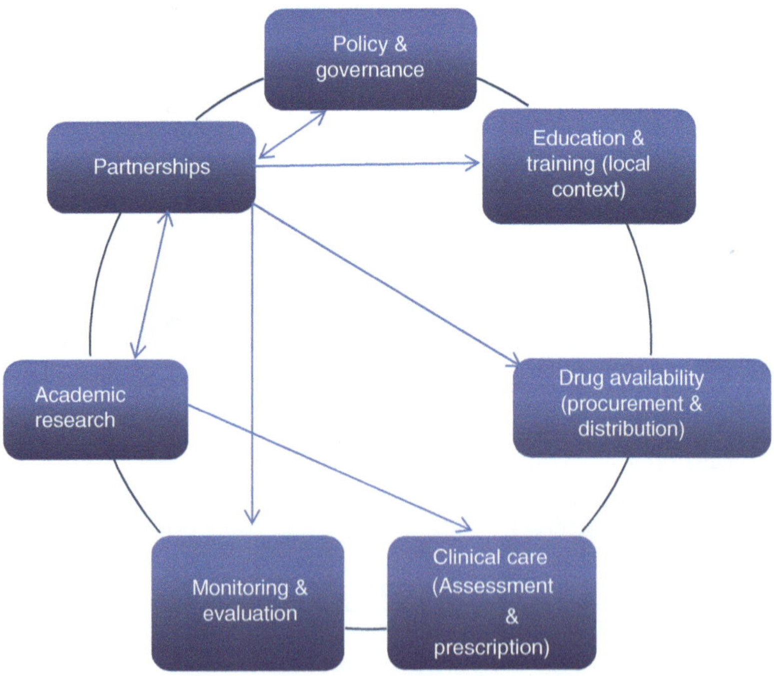

Fig. 4 Rwanda palliative care: a multisector collaborative approach

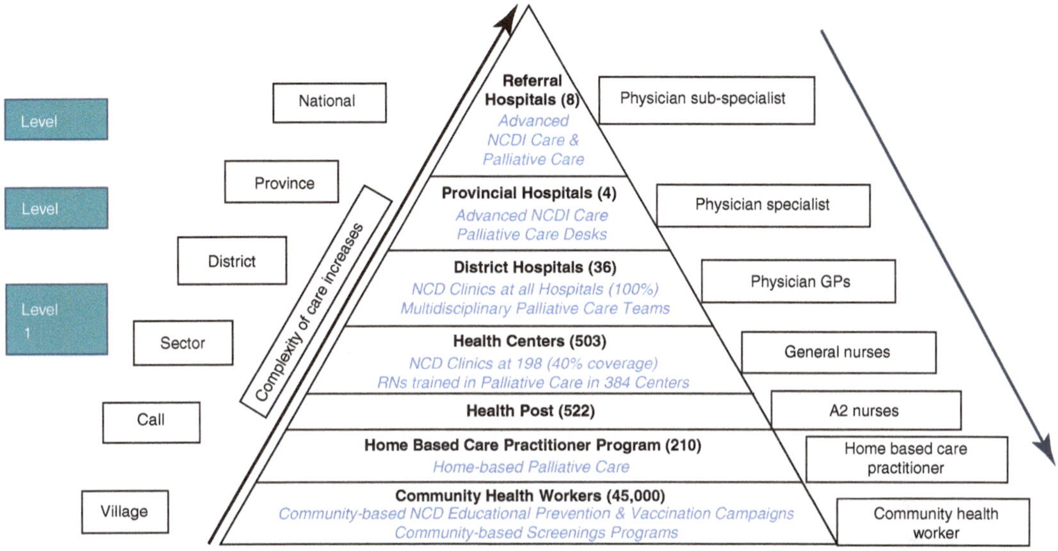

Fig. 5 Decentralized integration of the NCD model of care

chronic diseases. Figure 5 shows the NCD model in which palliative care is integrated at all levels of the public health system. It also shows the referral system and number of services available based on the complexity of care.

The Rwanda public health system has brought equity and social justice to all Rwandans via the classification of households by *Ubudehe*, an assignment of socioeconomic category that determines the level of patient cost for care according to income [66]. This policy brought equity to the population, along with satisfaction, responsibility, and sustainability. Those who are considered poor by the government receive 100% support in all health care services. The rest of the population pays 10% out-of-pocket, with 90% paid by the government through the *Mutuelle de Santé,* or Community-Based Health Insurance [67].

The decentralization of services has reduced unnecessary travel to referral health settings (district, provincial, and referral hospitals) for patients and families. The task-shifting system that empowers nurses and CHWs began in programs for HIV/AIDS, tuberculosis, malaria, and circumcision, with a positive response to services at the community level [68, 69]. The Rwandan government established an incentive program, Performance-Based Financing (PBF) [70], with clear indicators and a centralized reporting system. The PBF became a source of motivation for health care providers, improving clinical care as well as efficiency and productivity.

Future Trends in Rwanda

The Ministry of Health has prioritized the monitoring and evaluation of district-level NCD care and palliative care at the community level to understand the dynamics between the behavior of the population and diseases. The program of task shifting and capacity building in NCD treatment, including palliative care, at the district level will continue to expand local services, reaching the Rwandan population in every corner of the country. As the service package (NCD treatment along with palliative care) is well defined, full decentralization of NCD clinics to community Health Centers has become a priority for the government. For example, there could be a progressive decentralization through which expert district hospital staff will continue to mentor Health Center clinicians. The integration of palliative care services into NCD care highlights the holistic approach of the Ministry of Health to expand the HBCP program country-wide with the support of local and international partners. The government continues to collaborate with such partners to increase the number of trained health care professionals, strengthen the infrastructure for NCD interventions, as well as provide public awareness, prevention, and advocacy messages through educational campaigns and screening events.

Finally, existing palliative care services were adapted from models in the United States and the United Kingdom, which need to be customized for the post-genocide, culturally complex, rapidly developing society of Rwanda. It is imperative that African countries develop a model of care grounded in local context, socioeconomic burden, and cultural values.

References

1. Kübler-Ross E. On death and dying. New York: Macmillan; 1969.
2. Connor SR. Development of hospice and palliative care in the United States. Omega (Westport). 2007;56(1):89–99. https://doi.org/10.2190/om.56.1.h.
3. Anonymous. History of Hospice. NHPCO. Available via https://www.nhpco.org/hospice-care-overview/history-of-hospice/. Accessed 12 Feb 2020.
4. Anonymous. A controlled trial to improve care for seriously ill hospitalized patients. The study to understand prognoses and preferences for outcomes and risks of treatments (SUPPORT). The SUPPORT principal investigators. JAMA. 1995;274(20):1591–8.
5. von Gunten CF. Secondary and tertiary palliative care in US hospitals. JAMA. 2002;287(7):875–81. jel10002 [pii]
6. American Academy of Hospice and Palliative Medicine. Workforce Data and Reports. http://aahpm.org/career/workforce-study. Accessed 30 Jan 2020.
7. Lupu D, American Academy of Hospice and Palliative Medicine Workforce Task Force. Estimate of current hospice and palliative medicine physician workforce shortage. J Pain Symptom Manag. 2010;40(6):899–911. https://doi.org/10.1016/j.jpainsymman.2010.07.004.
8. Center to Advance Palliative Care. Growth of palliative care in U.S. hospitals: 2018 snapshot. 2019. Available via https://www.capc.org/mapping-community-palliative-care/. Accessed 20 Jan 2020.
9. TJC Palliative care certification. The Joint Commission. Available via https://www.jointcommission.org/en/accreditation-and-certification/certification/certifications-by-setting/hospital-certifications/palliative-care-certification/. Accessed 20 Jan 2020.
10. CAPC. Mapping community palliative care: a snapshot. Center to Advance Palliative Care; 2019.
11. TJC Certification options. Community-Based Palliative Care Certification. The Joint Commission. Available at https://www.jointcommission.org/accreditation-and-certification/certification/certifications-by-setting/hospital-certifications/palliative-care-certification/. Accessed 12 Feb 2020.
12. Parikh RB, Wright AA. The affordable care act and end-of-life care for patients with cancer. Cancer J. 2017;23(3):190–3. https://doi.org/10.1097/PPO.0000000000000264.
13. CMS. Report to the congress: medicare payment policy. Hospice services. Increase in total number of hospices driven by growth in for-profit providers. 2019. Available via http://www.medpac.gov/docs/default-source/reports/mar19_medpac_ch12_sec.pdf. Accessed 20 Jan 2020.
14. Fay M. Who pays for end of life care? debt.org. Available via https://www.debt.org/medical/hospice-costs/. Accessed 20 Jan 2020.
15. Avati A, Jung K, Harman S, et al. Improving palliative care with deep learning. BMC Med Inform Decis Mak. 2018;18(Suppl 4):122. https://doi.org/10.1186/s12911-018-0677-8.
16. Cross SH, Warraich HJ. Changes in the place of death in the United States. N Engl J Med. 2019;381(24):2369–70. https://doi.org/10.1056/NEJMc1911892.
17. Hiatt RA. New directions in cancer control and population sciences. Am Assoc Cancer Res. 2017;26:1165–9.
18. Temel JS, Greer JA, Muzikansky A, et al. Early palliative care for patients with metastatic non-small-cell lung cancer. N Engl J Med. 2010;363(8):733–42. https://doi.org/10.1056/NEJMoa1000678.
19. Hoerger M, Greer JA, Jackson VA, et al. Defining the elements of early palliative care that are associated with patient-reported outcomes and the delivery of end-of-life care. J Clin Oncol. 2018;36(11):1096–102. https://doi.org/10.1200/JCO.2017.75.6676.
20. Hui D. Palliative cancer care in the outpatient setting: which model works best? Curr Treat Options in Oncol. 2019;20(2):17–8. https://doi.org/10.1007/s11864-019-0615-8.
21. Committee for a Responsible Federal Budget. American health care: health spending and the federal budget. 2018. Available via https://www.crfb.org/sites/default/files/Health%20Care%20and%20the%20Federal%20Budget.pdf. Accessed 25 Aug 2020.
22. Anonymous Health Insurance Coverage in 2018. Current population survey. censusgov. Available via https://www.census.gov/data/tables/time-series/demo/income-poverty/cps-hi/hi.html. Accessed 22 Jan 2020.
23. Obama B. United States health care reform: progress to date and next steps. JAMA. 2016;316(5):525–32.
24. Tolbert J, Orgera K, Singer N, Damico A. Key facts about the uninsured population. 2019. kff.org. Available via https://www.kff.org/uninsured/issue-brief/key-facts-about-the-uninsured-population/. Accessed 15 Jan 2020.
25. Collins SR, Bhupal HK, Doty MM. Health insurance eight years after the ACA: fewer uninsured Americans

and shorter coverage gaps, But More Underinsured. 2019. Commonwealth Fund. Available via https://www.commonwealthfund.org/publications/issue-briefs/2019/feb/health-insurance-coverage-eight-years-after-aca. Accessed 25 Aug 2020.
26. Artiga S, Ubri P, Zur J. The effects of premiums and cost sharing on low-income populations: updated review of research findings. 2017. KFF (June 01, 2017). Available via https://www.kff.org/medicaid/issue-brief/the-effects-of-premiums-and-cost-sharing-on-low-income-populations-updated-review-of-research-findings/view/print/. Accessed 25 Aug 2020.
27. Siegel RL, Miller KD, Jemal A. Cancer statistics, 2018. CA Cancer J Clin. 2019;68(1):7–30. https://doi.org/10.3322/caac.21442.
28. American Cancer Society. Cancer treatment & survivorship facts & figures 2019–2021. 2019. Available via https://www.cancer.org/content/dam/cancer-org/research/cancer-facts-and-statistics/cancer-treatment-and-survivorship-facts-and-figures/cancer-treatment-and-survivorship-facts-and-figures-2019-2021.pdf. Accessed 25 Aug 2020.
29. Kirkwood MK. The state of cancer care in America, 2017: a report by the American Society of Clinical Oncology. Executive Summary. J Oncol Pract. 2016;13(6):256–60. https://doi.org/10.1200/JOP.2016.020743. Available via https://ascopubs.org/doi/pdfdirect/10.1200/JOP.2016.020743. Accessed 25 Aug 2020
30. Anonymous. NCI-Designated Cancer Centers. 2019. National Cancer Institute. Available via https://www.cancer.gov/research/nci-role/cancer-centers.
31. Anonymous. Treatment center directories and resources. 2020. American Cancer Society. Available via https://www.cancer.org/treatment/finding-and-paying-for-treatment/choosing-your-treatment-team/other-souces-of-information. Accessed 20 Jan 2020.
32. Temel JS, Shaw AT, Greer JA. Challenge of prognostic uncertainty in the modern era of cancer therapeutics. J Clin Oncol. 2016;34(30):3605–8. https://doi.org/10.1200/JCO.2016.67.8573.
33. Weeks JC, Catalano PJ, Cronin A, et al. Patients' expectations about effects of chemotherapy for advanced cancer. N Engl J Med. 2012;367(17):1616.
34. Yabroff KR, Gansler T, Wender RC, et al. Minimizing the burden of cancer in the United States: goals for a high-performing health care system. CA-A Cancer J Clin. 2019;69(3):166–83. https://doi.org/10.3322/caac.21556.
35. Bach P Center for health policy & outcomes: price & value of cancer drug | Memorial Sloan Kettering Cancer Center. mskcc.org. Available via https://www.mskcc.org/research-programs/health-policy-outcomes/cost-drugs. Accessed 14 Feb 2020.
36. Ramsey S, Blough D, Kirchhoff A, et al. Washington state cancer patients found to be at greater risk for bankruptcy than people without a cancer diagnosis. Health affairs (Project Hope). 2013;32:1143. https://doi.org/10.1377/hlthaff.2012.1263.
37. Altice CK, Banegas MP, Tucker-Seeley R, et al. Financial hardships experienced by Cancer survivors: a systematic review. J Natl Cancer Inst. 2017;109(2):djw205. . Available via https://www.ncbi.nlm.nih.gov/pmc/articles/PMC6075571/. Accessed 20 Jan 2020. https://doi.org/10.1093/inci/djw205.
38. Zafar SY. Financial toxicity of cancer care: it's time to intervene. JNCI-J Natl Cancer Inst. 2016;108(5):djv370. https://doi.org/10.1093/jnci/djv370.
39. Ganz P. Quality of care and cancer survivorship: the challenge of implementing the Institute of Medicine Recommendations. J Oncol Pract. 2009;5(3):101–5.
40. Chassin M. Health Care Issues Dominating the New Decade. 2019. jointcommission.org. Available via https://www.jointcommission.org/resources/news-and-multimedia/blogs/dateline-tjc/2019/12/Health Care Issues Dominating the New Decade. Accessed 15 Jan 2020.
41. Ferrell BR, Kravitz K. Cancer care: supporting underserved and financially burdened family caregivers. J Adv Pract Oncol. 2017;8(5):494–500.
42. van Ryn M, Sanders S, Khan K, et al. Objective burden, resources, and other stressors among informal cancer caregivers: a hidden quality issue? Psycho-Oncology. 2011;(1):44. https://doi.org/10.1002/pon.1703.
43. Wolff JL, Freedman VA, Mulcahy JF, et al. Family caregivers' experiences with health care workers in the care of older adults with activity limitations. JAMA Netw Open. 2020;3(1):e1919866. https://doi.org/10.1001/jamanetworkopen.2019.19866.
44. Schulz R, Beach S. Caregiving as a risk factor for mortality. JAMA. 1999;282(23):2215–9. Available via https://jamanetwork.com/journals/jama/fullarticle/192209. Accessed 20 Jan 2020
45. The Partnership for Solutions. Chronic conditions: making the case for ongoing care. 2004. In Family Caregiver Alliance (2016) Caregiver statistics: demographics. Available via https://www.caregiver.org/caregiver-statistics-demographics. Accessed 15 Dec 2020.
46. Farrell C. The shortage of home care workers: worse than you think. 2018. Forbes.com. Available via https://www.forbes.com/sites/nextavenue/2018/04/18/the-shortage-of-home-care-workers-worse-than-you-think/#1b8eb99c3ddd. Accessed 20 Jan 2020.
47. Berwick D, Nolan TWJ. The triple aim: care, health, and cost. Health Affairs (Millwood). 2008;27(3):759–69.
48. Anonymous. FY 2020 annual performance plan and report – goal 1 objective 1. 2019. Office of the Budget. HHS.gov. Available via https://www.hhs.gov/about/budget/fy2020/performance/performance-plan-goal-1-objective-1/index.html. Accessed 15 Dec 2020.
49. Casarett DJ, Fishman JM, Lu HL, et al. The terrible choice: re-evaluating hospice eligibility criteria for cancer. J Clin Oncol. 2008;27(6):953–9. https://doi.org/10.1200/JCO.2008.17.8079.

50. CMS. Medicare Care Choices Model. 2020. Center for Medicare & Medicaid Innovation. innovation.cms.gov. Available via https://innovation.cms.gov/initiatives/Medicare-Care-Choices/. Accessed 15 Jan 2020.
51. Valuck T MR. Innovation in serious illness care payment: progress to date and opportunities for the new administration. 2017. healthaffairs.org. Available via https://www.healthaffairs.org/do/10.1377/hblog20170308.059089/full/. Accessed 15 Jan 2020.
52. Haverhals LM, Manheim CE, Mor V, et al. The experience of providing hospice care concurrent with cancer treatment in the VA. Support Care Cancer. 2019;27(4):1263–70. https://doi.org/10.1007/s00520-018-4552-z.
53. Baquet-Simpson A, Spettell CM, Freeman AN, et al. Aetna's compassionate care program: sustained value for our members with advanced illness. J Palliat Med. 2019;22(11):1324–30. https://doi.org/10.1089/jpm.2018.0359.
54. Centers for Medicare & Medicaid Services. Medicare Value-Based Programs. 2020. Available via https://www.cms.gov/Medicare/Quality-Initiatives-Patient-Assessment-Instruments/Value-Based-Programs/Value-Based-Programs. Accessed 2 Feb 2020.
55. Engel EL. H.R.1676 – 115th congress (2017–2018): palliative care and hospice education and training act. 2018. congress.gov. Available via https://www.congress.gov/bill/115th-congress/house-bill/1676. Accessed 15 Jan 2020.
56. Myers RE, DiCarlo M, Romney M, et al. Using a health system learning community strategy to address cancer disparities. Learn Health Sys. 2018;2(4):1–7. https://doi.org/10.1002/lrh2.10067.
57. Anonymous. WHO | WHO Definition of Palliative Care. 2012. WHO. Available via https://www.who.int/cancer/palliative/definition/en/. Accessed 5 Jan 2020.
58. Ntizimira CR, Nkurikiyimfura JL, Mukeshimana O, et al. Palliative care in Africa: a global challenge. Ecancermedicalscience. 2014;8:493. https://doi.org/10.3332/ecancer.2014.493.
59. Binagwaho A, Farmer P, Nsanzimana S, Karema C, de Gasana M, Dieu N, et al. Rwanda 20 years on: investing in life. Lancet. 2014;384(9940):371–5. https://doi.org/10.1016/S0140-6736(14)60574-2.
60. Farmer PE, Nutt CT, Wagner CM, et al. Reduced premature mortality in Rwanda: lessons from success. BMJ Brit Med J. 2013;346(jan18 1):f65. https://doi.org/10.1136/bmj.f65.
61. Lu C, Mejía-Guevara I, Hill K, et al. Community-based health financing and child stunting in rural Rwanda. Am J Public Health. 2016;106(1):49–55. https://doi.org/10.2105/AJPH.2015.302913.
62. Lande A. Single convention on narcotic drugs, 1961, as amended by the 1972 protocol amending the single convention on narcotic drugs, 1961. New York: United Nations; 1977.
63. Knaul FM, Farmer PE, Krakauer EL, et al. Alleviating the access abyss in palliative care and pain relief—an imperative of universal health coverage: the lancet commission report. Lancet. 2018;391(10128):1391–454. https://doi.org/10.1016/S0140-6736(17)32513-8.
64. Connor SW, Sepulveda Bermedo MC, editors. Global atlas of palliative care at the end of life. 2014. Worldwide Palliative Care Alliance, World Health Organization. Available via https://www.who.int/nmh/Global_Atlas_of_Palliative_Care.pdf. Accessed 25 Aug 2020.
65. Mugeni C, Levine AC, Munyaneza RM, et al. Nationwide implementation of integrated community case management of childhood illness in Rwanda. Global Health Sci Pract. 2014;2(3):328–41. https://doi.org/10.9745/GHSP-D-14-00080.
66. Mitsunaga T, Mitsunaga T, Hedt-Gauthier B, et al. Data for program management: an accuracy assessment of data collected in household registers by community health Workers in Southern Kayonza, Rwanda. J Community Health. 2015;40(4):625–32. https://doi.org/10.1007/s10900-014-9977-9.
67. Rubagumya F, Costas-Chavarri A, Manirakiza A, Murenzi G, Uwinkindi F, Ntizimira C, et al. State of cancer control in Rwanda: past, present, and future opportunities. JCO Global Oncol. 2020;6:1171–7. https://doi.org/10.1200/GO.20.0028.
68. Hedt-Gauthier B, Amoroso C, Warugaba C, et al. Building equity in the global health research agenda: the partners in Health-Harvard Medical School research partnership in Rwanda. Ann Glob Health. 2015;81(1):151–2. https://doi.org/10.1016/j.aogh.2015.02.848.
69. Krakauer EL, Muhimpundu M, Mukasahaha D, et al. Palliative care in Rwanda: aiming for universal access. J Pain Symptom Manag. 2018;55(2):S77–80. https://doi.org/10.1016/j.jpainsymman.2017.03.037.
70. Klapwijk CJ, Bucagu C, van Wijk MT, et al. The 'one cow per poor family' programme: current and potential fodder availability within smallholder farming systems in southwest Rwanda. Agric Syst. 2014;131:11–22. https://doi.org/10.1016/j.agsy.2014.07.005.

Part XVII

West Africa: Cameroon

Palliative Care for Cancer Patients in Rural Central Africa: Experiences from Cameroon

Dina Bell Esther Hortense Murielle
and Catherine D'Souza

Introduction

Like most low-income countries, Cameroon is going through an epidemiological transitional period with the emergence of non-communicable diseases such as cancer. Providing early and quality palliative care for cancer patients improves the quality of life and overall survival [1]. With approximately 15,769 new cases of cancer per year, and an estimated number of deaths of 10,533 per year [2] (a lethality rate of 66.8%), cancer prognosis in Cameroon is still very poor; this is despite the availability of five medical oncology services and one radiotherapy service in referential hospitals. Living daily with cancer therefore constitutes a source of stress and chronic suffering for both patients and their families, due to: (i) the severe pain present in approximately 80% at advanced stage [3] (which sometimes cannot be handled due to the unavailability of strong opioids), (ii) deterioration of the physical aspect that may result from the disease or cancer treatments, and (iii) financial difficulties which arise from the expensive cost of treatments (chemotherapy, targeted therapies, radiotherapy and surgery) which are paid by patients and their families. Considering these observations, palliative care should be a priority for cancer patients in Cameroon.

D. B. Esther Hortense Murielle (✉)
Bonassama District Hospital,
Douala, Littoral, Cameroon

C. D'Souza
South Canterbury Hospice and District Health Board,
Timaru, New Zealand

Cameroon Baptist Convention and Hospice Africa,
Bamenda, Cameroon

The Story of Palliative Care in Cameroon

Cameroon is a country in Central Africa in the Gulf of Guinea, with an area of 475,442 km^2; it shares borders in the west with Nigeria, in the northeast with Chad, in the east with the Central African Republic and in the south with Congo, Gabon and Equatorial Guinea (Fig. 1). In the southwest, the country's coastline lies on the Atlantic Ocean. Cameroon is subdivided into ten regions; Yaoundé is the political capital and Douala is the economic capital. Cameroon is bilingual; English and French are spoken by 30% and 70% of Cameroonians, respectively [4].

The palliative care movement in Cameroon began in 2002 in the northwest region by Cameroon Baptist Convention Health Services (CBCHS). They were sensitized to the importance of setting up a palliative care program by Hospice Africa Uganda (HAU). Under the direction of Dr Jonah Wefuan, a physician and rheumatologist, and Mr Georges Ndinkintum Mbeng, a graduate of palliative care from HAU and the University of Makéréré, and with the support of the African Palliative Care Association (APCA),

M. Silbermann (ed.), *Palliative Care for Chronic Cancer Patients in the Community*,
https://doi.org/10.1007/978-3-030-54526-0_26

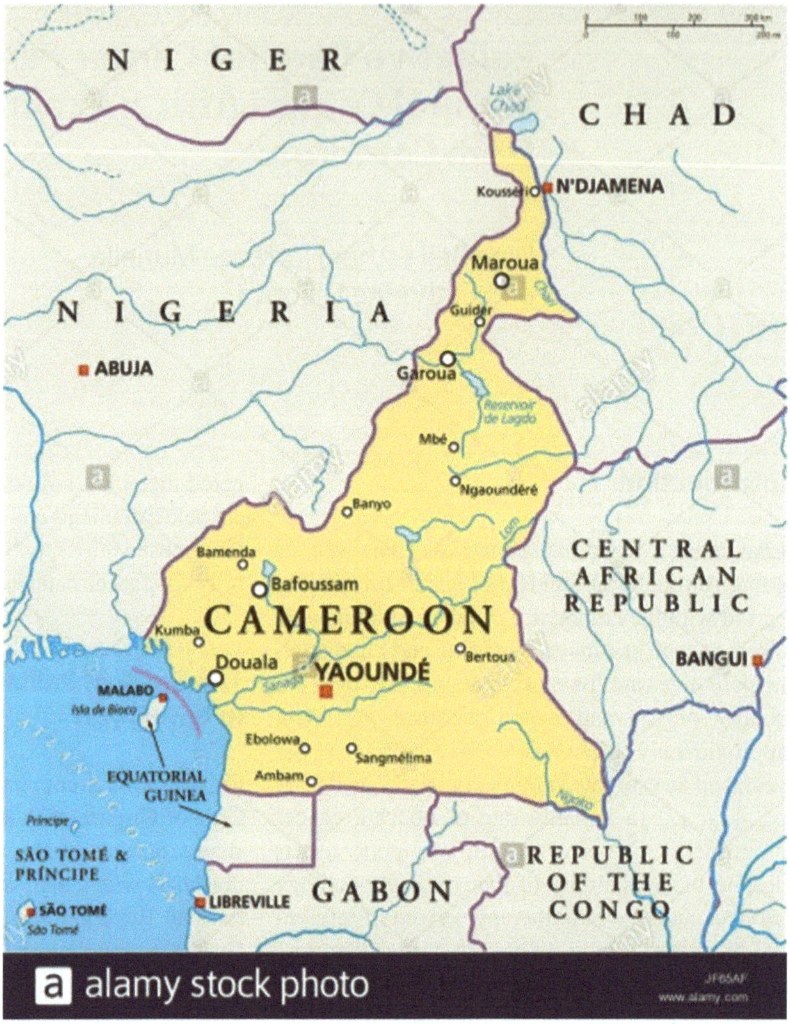

Fig. 1 Map of Cameroon [5]

Uganda, our national association named Hospice and Palliative Care Association of Cameroon (HPCAC) was created in 2009. In addition, strong advocates for improved access to morphine include doctors such as Paul Ndom, Jacqueline Ze Mikandè, Albert Mouelle Sone, Yomi Jean, Essomba Biwole Martin, Ekortarh Anncomy, Gérard Beyiha and Doh Anderson, as well as some civil society organizations such as Palliativos Sin Fronteras.

The first production of oral morphine solution was started in 2006 by CBCHS with the support of Dr Richard Fondoh, pharmacist and administrator of the Regional Funds for Health Promotion in the northwest region. A laboratory dedicated for this purpose was opened by CBCHS to produce and ensure the distribution of morphine oral solution in all their health centers. Unfortunately, only a few regions were supplied and, therefore, access to morphine remained difficult for cancer patients living in other regions of Cameroon.

In 2012, the first Francophone Palliative Care initiator's course was organized by Dr Catherine D'Souza and Supported by Hospice Africa Uganda and Hospice Africa France, in collaboration with the Cameroon Baptist Convention and HPCAC. Seven Cameroonians participated. After this training course, the development of palliative care took off in Cameroon. However, initiatives to develop palliative care in Cameroon remained the prerogative of some trained professionals, confessional or private hospitals, and civil society organizations (Palliativos Sin Fronteras, HPCAC, Santo Domingo SEG, Integrated Development Foundation and Volunteers for Palliative Care).

Cancer Statistics in Douala, Littoral Region, and the Need for Palliative Care in Cameroon

In order to contribute to the advocacy for the establishment of a palliative care community-based program, we needed data to convince decision-makers. To achieve this goal, we carried out a retrospective study from January 1 to December 31, 2013, in the medical oncology consultation unit of the Douala General Hospital, the first reference and cancer management center in the Littoral region. From the 376 clinical files of new cases of cancer received in consultation during the study period, socio-demographic, pathological, clinical (type of cancer, stage), therapeutic (therapeutic compliance, reasons for abandonment) and evolution (living, deceased, lost to follow-up) data were collected and analyzed. This work allowed us to make the following observations: the young population, particularly those whose age ranged from 31 to 45 years (34%), were the most affected by cancer as presented in Fig. 2 in the Appendix. The majority were women (66.27%) and breast and cervical cancers were the most prominent: 28.45% and 12.76%, respectively (see Fig. 3 in the Appendix). Approximately 48.4% of the patients were unemployed and therefore unable to assume the charges for cancer care. Ninety-five percent of the patients were received at an advanced stage (either generalization stage of cancer, or at the loco regional stage). The dropout rate among those who started was 35.38%, mostly due to financial reasons. As of December 31, 2013, 40% of patients were lost to follow-up, 11% died and 49% continued their medical follow-up. What had become of these patients, most of whom were lost to follow-up, at an advanced stage of the disease and jobless? The majority surely returned home or to their village and died without assistance and in severe pain. Following this study, it was clear that there was a need to set up a multidisciplinary palliative care team qualified to offer holistic management, to guarantee the uninterrupted availability of level III analgesics at affordable costs, to initiate a home-visit program for cancer patients and to disseminate palliative culture in order to extend the offer of palliative care in all regions of Cameroon.

In an advocacy process, assessing the need for palliative care is an essential aspect. In Cameroon, we can estimate the number of cancer patients in the general population needing palliative care based on the formula developed by Dr Anne Merriman, Emeritus Professor of Palliative Medicine. "This is based on the incidence of cancer in African countries before Independence, which was estimated at 0.1%. AIDS and other viral diseases have doubled this incidence to 2% and prevalence will include those cancer patients surviving from previous years, adding 1%. As palliative care is needed from the time of diagnosis of a life-limiting illness, it should be started immediately but, of course, many are unknown in communities. The prevalence for cancer alone in the population is 0.3%" [6]. Cameroon has a population of 24,348,251 inhabitants, and using this Merriman formula, the expected need for palliative care among cancer patients is $(24{,}348{,}251/100) \times (0.3) = 73{,}045$.

Advocacy for Oral Morphine at Douala General Hospital and the Beginning of a Home-Based Visit Program at Bonassama District Hospital

According to Benoît Burucoa, President of the FISP (Fédération Francophone Internationale de Soins Palliatifs), building a palliative home first requires four essential pillars: (i) the basic training in palliative care essential to practice it; (ii) practical training as an additional internship for future palliative care reference; (iii) an essential drug program, including the delivery of oral morphine solution; and (iv) a structural and funded program for palliative care (home visits, dedicated beds, mobile team, hospital unit, etc.). In order to offer palliative care to cancer patients followed at the General Hospital of Douala, it was first necessary to set up a unit for the production of oral solution of morphine to guarantee the management of severe pain. In 2014, the pharmacy department of the Douala General Hospital started producing oral solution of morphine dosed at 5 mg/5 ml, and thus made it possible to alleviate pain.

With the large number of patients lost to follow-up and discontinuation of treatment (in the majority of cancer patients for financial reasons), we chose to set up a home-based visit palliative care program in a district hospital (closer to the community and offering affordable health care). The idea was to follow patients at home with good psychosocial and spiritual support and, if needed, to receive oral morphine from the Douala General Hospital at a lower cost and other essential medicines from district hospitals.

Here, we present a summary of our activities serving cancer patients in the community during the past 28 months. In these 28 months, we have made 53 outings during which 273 homes were visited (see Table 1 in the Appendix). The average number of homes visited per month was 9.75. During this period, 146 cancer patients were enrolled in the home-visiting program, and the average age of our patients was 50.63 years with extremes from 10 to 85 years. The influence of three outlying variables (patients 85, 83 and 80 years old) explains the higher average age from the ones observed in the black African population by other authors [7]. Sixty-five percent of the patients resided in the suburbs of the city of Douala. The management of severe pain and other symptoms, coupled with psychological support, was the most frequent reason for intervention in patients' homes (33.56% of cases). Pain management alone represented 59.60% of the reasons for intervention in patients' homes, as presented in Table 2 in the Appendix, and was followed by the need for psychological support which was found in 58.90% of families. Breast (33.6%), cervical (8.3%) and prostate (6.3%) cancers were the most common (see Table 3 in the Appendix). This distribution is similar to the Yaoundé cancer registry [7]. The majority of patients were at the advanced stage of the disease (60% at stage IV, 37% at stage III and 3% at stage II).

This home-visit program, which has improved the quality of life for most of our patients, has not been without its challenges. Home visits were scheduled once a week (every Friday); however, these were sometimes canceled due to the unavailability of a patient or legal guardian, an exceptional calendar conflict with a hospital activity or the unavailability of the palliative care worker in charge for the day. The team used public transport to get to the patients' homes (taxi, motorbike taxi and, at times on, foot). At the beginnings of the program, the significant psychological distress of some team members required psychological support for the whole staff. This psychological care gave a new dynamic to the team to continue alleviating pain and suffering.

Extension of Palliative Care to Other Health Facilities in the Littoral Region

From the model developed at the Bonassama District Hospital, which made palliative care accessible to all strata of the population but had the geographical limitation of not reaching all patients in the Littoral region, we established a project to gradually extend palliative care to other district hospitals in this region. The project received the support of Dr Jean Dissongo, Regional Delegate for Public Health for the Littoral region, and was funded by The True Color Trust through the African Palliative Care Association. The project had three main objectives:

- Train at least two health professionals in palliative care in each of the 24 district hospitals of the Littoral region,
- Create palliative care units or mobile teams in these district hospitals and
- Disseminate palliative culture through the production of an awareness documentary film.

The Esop-Fosal project started in February 2018 with a 5-day training course in palliative care for health professionals (doctors and nurses). Among the 72 health professionals in attendance, 60 have been trained. Eight health facilities were able to start palliative care activities with mobile teams, and a palliative care unit was created at the Nkongsamba Regional Hospital as well as the Bonassama District Hospital. Hospitals that successfully completed the first phase of the project received quarterly technical support. A palliative care awareness film was produced and broadcasted on YouTube. Another home-visit program was then initiated by the Nkongsamba Regional Hospital, allowing palliative care to be offered in the department of Moungo.

Integrating a palliative care service in public hospitals is a challenge that can be taken on at the operational level to guarantee access to quality care for both patients and their families, in addition to end-of-life support, painlessly and with dignity. Through the Esop-Fosal model, the Littoral region has chosen a progressive and safe integrative approach for better care of cancer patients. A similar initiative has been successful in the West Cameroon region under the leadership of the Bafoussam Regional Hospital.

Conclusion

Palliative care for cancer patients is available in Cameroon and present in at least eight out of ten regions; it remains at its embryonic stage because it does not cover a large geographical area. The reverse sequence approach (decentralized services toward the top of the health pyramid) is the one by which palliative care makes its way into Cameroon. It is, therefore, important to continue advocating with relevant authorities for the uninterrupted availability of morphine to manage severe chronic pain, which is a fundamental human right. Palliative care should be integrated at all levels of the health pyramid, with a clear definition of the minimum package of palliative care services that each health facility is able to provide.

Acknowledgements *To palliative care advocates in Cameroon*

- Pr Anne Merriman
- Pr Paul Ndom
- Hospice Africa Uganda/France
- African Palliative Care Association
- Douala General Hospital palliative care team
- Volunteers For Palliative Care – Cameroon
- Esop-Fosal Project
- Bonassama District Hospital
- Hospice and Palliative Care Association of Cameroon
- ACA 2
- Palliativos Sin Fronteras
- Santo Domingo – Seg
- Bafoussam Regional Hospital
- Nkongsamba and Edéa Regional Hospitals
- Littoral Regional Delegation for Public Health
- Northwest Regional funds for health promotion
- Cameroon Baptist Convention
- The National Cancer Control Committee team
- Laquintinie Hospital
- Yaoundé General Hospital
- Faculty of Medicine and Pharmaceutical Sciences – Douala
- Faculty of Medicine and Biomedical Sciences – Yaoundé
- Adventist University Cosendai
- Chimissions
- Integrated Development Foundation
- Norwegian Hospital Ngaoundéré
- Faculty of Health Sciences-Buéa
- Cameroonians Palliative care providers

Appendix

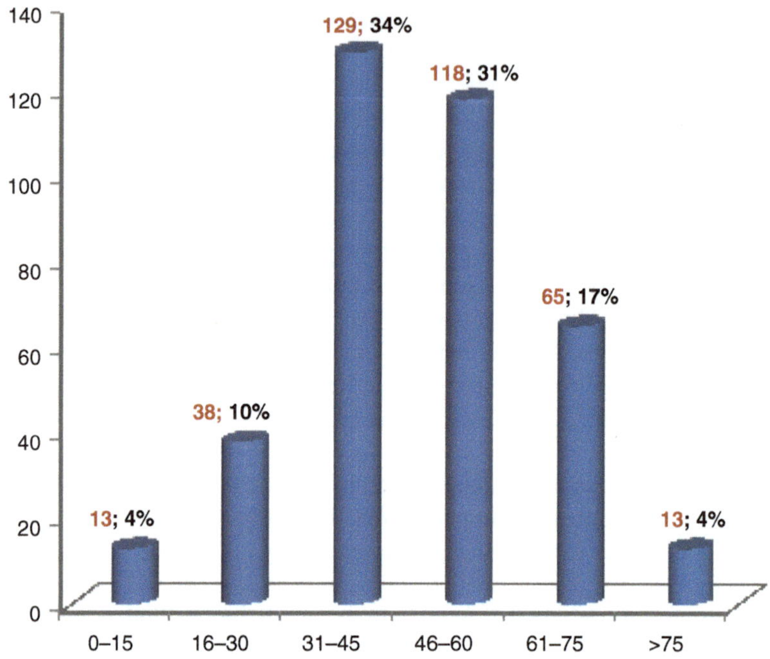

Fig. 2 Distribution of new cancer cases, by age groups. (Douala General Hospital, 2013) (Average age: 46 years ±15.97, Extremes: 2–86 years)

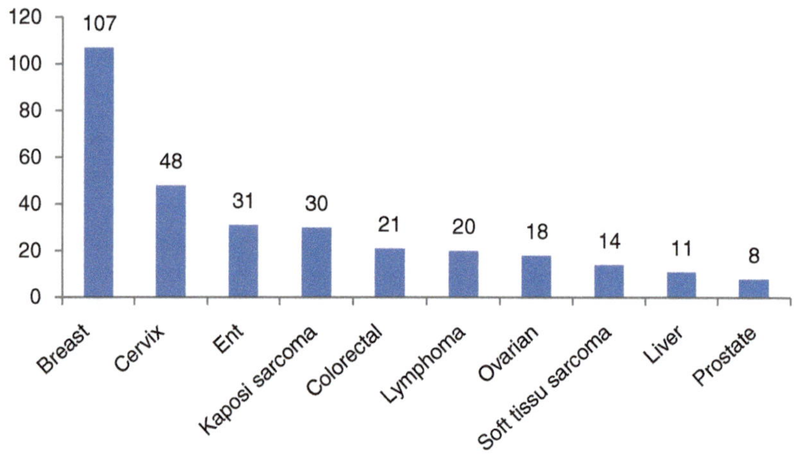

Fig. 3 The ten most prominent types of new cancer cases, listed by frequency. (Douala General Hospital, 2013)

Table 1 Monthly activity indicators of the Bonassama District Hospital Home-Visit Program, Douala Cameroon (August 2017 to December 2019)

Year	2017		2018		2019	
Month	Number of visited homes	Number of outings	Number of visited homes	Number of outings	Number of visited homes	Number of outings
January			15	3	18	3
February			11	2	11	2
March			10	2	6	1
April			5	1	11	2
May			13	3	9	2
June			11	2	8	2
July			8	2	5	1
August	6	1	5	1	6	1
September	12	2	17	3	13	3
October	12	2	7	2	5	1
November	10	2	11	1	11	2
December	15	3			5	1
Total	*55*	*10*	*113*	*22*	*108*	*21*

Table 2 Reasons for intervention (August 2017 to December 2019, Douala Cameroon)

Reasons for home visit	Effective	%
Pain + other symptoms management + psychological support	49	33.56
Symptoms management	25	17.12
Pain management + psychological support	21	14.39
Psychological support	16	10.95
Pain management	15	10.27
End of life care	13	8.9
Symptoms management + psychosocial support	3	2
Pain management + psychosocial support	2	1.36
Psychosocial support	2	1.36
Total	146	99.91

Table 3 Patient home visits according to the type of cancer (August 2017 to December 2019, Douala Cameroon)

Type of cancer	Effective	Percentage
Breast	49	33.6
Cervix	12	8.3
Prostate	9	6.3
Colorectal	8	5.5
Soft tissue sarcoma	7	4.86
Lymphoma	6	4.1
Cutaneous	5	3.42
Hepatocellular carcinoma	5	3.42
Ovarian	5	3.42
Vulvar	5	3.42
Lung	4	2.74
Cavum	3	2
Kaposi	3	2
Kidney	3	2
Oesophagus	3	2
Stomach	3	2
Anal	2	1.37
Brain	2	1.37
Osteosarcoma	2	1.37
Pancreas	2	1.37
Carcinoma of unknown origin	1	0.68
Gallbladder	1	0.68
Germ cell	1	0.68
Leukemia	1	0.68
Multiple myeloma	1	0.68
Salivary glands	1	0.68
Adrenal gland	1	0.68
Tongue	1	0.68
Total	146	100

References

1. Ambroggi M, Biasini C, Toscani I, et al. Can early palliative care with anticancer treatment improve overall survival and patient-related outcomes in advanced lung cancer patients? A review of the literature. Support Care Cancer. 2018;26(9):2945–53.
2. International Agency for Research in Cancer. (consulted on 01/20/2020). Cameroon (online). http://gco.iarc.fr/today/data/factsheets/populations/120-cameroon-fact-sheets.pdf.
3. Ovayolu Ö, Ovayolu N, Aytaç S, Serçe S, Sevinc A. Pain in cancer patients: pain assessment by patients and family caregivers and problems experienced by caregivers. Support Care Cancer. 2015;23(7):1857–64.
4. Plan National de dévelloppement sanitaire 2016-2020. (consulted on 01/28/2020). Ministry of Public Health (online). https://www.minsante.cm/site/?q=fr/content/plan-national-de-d%C3%A9veloppement-sanitaire-pnds-2016-2020.
5. Alamy. (consulted on 01/21/2020). Carte (online). https://www.alamyimages.fr/photo-image-l-afrique-l-amerique-centrale-cameroun-carte-atlas-carte-du-monde-voyage-afrique-147038711.html
6. Merriman A, Mwebesa E, Zirimenya L. Improving access to palliative care for patients with cancer in Africa: 25 years of Hospice Africa. Ecancermedicalscience. 2019;13:946. Available on https://doi.org/10.3332/ecancer.2019.946.
7. Enow Orock GE, Ndom P, Doh AS. Current cancer incidence and trends in Yaounde, Cameroon. Oncol Gastroenterol Hepatol Rep. 2012;1(1):58–63.

Part XVIII

Middle East: Cyprus

Collaboration Between Palliative Care and Oncology Services and Global Models of Integration

Haris Charalambous, Kyriakos Stylianides, and Sophia Nestoros

Introduction

According to the World Health Organization (WHO), palliative care (PC) aims to "improve the quality of life of patients and families who face life-threatening illness, through the prevention and relief of suffering by means of early identification and impeccable assessment and treatment of pain and other problems, physical, psychosocial and spiritual". Furthermore, the WHO recommends that PC becomes an integral part of health care for all patients affected by a life-threatening disease and that these patients should have access to PC services [1]. This statement is further supported by the European Association of Palliative Care [2] and is also in agreement with the guidelines of the European Council toward the European Union (EU) Member States [3]. Furthermore, evidence has been accumulating about the benefit of integrating PC within standard oncological care for patients with advanced or metastatic cancer resulting in improvement of patients' quality of life, decreased rates of depression, illness understanding, patient's satisfaction and even survival [4–7].

Progress and Limitations of the Service We Provide to Our Patients

Great progress has been achieved in both oncology and palliative care (PC) in the last 20 years. In oncology, we have witnessed the establishment of multidisciplinary teams and meetings, centralization of care and new radiotherapy (RT) techniques: intensity-modulated RT, image-guided RT and stereotactic RT, and the revolution of molecular biology, with the emergence of targeted therapy and immunotherapy with the use of checkpoint inhibitors [8]. In PC, essentially a new specialty was set up in many countries worldwide with major steps made in capacity building leading up to integration in a few countries [8–10]. Furthermore, there has been a recognition of the important role of PC in the palliation of patients with advanced illness, while more recently evidence for the earlier integration of PC in the disease trajectory has been adopted by major oncology organizations, including the American Society of Clinical Oncology (ASCO) and the European Society of Medical Oncology (ESMO) [11, 12].

H. Charalambous (✉)
Bank of Cyprus Oncology Center, Nicosia, Cyprus
e-mail: haris.charalambous@bococ.org.cy

K. Stylianides
Cyprus Association of Cancer Patients and Friends (PASYKAF), and Supportive Care Unit Bank of Cyprus Oncology Center, Nicosia, Cyprus
e-mail: kyriakos@pasykaf.org

S. Nestoros
Cyprus Anti-Cancer Society, Nicosia, Cyprus
e-mail: sophia.nestoros@anticancersociety.org.cy

M. Silbermann (ed.), *Palliative Care for Chronic Cancer Patients in the Community*,
https://doi.org/10.1007/978-3-030-54526-0_27

For oncology providers, it is sobering to reflect that in this process of exciting molecular biology and technological achievements, the American Society of Clinical Oncology in a statement titled "Toward individualized care for patients with advanced cancer" recognized that oncology care has become synonymous with disease-directed care, often without realistic conversations about prognosis, the potential benefits and limitations of disease-directed therapy and the potential role of PC, while often neglecting to address physical, psychological and spiritual consequences of disease and its treatment [13].

For palliative care (PC) providers, there is still the challenge to convince oncology providers, health care planners and stakeholders of the potential benefit of PC and the significant problems of a limited trained workforce and limited resources dedicated to PC Services. Finally, while steps are being made toward capacity building, this is not close to meeting potential demand for these services, and this is especially a problem in developing countries [14].

Symptom Control and Basic Palliative Care (PC) Skills of Oncologists and Referral Patterns to Palliative Care (PC)

Basic PC is provided by oncologists or primary care physicians addressing basic pain and symptom management, basic management of depression and anxiety, and basic discussion about goals, prognosis and suffering [15]. Specialist palliative care (SPC) is provided by a multidisciplinary PC team, that is, health care professionals with expertise in PC, and who are exclusively occupied in providing PC, dealing with management of refractory pain and other symptoms, complex depression, anxiety, grief and existential distress, and assistance with conflict resolution and in addressing futility issues [15].

Studies looking at the attitudes and knowledge of oncologists regarding symptom control management and providing basic palliative care suggest an obvious gap in knowledge and skills of oncologists in PC [16–21]. Two studies from the USA by Breuer [16] and Fisch [17] highlighted that US medical oncologists still lack the essential experience to provide good symptom control to the most basic of physical symptoms, that of pain. Furthermore, medical oncologists rated their specialty highly for the ability to manage cancer pain but rated their peers lower than themselves, while in response to two vignettes describing challenging clinical scenarios, 60% and 87%, respectively, endorsed treatment decisions that would be considered unacceptable by pain specialists [16]. Yet despite this suboptimal cancer pain management knowledge, frequent referrals to pain or palliative care specialists were reported by only 14% and 16%, respectively [16].

Equally, the European Society of Medical Oncology (ESMO) survey identified a major discrepancy between what we as oncologists think we know or do, and what we actually know or do [18]. For instance, while 88% of European medical oncologists felt that they should co-ordinate the care of their patients for all stages of disease including end-of-life care, only 43% did so, with only 39% commonly meeting with families of dying patients and only 11.8% managing delirium (despite this being a very common symptom in patients with advanced cancer). Furthermore, while over 60% of respondents claimed to be experts in the management of physical and psychological symptoms of patients with advanced cancer, only 37% reported that most oncologists they know shared similar expertise.

The problem may be even worse in recognizing and managing psychological or spiritual/existential distress symptoms. A similar survey of medical oncologists from Australia by Ward et al. [19] found that 92% oncologists felt confident in the management of physical symptoms, compared to only 61.7% for psychological symptoms and 53.9% for existential distress, while in the ESMO survey, respondents were involved more commonly in treating physical symptoms, such as pain (93%), fatigue (84%) and nausea/emesis (84%), than in managing psychological symptoms such as depression/anxiety (65%) and existential distress (29%). Finally, in a Canadian survey by Wendtland [20] and another Australian survey by Johnson [21], oncologists/cancer specialists were less likely to refer for psychosocial or spiritual problems, despite this being a domain that oncologists may have less expertise in.

The explanation for not referring for psychosocial or spiritual issues may relate to lack of experience in dealing with psychosocial problems along with lack of awareness about the potential of PC and multidisciplinary input to deal with these symptoms. It has been suggested that this results in "learned helplessness" and a misconception that nothing can be done about these issues [22]. On the contrary, previous experience of PC training or positive relationship/satisfaction with PC correlates with earlier referral to PC as shown in the Canadian survey by Wendtland [20].

Overall, in terms of oncologists' PC skills, in the Canadian survey by Wendtland [20], only 42% of physicians felt comfortable to provide PC to their patients, while 58% felt the need for additional training. In the ESMO survey [18], 42% of respondents felt that they had not received adequate training in PC during their training, while in the Australian studies by Ward [19], this was 26.1% and in the Johnson study 28% [21].

Relationship of Oncology and PC Services and Barriers to Referral to PC

There are many different settings and differences worldwide, in terms of the relationship of the two specialties, that may have a significant impact as to the way the two specialties collaborate, interact and work together. For instance, if both services are based in the same locality or have the same employer, if there are regular meetings and discussion of patients between specialists of both disciplines or if there is presence of palliative care physicians in the hospital or cancer center, these are important factors resulting in a better relationship, collaboration and referral patterns to PC. To the contrary, if services are run completely parallel, with little contact between the two specialties, then patients are traditionally moved from oncology care to palliative care for end-of-life care or perhaps may never be referred to palliative care, not even for end-of-life care. There may be other issues that have an impact on the collaboration and referral patterns between the two disciplines relating to availability of PC services and PC capacity. In cases where this PC availability is very limited, this makes collaboration very difficult.

Finally, it is important to consider that the collaboration and referral patterns to PC are influenced by significant barriers that are still present even today, including both patients' and oncologists' negative attitudes toward PC. In a recent European survey of lung cancer oncologists, up to 22% held negative attitudes regarding PC [23], and this was similar to the ESMO survey carried out 10 years earlier [18]. In terms of patient attitudes, even in countries with established PC, surveys of oncologists by Ward and Wendtland [19, 20] show that the biggest barrier for referral related to negative attitudes of patients to PC. This is thought to relate to "the misconception that PC is only for patients at the end-of-life and the death-defying mentality in our society" [24].

How to Improve Collaboration Between Oncology and PC Services

Both disciplines serve patients with advanced or metastatic cancer. In the paragraphs above, we outlined some limitations of standard oncology care, focusing on disease-directed therapy and some evidence from surveys of oncologists suggesting that there are deficiencies in providing basic PC to patients with advanced or metastatic cancer, and the finding that oncologists require more training in PC. Where oncology focuses on disease-directed care, PC focuses instead on patient's symptoms and quality of life, and evidence from randomized trials suggests that the approach that combines both specialties affords the best outcomes to patients with advanced cancer [11]. Within this context, it is even more important that oncology and PC providers collaborate to provide a more holistic care to patients with advanced incurable cancer. This can help to address issues like lack of time for oncologists to deal with patients' symptoms, lack of access to a multidisciplinary team especially useful for psychosocial and existential problems, lack of routine symptom scoring leading to underdiagnosis and undertreatment of patients' symptoms and, finally, lack of PC training. Furthermore, this collaboration, by bringing the two disciplines closer, can also work toward changing attitudes and eliminating barriers of referral to PC. We shall illustrate how collaboration can be improved between oncology and palliative care services, using the example of our own country, Cyprus, as was reported in previous publications [8, 25–27].

Cyprus is a small island in the Eastern Mediterranean with less than 1 million inhabitants. PC services are essentially provided by two non-governmental organizations (NGOs). The Cyprus Anticancer Society set up the Arodafnousa hospice and a home care team in 1976, while in 1986, PASYKAF (Pancyprian Association of Cancer Patients and Friends) set up a home care service for cancer patients. In the past, and up until 10 years ago, there was little collaboration between the PC and oncology teams. There were essentially only two PC physicians for a population of just under 1 million, and they both worked for one of the NGOs. They were based at the hospice, with no presence in either the main hospitals or the main oncology center in Cyprus [8, 26, 27]. Furthermore, in Cyprus the predominant oncology practice used to be of disease-directed therapy very much until the end of life, and then referral to the hospice for end-of-life care, hence making PC synonymous with end-of-life care. As a result, patients and families used to refuse to go to the hospice, as this was considered to be the place "where you go to die" [24–27].

How did change come about? About 10 years ago in 2010–2011, following a number of PC training courses organized by the Middle East Cancer Consortium (MECC) [25] and a course run by the Institute of Palliative Medicine from San Diego involving both PC and oncology staff, it was realized that there was a need for more collaboration between the oncology and PC providers and need for increased PC input within the main tertiary oncology center in Cyprus [26, 27]. As a result, a number of initiatives were set up:

- Firstly, a weekly specialist PC clinic was set up at the Oncology Center run by the two PC physicians, allowing for the referral of patients with difficult-to-control symptoms [8, 26, 27].
- On the day of the weekly PC clinic, the PC physician would also attend the daily ward-round in the Oncology Center, helping both with symptom control issues and also facilitating the referral of patients to the hospice [8, 26, 27].

How to Improve Collaboration Between PC and Onc Providers?

- Aim to bring the two specialties together
- Organize training courses to be attended by both specialties
- Provide increased presence of PC physicians within cancer center/hospital:
  - Regular (weekly) PC clinics in the cancer center/hospital
  - Review of ward patients by PC physician
- Set up weekly multi-disciplinary meeting jointly attended by both specialties
- Aim for joint audit/research projects and publications

- Joint training initiatives including weekly lectures for both oncology and PC staff were organized at the Oncology Center, while a residential communication skills course for staff from both oncology and PC was organized with the team of Professor Leslie Fallowfield from the UK [25–27].
- A daily supportive care/PC unit/drop-in center was set up at the Oncology Center to address urgent symptom control problems for cancer patients [26, 27].
- A weekly multidisciplinary team meeting involving both oncology and PC professionals (an oncologist, PC nurses, physicians training in PC, oncology nurses, pharmacists, psychologists and a Christian Orthodox priest) was set up at the Oncology Center [25–27].
- Finally, there have been a number of joint publications between oncologists and PC physicians [24–27], while an early PC intervention trial is being planned.

Following the success of these initiatives, encouraging earlier introduction of PC in patients with advanced or metastatic cancer, in 2012, the Board of the Oncology Center decided to fund the training of two physicians from the Oncology Center to receive post-graduate/specialist training in PC in the USA [8, 26, 27]. This was followed by both NGOs deciding to employ one additional physician each and train them within the same program in the USA. While one of the physicians from one of the NGOs subsequently dropped out of the training, the result of this initiative was to have three extra physicians with an interest in PC in Cyprus [8, 26, 27].

All the above initiatives resulted in a more comprehensive multidisciplinary care, by earlier involvement of the appropriate members of the multidisciplinary team in order to meet the complex needs of patients with advanced cancer and to improve collaboration and communication among the oncology and PC community and hospice teams [8, 26, 27]. As a result of the various initiatives in Cyprus, there has been a gradual change in terms of attitudes of oncologists and their approach to PC, resulting in increased referrals from oncologists to PC and earlier involvement of PC teams in patients' care in the community, evidenced by increased cancer patients receiving PC under the care of both NGOs in 2012 compared to 2010 [8, 26, 27].

Integration of PC and Oncology Care: Global Models

There is uniform consensus that the integration of PC into standard oncology care is beneficial to patients with advanced, incurable cancer. Randomized clinical trials on integration of oncology and palliative care [4–7], metanalyses and systematic reviews [28–31] point to significant health gains: improved symptom control, less anxiety and depression, reduced use of futile chemotherapy at the end of life, improved family satisfaction and quality of life and improved use of health care resources. A Lancet Oncology commission suggests that the combination of patient-directed care by specialist PC teams alongside disease-directed treatment promotes patient-centered care and affords the best outcomes [32]. This is also supported by the American Society of Clinical Oncology, which recently updated its previous Provisional Clinical Opinion into a Clinical Practice Guideline Update entitled "Integration of Palliative Care into Standard Oncology Care" advocating that patients with advanced cancer should receive dedicated palliative care services, early in the disease course, concurrent with active oncological treatment [11]. The European Society for Medical Oncology (ESMO) also strongly endorses the integration of oncology and palliative care [12] as does the American Cancer Society [33], and this is also supported by the NCCN Clinical Practice Guidelines [34].

However, there is no clear agreement on what constitutes integration, and in order to understand this better, Hui et al. undertook a systematic review on this topic which highlighted 38 clinical, educational, research and administrative indicators [35]. From a total of 101 selected relevant publications, process indicators of integration included the:

- presence of interdisciplinary PC teams ($n = 72$),
- simultaneous care approach ($n = 71$),
- PC guidelines ($n = 33$),
- routine symptom screening ($n = 25$),
- care pathways ($n = 11$), and,
- combined tumor boards ($n = 10$)

Similarly, in an international consensus of indicators on the integration of specialty PC and oncology programs for advanced cancer patients in hospitals with more than 100 beds, the panelists reached a consensus on 13 major and 30 minor indicators [36]. Major indicators included:

- Two (2) related to structure (consensus 95–98%), namely the presence of PC inpatient consultation team and outpatient clinics
- Four (4) on processes (88–98%): interdisciplinary team, routine symptom screening, routine documentation of advance care planning and early referral
- Three (3) on outcomes (88–91%): two on quality of end-of-life care relating to assessment of pain before death and emergency room visits during the last 30 days of life, and place of death consistent with patient's preference
- Four (4) on education (93–100%): oncology fellows to have PC training, continuing medical education for oncologists, combined PC and oncology educational activities for fellows and oncology fellows to have routine rotations in PC.

In 2003, the European Society for Medical Oncology (ESMO) started a process of accreditation for centers displaying integration of oncology and PC, resulting in an award of the status "Designated Centre of Integrated Oncology and Palliative Care" (ESMO-DC) using a list of 13 qualitative criteria related to program infrastructure, clinical processes, education and research [12] with over 200 institutions around the world having been accredited so far [37]. It is worth pointing out that this list of 13 criteria is different from the indicators on integration from the international consensus group [36]. The list of the ESMO criteria compared to the international consensus of indicators on integration of specialty PC and oncology programs can be seen in Table 1.

Due to studies of early PC driving the agenda for integration of PC into standard oncology care, great attention has been dedicated to the timing of referral to PC. Firstly, it is worth pointing out that in the international consensus of indicators on integration of specialty PC and oncology study, only half of the panelists agreed with using the 1–3 months from advanced cancer diagnosis as a cutoff for early PC referral, and in the end, this was defined as median time from referral to death >6 months before death [36]; see Table 1, item 5. Furthermore, the question of the timing of the referral of advanced cancer patients to PC was looked at in a Delphi consensus of 60 international experts, with most experts considering that >24 months to be too early, and identified the optimal timing as prognosis of 6–24 months [38]. It was also thought that the ideal timing for referral should be within 3 months of diagnosis of advanced cancer, if patients had a median survival of ≤1 year, had progressed through at least one line of systemic therapy and had Eastern Cooperative Oncology Group (ECOG) performance status ≥2 [38]. This reflects the concern that patients with metastatic disease for some cancers may have a median survival of several years, and for those patients, "the exact timing of 'early' PC may be a factor of need rather than any specific time point from diagnosis" [36]. Furthermore, it is worth pointing out that even within ESMO-designated centers of integrated Oncology and Palliative Care (ESMO-DC) and in a recent study in 2018, only 20% met the criterion for early referral to PC, with a median time from referral to death defined as >6 months before death [37].

Table 1 Criteria for ESMO-designated center and indicators of integration[a]

Criteria for accreditation as ESMO-designated center in integrated oncology and palliative care	Indicators of integration
1. The center is a cancer center which provides closely integrated oncology and palliative care clinical services	1. Presence of palliative care inpatient consultation team
2. The center is committed to a philosophy of continuity of care and non-abandonment	2. Presence of palliative care outpatient clinic
3. The center incorporates expert medical and nursing care in the evaluation and relief of pain and other physical symptoms	3. Presence of interdisciplinary palliative care team
4. The center incorporates expert care in the evaluation and relief of psychological and existential distress	4. Routine symptoms screening
5. The center provides routine patient assessment of physical and psychological symptoms and social supports and has an infrastructure that responds with appropriate interventions in a timely manner	5. Early referral to palliative care (>6 months)
6. The center provides emergency care of inadequately relieved physical and psychological symptoms	6. Proportion of routine documentation of advance care plan, median (IQR)
7. The center provides facilities and expert care for inpatient symptom stabilization	7. Proportion of outpatients with pain assessed before death, median (IQR)
8. The center incorporates programmatic support of family members	8. Proportion of patients with two or more emergency room visits in last 30 days of life, median (IQR)
9. The center provides high-level home care with expert back-up and coordination of home care with primary cancer clinicians	9. Proportion of place of death consistent with patient's preference, median (IQR)
10. The center provides respite care for ambulatory patients for patients unable to cope at home or in cases of family fatigue	10. Didactic palliative care curriculum

Table 1 (continued)

Criteria for accreditation as ESMO-designated center in integrated oncology and palliative care	Indicators of integration
11. The center provides facilities and expert care for inpatient end-of-life (terminal) care and is committed to providing adequate relief of suffering for dying patients	11. Continuing education in palliative care
12. The center participates in basic or clinical research related to palliative care and the quality of life of patients with cancer and their families	12. Combined palliative care and oncology educational activities
13. The center is involved in clinician education to improve the integration of oncology and palliative care	13. Routine rotation in palliative care for oncology fellows

[a]From Hui et al. [37]

Beyond indicators, integration between oncology and palliative care has been described in the following three levels or stages [39, 40]:

(a) *Linkage*: where oncologists just refer to PC
(b) *Coordination*: where there are established processes and pathways of interaction and pre-defined criteria for referrals
(c) *Full integration*: where there are pooled resources between oncology and palliative care

While the ideal level of integration may vary based on the individual health care system, resources, for example, PC workforce, and extent of PC provided by oncologists [39], it is desirable to aim to have either coordination or full integration, as this would avoid the scenario of very late referral to PC at the end of life and would thus provide more comprehensive care and allow for earlier input from specialized PC services in the disease trajectory.

Useful, especially for health care planners, is the study by Hui and Bruera [39], who describe conceptual models of integration between oncology and palliative care primarily to discuss the timing, selection of patients and criteria used to refer patients between oncology and palliative care. They describe four conceptual models:

(a) *Time-based model*: which uses chronological criteria in the disease trajectory for the referral/introduction of PC to cancer patients, for example, at the time of diagnosis of advanced disease or for end-of-life, the emphasis being on the timing of integration.
(b) *Provider-based model*: whereby oncologists and primary care physicians provide basic palliative care and specialized PC teams provide specialized PC. Hence, patients with more complex needs would need to be referred to PC.
(c) *Issue-based model*: which is focused on the individual symptoms and problems that patients have, and how those are being managed. Those can be managed as follows:
    (i) By the oncologist alone (the solo practice model).
    (ii) By the oncologist referring to various specialists (e.g. pain clinic and psychology); this is referred to as the congress model.
    (iii) By the oncologist referring to specialized PC, which is called the integrated model. The integrated model is recommended because it provides early concurrent PC with oncology care.
    (iv) System-based model: automatic referral based on predefined criteria (for instance, the National Comprehensive Cancer Network has issued guidelines for palliative care referral).

Global Level of PC Development
Level 1: No known hospice PC activity
Level 2: Capacity-building activity
Level 3a: Isolated PC provision
Level 3b: Generalized PC provision
Level 4a: Preliminary integration into mainstream service provision
Level 4b: Advanced integration into mainstream service provision [9].

Whichever model or indicators we consider for integration, of paramount importance is the level of PC services available; in order to be able to integrate PC into oncology care, there is a need for adequate PC services to be in place. In a 2013 report by the WHO and Worldwide Hospice Palliative Care Alliance (WHPCA), the global level of PC development was rated between 1 and 4 [9]. Based on this classification, the only countries that reached advanced integration were developed countries in Western Europe, North America, Australia and Japan, while all other countries had lower levels of PC development [9, 41].

Even in countries that have reached "advanced integration", there is evidence of large regional variation in PC provision [41]. A study of cancer centers in the USA showed that inpatient consultation teams, outpatient palliative care clinics, acute palliative care units and institution-run hospices were present in 92%, 59%, 26% and 31% of National Cancer Institute (NCI)-designated cancer centers, and 56%, 22%, 20% and 42% of non-NCI-designated cancer centers, respectively, while fewer than half of the cancer centers had PC fellowship training and research programs in place [42].

Collaboration and Integration: In Practice

There is now general agreement on the need for integration of PC with standard oncology care, hence "the question is no longer whether PC care should be offered, but what is the optimal model of delivery, when is the ideal time to refer, who is in greatest need of a referral, and how much palliative care should oncologists themselves be providing" [43]. Answers to these questions may differ for different countries and for different levels of PC development. Furthermore, it is worth considering that recommendations and indicators for integration have been produced from providers in PC resource-rich countries, and those may not apply to the majority of countries worldwide, where there is a huge shortage of PC specialist physicians and nurses [44]. It has furthermore been suggested that, given the differences in the availability of services, there is no "one-size-fits-all" approach that would work for every country, and instead we should be looking at solutions tailored to the individual centers'/countries' PC resources [44].

Hence in PC-rich settings, it is imperative that integration of PC into standard oncology care takes place early, perhaps at the time of diagnosis of advanced or metastatic disease, and certainly at a prognosis of greater than 6 months, and the indicators described before would provide standards against which this can be measured. For PC-poor settings though, where integration of the type described before is not possible, collaboration between the two specialties (starting with joint training courses and combined meetings and clinics, as shown by the example of our own country, Cyprus) can improve care and, over time, bring integration. Furthermore, collaboration between the two specialties can help to motivate oncology junior staff to train in PC, as happened in Cyprus, providing valuable physician workforce in PC in the long term and can also improve on the barriers of referral to PC. Moreover, the outcome resulting from a more efficient use of resources and the potential cost savings from PC services is unlikely to go unnoticed and may help convince health care planners and administrators to provide more resources to PC and allow, over time, PC capacity building.

We suggest that this progress of collaboration leading to integration can start even with a few PC physicians and nurses and a few oncologists. To the oncologists and PC physicians that would like to replicate the initiatives undertaken in Cyprus, we suggest that you form alliances with other health care professionals (oncologists and palliative care physicians and nurses) where you work, who share the same values as you about providing patient-centered care and concurrent oncology with PC [8]. When setting up common training courses for oncology and PC staff, help from other PC organizations from other countries may be needed [8, 45]. It is important that other physicians/surgeons and patients' negative attitudes and misconceptions toward PC are addressed, while cultural norms in the individual countries are respected [8, 46]. From joint training initiatives, the next step is to set up initiatives with clinical sessions, bringing the two disciplines together, as described with Cyprus (i.e. the importance of the physical presence of PC physicians within cancer centers or hospitals with oncology units as well as joint meetings).

Furthermore in PC-poor settings, we propose, depending on available PC capacity, a more flexible transition and a more targeted concurrent model of oncology and PC, where referral to specialized PC (SPC) should be tailored to patients with more complicated palliative care needs that cannot be met by their primary care physician or oncologist, that is, a way of rationing SPC services, until such time that there is adequate PC capacity to cope with the demand. Even colleagues from advanced health care systems in the USA and Canada propose that PC should be Targeted, Timely and Team based [43]. They describe "targeted PC that involves identifying patients most likely to benefit from specialist PC interventions, akin to the concept of targeted cancer therapies" and timely PC from the time of diagnosis of advanced incurable cancer as "preventative care to minimize crises at the end of life" [43].

In summary, we suggest that especially in PC-poor settings, the timing of referral should be dictated by available PC recourses and clinical need (patients having complex symptoms requiring SPC services) and ideally decided by a multidisciplinary board of oncology and PC professionals, rather than automatically at the time of diagnosis of advanced incurable cancer; this should be the aim of all countries with advanced PC services. Hence if, in your own country, you can set up a meeting whereby patients are being discussed, the patients more in need and more likely to benefit from specialist PC would be referred for PC input.

Finally, both in PC-rich and also in PC-poor resource settings, in addition to online and other methods of teaching, it is vital to provide more clinically based PC training to oncologists and oncology trainees [47], so that they can provide high-quality basic PC to their patients. In line with the specification for Oncology trainees for a dedicated clinical rotation in PC in the Global Core Curriculum for Oncology Training set by ASCO and ESMO, the aim is to acquire these valuable PC and communication skills as well as the understanding of when patients should be referred to specialist PC [48]. The closer collaboration and interaction among oncologists with PC physicians and nurses within cancer centers and hospitals can only further this goal.

References

1. World Health Organization. World Health Organization definition of palliative care. http://www.who.int/cancer/palliative/definition/en/. Accessed 14 April 2020.
2. Radbruch L, Payne S. White paper on standards and norms for hospice and palliative care in Europe: part 1 Recommendations from the European Association for Palliative Care. Eur J Palliat Care. 2009;16(6):278–89.
3. Council of Europe. Recommendation (2003) 24 of the Committee of Ministers to member states on the organization of palliative care. https://www.coe.int/t/dg3/health/Source/Rec(2003)24_en.pdf. Accessed 14 April 2020.
4. Temel JS, Greer JA, Muzikansky A, et al. Early palliative care for patients with metastatic non-small-cell lung cancer. N Engl J Med. 2010;14(8):733–42.
5. Bakitas MA, Tosteson TD, Li Z, et al. Early versus delayed initiation of concurrent palliative oncology care: patient outcomes in the ENABLE III randomized controlled trial. J Clin Oncol. 2015;33(13):1438–45.
6. Bakitas M, Lyons KD, Hegel MT, et al. Effects of a palliative care intervention on clinical outcomes in patients with advanced cancer: the project ENABLE II randomized controlled trial. JAMA. 2009;302:741–9.
7. Zimmermann C, Swami N, Krzyzanowska M, et al. Early palliative care for patients with advanced cancer: a cluster-randomized controlled trial. Lancet. 2014;383:1721–30.
8. Charalambous H, Silbermann M. The role of the Cancer Centre in Supporting Palliative Care Services Development. J Palliat Care Med. 2016;6(5):1000e139.
9. Lynch T, Connor S, Clark D. Mapping levels of palliative care development: a global update. J Pain Symptom Manag. 2013;45:1094–6.
10. Centeno C, Lynch T, Garralda E, et al. Coverage and development of specialist palliative care services across the World Health Organization European Region (2005-2012): results from a European Association for Palliative Care Task Force survey of 53 countries. Palliat Med. 2016;30:351–62.
11. Ferrell BR, Temel JS, Temin S, et al. Integration of palliative care into standard oncology care: American Society of Clinical Oncology clinical practice guideline update. J Clin Oncol. 2017;35(1):96–112.
12. Cherny N, Catane R, Schrijvers D, et al. European Society for Medical Oncology (ESMO) Program for the integration of oncology and palliative care: a 5-year review of the Designated Centers' incentive program. Ann Oncol. 2010;21:362–9.
13. Peppercorn JM, Smith TJ, Helft PR, et al. American society of clinical oncology statement: toward individualized care for patients with advanced cancer. J Clin Oncol. 2011;29(6):755–60.
14. Lamas D, Rosenbaum L. Painful inequities – palliative care in developing countries. N Engl J Med. 2012;366:1989–201.
15. Quill TE, Abernethy AP. Generalist plus specialist palliative care – creating a more sustainable model. N Engl J Med. 2013;368(13):1173–5.

16. Breuer B, Fleishman SB, Cruciani RA, et al. Medical oncologists' attitudes and practice in cancer pain management: a national survey. J Clin Oncol. 2011;29:4769–75.
17. Fisch MJ, Lee J-W, Weiss M, et al. Prospective, observational study of pain and analgesic prescribing in medical oncology outpatients with breast, colorectal, lung, or prostate cancer. J Clin Oncol. 2012;30:1980–8.
18. Cherny NI, Catane R, European Society of Medical Oncology Taskforce on Palliative and Supportive Care. Attitudes of medical oncologists toward palliative care for patients with advanced and incurable cancer: report on a survey by the European Society of Medical Oncology Taskforce on Palliative and Supportive Care. Cancer. 2003;98(11):2502–10.
19. Ward AM, Agar M, Koczwara B. Collaborating or co-existing: a survey of attitudes of medical oncologists toward specialist palliative care. Palliat Med. 2009;23(8):698–707.
20. Wentlandt K, Krzyzanowska MK, Swami N, et al. Referral practices of oncologists to specialized palliative care. J Clin Oncol. 2012;30:4380–6. https://doi.org/10.1200/JCO.2012.44.0248.
21. Johnson CE, Girgis A, Paul CL. Cancer specialists' palliative care referral practices and perceptions: results of a national survey. Palliat Med. 2008;22:51–7.
22. Abrahm JL. Integrating palliative care into comprehensive cancer care. J Natl Compr Cancer Netw. 2012;10(10):1192–8.
23. Charalambous H, Pallis A, Hasan B, O'Brien M. Attitudes and referral patterns of lung cancer specialists in Europe to Specialized Palliative Care (SPC) and the practice of Early Palliative Care (EPC). BMC Palliat Care. 2014;13(1):59.
24. Hui D, Finlay E, Buss MK, et al. Palliative oncologists: specialists in the science and art of patient care. J Clin Oncol. 2015;33:2314–7.
25. Silbermann M, Arnaout M, Daher M, et al. Palliative cancer care in Middle Eastern countries: accomplishments and challenges. Ann Oncol. 2012;3:15–28.
26. Charalambous H, Pitsillide B, Nestoros S. Palliative care in Cyprus: current status. In: Silbermann M, editor. Palliative care to the cancer patient. The Middle East as a model for emerging countries. New York: Nova Publishers; 2014. p. 1–21.
27. Silbermann M, Pitsillides B, Al-Alfi N, et al. Multidisciplinary care team for cancer patients and its implementation in several Middle Eastern countries. Ann Oncol. 2013;24:41–7.
28. Kavalieratos D, Corbelli J, Zhang D, et al. Association between palliative care and patient and caregiver outcomes: a systematic review and meta-analysis. JAMA. 2016;316(20):2104–14.
29. Gaertner J, Siemens W, Meerpohl JJ, et al. Effect of specialist palliative care services on quality of life in adults with advanced incurable illness in hospital, hospice, or community settings: systematic review and meta-analysis. BMJ. 2017;357:j2925.
30. Haun MW, Estel S, Rucker G, et al. Early palliative care for adults with advanced cancer. Cochrane Database Syst Rev. 2017;6:CD011129.
31. Kassianos AP, Ioannou M, Koutsantoni M, Charalambous H. The impact of specialized palliative care on cancer patients' health-related quality of life: a systematic review and meta-analysis. Support Care Cancer. 2018;26:61–79.
32. Kaasa S, Loge JH, Aapro M, et al. Integration of oncology and palliative care: a Lancet Oncology Commission. Lancet Oncol. 2018;19(11):e588–653.
33. https://www.cancer.org/treatment/treatments-and-side-effects/palliative-care.html. Accessed 14 April 2020.
34. Levy MH, Smith T, Alvarez-Perez A, Back A, Baker JN, Beck A, et al. NCCN clinical practice guidelines in oncology. Palliative Care. Available from URL: http://www.nccn.org/professionals/physician_gls/f_guidelines. Accessed 14 April 2020.
35. Hui D, Kim YJ, Park JC, et al. Integration of oncology and palliative care: a systematic review. Oncologist. 2015;20(1):77–83.
36. Hui D, Bansal S, Strasser F, et al. Indicators of integration of oncology and palliative care programs: an international consensus. Ann Oncol. 2015;26(9):1953–9.
37. Hui D, Cherny NI, Wu J, Liu D, Latino NJ, Strasser F. Indicators of integration at ESMO designated centres of integrated oncology and palliative care. ESMO Open. 2018;3(5):e000372.
38. Hui D, Masanori M, Watanabe S, Caraceni A, Strasser F, Saarto T, et al. Referral criteria for outpatient specialty palliative cancer care: an international consensus. Lancet Oncol. 2016;17(12):e552–9.
39. Hui D, Bruera E. Models of integration of oncology and palliative care. Ann Palliat Med. 2015;4(3):89–98.
40. Leutz WN. Five laws for integrating medical and social services: lessons from the United States and the United Kingdom. Milbank Q. 1999;77:77–100.
41. Hui D, Bruera E. Integrating palliative care into the trajectory of cancer care. Nat Rev Clin Oncol. 2016;13(3):159–71. https://doi.org/10.1038/nrclinonc.2015.201.
42. Hui D, et al. Availability and integration of palliative care at US cancer centers. JAMA. 2010;303:1054–61.
43. Hui D, Hannon BL, Zimmermann C, Bruera E. Improving patient and caregiver outcomes in oncology: team-based, timely, and targeted palliative care. CA Cancer J Clin. 2018;68(5):356–76.
44. Verna L, Giusti R, Marchetti P, et al. Integration between oncology and palliative care: does one size fit all? Ann Oncol. 2016;27(3):549. https://doi.org/10.1093/annonco/mdv582.
45. Pantilat SZ, Kerr KM, Kutner JS, et al. Leveraging external resources to grow and sustain your palliative care program: a call to action. J Palliat Med. 2012;15(1):25–8.
46. Silbermann M, Epner DE, Charalambous H, et al. Promoting new approaches for cancer care in the Middle East. Ann Oncol. 2013;24(Suppl 7):vii5–10.
47. Charalambous H, Silbermann M. Clinically based palliative care training is needed urgently for all oncologists. J Clin Oncol. 2012;30(32):4042–3.
48. Dittrich C, Kosty M, Jezdic S, et al. ESMO/ASCO recommendations for a global curriculum in medical oncology edition 2016. ESMO Open. 2016;1:e000097. https://doi.org/10.1136/esmoopen-2016-000097.

Part XIX

Middle East: Iran

The Role of the Nurse in the Community in Running the Palliative Care Interdisciplinary Team: The Iranian Experience

Maryam Rassouli, Leila Khanali Mojen, Azam Shirinabadi Farahani, and Samira Beiranvand

Introduction

The global health system has undergone many changes in the past 20 years [1–4] and has encouraged countries to develop new models for primary health care provision [5]. One of the most important factors that have made health care reform inevitable is the increasing costs of this sector [6]. Changing lifestyles have led to increased life expectancy and subsequently the increased incidence and prevalence of non-communicable diseases (NCD), which in turn increases the need for health care and services [6–13]. NCDs are now considered a threat to the health and longevity of people in developed and developing countries [14, 15]. More than 76% of disease burden in Iran is associated with these diseases. The increasing prevalence of these diseases and their chronic, progressive and disabling nature puts the productive force of societies in danger of death, disability and incapacitation. Due to the costs of long-term treatment and high out-of-pocket expenses, these diseases can lead to heavy costs of health care and, subsequently, poverty. Therefore, NCDs are among the major barriers to the development of countries, and the high costs of these diseases bring up many challenges for any health systems [16].

In 2013, the World Health Organization (WHO) introduced the Global Action Plan (2013–2020) to the world, which included 9 goals and 25 indicators to control 4 major NCDs including cardiovascular disease, diabetes, cancer and respiratory diseases, and also to reduce the four risk factors of smoking, inactivity, poor diet and alcohol abuse, and recommended practical measures that can help countries all around the world accomplish these goals. Going by the motto "PHC- Now More Than Ever", the most important goal of this organization was to implement PHC in order to prevent and control these diseases. To this end, PHC should be reoriented appropriately [16].

M. Rassouli (✉)
Cancer Research Center, Shahid Beheshti University of Medical Sciences, Tehran, Iran

L. Khanali Mojen
Medical-Surgical Nursing Department, School of Nursing & Midwifery, Shahid Beheshti University of Medical Sciences, Tehran, Iran

A. Shirinabadi Farahani
Pediatric Nursing Department, School of Nursing & Midwifery, Shahid Beheshti University of Medical Sciences, Tehran, Iran

S. Beiranvand
Department of Nursing, Student Research Committee, School of Nursing and Midwifery, Ahvaz Jundishapur University of Medical Sciences, Ahvaz, Iran

M. Silbermann (ed.), *Palliative Care for Chronic Cancer Patients in the Community*,
https://doi.org/10.1007/978-3-030-54526-0_28

WHO's essential intervention package for NCDs in PHC is a set of prioritized effective interventions that can be provided with an acceptable quality, leading to the improvement of health system. The current programs integrated into PHC only focus on one risk factor such as high blood pressure or diabetes, but the integrated look into risk factors and diseases, and the integrated prevention and treatment of them result in accomplishing goals at lower costs, with higher effectiveness. Influential approaches to reducing the burden of NCDs included a combination of community-level interventions and individual interventions. Such low-cost and highly-effective interventions are currently available and include the detection and early diagnosis of NCDs using inexpensive technologies, pharmacological and non-pharmacological approaches to removing the risk factors in NCDs and available medicines for preventing and treating myocardial infarction, stroke, diabetes, cancer and asthma. If these interventions are effectively applicable through inexpensive technology and in the form of PHC, they can lead to reduced medical costs and improved quality of life and productivity in people [16].

As the health systems expand, the importance of PHC as the basis of an efficient health system becomes more apparent. Since all members of society must be able to use the health system's full capacity fairly, the implementation of PHC strategies can play a key role in the health system at local, national and international levels [17, 18], and it continues to be a key strategy for promoting justice in health care [19]. Since 2010, universal health coverage has been widely accepted worldwide and is now recognized as one of the major components of Sustainable Developmental Goals, and governments are obliged to implement it [20]. Universal health coverage means having access to a variety of nationally approved health services (including health promotion, prevention, and health care, rehabilitation and palliative care services) whenever necessary, with appropriate quality and financial support. Iran has a long history of implementing interventions to achieve universal health coverage [3]. Since 1973, about 5 years before the international Declaration of Alma-Ata, Iran has been taking actions in the field of PHC provision, which are considered as successful programs and experiences in achieving universal health coverage [21].

One of the strategies for managing and providing services to NCD patients is the intersectoral cooperation (hospitals and community health centers) and rigorous community-based planning. The WHO has also developed a patient-centered health care strategy at the community level [22, 23]. The aim of this strategy is to reduce health care costs, improve the quality of care, decrease the length of hospital stay, move toward community care and utilize non-hospital resources, as well as providing appropriate and quality home care [24].

Changes in policy priorities, use of community-based approaches to solve care problems, demographic changes and the increased need for long-term care, shifts in the family structure from extended to nuclear, more participation of women in society as workforce, changes in people's attitudes toward and expectations from health care services and the increased demand for private services in society have led health policymakers to address these needs and replace the traditional approaches to hospital care with community-based care, in regard with NCDs [25, 26].

Community-based care has a unique place in the field of care provision due to reasons such as reducing costs, increasing patient's satisfaction, minimizing the need for hospitalization, providing comprehensive services, controlling chronic diseases, adherence to treatment, improving the quality of life, increasing the patients' knowledge of their disease, self-management and social engagement [27–30].

Cancer as a Non-communicable Disease

Cancer is a chronic disease with an increasing incidence that has risen to 18.1 million cases globally, according to the 2018 WHO report. In addition, according to this report, the latest cancer death rate is around 9.6 million, known as the second leading cause of death worldwide [31].

In Iran, the prevalence of cancer is increasingly on the rise and is recognized as the second leading cause of death. In 2016, 82% of deaths in Iran were due to chronic diseases, with cancer accounting for 16% of the total cases [32]. As the WHO predicts, in 2020, cancer incidence in Iran will increase to 85,653 cases and would cause 62,897 cases of cancer death [33].

In recent years, rapid advances in the early diagnosis and treatment of cancer have led to an increased number of cancer survivors. In some studies, cancer survival rate has been reported to be up to 85% in Iran [24, 34]. The mean age of patients with several types of cancer in Iran is lower than that in other countries. The age of onset is an influential factor in the survival rate of these patients. Cancer at an earlier age is associated with an increased survival time. Therefore, it can be said that Iranian cancer patients are mostly younger and exposed to complications for a longer period of time [35]. However, older survivors experience more complex conditions due to underlying problems and comorbidities [24]. Cancer survivors, on the other hand, face unique challenges in both short- and long term [36] that are related to their physical, mental, social and functional health, and lifestyle changes [37]. These patients are exposed to a wide range of complications caused by the disease and its treatment, as well as physical, emotional, mental, social and lifestyle changes that can lead to a reduced quality of life [38, 39]. Given the family's key role in providing care for these patients, family members also face many problems and challenges that can lead to a decreased quality of life, and thus decreased quality of patient care [40, 41].

Therefore, patients and their families need complex health care at all stages of the disease, from the diagnosis to treatment, follow-ups and end-of-life care as a comprehensive care [42].

Comprehensive care is an approach that addresses all the patient's needs and usually requires a coordinated multidisciplinary care team. The main goal is to help improve the quality of life in the patient and his/her family [43, 44].

A large part of cancer care is provided in the form of supportive and palliative care for patients. There are different structures for providing this care, varying in each country depending on the structure of the health system. In 2014, the World Health Organization identified the access to palliative care as a key component in any health care system and emphasized the provision of these services, especially at the level of primary care and home care [28, 44].

The by-laws for the Development of Cancer Supportive and Palliative Care in Iran are formulated in seven chapters, based on which the levels of supportive and palliative care provision, hospital unit, counseling team, clinic and home care team are defined [45], in line with the levels recommended by the WHO guidelines [46].

Since palliative care clinics, home care, long-term care facilities and hospices are defined as out-of-hospital settings of palliative care provision, that is, at the community level, this chapter presents a review of the *status quo* of service provision in these settings in Iran.

Palliative Care Clinics

The availability of supportive and palliative care for all patients is an ethical and legal obligation in the field of health. In Iran, the National Cancer Management Plan begins inclusively and comprehensively in various areas of fighting cancer in the form of diagnosis and screening programs, and ends with supportive and palliative care plans. One of the components of this program is the development of palliative care management instruction, which includes the development of a service delivery network, infrastructures, manpower, facilities, as well as pathways for service delivery, monitoring and evaluation [47].

Palliative care requires a well-structured design and varies based on the circumstances and the resources of each country [48]. Although in recent years, these services have not been systematically provided in Iran, the most common structures for providing them were hospital sectors [30]. However, due to changes in the levels of needs and public awareness, receiving outpatient or home-based palliative care is considered a priority for patients, families and caregivers, and the World Health Organization also emphasizes the provision of these services at the community level [49].

Although in the current situation, health policymakers are aware of service shift from hospital to home, adding these services to the Iranian health system structure requires some changes, which most notably includes focusing on treatment at the level of treatment centers and the absence of nurses at the community [12]. Due to the weakness of community-based service delivery structures, cancer patients receive most services at the hospital and are mostly referred to doctor's offices and various hospital wards. Perhaps one of the major challenges faced by the current health system is how to create a link between the primary level, that is, community-based services, and secondary level, the health-care services [12, 50].

Some Iranian studies have shown that palliative care clinics are the most appropriate setting for hospital care. Therefore, health policymakers address this challenge by designing and establishing a link between the primary and secondary levels through establishing hospital-based palliative care clinics [51]. Numerous studies have also shown that the end-of-life care in outpatient consultations provided at these clinics has higher quality than inpatient services do. According to the qualitative study conducted by Khanali Mojen et al., based on the experts' opinions and viewpoints, this structure has the highest priority [52].

At present, the current structures for providing community-based health services, home care centers and public clinics as well as health centers and health homes are facing challenges such as insufficient expert staff, and in other cases, high costs due to the lack of insurance coverage and lack of easy access, which diminishes the provision of these services at the community level [50, 53, 54].

In advanced countries, palliative care service provision is considered as a triangle, with the base being community-based services, and specialty services gradually move toward the top of the pyramid, indicating the classification of palliative care services [55, 56]. In Iran, this triangle is inverted due to the provision of specialty services at the third level, known as tertiary hospitals, and most patients are referred to this level. Therefore, these patients are linked to the community level only through hospital clinics in order to facilitate the shift from hospital to home.

Therefore, in response to this need and also according to the World Health Organization's recommendation regarding the necessity of service delivery at PHC level, health policymakers have considered it necessary to establish hospital clinics and have implemented programs to make them executable. In 2018, the Ministry of Health imposed the establishment of hospital clinics to 14 universities of medical sciences, and also trained the necessary workforce for this purpose at the national level. Based on this program, 18 specialty hospitals with oncology, radiotherapy and chemotherapy departments were selected, from each of which two to four general practitioners and also oncology nurses were introduced. The program was approved and implemented as two theoretical and practical courses during 240 educational hours [55, 57–59].

In order to execute this program and to achieve the goals of the Cancer Centers Classification Program in the National Cancer Preparation Program, the by-law of establishing these clinics is also being drafted and approved [60]. According to the by-law, these centers, which are established in hospitals and preferably near the emergency departments, are required to provide outpatient and consulting services by trained physicians and nurses. In response to the different needs of patients at different levels, these clinics are connected with the three sectors, *home care, inpatient wards and specialty clinics*, to facilitate access to services, in case patients need each of these levels. Service delivery pathway at these clinics begins with an assessment done by trained nurses and physicians, and if more specialized services are necessary, it is referred to other departments and followed up by the nurse.

An overview of the proposed clinic and the pathway of service delivery is presented in Fig. 1.

In Iran, these clinics were designed in cancer centers in Type-II and Type-III in the cancer regionalization program. When these clinics are combined with inpatient consultation services,

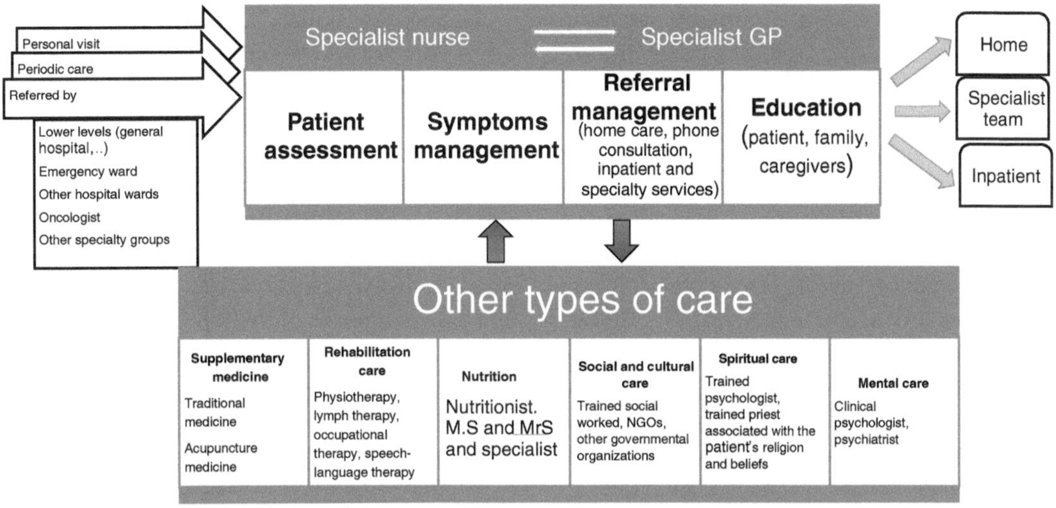

Fig. 1 The proposed clinic and the pathway of service delivery

according to WHO's recommendation, this would be the best model in case the start-up funding and resources are limited, and since most of the expert workforce in the Iranian health system is associated with the third-level care, it would be reasonable and also cost-effective to establish palliative care clinics at this level in specialist hospitals.

Home Care

Investigations done by a panel of experts on palliative care structures in Iran, focusing on criteria such as health infrastructures, social and cultural status, economic conditions and the availability of equipment and facilities in the country, indicated that some approaches, especially community-based models such as home care, have seemingly higher priorities [60].

In a study with the aim of prioritizing research goals in the field of cancer from nurses' point of view, finding strategies to ensure the continuation of hospital care at home as community-based services has been one of the top five research priorities [61].

The WHO recommends the provision of palliative home care for patients in the form of primary health care, so that all patients can access this care and benefit from it in the shortest possible time, regardless of its costs [46]. This care has been considered a desirable care approach in the twenty-first century and is divided into two types: Specialized and General. The overall goal of this approach is to provide appropriate, cost-effective and quality care to maintain individuals' ability and independence in life. However, its nature may be different from those of primary health care, secondary level of health care and even rehabilitation [46, 62]. This type of care, which is one of the major models of community-based care, is important in the management of limited resources and is aimed at reducing the length of hospital stay and treatment costs [63].

Providing such services by formal or informal caregivers at home in order to promote, restore and maintain the maximum comfort, performance and health as well as respecting the dignity of the patient and his/her family until death, which can be offered as services, associated with prevention, health promotion, treatment, rehabilitation, palliative and long-term care [64]. Among the other benefits of its implementation are the empowerment of the patient and his/her family [54], a decrease in the patient's frequent hospital admissions due to the disease-related complications and problems [65], reduced emergency visits [66], as well as reduced costs [67] and length of hospital stay [68].

This approach prevents the patient and his/her family to be left with unfinished care and also the possible complications associated with it by monitoring and following up the patient and his/her family, as well as examining his/her care situation after discharge, and ultimately, will lead to the patient and family's satisfaction as an outcome of care [69]. As a result, home care has the best outcome and the lowest cost compared with hospital care and is particularly preferable for the elderly, chronic patients and end-of-life care [70].

Today, home care is one of the most urgent needs of developing societies, including Iran, and plays an important role in the provision of health services by using capabilities and the capacity of families, the community and NGOs [63].

The Iranian Palliative Care Association encourages families to provide end-of-life patient care. The most important goal of this association is to reduce the costs of unnecessary hospitalizations and futile care for such patients. On the other hand, according to Iranian culture, dying at home beside one's family members and loved ones is everyone's wish. Moreover, the dominant religious values of Iran also emphasize caring for patients and the elderly at home and advise everyone to participate in care provision for the elderly and the disabled. Therefore, home care is in line with the prevailing culture of Iranian society and can highlight the need to establish this care model. The family is considered a social foundation in the Islamic society and Iran's constitution, and using this potential in care helps facilitate and provide health care services at the patient's own home, with a minimum rate of referrals to medical centers. In such a situation, the duty of care provision falls on the first-degree relatives (spouse, children and siblings). Male family members are usually responsible for the financial, practical and logistical aspects of care, while females provide care and nursing, feed patients and give them hope. Usually, the elder member of family, larger family member, preferably the patient's eldest son, is considered to be the leader or the head of the support team [25, 29, 58].

In Iran, few studies have been conducted on home care [25]. In a study conducted by Barati et al in 2010 on investigating policymakers' views regarding the benefits of home care development in Iran [71], the socioeconomic advantages, and the benefits for the patient, the family and the health system were highlighted by the experts, and it was concluded that the development of this type of care is one of the significant and essential needs of the Iranian health system which can contribute to the enhancement of community participation in primary health care in Iran through utilizing the capacity of individuals, community, volunteers and NGOs [63]. In a qualitative study, the managerial aspects of home care including infrastructure and policy-making were investigated [72].

Focusing on treatment rather than care, the lack of appropriate infrastructure [27], the lack of access to palliative care services at home and hospice, as well as the lack of educational opportunities for nurses are among the barriers to home care, despite its social acceptance [73]. Thus practically, providing care services for cancer patients is generally hospital-based. In other words, most patients receive their required care in hospitals [74, 75].

In order to solve this problem, in accordance with the Article 22 of the by-law on the establishment of counseling centers and the provision of nursing home care, approved on July 5, 2016, under the code D/101/691 and communicated by the Minister of Health with the aim of organizing "home care" and ensuring the continuity of treatment after discharge, home care units were established in hospitals and medical centers across the country.

According to the by-law, home care is hospital-based, and the home care units based in the hospital are responsible for the patient's referral to home care centers [76]. These units aim to organize, maintain and coordinate patient care after discharge, provide safe and cost-effective home care in order to reduce the length of stay at hospitals and treatment centers, reduce care costs, reduce recovery time, control and decrease hospital-acquired infections, rehabilitate and improve the quality of nursing services, and ultimately increase the satisfaction of patients and families [77].

After referring the patient to the home care center, the initial examinations will be performed by the center's physicians and the necessary care will be provided as a care plan by physicians and nurses depending on the patient's status, documents and medical tests. This plan will be implemented by the nurse at home. Any changes to the initial plan (such as the need to increase the narcotic dose for pain relief) should be made based on the discretion of the center's physician. The possibility of consulting an oncologist or a fellow palliative care specialist of the center should also be considered by the home care center. If necessary, the patient should be visited by a physician at home [78].

Hospitals and medical centers can conclude a contract with one or several centers. Centers should introduce representatives to be present at the location of the unit in order to report to the home care unit after the completion of home care. Patients in need of nursing home care are identified by the nurse and the treating physician and are referred to the unit with the patient and the guardian's consent. The unit should also submit a monthly report of its performance to the university and hospital's nursing management [79].

The number of these centers is also explicitly stated in the Standard Manual of Style for the Number and Distribution of Counseling Centers and the Provision of Nursing Home Care and the Instruction for its Physical Conditions, Facilities and Equipment, which is approved by the Nursing Deputy of the Iranian Ministry of Health. In this regard, medical universities across the country can grant licenses for the establishment of one center for covering every 50,000 people.

In order to properly distribute the centers across the city, universities can determine the number of the centers required in each district of municipality and issue licenses accordingly. In cities with a population under 50,000, it is also possible to grant licenses to two centers. Meanwhile, the Deputy of Nursing declares the criteria and the standard number of centers annually.

Monitoring the Performance of Home Care Unit

The performance of home care unit is monitored by the hospital's nursing management. The nursing manager of university, in collaboration with the hospitals and university authorities, is responsible for following, setting up and monitoring the performance of units in hospitals and the affiliated medical centers [79]. To this end, monitoring is carried out in several areas including legal licenses, physical space, equipment (office/medical), documentations and performance [79].

Necessary Specialists for Home Care Provision

Teamwork and cooperation are essential in providing quality home care. To this end, a team of nurses, nursing assistants, physicians, support experts and finally an individual as the technical expert of the center should cooperate:

- Nurses: nurses providing this type of care are chosen based on the criteria including having a valid professional license, having a B.S degree with at least 5 years of clinical experience and at least 2 years of job experience in oncology and palliative care wards, at least 10 successful home visits along with the care team, passing palliative care and home care professional courses with a valid professional certificate, and passing courses such as pain and wound management over the past 2 years.
- Fellow ranks, including nursing assistants
- A general practitioner trained in the field of palliative care and available 24 hours a day
- Support staff
- The Center's technical officer is responsible for addressing, monitoring and responding to the needs of patients and the technical staff of the center, and requires meeting the criteria such as passing palliative care and home care training courses, having at least 5 years of job experience in oncology and palliative care wards and at least 6 months of providing home care in cancer care services center [79, 80].

There are also social criteria for receiving home care, the most significant of which are the trainability of family members or companions and their taking the responsibility of caregiving. It is also important for the family to have awareness of the disease, and their ability to provide home care for the patient should also be approved. Family involvement in patient care planning is one of the important issues that can affect the quality of services. During this process, the family must receive the necessary training. The patient–family relationship with the specialist physician should continue at the time of the diagnosis of malignancy until the patient's death, and this relationship should be mutual [79, 81].

In this regard, in Iran, due to the chronic and recurrent nature of cancer on the one hand, and the need for symptom management and the treatment of the disease on the other hand, the end-of-life care standard service package for cancer home care is classified into two types of services:

- Public services that can be generalized to other chronic diseases
- Specialized services designed specifically for cancer patients in the form of supportive and palliative care [78].

In order to determine the care level and consequently providing the appropriate and quality home, it is necessary to estimate the severity of the disease. Two tools are used to determine the severity of cancer:

Edmonton Symptom Assessment System-revised (ESAS-r) is a symptom screening tool the utilization of which is necessary, because not controlling these symptoms can exacerbate the negative effects on the quality of life in these patients and may threaten the continuity of care and treatment due to increased costs of complications. This tool can be completed by the patient, the caregiver and the professional staff. The ESAS-r consists of nine visual items as follows, and one blank item based on the patient's opinion:

Anxiety, Depression, Drowsiness, Lack of Appetite, Nausea, pain, Shortness of Breath, Tiredness and Overall well-being

This criterion is scored on a scale of 0–100. A higher score indicates the severity of symptoms. A score above 7 in one or more cases indicates the severity of complications.

Palliative Performance Scale (PPS) also focuses on the movement, activity, the evidences of disease, self-care, intake and the level of consciousness. PPS $\leq$ 40 is an indication of end-of-life, palliative and specialized care [78, 82–85].

Based on the above criteria (e.g. PPS: 100-40), in regard with the instructions for the establishment of home care unit for patients during the active phase of cancer treatment, and after the treating physician's approval, the most significant services provided at home are as follows:

Simple wound management, nutritional care, ostomy care and care training, examining the patient and the family's adherence to treatment, types of injections according to the physician's instruction, urinary catheter insertion and maintenance, pain management (pharmacological and non-pharmacological) based on existing guidelines and blood sampling according to physician's instructions.

In cases where it is not possible to manage the patient at home after the nurse visits, the consultant contacts with a fellow physician of the service center or the referring physician, and can refer the patient to the hospital in coordination with the physician and the hospital [79].

Discharge

Based on the available evidences and documents of the patient's health status, formulated criteria, and the patient and the family's opinions, decisions are made about the patient's discharge by the treatment team. The most important discharge criteria are:

Changes in the patient's medical condition, the lack of improvement and the need for referral to the hospital, change in the patient's social condition, services disproportionate to the patient's problems, the achievement of care goals set in care plan and death.

Transferring the patient to the hospice and long-term care services is recommended in case home care conditions are not met (the lack of caregiver at home, abandoning, neglecting or abusing the patient). Although there are no such centers in Iran yet, and currently, the by-law for their establishment has been developed and submitted to the relevant authorities for legislation and legal reviews [78, 79].

Charitable Organizations

Iran is a vast country with different ethnicities, with a 99% of the population constituted by Muslims and different minorities such as Christians, Armenians and Jews [86] living in it. In addition, the Iranian health system follows the referral and classification system, and its services are provided as primary health care services for the community. The system is structured in a way that comprehensive urban and rural health centers are each responsible for delivering health services to a specific area [87].

In home care provision as a modern care approach, private centers and charitable organizations also provide scattered home-based palliative care services to the covered population [44].

In other words, in addition to the cooperation and coordination of government organizations, non-governmental charitable organizations and institutions also play an important role in fighting cancer. Since the costs of cancer diagnosis, treatment and control are so high, it is predicted that even middle-class people of the society will not be able to afford them. Therefore, non-governmental charitable organizations play an important role in supporting cancer patients, and governments do not see themselves needless of receiving aid from such organizations. Thus, governments facilitate the establishment, development and delivery of services to patients by providing the necessary conditions through NGOs [88].

In this way, the high costs of cancer patients are partly covered by charitable organizations which can reduce the financial burden of cancer patients and help them manage their disease. For many patients, the initial diagnosis of cancer is shocking, and more than a third of patients experience anxiety and depression. Cancer is equally stressful for the patient's family and profoundly affects the economic situation and daily functioning of the patient's relatives. The economic shock often includes reduced income and the expenses associated with the costs of health care [89].

The activities of institutions located in different Iranian provinces [28] mostly include socio-economic (care and treatment funding), preventive and educational (publishing books and magazines to improve people's knowledge and awareness), research (providing databases and assisting researchers), therapeutic (physical, mental) and rehabilitation (providing facilities, establishing cottage hospitals) supports.

Depending on the type of the service provided, these centers can be divided into two major categories of child care and adult care.

- Service Delivery to Children

Various centers across the country provide services for children and their families. The major goal of all of them is to prepare the necessary facilities for the child's health to be restored, as well as providing subsidiary support. In addition to providing financial support, these institutions have directly made extensive cooperation in providing appropriate care. Mahak Charity is an example of such institutions in the field of therapeutic and palliative care services for cancer children. However, this institute does not offer home care services and has only a temporary residence for families who have brought their children to other cities to the institute for treatment.

- Service Delivery to Adults

The centers seek to educate, prevent, treat and provide care for adult cancer patients. Raising awareness on common cancer symptoms, the complications of some treatment approaches, such as radiation therapy and chemotherapy, and acquaintance with pharmaceutical centers across Iran are also among the important goals of these centers. However, since many years ago, privately managed institutions under the supervision of the Ministry of Health have also provided medical and paramedical home services for patients, and part of their job description is to provide education and consultation for the patient and the family in the field of self-care and following the instructions prescribed by the physician. Noticing these issues after service provision indicates that although in the past the Ministry of Health focused on the secondary level of care, that is, treatment in hospital settings, statistics show that today focuses are on the primary level of care. There are currently two home care plans being executed across the country: a neonatal home care plan in Isfahan and an elderly care plan in the suburban areas and cities with less than 50,000 people.

In charity and private sectors, there are two home care centers active in Isfahan and Tehran for cancer patients run by the Ala Charity Foundation, which were established in 2010 and 2016, respectively.

Although many centers seek to help cancer patients and their families voluntarily without government supports, these patients and their families are still under the burden of the disease and its consequences. One of the items that can be effective in enhancing and improving patient service is interprofessional and intersectoral collaboration. In other words, there should be proper coordination and collaboration between the health service settings such as home, hospital, primary health care practitioners and health centers, and different levels of health system from health homes to specialty hospitals, NGOs and volunteers can help patients [66].

Today, it is hoped to increase the satisfaction of patients and families and reduce their problems by the development of home-based and community-based care as one of the important and urgent needs of developing communities such as Iran, carried out through the proper provision of this type of care with the aim of organizing, maintaining and coordinating care provision for patients after their discharge from hospital, and also utilizing the capacity and potential of NGOs and charitable centers and organizations [63] which are voluntarily operating in large numbers at the community level.

Barriers to the Provision of Home Care

Providing home care seems to gradually become an alternative to hospital service delivery [25] due to greater satisfaction in patients and their families, and the use of advanced technology, and research results continue to approve home-based hospital care and refer to it as something accepted in today's Iranian society [61, 73].

However, given the prevailing traditional attitude of the Iranian society [28], the economic and social situation conditions of the country and the level of access to various resources, the possibility to provide home care should be investigated. In other words, it is necessary to study the barriers to this type of care. According to the results of many researches, the best approach to the provision of this type of care for cancer patients is to remove some of the main barriers, the most important of which are cultural, spiritual and religious beliefs affecting care, insufficient education of staff, the shortage of specialist staff, the lack of social awareness about the services provided, insufficient funding, the lack of instructions and guidelines and time constraints [73, 90].

Iran has a traditional culture and a religious atmosphere [58] which can have effects on providing home care. Cultural and social factors influence the approach to providing care for patients. In other words, the type of care depends on the context in which the nurse is serving. Even the legal and ethical issues that nurses may face when entering the patient's home depend on the cultural and social background of patients and their families. Therefore, social acceptability is considered a major factor in the development of any plan [91].

On the other hand, the level of knowledge and skills of the care team members is of great importance. These people must receive professional trainings and become qualified to enter patients' homes. In fact, education, necessary competencies and, as a result, social acceptability are among the most important issues to be considered; if not addressed, they will be a barrier to the implementation of home care. Therefore, the lack of educational programs with the aim of empowering professional staff in providing these services has been referred to as an important challenge in Iran [44, 92].

In order to provide specialized staff for home care provision in Iran, experts with Master's degrees in the field of community health nurse were started to be trained. However, despite years of professional training, there is still no skilled nursing force for home care provision, which may be due to the lack of a definition for their position at the community level and the lack of job descriptions for them [93]. In advanced countries, efforts have been made to solve this problem by training nurses in specialist roles and primary care roles, the first one for providing clinic-based care, and the second to provide community-based care. However, given the complexity of providing home care and community-based care, sufficient evidences are not available in this regard [94, 95].

Due to the fact that the society's population is growing older, and subsequently, the prevalence of various chronic diseases, home care is considered as a care delivery model and an important and significant need of the Iranian health system.

Although the implementation of this type of care may be disturbed due to the above barriers, it is possible to establish home care in the best way possible and to overcome these barriers by utilizing the existing potentials, applying functional changes in the nursing education curriculum and using the experiences of leading countries in this regard, as well as conducting appropriate researches.

Long-Term Care Facilities and Hospices

In recent years, rapid advances in the field of early diagnosis and treatment have led to an increase in the number of cancer survivors. In some studies, the survival rate of cancer patients in Iran has been reported to be 85% [24, 34]. The mean age of patients with different types of cancer in Iran is lower than that of other countries. The age of onset is an important factor in the survival rate of these patients. Cancer at an earlier age is associated with increased survival time. Therefore, it can be said that in Iran, cancer patients are mainly younger and experience complications for a longer period of time [3]. However, older survivors experience more complex conditions due to the underlying problems and comorbidities [24].

Cancer survivors, on the other hand, face many unique challenges both short and long term [36], that are related to their physical, mental, family, as well as functional health and lifestyle changes [37]. These patients are exposed to a wide range of complications caused by the disease and treatment, and physical, emotional, mental, social and lifestyle changes that can result in a decreased quality of life [38, 39].

Given the family's vital role in caring for these patients, family members also face many problems and challenges that can lead to a decreased quality of life in them, and thus a decrease in the quality of patient care [40, 41]. Therefore, cancer is considered a chronic disease today, and the main focus is on providing long-term care for cancer patients [96].

In addition, universal health coverage (UHC) is one of the major goals of the World Health Organization and is defined as everybody's having access to health services with the necessary quality, without experiencing financial pressure. It also encompasses a wide range of quality primary health services in the field of prevention, treatment, rehabilitation and palliative care [97]. Since chronic diseases such as cancer can only be managed by providing long-term care [98], it is also necessary and increasingly urgent to establish long-term care systems in Iran [98, 99].

Long-Term Care Facilities

Long-term care includes a variety of services designed to address the health or care needs of an individual either short or long term. These services help the individuals who are unable to carry out their daily activities on their own, need constant care after being discharged from the hospital and need to be provided with care in specific circumstances. The purpose of these services is to help people live as independently and safely as possible. This type of care is provided in different settings, such as homes, nursing homes, day care centers and on the community level, and by different caregivers, formal and informal, depending on the individual's needs [100].

In these systems, appropriate, cost-effective and long-term integrated care is provided for people. Depending on the funding and the national context, care may be provided by families, the civil society, the private sector and/or the public sector. Governments are not obliged to carry out all the activities in this area, and their general responsibility is to ensure the proper functioning of the system [101]. Long-term care systems, including hospices, are necessary in all countries to help improve well-being and to address the needs of the individuals whose capabilities and capacities are reduced. In addition to this need, the available data indicate a large gap between the provision and access to these services in many low- and middle-income countries [102].

The Context of Long-Term Care in Iran

Various studies have emphasized the importance of inpatient care centers, outpatient clinics and home care programs for cancer patients [103, 104]. Literature review shows that in other countries, a variety of care settings are designed and developed to provide long-term care. In Iran, the most common formal pattern of long-term care is nursing homes. In these centers, various groups of people with disabilities and different physical and cognitive conditions, especially the elderly, are accommodated. Many of these centers do not meet the required standards and usually do not provide quality care [105, 106].

However, in Iran, the first legislation in the field of home care dates back to 1999, and these services were initially launched almost 20 years ago. However, an overall assessment shows that these services are not sufficiently and appropriately provided in Iran, and like many other countries, Iran faces many challenges such as care problems, insufficient nursing capabilities (workforce), inappropriate management, the lack of proper infrastructures, cultural issues, improper payment patterns, poor interprofessional coordination and cooperation, and job dissatisfaction [23, 25, 28].

In addition, Iran lacks formal programs and structure to provide palliative services. However, in recent years, few centers have provided palliative care services for cancer patients sporadically, at home and in in-patient wards, mainly in major cities. These services are provided without reference to clinical guidelines and merely based on the caregivers' experience and knowledge [28, 29, 58].

A major challenge in providing long-term care is the provision of stable financial resources [107]. In Iran, no types of long-term care services are currently covered by social insurances, and the costs of these services are paid by families [3]. Moreover, there is no specific insurance coverage such as long-term care insurances, and health and social insurance coverage is subject to the individual's occupational status. In the case of supportive and semi-supportive insurance, only certain social strata are covered. Iran's demographic and economic outlook over the next two decades emphasizes the importance and the necessity of strengthening and expanding insurance plans, given the limited government resources.

It can be said that the infrastructure of long-term care services and programs encompasses all the facilities, policies and laws required in the field of chronic diseases and palliative care [21]. Recently, in regard with the establishment of these services, regulations for the establishment and operation of long-term care and treatment centers, and standard care service packages of care provision for cancer patients and end-of-life patients have been formulated by the Deputy of Nursing of the Ministry of Health and Medical Education for insurance coverage [108], the implementation of which will depend on the pricing of services.

Hospice Care

Due to the significant advances in medicine and an increasing access to various therapeutic and care services, patients with chronic diseases in the advanced and terminal stages also undergo highly invasive treatments. However, these measures are not accompanied by better quality of life and outcome for the patient and family, and are usually in conflict with their preferences. In fact, when long-term treatments are not helpful and death is inevitable, these patients will need to receive special end-of-life care [109, 110].

Patients in end-of-life stages have special and complex physical, social, psychological, spiritual and supportive needs, which if not addressed can make patients and their families uncomfortable and distressed. Some of these needs include the need for pain control, symptom management, a peaceful passing in an environment similar to their own homes, support and serenity, and dealing with disease-related problems [111, 112].

Investigations show that in Iran, the majority of expected deaths occur in hospitals, especially in the intensive care units, while these patients do not receive quality care in the end-of-life stages despite spending high amounts of money [19, 113, 114]. The quality of end-of-life care is a major challenge for patients and their families, and for the health policymakers and professionals to the same extent, and must be provided equally [115]. Therefore, the attention of patients and their families is of particular importance at this stage. Nowadays, the main approach to providing care for patients who are not able to receive homecare is to provide hospice services [115].

Hospice care is considered as a part of long-term care [116] and is a special type of care in which patients with life-threatening and terminal diseases and also those in end-of-life stages benefit from the mental, spiritual and therapeutic support of professional health teams and non-professional teams, such as service volunteers and priests. This type of care focuses on controlling pain and other symptoms of the disease, so that patients can experience more comfort as they approach end of life. Such care is also provided for patients' families [117]. The aim of providing end-of-life care, which is generally ignored in the health system, is to increase the quality of care and the quality of death for patients and support families and caregivers [4].

The Background of Hospice Care in Iran

It can be said that the first Iranian hospice centers were established in the early 1920s to provide care for patients with terminal diseases such as leprosy, tuberculosis and mental illnesses in some cities. However, it was not until 2000 that modern palliative care was first launched in Iran, and the first palliative care center was established in 2006 at the Cancer Institute of Tehran University of Medical Sciences, and service provision mostly began in 2009. Along with the opening of new centers in Tehran, others were launched in cities such as Isfahan and Zanjan [118]. Iran lacks formal plans and structures for providing hospice services and end-of-life services [28, 29, 58].

However, the regulations for the establishment and operation of long-term care and treatment centers also consist of hospice services [108]. Based on the national action plan for non-communicable diseases, plans for the next two decades should focus on the specific needs of patients with the most common chronic diseases, especially cancer. Moreover, studies done in recent years have shown that demand for end-of-life care is increasing and that patients and their families are seeking optimal care [119]. Meanwhile, due to the increasing rate of chronic diseases especially cancer and ageing population, while considering the successful experiences of the developed countries, it is necessary to design and develop hospice services in Iran. However, providing these services depends on various factors such as the cultural and social status of the community [115].

Challenges to the Establishment of Hospice Centers in Iran

In the establishment and development of hospice centers in Iran, important issues should be taken into consideration, which may have facilitating or inhibiting roles in many aspects and lead to the acceptance or rejection of these types of care and centers.

Legal and Ethical Considerations

There are also legal and ethical problems and limitations which need further inconsideration prior to designing and developing hospice centers in Iran. For example, the necessity of performing resuscitation operation despite the patient's irreversibility, due to the lack of written DNR instructions for the end-of-life patients and religious barriers, the need to carefully record measures during resuscitation from the fear of complaints and legal accountability, and the lack of clinical guidelines and protocols regarding the end-of-life care [120].

In addition, in the Iranian health system, patients and families usually play no role in deciding whether to continue or stop the treatment [119]. The major challenge in this regard is the opposing opinions and points of disagreement between the medical staff and the patient's relatives concerning treatments that are medically useless or ineffective according to the physicians, but is requested by relatives. On the contrary, there are medical suggestions and treatments that are considered useful by the medical staff, but are not accepted by the patient or relatives due to treatment costs or other reasons. In such cases, legal and ethical challenges increase when the patient is willing to undergo these measures, but the relatives are reluctant to accept or to take action after only apparently accepting it [110, 121].

Finally, any of the above cultural-religious, ethical and legal issues can be considered as either an opportunity or a threat to designing and development of hospice services in Iran. However, in the Iranian society, culture and religion are obviously the two important factors in the social perception of end-of-life issues [122]. Moreover, the key role of families in providing hospice services cannot be ignored [123]. It is also necessary to fill the legal and ethical gaps before designing and developing hospice centers.

Cultural and Religious Issues

Over 98% of the Iranian population are Muslims and Iran is considered a religious country. The issue of death and the end-of-life stage is strongly and explicitly linked to religious beliefs. From Quran's perspective, Muslim's holy book, the afterlife world is the real world, and death is unpredictable and inevitable [124]. On the contrary, Islam has mentioned the inherent values and the sanctity of life, and regarded the worldly life as a worthwhile opportunity for mankind to move toward a better future in the eternal world of the afterlife, and the preservation of life as a duty. Humans need time and should pass the stages of spiritual journey in this world to reach the ultimate perfection. Thus, paying attention to the worldly life is of great importance, and many Muslim prayers focus on seeking prolonged life from God [122].

Accordingly, every type of care with the aim of meeting this necessity in life is considered sacred. Therefore, the most important right of a dying person, like other living individuals, is to keep hope and be provided with care until death, by those who can keep his/her hopes alive. Dying individuals should be able to express their feelings and attitudes toward the proximity of death in their own way and must not be deceived. They should be supported by their families, be helped to accept death and pass away in peace and with dignity. They should not be judged by others, and their personalities should be respected. They must participate in decision-making regarding their own care, must not die alone and must be relieved from pain. Their questions should be answered correctly, and their bodies should be cleaned and respected. Moreover, in all cultures and particularly Islam, there is valuable and profound religious advice for patients and their relatives to manage this period of life [18].

Therefore, the acceptance of hospice care in Iran is considered a paradox. In the Iranian society, given the human values concerning life and death, the importance of religion, and the society and the public believing that their loved ones should be provided with the end-of-life care as well as possible, it seems that these services will be welcome. In addition to these issues, the problems and concerns of families regarding the provision of end-of-life care for their patients, such as lack of knowledge and insufficient time, duplicate the need for these centers. However, on the other hand, in the traditional society of Iran, the religious and cultural beliefs and issues of patients and their families may lead to the rejection of these types of services in hospice centers [125].

According to the studies conducted, caring for end-of-life patients, despite being irreversible, requires to be continued until the last moment, in spite of the imminent death. This commitment is rooted in religious attitudes and the caregivers and families' belief in miracles and the possibility of unexpected return to life until the last moment. Additionally, based on Iranian Muslim's particular value system concerning death, caregivers and patients consider end-of-life care as a valuable opportunity offered by God, and believe that they have been given a special privilege which will have good results and leave valuable experiences in their lives [119].

One of the most important parts of end-of-life care is religious care, which is mainly provided by the patient and his/her family [126]. Furthermore, the cultural and religious structure of the country has led even health professionals to have a negative attitude toward euthanasia and the end of life, despite the patient's being untreatable [125].

On the other hand, culture is considered to be a determining factor in health care due to its impact on lifestyle, beliefs and values, the individuals' perception of quality of life and palliative care, the interaction with the health care system, and decision-making during the illness and end-of-life stages [123]. Numerous studies have shown that individuals' cultural background and their ethnicity/race have a relationship with their end-of-life preferences. Therefore, along with the facilities and resources available in the health system of each country in designing a specific service delivery structure, patients' choice is also of significant importance [123, 127]. Choosing a place for care and going through the end-of-life stages and also the place of death are influenced by the social and demographic characteristics of patients and their caregivers [123] and are rooted in culture [128].

Many Iranian families still want to receive services in their homes [129], despite the fact that the results of some studies in Iran emphasize the establishment of centers dedicated to end-of-life care and hospice service provision [119, 130]. The participants in the study conducted by Heidari et al. preferred to receive end-of-life care first at home and then in hospital rather than hospice centers [131]. In addition, Estebsari et al. have considered home care and being with the family in the familiar environment of home as factors affecting the patient's quality of life in the end-of-life stage [132].

In Iranian culture and society, extended families with traditional structures mostly tend to provide care for patients, especially in the end-of-life stage, and prefer to care for their dying patients at home [133]. However, some recent studies have also indicated that Iranian families face issues and have concerns about providing end-of-life care due to economic and livelihoods problems, family nucleation and being too busy [125, 131]. Therefore, the patient's and his/her family's preference to receive palliative home care, especially in the end-of-life stage, needs further investigation [123, 128, 129].

Early discussion of the prognosis of disease and end-of-life care options will contribute to faster acceptance of palliative care at these stages. The tendency to tell or know the truth about the disease or death is considered a value in Western cultures, and every patient has the right to know about his/her condition, so that he/she can make decisions about the end-of-life care. However, in some societies, talking about the diagnosis, prognosis and death is a taboo, as it kills hope and leads to concerns of reduced adherence to treatment [134].

In Iranian culture, it is also common to hide the truth about the disease and death from the patient, and these cases are only told to the patient's family, mostly at the family's request, which is because it is believed that the truth will cause hopelessness and increased suffering and discomfort in the patient. However, in some cases, studies have suggested that patients prefer to know about the disease, its diagnosis and its prognosis [120, 134]. In addition, the Iranian society has a variety of ethnicities and subcultures that have impacts on their health behaviors and beliefs [121]. The results of some studies have indicated that cultural differences have had a major impact on the acceptance and the use of hospice services. These differences should be taken into account while designing and developing these services in each society [135].

Ethical Challenges to Providing Community-Based Services

The expansion of palliative care in the community is a symbol of respect for the dignity and heeding the wishes of every single patient for the rest of his/her life, and has been raised as an ethical responsibility. Since palliative care is more focused on the patient's life and death, most care teams are faced with the question "What is the right decision?" Thus, the ethical challenges increase in this type of care. The following are some of these challenges considering ethical principles.

The Principle of Autonomy

In Iran, due to the stigma of cancer which is a reflection of mortality and death, and also due to the types of family relations and emotional bonds, physicians choose not to tell the truth to patients. However, in recent years, patients' right to receive information and make free decisions while receiving health services has been one of the five principles of the patient's bill of rights, which is imposed by the Health Deputy of the Ministry of Health and Medical Education to health centers, and has been considered an indicator in the evaluation of health centers in recent years [136]. In addition, the formulation of a palliative care ethical guideline is another action taken in Iran, according to which, the patient is the primary decision-maker [137]. In addition, the codes of ethics approved by the Ministry of Health have been communicated to universities, and the establishment of ethics committees in hospitals and universities is emphasized, in order to prevent arbitrary reactions to ethical challenges in providing care for cancer patients.

Benefit and Do-No-Harm Principle

When a patient's condition is deteriorating and the treatment is ineffective, end-of-life care plans are brought up in order to avoid futile care, leading to medical, legal and ethical challenges [138]. Futile treatments increase the quantity by prolonging the patient's life while ignoring the quality of the remaining life which is the ultimate goal of palliative care [139]. Although AAP has prohibited heavy treatments in order to maximize the quality of life at the end of life, there are still different opinions surrounding this issue. The attitude of the treatment team is an important factor in end-of-life care [140]. The results of another study in Iran showed that 78% of patients and 63% of physicians agreed with performing at least one case of euthanasia. Voluntary active euthanasia and voluntary passive euthanasia, in which the treatment is withdrawn, were the types of euthanasia upon which patients mostly agreed [141].

However, according to the principles of Islamic jurisprudence, Do-Not-Resuscitate, that is, ending one's life, is unacceptable and there is no official law for this purpose in the country. According to Islam, human life is a divine blessing that one must strive to preserve, and no one can even decide about ending his/her life. Therefore, helping to end one's life and active euthanasia are rejected, in any form [142].

Since there are no approved ethical and clinical guidelines for DNR in Iran, decisions for DNR are made by the treating physician and, in many cases, without the patient or family's awareness. In line with the increasing public pressure for the legal recognition of euthanasia in order to end the suffering caused by terminal diseases, it is increasingly necessary to pay more attention to the ethical issues for improving palliative care. To this end, Peimani et al. have suggested to formulate a national NDR guideline in accordance with the ethical principles, scientific standards and Iranian native culture [143].

The Principle of Justice

Discrimination in accessing health care, along with a significant increase in the costs of treatment, has caused challenges on the way of establishing social justice as an ethical principle. In Iran, according to the studies on the palliative care, the fair distribution of resources, as well as easy access to services are reported as patients' basic needs [52, 54]. Studies on the classification of palliative care services as well as designing a palliative care model in hospice and home care structures would address the need for the provision of community-based services [144].

At present, economic problems have been reported as a cause to impose burden on families [145]; thus, some patients may not be able to afford the costs due to financial problems and are deprived of these services. Therefore, protecting this vulnerable group is an ethical responsibility that requires easy access to palliative care services. Policymakers are bringing up and developing palliative care packages, in response to this need in cooperation with the Deputy of Treatment and Deputy of Nursing of the Ministry of Health, and insurance companies.

Challenges to Providing Community-Based Services

UHC needs fair, effective and efficient health systems that address priority health care needs through integrated and people-centered care. The quantitative and qualitative availability of health care workers is an essential factor in achieving UHC [146]. In line with accessing human resources, nurses, as the frontline health workers, play a vital and key role in achieving the goal of universal health coverage [147]. The 66th Session of the WHO's Regional Committee for the Eastern Mediterranean Health Ministers has emphasized the designing plans to promote and enhance community health nursing, with regard to the importance of nursing services in health service systems and its role in the universal health coverage. Additionally, with the beginning of 2020, designated by the WHO as the "Year of Nurses and Midwives", this organization has compelled governments to empower nurses and midwives at various levels of service provision, including community-based care provision [148].

However, community health nurses are currently facing barriers and challenges in providing specialty services in the form of specialized job descriptions developed by the Ministry of Health [24], and these nurses offer services in hospitals rather than in the community. The attitude of most Iranian health policymakers revolves around the employment of nurses at the secondary level of prevention, that is, clinical care in hospitals [10, 12].

The nurses' role in providing quality primary health care and universal health coverage is of great importance. Therefore, policies should be made for training and recruiting nurses in the field of PHC [149, 150].

Heydari et al. (2017), in a qualitative study with the aim of investigating the position of community-based nursing in Iran, showed that there were no job opportunities to hire community health nurses in comprehensive health centers, that policymakers' attitude toward the community-based nursing is not positive and that the community is not yet prepared to accept community-based nursing services [151].

According to the World Health Organization's report, physician-based management is one of the threats to the Iranian health system [27]. Therefore, despite the fact that educating and training community health nurses with Master's degrees is costly for the government, their expertise is of no use [151, 152].

Conclusion

In regard to the increasing need for UHC and the necessity of receiving cost-effective, available and fair services, the primary level of the health system is considered an appropriate context for the provision of palliative care services. However, given the absence of a referral system, there is virtually no link between the primary level of service delivery, that is, community-based care, and the secondary level, that is, hospital-based services. Therefore, shifting care settings from hospitals to the community level faces serious challenges.

Despite the importance of community-based services, barriers such as the community's ignorance of these services; cultural, religious and social barriers; the lack of insurance coverage for these services; the lack of employment of appropriate forces at the community level as well as the lack of a referral system and relationship between first and second levels of service delivery are also influential in shifting the palliative care services to the community.

Given that the preliminary structures for the establishment of community-based palliative care system are already in place, and given the potentials, such a system can be established in the not-too-distant future.

Acknowledgement The authors would like to express their gratitude to Professor Michael Silbermann for his efforts at establishing a palliative care system in Middle East countries and to Professor Mohammad-Esmaeil Akbari, the Head of the Cancer Research Center of Shahid Beheshti University of Medical Sciences, for his support and guidance.

References

1. Fernanda Raphael Escobar Gimenes, Faleiros F. Nursing challenges for the 21st century. J Nurs Care. 2014;3:1. https://doi.org/10.4172/2167-1168.1000143.
2. Koponen P. Community nursing in Finland: the division of fields of activity and patterns of care: comprehensive or specialized care? Scand J Caring Sci. 1995;9(4):203–8.
3. Kashef R. Long-term care, occupational illnesses and work-related accidents in social health insurance. Q J Soc Secur. 2007;9(4):81–98.
4. Khanali Mojen L. Palliative care in Iran: the past, the present and the future. Support Palliat Care Cancer. 2017;1(1):8–11.
5. Laurant M, van der Biezen M, Wijers N, Watananirun K, Kontopantelis E, van Vught AJ. Nurses as substitutes for doctors in primary care. Cochrane Database Syst Rev. 2018;7:CD001271.
6. Shariati M. Why health reform? and how? J Knowl Health Basic Med Sci. 2010;5(Summer 2010: Supplement):20–1.
7. World Health Organization ROfS-EA. Comprehensive community- and home-based health care model. New Delhi: WHO Regional Office for South-East Asia; 2004.
8. Underwood J. Maximizing community health nursing capacity in Canada: a research summary for decision makers. Canadian Health Services Research Foundation Health Canada. 2010. https://www.cfhi-fcass.ca/Migrated/PDF/ResearchReports/11510_Reiss_report_en_FINAL.
9. Sadat Hosseini A, Cheraghi M, Shali M, Javaheri F. Neuman theory application in solution of Iranian nursing Education and care challenges. Iran J Syst Rev Med Sci. 2017;1:1–14.
10. Yazdani S, Nikravan Mofrad M, Ahmadi S, Zagheri Tafreshi M. An analysis of policies of the Iranian health care system in relation to the nursing profession. J Qual Res Health Sci. 2016;5(2):211–20.
11. Ahmadian S, Mokhtari J. A review of the evolution and challenges in nursing role development. Iran J Med Ethics Hist Med. 2017;9(6):48–60.
12. Heidary A, Mazlom SR, Ildarabadi E. Nursing's position in health care delivery system in Iran. Iran J Nurs Res. 2012;7(25):37–44.
13. NHS England/Nursing. Framework for commissioning community nursing. 2015. https://www.england.nhs.uk.
14. Karimi S, Javadi M, Jafarzadeh F. Economic burden and costs of chronic diseases in Iran and the world. Health Inf Manag. 2012;8:984–96.
15. Nugent R. Chronic diseases in developing countries: health and economic burdens. Ann N Y Acad Sci. 2008;1136:70–9.
16. WHO. Package of essential noncommunicable (PEN) disease interventions for primary health care in low-resource settings. 2010. https://www.who.int.
17. Bahramnezhad F, Askari P, Shiri M, Sanaie N. Concept of palliative care of the end of life from the perspective of the Quran and Hadith. Quran Med. 2018;3(4):193–8.
18. Cheraghi MA, Payne S, Salsali M. Spiritual aspects of end-of-life care for Muslim patients: experiences from Iran. Int J Palliat Nurs. 2005;11(9):468–74.
19. Feizi E, Eydi M, Ansar IM. Mortality rate and effective factors of patients in intensive care unit. J Ardabil Univ Med Sci. 2008;8(4):420–3. (Persian).
20. Kruse C, Mileski M, Vijaykumar A, Viswanathan Vishnampet S, Suskandla U, Chidambaram Y. Impact of electronic health records on long-term care facilities: systematic review. JMIR Med Inform. 2017;5:e35.
21. Safdari R, Sadeghi F, Mohammadiazar M. Aged care and services programs in Iran: looking at the performance of relevant organizations. Payavard Salamat. 2016;10(2):155–66.
22. Nikbakht Nasrabadi A, Shabany HM. Providing healthcare services at home-A necessity in Iran: a narrative review article. Iran J Public Health. 2016;45(7):867–74.
23. Fatemi NL, Moonaghi H, Heydari A. Perceived challenges faced by nurses in home health care setting: a qualitative study. Int J Community Based Nurs Midwifery. 2019;7:118–27.
24. Maajani K, Khodadost M, Fattahi A, Shahrestanaki E, Pirouzi A, Khalili F, et al. Survival rate of colorectal cancer in Iran: a systematic review and meta-analysis. Asian Pac J Cancer Prev. 2019;20(1):13.
25. Nikbakht-Nasrabadi A, Shabany-Hamedan M. Providing healthcare services at home-a neces-

sity in Iran: a narrative review article. Iran J Public Health. 2016;45(7):867.
26. Genet N, Boerma WG, Kringos DS, Bouman A, Francke AL, Fagerstrom C, et al. Home care in Europe: a systematic literature review. BMC Health Serv Res. 2011;11:207.
27. Heydari H, Shahsavari H, Hazini A, Nasrabadi AN. Exploring the barriers of home care services in Iran: a qualitative study. Scientifica. 2016;2016:2056470.
28. Rassouli M, Sajjadi M. Palliative care in the Islamic Republic of Iran. In: Silberman M, editor. Palliative care to the cancer patient: the Middle East as a model for emerging countries. New York: Nova; 2014. p. 39–52.
29. Abedi M. Palliative care within the Iranian context: re-defining palliative care, deploying spirituality as a support measure and need for cultural sensitivity. 2012. Available at: http://www.inter-disciplinary.net.
30. Rassouli M, Sajjadi M. Palliative care in Iran: moving toward the development of palliative care for cancer. Am J Hosp Palliat Med. 2016;33(3):240–4.
31. Bray F, Ferlay J, Soerjomataram I, Siegel RL, Torre LA, Jemal A. Global cancer statistics 2018: GLOBOCAN estimates of incidence and mortality worldwide for 36 cancers in 185 countries. CA Cancer J Clin. 2018;68(6):394–424.
32. World Health Organization. Noncommunicable diseases (NCD) country profiles. 2018. Available from: http://www.who.int. Accessed 28 Oct 2018.
33. Iran's Cancer Registry System. 2013. Avilable at: August 2013.
34. Fallahzadeh H, Momayyezi M, Akhundzardeini R, Zarezardeini S. Five year survival of women with breast cancer in Yazd. Asian Pac J Cancer Prev. 2014;15:6597–601.
35. Rahimzadeh M, Pourhoseingholi MA, Kavehie B. Survival rates for breast cancer in Iranian patients: a meta-analysis. Asian Pac J Cancer Prev. 2016;17:2223–7.
36. Shirinabadi Farahani A, Rassouli M, Salmani N, Mojen L, Sajjadi M, Heidarzadeh M, et al. Evaluation of health-care providers' perception of spiritual care and the obstacles to its implementation. Asia Pac J Oncol Nurs. 2019;6(2):122–9.
37. Abdollahimohammad A, Firouzkouhi M, Naderifar M. Lived experiences of Iranian cancer patients after survival: a phenomenological research. J Patient Exp. 2019;6(2):164–8.
38. Faghani S, Mohammadian R, Rahmani A, Mohajjel-Aghdam A, Hassankhani H, Azadi A. Supportive care needs of Iranian cancer survivors and relationships with social support. Asian Pac J Cancer Prev. 2015;16(15):6339–45.
39. Naughton M, Weaver K. Physical and mental health among cancer survivors: considerations for long-term care and quality of life. N C Med J. 2014;75:283–6.
40. Nemati S, Rassouli M, Ilkhani M, Baghestani AR. Perceptions of family caregivers of cancer patients about the challenges of caregiving: a qualitative study. Scand J Caring Sci. 2018;32(1): 309–16.
41. Torkzahrani S, Rastegari L, Khodakarami N, Akbarzadeh-Baghian A, Alizadeh K. Quality of life and its related factors among Iranian cervical cancer survivors. Iran Red Crescent Med J. 2013;15: 320–3.
42. Sajjadi M, Rassouli M, Abbaszadeh A, Alavi Majd H, Zendehdel K. Psychometric properties of the Persian version of the Mishel's Uncertainty in Illness Scale in patients with cancer. Eur J Oncol Nurs. 2014;18(1):52–7.
43. www.cancer.org/treatment.
44. Rassouli M, Shirinabadi Farahani A, Khanali Mojen L. Palliative care perspectives and practices in the Islamic republic of Iran, and their implication on patients' quality of life. In: Silbermann M, editor. Palliative care: perspectives, practices and impact on quality of life. New York: Nova Scientific; 2017.
45. Cancer Research Center. Development of a comprehensive national program for palliative and supportive cancer care project [Persian]. 2014. Available at: http://crc.tums.ac.ir/Default.aspx?tabid=519. Accessed November.
46. World Health Organization. Why palliative care is an essential function of primary health car. 2016. Available from: https://www.who.int.
47. Health mo. Cancer Care Development Network. Available from: http://behdasht.gov.ir.
48. Mojen LK, Rassouli M, Eshghi P, Sari AA, Karimooi MH. Palliative care for children with cancer in the Middle East: a comparative study. Indian J Palliat Care. 2017;23(4):379.
49. Farahani AS, Rassouli M, Mojen LK, Ansari M, Ebadinejad Z, Tabatabaee A, et al. The feasibility of home palliative care for cancer patients: the perspective of Iranian nurses. Int J Cancer Manag. 2018;11(8):e80114.
50. Nasiripour AA, Rezaei B, Yarmohammadian MH, Maleki MR. A comparative study of primary health care management in selected countries and designing a model for Iran. Iran J Nurs Midwifery Res. 2009;14(3):137–42.
51. Deputy of Nursing MoH. Palliative care. Available from: http://behdasht.gov.ir/news.
52. Mojen LK, Rassouli M, Eshghi P, Zendedel K, Sari AA, Karimooi MH, et al. Pediatric palliative care in Iran: applying regionalization of health care systems. Asian Pac J Cancer Prev. 2018;19(5):1303.
53. Davari M. Economic challenges of the Iranian health system. J Health Inf. 2012;8(7):915–8.
54. Khoshnazar TA, Rassouli M, Akbari ME, Lotfi-Kashani F, Momenzadeh S, Haghighat S, et al. Structural challenges of providing palliative care for patients with breast cancer. Indian J Palliat Care. 2016;22(4):459–66.
55. Palliative Care in NSW. What are "end of life care" and "palliative care"? https://www.health.nsw.gov.au/palliativecare.

56. Bycroft K, Drake R, Glavish N, et al. Guidance for integrated paediatric palliative care services in New Zealand. Report to the Ministry of Health. 2012.
57. www.hamshahrionline.ir/news.
58. Rassoul IM, Sajjadi M. Cancer care in countries in transition: the Islamic Republic of Iran. In: Silbermann M, editor. Palliative care in countries & societies in transition. Cham: Springer; 2016.
59. http://ino.ir/TabId/8563/ArtMID.
60. http://behdasht.gov.ir.
61. Ghanbari Khanghah A, Baghfalaki M. Nurses' perspectives of nursing research priorities about cancer patients. Iran J Nurs. 2009;22(57):87–97.
62. Ferrell BR, Coyle N, Paice J. Oxford textbook of palliative nursing. New York: Oxford University Press; 2015.
63. Barati A, Janati A, Tourani S, Khalesi N, Gholizadeh M. Iranian professional's perception about advantages of developing home health care system in Iran. Hakim Health Syst Res J. 2010;13(2):71–9.
64. Department of Health. National guideline on home-based care and community-based care. Pretoria: Government Printers; 2001. https://www.western-cape.gov.za. Accessed 21 Feb 2019.
65. Adib-Hajbaghery M, Maghaminejad F, Abbasi A. The role of continuous care in reducing readmission for patients with heart failure. J Caring Sci. 2013;2(4):255.
66. Seow H, Bainbridge D. A review of the essential components of quality palliative care in the home. J Palliat Med. 2017;21(S1):S37–44.
67. Kok L, Berden C, Sadiraj K. Costs and benefits of home care for the elderly versus residential care: a comparison using propensity scores. Eur J Health Econ. 2015;16(2):119–31.
68. O'Connor M, Hanlon A, Naylor M, Bowles K. The impact of home health length of stay and number of skilled nursing visits on hospitalization among Medicare-reimbursed skilled home health beneficiaries. Res Nurs Health. 2015;38(4):257–67.
69. Abusalem S, Myers JA, Aljeesh Y. Patient satisfaction in home health care. J Clin Nurs. 2013;22(17–18):2426–35.
70. Carpenter I, Gambassi G, Topinkova E, Schroll M, Finne-Soveri H, Henrard J-C, et al. Community care in Europe. The aged in home care project (AdHOC). Aging Clin Exp Res. 2004;16(4):259–69.
71. Rassouli M, Shirinabadi Farahani A, Khanali Mojen L. Palliative care research in Iran: a review of current status. In: Silbermann M, editor. Palliative care: the role and importance of research in promoting palliative carecpractice, vol. 3. New York: Nova Scientific Publisher. A Global View; 2019. p. 273–308.
72. Shahsavari H, Nasrabadi A, Almasian M, Heydari H, Hazini A. Exploration of the administrative aspects of the delivery of home health care services: a qualitative study. Asia Pac Fam Med. 2018;17(1):1.
73. Shirinabadi Farahani A, Rassouli M, Khanali Mojen L, Ansari M, Ebadinejad Z, Tabatabaee A, et al. The feasibility of home palliative care for cancer patients: the perspective of Iranian nurses. Int J Cancer Manag. 2018;11(8):e80114.
74. Davari M, Haycox A, Walley T. Health care financing in Iran; is privatization a good solution? Iran J Public Health. 2012;41(7):14–23.
75. Mehrdad R. Health system in Iran. JMAJ. 2009;52(1):69–73.
76. Home Care Unit 2016 1/101 /D [Internet]. Podcast.
77. Home Base Care Unit. http://dn.behdasht.gov.ir.
78. Standard End of Life Care Service Package. https://www.isna.ir.
79. http://dn.behdasht.gov.ir.
80. Eshaghian-Dorcheh A, Zandi M, Rassouli M, Tahmasebi M. The lack of systematic training for health care providers, a challenge for providing pediatric palliative home care: a comparative study. Int J Pediatr. 2019;7(5):9481–96.
81. European Society for Medical Oncology. A guide for patients with advanced cancer. Lugano: ESMO; 2011. Available from: https://www.esmo.org. Accessed 9 Mar 2019.
82. Kitreerawutiwong N, Mekrungrengwong S, Keeratisiroj O. The development of the community-based palliative care model in a district health system, Phitsanulok Province, Thailand. Indian J Palliat Care. 2018;24(4):436–45.
83. Aqabrary A, Ahmadi F, Mohammad AA, Hajizadeh A, Farahani A. Dimensions of physical, psychological and social quality of life in women with breast cancer the chemotherapy. Nurs Res. 2007;1(3):55–65.
84. Cai J, Guerriere DN, Zhao H, Coyte PC. Correlation of palliative performance scale and survival in patients with cancer receiving home-based palliative care. J Palliat Care. 2018;33(2):95–9.
85. Weng LC, Huang HL, Wilkie DJ, Hoenig NA, Suarez ML, Marschke M, et al. Predicting survival with the Palliative Performance Scale in a minority-serving hospice and palliative care program. J Pain Symptom Manag. 2009;37(4):642–8.
86. Danaei G, Farzadfar F, Kelishadi R, Rashidian A, Rouhani OM, Ahmadnia S, et al. Iran in transition. Lancet. 2019;393(10184):1984–2005.
87. Zanganeh Baygi M, Seyedin H, Salehi M, Jafari Sirizi M. Structural and contextual dimensions of Iranian primary health care system at local level. Iran Red Crescent Med J. 2015;17(1):e17222.
88. Kheshabi J. Abstract book of first national cancer seminar. Sanandaj [Persian]. 2011. Available at: http://www.iausdj.ac.ir. Accessed 30 July 2014.
89. National Cancer Control Programs. https://phc.umsu.ac.ir.
90. Brant JM, Fink RM, Thompson C, Li YH, Rassouli M, Majima T, et al. Global survey of the roles, satisfaction, and barriers of home health care nurses on the provision of palliative care. J Palliat Med. 2019;22(8):945–60.
91. Skovdal M, Mushati P, Robertson L, Munyati S, Sherr L, Nyamukapa C, et al. Social acceptability and perceived impact of a community-led cash trans-

fer programme in Zimbabwe. BMC Public Health. 2013;13(1):342.
92. Irajpour A, Alavi M, Izadikhah A. Situation analysis and designing an interprofessional curriculum for palliative care of the cancer patients. IJME. 2015;14(12):1047–56.
93. Sajjadi M, Rassouli M, Khanali Mojen L. Nursing education in palliative care in Iran. J Palliat Care Med. 2015;54(1):1–5.
94. Koy V. Policy recommendations to enhance nursing education and services among Asean member countries. IJAM. 2017;2(3):6.
95. Elliott L, Kennedy C, Raeside R. Professional role identity in shaping community nurses' reactions to nursing policy. J Nurs Manag. 2015;23(4): 459–67.
96. Lin C-C. When cancer care becomes a long-term care issue: are we ready? Cancer Nurs. 2017;40:341–2.
97. Sarah LB, Megumi R. Aging and universal health coverage: implications for the Asia Pacific region. Health Syst Reform. 2017;3(3):154–8.
98. Sloane P, Zimmerman S, D'Souza M. What will long-term care be like in 2040? N C Med J. 2014;75:326–30.
99. Rahimi M, Fadayevatan R, Abedi H. Care instability in nursing homes; A qualitative study. Innov Aging. 2017;1(Suppl 1):628–9.
100. Douglas AS. Effective management of long-term care facilities. 3rd ed. Burlington: Jones & Bartlett Learning; 2014.
101. WHO. Long-term-care systems. 2019. Available at: https://www.who.int/ageing/long-term-care/en/. Accessed 23 Oct 2019.
102. Tahmasebi M. Palliative care in Iran: a long, long way to go. Basic Clin Cancer Res. 2018;10(3): 34–7.
103. Ashrafian S, Feizollahzadeh H, Rahmani A, Davoodi A. The unmet needs of the family caregivers of patients with cancer visiting a referral hospital in Iran. Asia Pac J Oncol Nurs. 2018;5:342–52.
104. Hashemi M, Irajpour A, Taleghani F. Caregivers needing care: the unmet needs of the family caregivers of end-of-life cancer patients. Suppor Care Cancer. 2018;26(3):759–66.
105. Nasiri M, Foroughan M, Rashedi V, Makarem A, Mourjan B. Compliance to universal design criteria in nursing homes of Tehran. Iran J Ageing. 2016;11:340–7.
106. Regulations the Ministry of Health. Laws of establishment to provide clinical services and health care at home medcare. 2013. Available from: http://darman.umsu.ac.ir.
107. Kruse C, Mileski M, Vijaykumar AG, Viswanathan SV, Suskandla U, Chidambaram Y. Impact of electronic health records on long-term care facilities: systematic review. JMIR Med Inform. 2017;5(3):e35.
108. Ministry of Health and Medical Education. Setting the regulation of the long term care centers establishment [Online]. 2019 July 20 [cited 2019 July]. Available from: http://dn.behdasht.gov.ir/news.
109. Ghaljeh M, Rezaee N. Experiences of nurses about end-of-life care for cancer patients in Iran: a qualitative study. Iran J Nurs. 2018;31(114): 65–75.
110. Mobasher M, Aramesh K, Zahedi F, Nakhaee N, Tahmasebi M, Larijani B. End-of-life care ethical decision-making: Shiite scholars' views. J Med Ethics Hist Med. 2014;7:2.
111. Hatamipour K, Rassouli M, Yaghmaie F, Zendedel K, Alavi Majd H. Spiritual needs of cancer patients: a qualitative study. Indian J Palliat Care. 2015;21(1):61–7.
112. Sotoudeh S, Mahdav IH, Tahmasebi M. Crises in caring for dying patients regarding cancer within Iranian cultural backgrounds: a systematic review of qualitative studies. Int J Cancer Manag. 2019;12(2):e87245.
113. Ziloochi MH, Pourreza A, Akbari F, Rahimi-Foroshani A. Evaluating the hospitalization costs for elderly patients in teaching hospitals of Kashan university of medical sciences during 2009-10. Feyz J Kashan Univ Med Sci. 2012;16(1):86–94.
114. Amiresmaili MR, Imani E, Amin JS. Evaluation of terminal life cost for patients admitted in teaching hospitals affiliated with Kerman University of Medical Sciences in 2014. J Health-Based Res. 2015;1(2):133–43. (Persian).
115. Aghdam A, Aghaei M, Hassankhani H, Rahmani A. Awareness and attitude of nurses in regard to providing hospice care. Asian Pac J Cancer Prev. 2015;16(16):6941–5.
116. Hui D, Cruz M, Mori M, Parsons H, Kwon JH, Torres-Vigil I, et al. Concepts and definitions for "supportive care," "best supportive care," "palliative care," and "hospice care" in the published literature, dictionaries, and textbooks. Support Care Cancer. 2013;21:659–85.
117. National Hospice and Palliative Care Organization. NHPCO's facts and figures on hospice [Online]. 2019 May 4 [cited 2018 April 10]. Available from: https://www.nhpco.org/hospice-statistics-research-press-room/facts-hospice-and-palliative-care.
118. Borhani F, Hosseini S, Abbaszadeh A. Commitment to care: a qualitative study of intensive care nurses' perspectives of end-of-life care in an I slamic context. Int Nurs Rev. 2014;61(1):140–7.
119. Mogadasian S, Abdollahzadeh F, Rahmani A, Ferguson C, Pakanzad F, Pakpour V, et al. The attitude of Iranian nurses about do not resuscitate orders. Indian J Palliat Care. 2014;20:21–5.
120. Motlagh A, Yaraei N, Mafi AR, Hosseini Kamal F, Yaseri M, Hemati S, et al. Attitude of cancer patients toward diagnosis disclosure and their preference for clinical decision-making: a national survey. Arch Iran Med. 2014;17(4):232–40.
121. Zamani A, Shahsanai A, Kivan S, Hematti S, Mokarian F. Iranian physicians and patients attitude toward truth telling of cancer. J Isfahan Med Sch. 2011;29(143):752–9.

122. Banazadeh M, Azizzadeh Foroozy M, Iranmanesh S. Assessment of Barriers in providing end of life care to terminally ill pediatric patients from the perspective of nursing staff. Iran J Pediatr Nurs. 2015;1(2):74–85.
123. Azami-Aghdash S, Ghojazadeh M, Aghaei M, Naghavi-Behzad M, Asgarlo Z. Perspective of patients, patients' families, and healthcare providers towards designing and delivering hospice care services in a middle income country. Indian J Palliat Care. 2015;21(3):341–8.
124. Kazemi A-o-h, Kazemi M, Abbasi M, Kiyani M, Feyzollahi N, Ataloo S, et al. Assessing end of life support. J Med Ethics Hist Med. 2012;5(2):45–57.
125. Bahramnezhad F, Askari P, Shiri M, Sanaie N. Concept of palliative care of the end of life from the perspective of the Quran and Hadith. J Quran Med. 2018;3(4):193–8.
126. Hatamipour K, Rassouli M, Yaghmaie F, Zendedel K, Majd HA. Spiritual needs of cancer patients: a qualitative study. Indian J Palliat Care. 2015;21(1):61–7.
127. Alborzi J, Sabeti F, Baraz S, Miladinia M, Saidkhani V, Sharhani A. Investigating of moral distress and attitude to euthanasia in the intensive care unit nurses. Int J Pediatr. 2018;6(11):8475–82.
128. Park NS, Jang Y, Ko JE, Chiriboga DA. Factors affecting willingness to use hospice in racially/ethnically diverse older men and women. Am J Hosp Palliat Med. 2016;33(8):770–6.
129. Slomka J, Prince-Paul M, Webel A, Daly B. Palliative care, hospice, and advance care planning: views of people living with HIV and other chronic conditions. J Assoc Nurses AIDS Care. 2016;27:476.
130. Razzak R, Smith T. Palliative care: a new and emerging paradigm. In: Silbermann M, editor. Palliative care to the cancer patient: the Middle East as a model for emerging countries. Hauppauge: Nova Science Publishers, Inc; 2014. p. 223–38.
131. Heidari M, Hoseinkhani N, Norouzzadeh R. Education for nurses about end-of-life concerns of the elderly. J Nurs Educ. 2018;7(2):35–44.
132. Estebsari FF, Taghdisi MH, Mostafaei D, Latifi M, Estebsari K. A qualitative study on affecting factors on quality of life in end-stage patients. Iran J Health Educ Health Promot. 2015;2(4):290–302.
133. Fallahi S, Rassouli M, Mojen L. Cultural aspects of palliative cancer care in Iran. Palliat Med Hosp Care Open J. 2017;SE(1):S44–50.
134. Senel G, Silbermann M. Cultural challenges in implementing palliative programs in emerging countries. Palliat Med Hosp Care Open J. 2017;SE(1):S1–3.
135. Aseyedali M, Sadeghi Mahalli N, Norouzi Tabrizi K. A review on adult daycare centers in the world. Iran J Ageing. 2019;13(4):518–29.
136. Parsapoor A, Bagheri A, Larijani B. Review of revolution of patient's right charter. IJME. 2010;3(1):39–47.
137. Department of Medical Ethics IoEaM, Tehran University of Medical Sciences, Tehran, Iran. National ethical guidelines on palliative care in end-of-life patients. 2019. Available from: http://file.qums.ac.ir.
138. Yekefallah L, Ashktorab T, Manoochehri H, Alavi Majd H. Causes of futile care in end of life patients in intensive care units from the viewpoints of nurses. J Health Care. 2018;20(2):105–13.
139. Hospice Palliative Care Association of South Africa. Legal aspects of palliative care. Pinelands: Hospice Palliative Care Association of South Africa; 2009.
140. Bayat ZS, Borhani F, Nasiri M, Mokhtari P. Correlation between nurses' attitude towards death and the quality of nursing care to patients at the end stages of life in the ICU: a systematic review. J Res Med Dent Sci. 2018;6(6):135–40.
141. Taghadosi Nejad F, Okazi A, Maghareh Zade Esfehani M, Yousefi Nejad V. Comparison of attitude of physicians and patients about euthanasia in Tehran's University of Medical Sciences Hospitals in 2012–2013. 2014. https://www.semanticscholar.org.
142. Salimi E, Fathi MJ. A legal analysis of euthanasia in the Islamic criminal code of 2011. IJME. 2013;6(4):17–28.
143. Peimani M, Zahedi F, Larijani B. Do-not-resuscitate order across societies and the necessity of a national ethical guideline. Iran J Med Ethics Hist Med. 2012;5(5):19–35.
144. Ansari M, Rassouli M, Akbari ME, Abbaszadeh A, Akbarisari A. Palliative care policy analysis in Iran: a conceptual model. Indian J Palliat Care. 2018;24(1):51–7.
145. Hassankhani H, Eghtedar S, Rahmani A, Ebrahimi H, Whitehead B. A qualitative study on cancer care burden: experiences of Iranian family caregivers. Holist Nurs Pract. 2019;33(1):17–26.
146. World Health Organization. Facts sheet on universal health coverage. 2015. https://www.who.int/news-room/fact-sheets.
147. World Health Organization. Global strategic directions for strengthening nursing and midwifery 2016–2020. 2016. https://www.who.int.
148. http://www.emro.who.int/media.
149. Naylor MD, Kurtzman ET. The role of nurse practitioners in reinventing primary care. Health Aff. 2010;29(5):893–9.
150. https://www.who.int.
151. Heydari H, Rahnavard Z, Ghaffari F. Exploring the position of community-based nursing in Iran: a qualitative study. Int J Community Based Nurs Midwifery. 2017;5(4):386.
152. Masters exam registration manual. Ministry of Health Medical Education Assessment Center. 1398.

Part XX

Middle East: Iraq

The Current Situation of Palliative Care Services in Iraq

Samaher Abdulrazzaq Fadhil
and Hasanein H. Ghali

Introduction

Background

Iraq is one of the easternmost countries of the Arab world. In ancient times, it was known as the region of Mesopotamia, which means "the land between the rivers". It is the land of some of the earliest-known civilizations, namely Sumer, Akkad, Babylon, and Assyria. This affluent area later progressed to become an essential part of future larger nations, including Persia, Greece, and Rome, and after the seventh century it constituted a nucleus to the Islamic world. Later, in the eighth century, Iraq's capital, Baghdad, became the capital of the Abbasid caliphate.

Demography, Religion, and Economy

Iraq is 168,754 square miles (437,073 square kilometers), bordering Turkey on the north, Iran on the east, Syria and Jordan on the west, and Saudi Arabia and Kuwait on the south. Iraq is a middle-income country, estimated by the World Bank to have a gross domestic product of 197 billion US dollars. The economy relies mainly on income from the production and sale of oil. The total population of Iraq was estimated at 38.3 million in 2017 – Arabs comprise about three-fourths of the population and Kurds comprise about one-fifth. The remaining population is divided into several ethnic groups, including Assyrian, Turkoman, Chaldean, Armenian, Yazidi, and others. Islam is the officially recognized religion of Iraq and is practiced by 95% of the population. A small percentage of the population is Christian, Yazidis, and other religions.

For the last three decades, Iraq has experienced almost continuous conflict including multiple wars, an invasion in 2003, and economic sanctions and sectarian tensions that have left the country in a state of chaos. This has led to political, economic, and social instability, and a poor quality-of-life for the Iraqi people, despite Iraq being one of the richest countries with an abundance of natural and human resources.

Desperate Living Conditions

Since 2014, approximately 3 million people have been displaced from their homes and regions following the ISIS (Islamic State of Iraq and al-Sham) invasion of about one-third of Iraq's land, including the northern and western regions. This resulted in further setbacks on all levels and was

S. A. Fadhil (✉)
Children Welfare Teaching Hospital, Medical City, Baghdad, Iraq

H. H. Ghali
Department of Pediatrics, College of Medicine, University of Baghdad, Children Welfare Teaching Hospital, Medical City, Baghdad, Iraq

M. Silbermann (ed.), *Palliative Care for Chronic Cancer Patients in the Community*,
https://doi.org/10.1007/978-3-030-54526-0_29

followed by a government endeavor to regain these areas using military force which further resulted in increasing infrastructural damage. Consequently, many Iraqis sought better living conditions within Iraq and sought asylum in camps or specially-designed temporary shelters safer governorates leaving them in a desperate need of food and health services. Many others looked for help outside of Iraq in neighboring countries and in Europe. Following the liberation from ISIS in most regions, many are coming back home; however, approximately 700,000 Iraqis are still living in camps, which offer limited opportunity to earn a living wage, and struggle to provide food for them and their families.

Additionally, current figures indicate that the unemployment rate in Iraq is highest compared with other Arab countries. This, along with increasing illiteracy among young people, limited economic prospects, and political and social instability has had an extremely negative impact on the health and well-being of many people.

Iraqi Culture and Society

Iraq has one of the world's oldest cultural histories, evolving into a multi-cultural society with a rich heritage. Modern Iraq lies between two rivers, the Tigris and the Euphrates (anciently named *Mesopotamia*) and was an important hub in early civilization, witnessing the rise and fall of many empires and related cultures.

Seventy-five percent of the population are Arabs, 15–20% are Kurds, and smaller groups (5%) include Turkmen, Jews, Armenians, and Assyrians. Arabic is the official language and Islam is the official religion (96%); others are Christians (3%) and small religious and ethnic minorities such as Yazidis and Mandaeans.

Loyalty and honor to extended family and the tribe are of great importance in Iraqi society. There is immense respect for the elderly and their opinions are considered very important, regardless of the topic; women are to be protected but are usually subservient to men, although many Iraqi women have received degrees in higher education and are professionals; children, although coddled, are subjected to strict punishment for misbehaving. In most cases, death and illness are accepted as God's will, and family and friends often hold social events for moral and financial support, especially in times of trouble and at the time of death.

Iraq was well known and admired for its quality educational and health system in the 1960s and 1970s. Academic degrees were one of the higher priorities that families tried to guarantee for their children. A free education and a free healthcare system were introduced in the 1970s and, as of today, both are free and accessible to all people.

The last three decades of inappropriate and chaotic policies have led to a dramatic decline in Iraq's social and economic development, and the economic situation is currently complicated; many years of violence, tensions, and the displacement of its people due to security and economic conflicts have had a negative impact on the quality of life, people's priorities, and the educational and health systems.

Iraqi Health Care System

A system of free health care was developed in the 1970s by the Iraqi Ministry of Health (MOH) and is the cornerstone of the health system and the main health care provider. The private sector also provides medical services for wealthy people and has grown in the last few years. The Iraqi MOH is centrally funded by the government and, despite its good reputation during the 1970s and early-1980s, when Iraqi healthcare services were considered the best in the Middle East, it witnessed serious setbacks in the following years, causing it to progressively deteriorate. The subsequent and prolonged civil conflicts following 2003 had a major impact on the provision of health services and many health care professionals started fleeing from the country searching for a better, safer, and more reliable place to work. Despite this gloomy picture, efforts to rebuild and restore the infrastructure continue.

The Ministry of Health struggles to overcome challenging obstacles and sometime sends patients abroad for difficult surgical procedures, radiotherapy, and bone marrow transplantation through special committees in the MOH that evaluate patients' records and make the ultimate confirmation as to whether adequate care can be provided at an Iraqi health facility. If the case requires specialized care beyond the local facilities' capabilities, the case file is then forwarded to another committee for financial assessment and processing of the necessary travel arrangements.

There have been cases of health care professionals from various disciplines being sent to train abroad through contracts with more developed centers. Still, local heath institutions and heath care providers work hard to provide free medical care in governmental hospitals and primary health care centers.

In recent years, non-communicable diseases (NCDs), such as cardiovascular diseases (CVD), diabetes, chronic obstructive pulmonary diseases (COPD), and cancers have become pandemic at a disproportionately higher rate in developing countries. The World Health Organization (WHO) estimates that NCDs account for 80% of the global burden of disease, causing seven out of every ten deaths in developing countries, about half of them being premature death under the age of 70 [1].

Following quite a while of disengagement, Iraq must now strive to regain worldwide standards of health. Hospitals do not have the adaptability to successfully deal with their administrations. Significant general medical issues such as smoking, weight issues, and NCDs are not being adequately addressed. Cancer has become a major medical issue in Iraq, and the incidence of cancer has increased as the population continues to grow.

Palliative Care in Iraq: Current Services

The term "palliative care" (PC) is a relatively new concept throughout medical practices in Iraq, and there are currently no clinical disciplines in the curriculum of medical and nursing schools; in addition, no national program has been established to provide for palliative care.

The improvement in the awareness of palliative care terminology is attributable to the Middle East Cancer Consortium (MECC), who invited two pediatric oncologists (Prof. Salma Al-Hadad and Assistant Prof. Mazin F. Al-Jadiry) to preside over a workshop that took place in November 2011 in Larnaca, Cyprus. Dr. Salma Al-Hadad, who heads the pediatric hematology oncology unit in Children Welfare Teaching Hospital (CWTH) in Baghdad, was one of the first to introduce palliative care philosophy and launched PC practices into the pediatric oncology unit in Baghdad.

This was followed by a few short training courses and lectures on PC which were delivered to pediatric oncologists, residents, and nurses working in the Baghdad Medical City complex. Major efforts to introduce PC were carried out by the MECC and Prof. Michael Silbermann, its Executive Director, as it introduced and supported PC programs for low-resource countries in the region.

Thereafter, there were rising concerns and discussions regarding the sub-optimal supportive care services and inadequate pain management for pediatric oncology patients in these countries, with an emphasis on the compassionate care provided by nurses and physicians. Meetings and workshops on PC took place from 2012 to 2016, with the participation of five pediatric oncologists and four nurses.

CWTH is one of two main centers for treating childhood cancer in Iraq, with an average of 300 new cases per year. CWTH is a public referral and teaching hospital with 240 beds managed by the Ministry of Health (MOH) and the staff members who are all government employees. The oncology unit in CWTH has a capacity of 56 beds, but the number of actual inpatients ranges from 60 to 90. The medical staff includes 8 oncologists, 1 fellow (the number varies annually), 6 residents (changing every 2 months) and 25 nurses. A large number of pediatric oncology patients are diagnosed with advanced stage disease or referred with progressive disease because of poor resources and limited diagnostic facilities, presenting a burden to the health system, the patients, their families, and caregivers. The latter often experiences psychological, behavioral, and physiological issues that affect their daily lives, and palliative care stands out as an essential tool in reducing the impact that cancer has on patients and their families, alleviating suffering and improving quality of life.

There is no structured or organized training for physicians and nurses in the oncology unit for delivering PC nor is there training in the field of pain management. The only available information can be found on the internet and in published articles. No local guidelines are available. Current practices focus primarily on the field of pain management, and families' and caregivers' skills are based on individual abilities rather than acting as a collaborative group. The pediatric oncologists provide some degree of psycho-social support and pain management with their routine clinical duties but there is no designated professional team responsible for PC. The game players consist of the patient, the oncologist, and the patient's loved ones. No specialized PC physician, PC nurse, social worker, pharmacist, physical therapist, chaplain, sheik, or dietician is assigned to any case.

In Iraq, there are no special units or outpatient clinics. In 2013, a pediatric oncologist with no basic qualifications in PC took responsible for palliative care services in her unit; she is a member of the Pediatric Oncology East Mediterranean (POEM) PC group. No spiritual advisers, occupational therapists, or psychotherapists are available, and there is no significant role for pharmacists in pain management.

There is no official funding for PC or cancer care; financial contributions come from a few non-governmental organizations and individuals. Volunteer work is rudimentary and undeveloped, however, sometimes entertainment, parties, and arts and crafts are arranged by non-funded social workers, on an irregular basis.

There is no home or hospice care; terminal patients are isolated in a private room, if available, to give them time with their families and to limit contact with other patients who can become fearful and disappointed by witnessing the disease progression or death of other children. Due to the parents' difficulty to cope alone with the death process of their child, pediatric patients usually die in the hospital, unlike the elderly who prefer to die at home.

Iraq is still recovering from a long gloomy period of political and economic conflicts. While there is a global shift toward improving quality of life and alleviating the burden of cancer and chronic illness, the philosophy of PC is still considered "luxurious". As health institutions struggle to provide basic management and lifesaving tools, most patients and their families are uncertain about what PC is, and they resist the idea of palliation preferring to continue treatment even in hopeless cases. Furthermore, the term PC is not well-understood even by many health care professionals and providers.

For all these reasons, humble steps were taken to establish the first PC Unit in Baghdad Medical City at the end of 2017, which is currently run by two anesthesiologists; however, it is still in its early stages and mainly provides pain management, which is also inadequate due to the shortage and limited availability of various type of narcotics.

Pediatric Oncology Units in Iraq

In an August 2011 email, Dr. Mazin Al-Jadiry (Fig. 1), a pediatric oncologist at Children's Welfare Teaching Hospital in Medical City Baghdad wrote: *Really, I'm asking my/ourselves if we have the power to continue as the circumstances around us are not improving, but deteriorating on levels that we could never-have-imagined: chaos, corruption and a loss of principles which were already declining over the last 30 years. There is continuity of the obstacles. And, the number of patients is increasing. We feel we should/cannot be static, that we must improve our abilities and expand our capacities. This puts even more of a burden on us, both physically and mentally* [2].

In Iraq, childhood cancer and leukemia continue to be a long-term health dilemma. Before 2005, pediatric tumors were treated in the three main oncology units in the large cities (Baghdad, Basra, and Mosul). After 2005, many small units

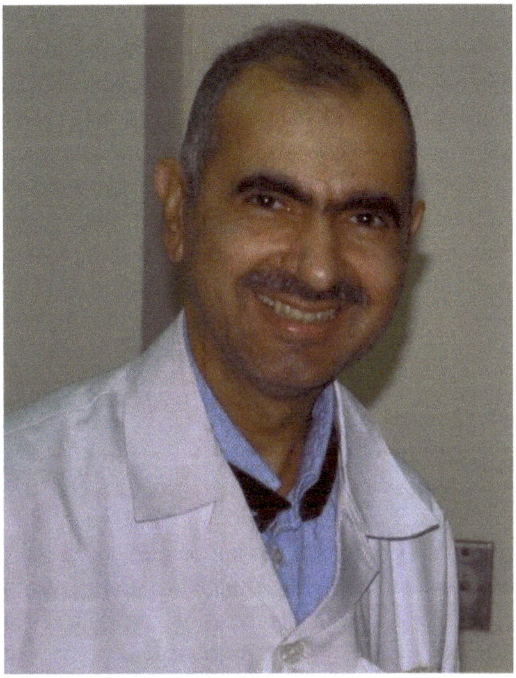

Fig. 1 Dr. Mazin F. Al-Jadiry; Pediatric Oncologist at CWTH, Medical City, Baghdad, Iraq

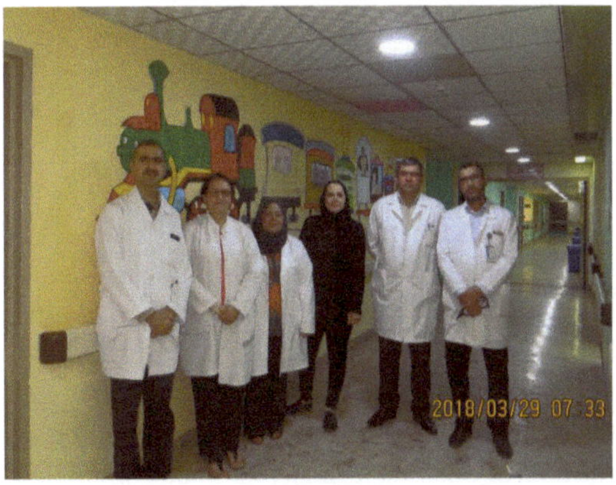

Fig. 2 Oncology team in CWTH, Medical City, Baghdad, Iraq

in other cities were established in other parts in Iraq; Erbil, Sulaymaniyah, Wasit, and in the last 3 years, the number of units have increased to include other cities such as Kerbala, Babil, and Najaf. Currently, there are 30 Pediatric Oncologists working in the country (having earned board certification or a diploma in pediatrics with variable structured training in pediatric oncology), and the number is increasing annually.

The pediatric oncology unit at CWTH is one of two main units in Baghdad, receiving the bulk of their cases from Baghdad and the center, south, and north of Iraq (excluding Kurdistan) with significant evidence of limitations in cancer management, including surgical and radiation oncology facilities. There is no multidisciplinary team, and physicians have inadequately structured training in pediatric hematology/oncology. Nurses also lack the training needed to meet the demands of children with cancer. The shortage of effective chemotherapy medications and medicines required for supportive care (antibiotics, anti-emetics, pain medications, etc.), a lack of other supportive care facilities, and lack of infection-control teams and policies have caused an increase in morbidity and mortality rates and have impacted negatively on the quality of care. Blood bank services also have their difficulties with the shortage of bags, kits for screening, and cell separator kits. Transferring blood from the bank to the hospital is done by the parents without proper storage conditions during transportation.

Delay in referring newly diagnosed cases further impedes the management plan as patients present with an advanced stage of disease and there is no established PC program. Most children with cancer die with a DNR, which is commonly accepted by most families.

Currently, in CWTH, there are 7 pediatric oncologists (Fig. 2); they are working full-time (8:00 a.m. – 03:00 p.m.), with 1 fellow and 27 nurses. The oncologist/new patient ratio is 1:4; nurse/inpatient ratio is 1:6 in the earlier shift (8:00 a.m. – 03:00 p.m.) and 1:15 at night (03:00 p.m. – 8:00 a.m.).

All cases of pediatric tumors (including those with very advanced tumors) are admitted to and treated in the oncology unit of CWTH. At the end of 2017, pediatric brain tumors were added to the responsibilities of the oncology unit of CWTH.

The average registered mortality rate has ranged from 10% to 20% over the last 10 years. Two-thirds of these deaths occurred during hospitalization and resulted from the lack of optimal supportive care. About the same percentage, two-thirds of patients, arrived at CWTH in an advanced stage of disease. The median total diagnosis delay was 55 days (from 3 days to 36 months). The median physician delay was 43 days, which is more than double the longest doctor delay mentioned in the literature; the average patient's delay in seeking diagnosis/treatment is comparable with that mentioned in publications. This late diagnosis, along with iatrogenic complications, can make for a poor prognosis [2].

Pain Management for Cancer Patients

Many countries in the Middle East still have low opioid consumption. While the global consumption of opioids has increased throughout the past 30 years, there has been little increase in opioid consumption in the Middle East, despite increasing economic and health care development in some countries of the region [3].

In Iraq, there is a strong evidence of inappropriate pain assessment and suboptimal pain management, mostly due to the shortage and limited regulations of use of opioids and lack of proper training of health care providers. Unfamiliarity with the use of pain medicine has had a negative effect on the quality of life of patients.

Pain killers such as propoxyphene, codeine, and acetaminophen are used to treat mild to moderate pain. For severe pain, oral and parenteral tramadol are available, and there is limited use of injectable (but no oral) morphine and transdermal fentanyl (on an irregular basis). Opioids for outpatients have never been allowed in Iraq and, even for inpatients, prescriptions require strict documentation and is only allowed by two physicians, according to the hospital regulations. The lack of adequate management of opioids by nurses and medical staff along with the cultural fears from addiction are the major problems associated with opioids prescription.

Generally, the communication between the patients and medical staff regarding pain is poor, as they have little experience in pain assessment, which can lead to random treatments instead of following the pain management guideline. Many families interfere with pain management, the majority being resistant to opioids, as they prefer for their child to be awake and talking with them in the terminal stages rather than being sleepy.

Inadequate knowledge of and inadequate training in pain management in undergraduate curriculum and postgraduate education lead to popular myths about opioids at both the medical and individual levels. Improper pain management instruction negatively affects patients' mental, physical, and psychosocial lives and, hence, their quality of life.

Additionally, some beliefs in Iraq's culture is that Islam, being the religion of the majority, discourages people from taking opioids. For example, Layla, a middle-aged female with metastatic breast cancer reaching the vertebrae, refused to take any opioids for her intractable bone pain to alleviate her suffering as she believed that pain will bring her closer to God.

Attitudes Towards Palliative Care Among Health Professionals

In the current frame of health services in Iraq, no information is available in the curricula or in the guidelines. Many medical health workers are not familiar with the terminology, and they do not know what PC is about. Those who are familiar with terminology think that PC is about comforting patients with terminal cancer before their death. Most of the awareness in this field lies in the area of oncology, and a remarkable number of professionals who have knowledge regarding PC practices believe that it is luxurious care in Iraq's current situation where the health care providers are struggling to provide basic and lifesaving diagnostic and therapeutic measures. PC is a developing medical specialty and effective PC service delivery requires a strong health system, with health care providers who have the awareness, positive attitude, and desire to provide compassionate care to those who are suffering and dying. They should be enthusiastic and eager to deliver PC services.

Education and training in palliative care influences not only the level of care provided but also the level of team participation among health care professionals [4]. Medical students and other health care professionals across the globe are still uncomfortable facing death and dying, despite its growing scientific base, yet often perceive PC as not important [5].

Next Step Forward

An important question to ask is: how can we apply a PC program to our setting? Of course, all people have the right to receive the best possible health care when they are suffering from chronic disease and terminal illnesses, along with optimal and adequate treatment for their pain and other symptoms. The first step forward is to formally recognize Palliative Medicine as a specialty and PC as a medical specialty, as it is in most developed countries, in neighboring countries like Jordon and Lebanon. This could be achieved in the next few years in Iraq if the stakeholders and those in power have the intention to do so. Introducing PC to the curriculum of medical and nursing schools at the undergraduate level will enhance its chances.

Few steps have been taken by academic professionals to promote this issue, as the main practice of PC has been in the field of pediatric oncology. Many lectures and presentations on this subject were given by oncologists and nurses in local meetings and as part of the hospital's educational lectures, which led to better awareness of PC among local health care providers. The subjects included different aspects of PC, such as helping people to die with dignity, to focus on reducing the families' stress, and managing pain and other symptoms.

Further research and surveys pertaining to the present-day knowledge and practices of palliative care in our health institutions are crucial to close the gap left by the deficiency of these terms and to figure out what steps are required to improve it. Awareness of the constraints and obstacles will be important when applying these steps.

Researching PC in Iraq is confined to models assessing physicians' and nurses' knowledge regarding PC and pain management by answering written questionnaires about the definition and main terminologies of PC. Most of these surveys are carried out as part of a collaboration with international organizations and institutions. Still, these simple steps represent a step forward to highlighting the importance of palliative and compassionate care, with the goal of recognizing PC as a key and valuable medical discipline.

Palliative Care Barriers

Cultural Barriers

Culturally, health care providers struggle to tell the truth to the patient's family, as this can cause psychological trauma; there is a risk that the family will decide to abandon treatment and seek other health professionals who might deceive them. Discussion with the family about palliative care issues is a difficult task and depends on the beliefs of the physician and the family. The perception of palliative care is almost always affected by these beliefs. Education plays another role in understanding the PC issue. In Iraq, as in many other regional countries, the health care system seems to be ill-equipped to deal with a dying cancer patient [6].

Parents continue to consult with health care professionals about the role of adding more chemotherapies to the treatment of their sick children with terminal malignancies and even sometimes refuse the use of strong analgesics, as this could be a sign of reaching the end of the story of their child, the death, which they do not want to believe. They, as well as many other health care professionals, cannot understand that PC helps improve the quality of life by decreasing the suffering of their terminally ill child. Discussing the eventual death of their patients could be understood as the physician's failure to treat their patients.

Awareness of one's own culture, and the cultural practices of others, plays an important role in providing compassionate and competent care.

System Barriers

The health system in Iraq is fragile, and is now emerging from the disheartening period following many years of political sanctions and internal conflicts. There are significant disparities between developed and developing regions in the provision of PC services for individuals with life-limiting illnesses, particularly with regard to the awareness and attitude toward PC. There is a lack of awareness on the part of policymakers, and even many health professionals, of what PC is about and the benefits it can offer to patients and health systems. Other barriers to pain management include (a) the culture's fear of opioid addiction; and (b) absence of government policies, education, and access to essential medicines (particularly opioids).

A Story from Anbar – West of Iraq

Noor, from the west of Iraq (Anbar), was 12 years old when she was diagnosed with acute lymphocytic leukemia (ALL) in April 2010 and underwent treatment at CWTH for 2.5 years until August 2012. She abandoned follow-up after the al-Qaeda invasion in November 2013, followed by the presence of ISIS in her area. In July 2017, Noor presented with a relapse of the disease. Her family could not leave the city for medical advice and her vision deteriorated. One night in August 2017, her parent managed to escape from their city to reach CWTH in Baghdad, leaving four children behind. Noor refused treatment and said: *I am blind, why should I receive chemotherapy treatment?*

Physicians working in CWTH convinced her that, although they cannot make her see again, they can help her to improve and to feel less pain. Financial support was offered to her family to rent a house. She was treated again at CWTH but, this time, she was blind. The parents were strong despite not knowing the fate of their children left behind. They stayed for several weeks, but unfortunately, Noor died from the progression of disease, away from her city, her brothers, and sisters. The strength of Iraqi community lies in the notion that friends and relatives will provide psychosocial, spiritual, financial, and moral support to the patient and family.

Conclusion

Eighty percent of people with cancer in low- and middle-income countries present with advanced stage disease [7]. In our setting, many cases presented with delay in referral, leaving patients and their families to struggle with the consequences of progressive illness. Distressing symptoms and severe pain have profound psychological impact on patients and their families. The integration of PC into a standard form, which provides evidence-based guidance and recommendations for symptom management, emotional support, and stress management starting at the time of diagnosis through the treatment and coordination of care to the end of life, will provide a realistic solution to our problems. Exhibiting the disparities between developed and developing regions regarding the punctual recognition of cancer and other chronic diseases will help policymakers set their priorities. Finally, emphasis should be put on the importance of research in PC, increasing awareness and directing national healthcare policies and guidelines to increase government-sponsored programs for PC.

References

1. Islam SM, Purnat TD, Phuong NT, Mwingira U, Schacht K, Fröschl G. Non-communicable diseases (NCDs) in developing countries: a symposium report. Glob Health. 2014;10:81. Published 2014 Dec 11. https://doi.org/10.1186/s12992-014-0081-9.
2. Al-Hadad SA, Al-Jadiry MF, Lefko C. Paediatric cancer care in a limited-resource setting: Children's Welfare Teaching Hospital, Medical City, Baghdad. Ecancermedicalscience. 2016;10:ed55. Published 2016 May 24. https://doi.org/10.3332/ecancer.2016.ed55.
3. Cleary J, Silbermann M, Scholten W, Radbruch L, Torode J, Cherny NI. Formulary availability and regulatory barriers to accessibility of opioids for cancer pain in the Middle East: a report from the Global Opioid Policy Initiative (GOPI). Ann Oncol. 2013;24(Suppl 11):51–9. Available from https://doi.org/10.1093/annonc/mdt503.

4. Rajgopal MR, Venkateswaran C. Palliative care in India: successes and limitations. J Pain Palliat Care Pharmacother. 2003;17:121–8.
5. Jahan F, Al Shibli HS, Qatan RS, Al Kharusi AA. Perception of undergraduate medical students in clinical years regarding palliative care. Middle East J Age Ageing. 2013;10(2):22–31.
6. Ghali HH. Cultural challenges in implementing palliative care services in Iraq. Palliat Med Hosp Care Open J. 2017;SE(1):S19–23. https://doi.org/10.17140/PMH-COJ-SE-1-105.
7. Cazap E, Magrath I, Kingham TP, et al. Structural barriers to diagnosis and treatment of cancer in low- and middle-income countries: the urgent need for scaling up. J Clin Oncol. 2016;34:14–9.

Dr. Samaher Abdulrazzaq Fadhil is a hematology-oncology specialist at Children Welfare Teaching Hospital/Medical City, Baghdad, with MD, FICMS and CABP (ped), FICMS (pediatric hemonc). She graduated from the Medical School, University of Al-Mustansiriya in 2000 and got a fellowship degree in pediatrics in 2009 and a subspecialty degree in pediatric hematology/oncology in 2013. Her postgraduate training was at Children Welfare Teaching Hospital, Medical city. She got training opportunities in pediatric hematology/oncology in Jordan (KHCC) and USA (BCH/DFCI); her field of activity is neuroblastoma and neuro-oncology, and she has special interest in palliative care, spirituality, and medical ethics.

Dr. Hasanein H. Ghali is a consultant pediatric hematologist-oncologist at Children Welfare Teaching Hospital/Medical City, Baghdad, with MD, DCH, FICMS (ped), FICMS (hemonc) graduated from Medical School, University of Baghdad in June 2002 and was assigned as a faculty member in 2003, got a fellowship degree in pediatrics in 2009 and a subspecialty degree in pediatric hematology/oncology in 2012. His postgraduate training was in Children Welfare Teaching Hospital, Medical city. He got training opportunities in Pediatric hematology/oncology in Japan (Shinshu Hospital), Jordan (KHCC) and USA (BCH/DFCI). Currently, he is an assistant professor of pediatric in the department of pediatric in Baghdad college of Medicine.

Part XXI

Middle East: Israel

The Current Status of Pediatric Palliative Care at Home – The Israeli Perspective

Sergey Postovsky and Myriam Weyl-Ben-Arush

Introduction

Every year approximately 450–500 new pediatric patients are diagnosed with various types of cancer in Israel. The incidence of pediatric cancer is not uniformly distributed throughout the country and depends on the geographical region of Israel. Thus, the highest incidence is observed in the metropolitan area of Tel Aviv (180.2 per 1,000,000 of pediatric population up to age 19, whereas the lowest incidence was registered in the north of Israel with 150.8 cases per 1,000,000) (Fig. 1) [1]. In Israel today, approximately 80% of these children are regarded as long-term survivors and even cured. On the other hand, however, it means that approximately 90–100 children with cancer will ultimately succumb to their disease every year.

There are six major pediatric oncology departments functioning within large hospitals in Israel: Ruth Rappaport Children's Hospital located within Rambam Medical Center in Haifa; Hadassah Ein Kerem in Jerusalem; Dana Children's Hospital integrated into Sourasky Medical Center in Tel Aviv; Safra Children's Hospital within Sheba Hospital in Tel Ha-Shomer; Schneider Children's Hospital in Beilinson Medical Center in Petach Tikvah; and Saban Children's Hospital within Soroka Medical Center in Beer Sheba. Along with these major medical centers, there are several smaller hospitals with small pediatric oncology units which provide oncology treatment to a relatively small number of children with cancer diagnoses.

Although the number of childhood deaths each year may seem small, the emotional, social, and financial impact is extraordinary.

In Israel, as in other Western developed countries, pediatric oncology patients who need palliative care (PC) at the end of life occupy the third place (after children with incurable genetic/congenital and neuromuscular disorders) [2]. The pediatric cancer patients who become subjects for palliative care services comprise only about 20% of all pediatric patients who need and receive PC from various providers [2].

Pediatric palliative care (PPC) in Israel exists and functions on three levels:

- Hospital level
- Community level
- Pediatric hospice

All these three levels of PPC are connected to and dependent on each other and deliver their services to pediatric oncology patients who spend most of their time at home after being regarded as incurable.

S. Postovsky · M. Weyl-Ben-Arush (✉)
Pediatric Hematology Oncology and Bone Marrow Transplantation Division, Ruth Rappaport Children's Hospital, Rambam Health Care Campus, Haifa, Israel
e-mail: s_postovsky@rambam.health.gov.il; m_benarush@rambam.health.gov.il

M. Silbermann (ed.), *Palliative Care for Chronic Cancer Patients in the Community*,
https://doi.org/10.1007/978-3-030-54526-0_30

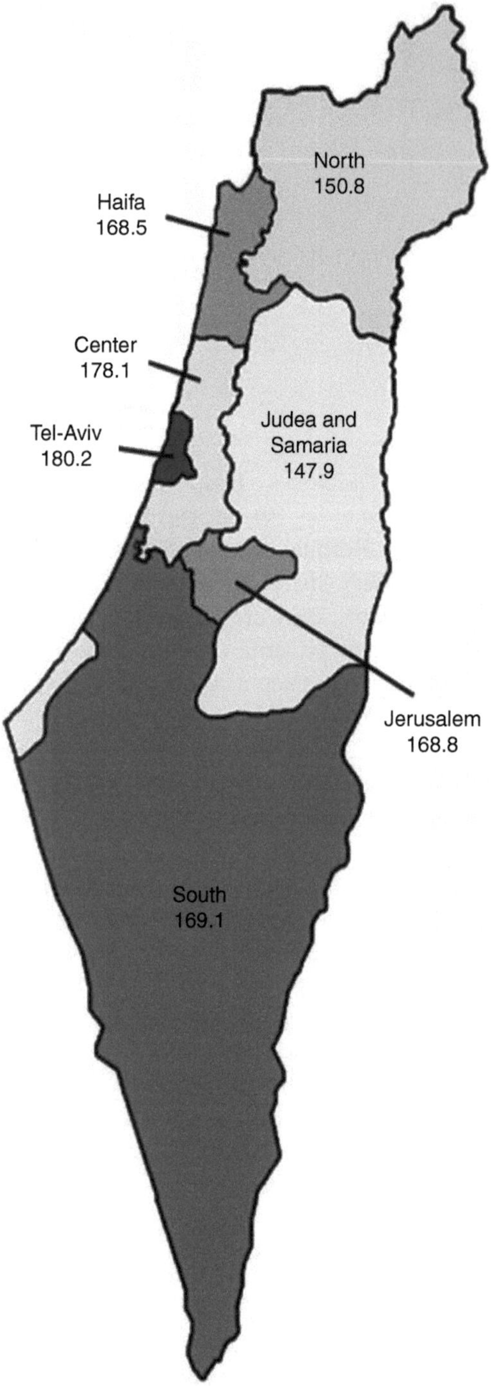

Fig. 1 Childhood cancer incidence rates (0–19 years) in seven districts of Israel from 1998 to 2007

Hospital Level

It is generally agreed that most people would prefer to die at home surrounded by close family members and friends, and it is logical to assume that children are not exempt from this general rule. Despite this assumption, we seldom witness the death of a child dying from cancer at home [3–5]. Among pediatric cancer patients who were followed and assisted by one of six major PPC services in USA and Canada, only 45.3% died at home. Others died either in hospital or in hospice facilities [2]. In a study evaluating the place of death of pediatric patients with complex chronic conditions in 11 different countries, it was shown that, in a majority of these countries, less than half the cases of children with cancer died at home [5]. In South Korea, for example, the percentage of children with cancer who died at home was extremely low (1.8%). A low percentage of pediatric cancer patients dying at home was also reported in the Czech Republic (17.0%) and in France (17.9%). In North America, the proportion of children dying of cancer at home is higher but still does not reach the 50% level (USA – 39.4%, Canada – 21.8%). In the study by Hakanson et al. [5], there were only two countries that reported percentages of pediatric oncology patients' deaths at home by more than 50% (Belgium – 60.8% and New Zealand – 52.6%).

In Israel, an absolute majority of children with chronic and life-limiting conditions, including cancer, die in hospitals.

There are several possible explanations for this. First, the nature of progressive cancer with its accompanying multiple symptoms, which are sometimes difficult to control, needs the hospitalization of a dying child [6]. Second, the immense psychological impact that imminent death poses for other family members may preclude keeping an ill child at home. Third, at times there are human, financial, and/or other shortages that limit or even completely preclude the possibility of managing the terminal phase of cancer in an ill child at home. Many families spend a significant part of time in pediatric oncology departments during the course of their children's disease. It is a rule that during this time, which is measured usually by months and even years, tight and non-formal relationships are established between patients, their parents, and the departmental staff. Many families see pediatric oncology departments as their "second homes". Therefore, it is understandable that many such families will decide to come to hospital when the child's death becomes imminent and the psychological burden is great, despite the fact that there are proper conditions for ending the child's life at home. It is also worth noting that Israel is a relatively small country where a majority of the population lives in several large urban centers with a well-developed health system including large hospitals. It means that practically all pediatric oncology patients with advanced and incurable cancer live within short distances of their corresponding pediatric oncology departments, making it is very tempting and easy to arrive at these facilities in the event of any crisis and, especially, when the death of a child with cancer becomes imminent.

Community Level

Two models for providing PPC at the community level exist in Israel:

- Medical insurance providers that have their own palliative care services – "home hospice" and "continuation treatment" units. There are four major such providers: Clalit (largest), Maccabi, Meuchedet, and Leumit (smallest).
- External services provided by free-standing firms specializing in palliative care, such as "TSABAR" organization.

All these palliative services have no specialists certified in pediatric palliative care. The only palliative care specialist who has been certified in PPC and works in such a capacity outside any hospital provides her services privately (free-lance), mainly in the center of country.

Summarizing all the above, PPC services in the community is provided by "adult" specialists without special knowledge and/or experience in pediatrics.

Pediatric Hospices

There is only one dedicated pediatric hospice in Israel – Beit Wiesel in Tel Hashomer (one hospice per more than 2.8 million children living currently in the country). This hospice is located within a large general hospital (Sheba Medical Center) and is designated only for children with cancer who were almost exclusively treated in that hospital [7].

Children with likely incurable cancer who receive oncology treatment are introduced to this place from the very early stages of their treatment and are supposed to become acquainted with the hospice from the very beginning. Therefore, beds in this hospice may both serve as hospital and hospice beds, depending on the stage of disease and goals of treatment. The children are treated by the same medical personnel (both nurses and doctors), irrespective of the stage of cancer. This makes it unnecessary to introduce new staff as the disease progresses, and palliative care is delivered by the same specialists who have long since become familiar with the child, his/her parents, and other family members. Such familiarity and well-established contacts that are created between PPC providers and an ill child and family become especially important at the end of life and facilitate better management of many problems which are encountered in a pediatric oncology patient as death approaches.

There are several general hospices operating in Israel that potentially may provide palliative care for children with cancer at the end of life in their homes. Authors have described positive experiences in cooperation with the hospice of the Upper Galilee. The staff of this hospice provides palliative care to a variety of patients with different diagnoses across practically all age groups. The services of this hospice cover a large part of northern Israel, including population living not only in the upper Galilee as its name suggests, but in the whole territory of the Israeli Golan Heights as well. Close collaboration with this hospice has allowed us to successfully manage difficult symptoms of several of our patients in their homes until the very end of their lives.

Rational organization and close collaboration between the medical staff of pediatric oncology departments and various PC providers at the community level frequently suffice to successfully manage complex problems in children with advanced forms of cancer. It has become common reality to manage pain in children at home, using not only orally or transcutaneously administered forms of opioids but to deliver parenteral morphine via patient- or parent-controlled analgesia, practically to every child after his/her condition is stabilized in a pediatric oncology department and she/he was discharged home for continuation of palliative care. It is also possible to arrange oxygen supply to patients with respiratory distress practically in all cases. Many patients receive a variety of nutritional support, including total parenteral nutrition while receiving PC at home. Such collaboration and involvement of medical and psycho-social staff at the community level optimizes maximally the time spent by the child and his parents at home, minimizes the duration of the hospital stay and, related to it, patient and family stress and associated financial and other costs. All this ultimately leads to improved quality of life, which becomes an especially important issue when the child is regarded as incurable and his/her death approaches. Hence, we can conclude that, despite that the absolute majority of pediatric cancer patients ultimately dying in hospital, many of them may spend a considerable amount of time at home during the last phases of their diseases, provided that adequate palliative care is properly delivered by medical and psycho-social staff at the community level.

Before discharge of pediatric oncology patients with incurable cancer from hospital to their homes for continuation of palliative treatment provided by medical services in the community, we usually discuss with the parents the future probable situations when the general condition of their child will deteriorate, and there will be a need to decide whether or not resuscitative actions will be applied. During these discussions, we explore such issues as place of death and "do not resuscitate" (DNR) orders. If the parents are not interested in resuscitation and placement of their child in an intensive care unit, we provide them with a special letter that indicates that the family prefers not to perform resuscitation at home. This letter does not have any obligatory power and the parents may change their minds at any moment and just not show the letter to the ambulance team. In such cases, the child will undergo all necessary life-sustaining interventions according to his/her condition and will be delivered to the hospital. From the experience accumulated during several years of writing such letters, we may conclude that more than 90% of families prefer not to proceed to artificial ventilatory support or full cardiopulmonary resuscitation, but still the absolute majority of them prefer to spend the last hours or days in hospital in the pediatric oncology departments.

Palliative care does not end at the time of the child's death. Parental and other family members' stress should be addressed properly to minimize long-term consequences of unattended and unresolved grief [8–10]. Although home visits by members of medical and psychosocial staff are not reimbursed by current regulations in Israel, in practically all instances when a child with cancer dies, representatives of the treating hospital team go to the deceased child's home. Such visits facilitate better adjustment to the new reality for family members and help medical personnel deal successfully with their own stress and frustration.

In conclusion, PPC in Israel is not comprehensive (it exists mainly at the hospital level and pediatric oncology departments). PPC in Israel is fragmentary geographically with scarcity of human, material, and other resources, especially both in the north and south of the country. Additionally, there is a lack of PC certified specialists (currently there are only three) who have certification in pediatrics. For better development of PPC at the home of children with advanced and progressive cancer, many improvements in such fields as continuous professional education and creation of financial mechanisms directed at a stimulation and reimbursement policy should be considered and implemented.

References

1. Rabinowicz R, Barchana M, Liphshiz I, Futerman B, Linn S, Weyl-Ben-Arush M. Cancer incidence and survival among children and adolescents in Israel during the years 1998 to 2007. J Pediatr Hematol Oncol. 2012;34:421–9. https://doi.org/10.1097/MPH.0b013e31826157ce.
2. Feudtner C, Kang TI, Hexem KR, Friedrichsdorf SJ, Osenga K, Siden H, Friebert SE, Hays RM, Dussel V, Wolfe J. Pediatric palliative care patients: a prospective multicenter cohort study. Pediatrics. 2011;127:1094–101. https://doi.org/10.1542/peds.2010-3225.
3. Gao W, Verne J, Peacock J, Stiller C, Wells C, Greenough A, Higginson IJ. Place of death in children and young people with cancer and implications for end of life care: a population-based study in England, 1993–2014. BMC Cancer. 2016;16:727. https://doi.org/10.1186/s12885-016-2695-1.
4. Feudtner C, Christakis DA, Zimmerman FJ, Muldoon JH, Neff JM, Koepsell TD. Characteristics of deaths occurring in children's hospitals: implications for supportive care services. Pediatrics. 2002;109:887–93. https://doi.org/10.1542/peds.109.5.887.
5. Håkanson C, Öhlén J, Kreicbergs U, Cardenas-Turanzas M, Wilson DM, Loucka M, et al. Place of death of children with complex chronic conditions: cross-national study of 11 countries. Eur J Pediatr. 2017;176:327. https://doi.org/10.1007/s00431-016-2837-0.
6. Postovsky S, Ben Arush MW. Care of a child dying of cancer: the role of the palliative care team in pediatric oncology. Pediatr Hematol Oncol. 2004;21:67–76.
7. Golan H, Bielorai B, Grebler D, Izraeli S, Rechavi G, Toren A. Integration of a palliative and terminal care center into a comprehensive pediatric oncology department. Pediatr Blood Cancer. 2008;50:949–55. https://doi.org/10.1002/pbc.21476.
8. Lövgren M, Sveen J, Nyberg T, Eilegård Wallin A, Prigerson HG, Steineck G, Kreicbergs U. Care at end of life influences grief: a nationwide long-term follow-up among young adults who lost a brother or sister to childhood cancer. J Palliat Med. 2018;21:156–62. https://doi.org/10.1089/jpm.2017.0029.
9. Mulhern RK, Lauer ME, Hoffmann RG. Death of a child at home or in the hospital: subsequent psychological adjustment of the family. Pediatrics. 1983;71:743–7.
10. Lauer ME, Mulhern RK, Wallskog JM, Camitta BM. A comparison study of parental adaptation following a child's death at home or in the hospital. Pediatrics. 1983;71:107–12.

Part XXII

Middle East: Jordan

Community-Based Palliative Care in the Arab Region: Current Status and Future Directions

Loai Mohammad Abu Sharour, Huda Al-Noumani, Suleiman Al Sabei, Iman Al Hashmi, Maryam Al Harrasi, and Basma Al-Yazidi

Introduction

Community palliative care is a main component in health systems. The complex care needs of older adults and people requiring palliative care are increasing due to the increase in life expectancy [1]. The rapid change in lifestyle in recent decades has left health-care systems unable to accommodate this gap and meet the care needs of older adults with chronic illness [2].

Palliative care is defined as relieving pain, managing associated symptoms, providing care during the dying process, offering psychological and spiritual care, and maintaining quality of life (QOL) [3]. However, it remains limited in the Middle East, which has Muslim-majority populations [1]. The meaning of community palliative care, access, national drug laws and regulations, the issue of addiction, knowledge deficit among health-care professionals, the structure of health-care systems and the perception of Muslim families toward palliative care are all factors that might limit the development of community palliative care in the Arab region.

This chapter discusses community-based palliative care in Arab countries, the decision-making process, autonomy and disclosure of information, the role of palliative care nurses in the community, paediatric palliative care (PPC) and research on palliative care in Arab countries.

Community-Based Palliative Care in Arab Countries

Nowadays, palliative care practice has shifted toward community-based palliative care. This change is thought to overcome challenges to palliative care and bridge the gap in practice between hospital care and community needs. Access to community-based palliative care has been linked to reduction in cost, utilisation of hospital and emergency departments, length of inpatient stay and unplanned admission, especially for patients requiring end-of-life care [4, 5]. One of the major barriers to optimal palliative care is a lack of home care services [6].

Palliative care in Arab countries is dominantly hospital-based and physician-led [7]. Currently, palliative care faces various challenges in its implementation by health care providers and the accessibility by the public [8]. Moreover, the infrastructure of Arab countries is not well-established enough to allow development of

L. M. Abu Sharour (✉)
Faculty of Nursing, AL-Zaytoonah University of Jordan, Amman, Jordan
e-mail: Loai.S@zuj.edu.jo

H. Al-Noumani · S. Al Sabei · I. Al Hashmi
M. AlHarrasi · B. Al-Yazidi
College of Nursing, Sultan Qaboos University, Muscat, Oman
e-mail: hudasn@squ.edu.om; alsabei@squ.edu.om; eiman@squ.edu.om; maryam22@squ.edu.om; basma84@squ.edu.om

M. Silbermann (ed.), *Palliative Care for Chronic Cancer Patients in the Community*,
https://doi.org/10.1007/978-3-030-54526-0_31

qualified community-based palliative care programs that could operate independently with the support of governmental and non-governmental sectors. Patients with cancer who require palliative care are commonly managed at emergency departments, outpatient clinics and inpatient palliative care settings [8, 9].

Arabs are characterised by an extended family structure. In their culture, Arabs prefer to care for their terminally ill relatives at home, and patients who require end-of-life care prefer to die in their own homes. Extending palliative care to community settings would be preferred by families, especially those in rural areas where access to palliative care is a challenge [10, 11].

Status of Community-Based Palliative Care in Arab Countries

In Oman, there are two main cancer centres. Palliative care in Oman is still in its infancy stage, and the country is now in the process of palliative care capacity building. In 2012, an introductory course on palliative care for community nurses was started in collaboration with the United States Oncology Nursing Society in Pittsburgh (USA) [8, 12]. Approximately 24 community nurses have been trained to provide palliative care at primary health centres, but not at a community level [13].

In Jordan, the King Hussein Cancer Centre (KHCC) started palliative care in 2004 and became the first comprehensive cancer centre in the Middle East, providing cancer management and palliative care. The palliative care program at KHCC has a home care program consisting of two teams led by community nurses, who conduct home visits to provide palliative care to patients with cancer. Despite its huge services to the country, home-based palliative care is limited to Amman, the capital city, and to patients residing within a 100-mile radius [8, 14]. Currently, the focus of KHCC is directed toward shifting from hospital or hospice care to community-based palliative care for the adult population, and care for the paediatric population as a home care service is not yet adequate [8].

In 1995, through the National Cancer Control Workshop, Lebanon initiated its initiative toward palliative care by Professor Michael Silbermann and the Middle East Cancer. Since then, Lebanon has been working toward adopting and achieving gold standards and goals of palliative care, of which advancement of home-care palliative care and social assistance is one of the key emphases. In 2003, a symposium was conducted to highlight the role of community nurses in home-based palliative care. Recently, palliative care concepts have been introduced in undergraduate and postgraduate nursing education but palliative care, including community-based practice, is still not at the optimal level [8, 12].

In Egypt, the first initiative toward providing palliative care services was in 1981. Until recently, community-based palliative care has been a challenge in Egypt, and there is no well-established system to provide community palliative care to the public taking into consideration the large population of Egypt [8].

Until 2008, Palestine had no palliative care facilities nor a community-based palliative care system. In 2008, the first non-governmental initiative (Al-Sadeel Society) was begun to establish palliative care at home and at the community level. However, this initiative is based on volunteerism only, in which nurses and other health-care providers raise awareness about palliative care and its significance at the community level [8].

In Saudi Arabia, there is a well-developed system of inpatient care of patients with cancer at tertiary level hospitals. However, primary level settings and their networks have a poorly developed system providing palliative care with family practitioners and community nurses [15]. In 1990, Saudi Arabia piloted a community palliative care nursing program with 12 patients who were terminally ill. Community nurses, under the supervision of referral hospitals, provided palliative care at home settings. In 1992, the King Faisal Specialty Hospital and Research Centre officially established a palliative care unit; this unit extends its services to home-based care for patients with cancer through its home care program [8]. In 2010, about 15 well-established palliative care centres were available in Saudi

Arabia with home-based services [12]. However, until recently, only patients living close to the centres could benefit from the home-based palliative care program [9, 12].

In Bahrain, the first official palliative care unit opened in 2010. The unit serves patients with cancer through follow-up clinics and hotline services. Palliative care has not yet extended to community or home-based care [12].

Qatar's main cancer centre (Al-Amal Hospital) started its palliative care services in 2008. Qatar is another country where palliative care is in the process of capacity building, indicating that community-based palliative care programs have not yet been established [12].

The United Arab Emirates started its first palliative care services in 2007 through Abu-Dhabi Tawam Hospital, and palliative care has yet to be extended to the community level [12].

In Iraq, despite the large number of cancer cases, palliative care has not yet begun, while Yemen and Syria were reported to be the two Middle Eastern countries without any known activities in palliative care [12].

Key Components of Best Practice in Community Palliative Care

Community-based palliative care is an essential practice for extending palliative care from the hospital setting, where the majority of resources are available in the community setting, and where more coordination of care and qualifications of multidisciplinary professionals are required. Therefore, community-based palliative care should maintain the quality of palliative care practice in the community. The Table 1 below summarises key components of ensuring best practice in community-based palliative care [16–19].

Table 1 Key components of best practice in community palliative care

1. *Interprofessional teamwork* with the right people on the team
2. *Strong partnership and linkage* between community health-care providers and other health-care organisations and hospitals to facilitate transition of patients' care and medical records
3. *Capacity building* and training of community care providers regarding essential skills for palliative care, specifically pain and symptom management strategies under direct supervision of palliative care specialists
4. *Holistic care approach* that includes physical, psychosocial, spiritual, mental and end-of-life needs. This requires a competent multidisciplinary team with effective teamwork skills.
5. *Continuity of care* even outside of working hours
6. Presence of *timely and responsive care* in cases of crisis and exacerbation
7. *Care coordination and transition* between and among different sectors at the community, primary care and hospital levels
8. Proper *identification of patients* requiring community-based palliative care
9. *Patient and family support/empowerment* to make them important contributors toward high-quality palliative care
10. *Appropriate care plan in the dying phase*
11. *Political support* in implementing national and international policies related to community-based palliative care
12. Availability of *safe environments, communication, transportation* and care kit storage

Patients' Priorities in Palliative Care

There has been a great emphasis on key priority topics that should be available in every palliative care program. At the patient level, the following priority topics need to be considered when assessing and evaluating hospital-based or community-based palliative care programs: pain and symptoms (e.g. nausea, vomiting, bowel obstruction, delirium, nutritional deficiencies) management, shared decision-making, patient and family support, reduction of despair and suffering, easy accessibility to human and community resources, continuity of care, availability of palliative sedation therapy and medical assistance in dying and end-of-life processes [20]. In Arab countries, these patient-related priorities should be highly considered for effective planning and coordination of care and services, taking into consideration that community-based palliative care is still growing.

Barriers to Community-Based Palliative Care in Arab Countries

The literature among Arab communities has reported various barriers to the successful establishment of palliative care services in community settings. These barriers can be linked to individual communities, health-care professionals, organisations, or health policy and legislation. The following are barriers to the establishment of community palliative care:

1. Limitation of human, educational, infrastructural and financial resources supporting palliative care in some Arab countries [6, 12, 14].
2. Limitation in funds allocated to palliative care programs, which affects the application of community-based palliative care programs. Limitation of funds could be related to under-recognition of the significance of such programs, leading to scarce distribution of resources. Additionally, the Arab region is still influenced by the Arab Spring, which was the reason for the instability, financial crises and insufficient development of the region's infrastructure [14].
3. Limitation in accessibility of palliative care medications (e.g. opioids) and specialists in particular settings, areas and even countries [9, 12, 14].
4. Insufficient supply of equipment and medications [6].
5. Lack of legislation, policies and regulations for palliative care [8, 12, 14].
6. The majority of organisations providing palliative care at the community level are non-governmental organisations (NGOs) with limited support from the government [8].
7. Unsatisfactory relationship between patients with cancer and their treating team [15].
8. The palliative care community team is not well-supported in terms of constant training, education and resources which is the main reason for burnout. In addition, a lack of appropriate training and qualifications of community nurses creates a huge challenge to establishing a strong, well-organised community-based palliative care system [6, 8, 10, 12, 14]. Providing the public with community nurses who are affiliated with community health-care providers or a cancer centre can minimise this challenge and ensure the provision of community-based palliative care services [6, 8].
9. Poor coordination of care between community-health nurses and hospital settings, which will influence the continuity of care in community settings [6, 8, 12, 14].
10. The community lacks awareness of the meaning and importance of palliative care, specifically community-based palliative care [6, 8, 12, 14]. For instance, palliative care is generally misunderstood and confused with euthanasia, which makes it hard to accept palliative care in community settings. Additionally, people perceive that morphine is a medication used to facilitate euthanasia instead of improving QOL by easing pain [15].
11. The culture could impose a barrier to home-based palliative care because, in some cultures, families (especially females) forbid health-care practitioners from entering their homes to provide care [6, 15].
12. Death and dying are considered taboo subjects, and the public refuses to discuss issues related to death and dying [14, 15].

Coordination Services in Community-Based Palliative Care

Shifting palliative care from hospital-based to community-based requires effective coordination services of the care. The implementation of successful coordination services between various entities (e.g. organisations, hospitals, hospice care, multidisciplinary health-care providers, community workers and volunteers, families and patients themselves) necessitates comprehensive planning and collective effort. Effective coordination of palliative care services at the community level: (1) is key to a successful multidisciplinary work, (2) reduces confusion and redundancy of patients' care, (3) reduces role conflicts within the team, (4) improves communication and (5) facilitates the provision of comprehensive care [20]. Well-established coordination services also have a great impact on care transition from hospitals to the community.

Future Direction and Recommendations

In summary, palliative care is a growing field in cancer and end-of-life management in Arab countries. Currently, palliative care in Arab countries is hospital-focused, with less attention given toward community-based palliative care. To improve the services of palliative care in general and community-based palliative care in particular, significant attention should be given by governments of Arab countries to the following recommendations:

1. The principle of palliative care should be highlighted as a main standard in postgraduate education programs, such as paediatrics, community nursing and family practitioners [8].
2. Ongoing training programs need to be offered to health-care providers such as oncologists, community nurses, pharmacists and social workers [21].
3. Enhancing community-based palliative care through the qualifications of a multidisciplinary health-care community team, including community nurses, to provide qualified and scientific palliative care [8].
4. Supporting community nurses and other family practitioners to adopt a new palliative care model that focuses on preparing family members to be a functional unit to provide palliative care at home. This will strengthen the provision of quality palliative care at the community level [8].
5. Establishment of educational and training programs for family caregivers and the public to empower care provided in areas where access to hospitals and community palliative care programs is inadequate [21].
6. Increase governmental support toward NGOs to improve community-based palliative care [8].
7. Establishment of constant governmental and non-governmental funds to maintain a well-developed and qualified palliative care system to serve the community [8, 12].
8. Development of national and/or regional policies and programs related to community-based palliative care [8, 12].
9. Establishment of home and hospice care programs taking into account that some patients have limited access to palliative care services, while others have no palliative care programs provided in their countries [12].
10. Strengthening the liaison between hospital teams and community nurses to improve palliative care provision in community settings [8].

The Decision-Making Process: Autonomy and Disclosure of Information

Patients' autonomy and self-determination are well-preserved rights in Arab communities. Patients have the right to determine the type and course of care that is best for them as long as they have the decision-making capacity [22]. When patients lack the capacity to make healthcare-related decisions, surrogate decision-makers give the necessary support [23].

However, the level of patients' autonomy varies significantly around the nation, especially among patients requiring palliative care. The concept of 'communicating bad news' makes the decision-making process more complicated. As we live in a culturally diverse world, there are certain Middle Eastern societies that do not disclose the disease diagnosis or the prognosis to patients, especially if the patients are old, uneducated or at an advanced stage of cancer [24]. Findings from a study conducted in Saudi Arabia revealed that family members prefer withholding detailed information about patients' cancer status and prognosis, as this information may result in fear and loss of hope [25]. As a result, the family often knows more about the diagnosis and treatment plan than the patients themselves [26].

Studies indicate that the majority of patients prefer to be well-informed about their disease and want disclosure of related information [25, 27]. While, in Western communities, patients are usually the first to know and agree to the treatment plan, in many Middle Eastern communities patients prefer that their families be the first to know about the disease condition and to agree to the treatment plan [28]. Thus, health-care professionals should be aware of the socio-cultural aspects and accept different practices to preserve patients' dignity and faith and provide high-quality care [29].

The Role of Family and Belief Systems in the Palliative Care Process

Patients' culture, belief system and morals are fundamental aspects of their palliative care process. Although the need for comfort, dignity and improvement in the quality of living at the end of life are universal concepts, there are still unique aspects of culture and religion that make the end-of-life decision-making process vary from nation to nation. In Arab communities, the family support system plays a significant role in decision-making. Close family members are more often directly involved in palliative care decision-making. Parents, spouses and older children have the greatest decision-making power compared with other members [30].

Another factor that plays a role in the palliative care decision-making process is the spiritual belief system. In Middle Eastern countries, Islam is the dominant religion. Muslims believe that having an illness represents an opportunity to expiate personal sins and that there is a treatment for every sickness. Yet, people should seek treatment to relieve suffering. Such an attitude has an impact on how patients and their families make their end-of-life choice of treatment. For example, unlike some Western countries, euthanasia is ethically not an acceptable practice in Middle Eastern countries. In addition, the use of opioids that affect consciousness is strictly prohibited. However, administering medically prescribed analgesics is acceptable as a pain management strategy and can be tolerated from Islamic ethical perspectives. It is very important for the health-care providers to discuss the possible side effects, such as drowsiness, with the family members prior to administration [22].

View of Policymakers and Future Direction of Palliative Care in Arab Communities

Access to palliative care should be part of the patient's bill of rights. As the demand for palliative services is increasing worldwide, policymakers and health-care organisations should expand palliative care services and training in Middle Eastern communities. Furthermore, access to palliative care needs to be an explicit right for people to plan for their end of life.

Raising community awareness about palliative care is highly recommended. Because patients and their families are an integral part of the decision-making process, increasing their awareness about palliative care would help to make their decisions more informed. Arab communities should be educated that their treatment preferences can be exercised using certain mechanisms, such as the advanced directives and living wills. Although these documents are considered legal in several Western countries, they are seldom used in Arab communities [31]. However, to provide patients and their families with more autonomy, these documents should be given legal status.

Because of the lack of palliative care laws and national policies and guidelines, health-care professionals working in Muslim-majority countries might be more vulnerable to malpractice and liability charges [22]. Therefore, patient autonomy should have an influence on the clinical practice, and policies should be developed for disease disclosure and proper information communication between patients and their care provider [32]. In addition, health-care providers should be educated and trained to cope with patients' sensitivities and different socio-cultural practices. The family-centred decision should be emphasised while providing palliative care for Arab patients.

The Role of Community Nurses in the Palliative Care Decision-Making Process

Community nurses should collaborate with other health-care team members to provide comprehensive end-of-life palliative care. Nurses should establish a decision-making process that reflects patients' preferences and religious and cultural values and addresses patients' psychosocial needs. In Arab countries, families play a significant role in the decision-making process, so nurses need to attend to patients' preferences and advocate for patient–family-centred care.

Patients' religious affiliation represents a key component of the value system and medical decision-making, particularly in issues involving end-of-life decisions such as withholding or withdrawing of treatment, medical futility and do-not-resuscitate orders [33]. Awadaei, Almoosawi, Humaidan and Dovey (2019) interviewed 12 Western-educated Bahraini doctors whose medical practice often included end-of-life decision-making [34]. Participants revealed differences between their palliative care practice in Bahrain, a Middle Eastern country, and previous work in Western countries, recognising the influences of religious and cultural beliefs on their practice in Bahrain. In Middle Eastern communities, it is very common for Muslim patients to consult and seek guidance — formally known as a *fatwa* — from an imam regarding some medical treatments [35]. An imam is a knowledgeable person educated about Islam's rules and regulations. Thus, health-care providers, including local and expatriate community nurses, should be sensitive to patients' varying religious beliefs, local cultural values and ethical standards.

Another important role of community nurses in palliative care decision-making is to assess and address psychosocial needs of patients, their families and care givers. Psychosocial care within palliative care is defined by the British Council for Palliative Care as being concerned with the psychological and emotional well-being of the patient and his or her family/care providers, including issues of self-esteem, insight into an adaptation to the illness and its consequences, communication, social functioning and relationships. Patients with terminal illnesses undergo a very stressful event. Hence, nurses should provide emotional support and facilitate spiritual support for patients and their family members [36].

The Role of Palliative Care Nurses in the Community

In the community, the role of palliative care nurses can be divided into two primary roles: direct patient care and indirect patient care [37].

Direct Patient Care

Besides conventional nursing care, such as assessment of symptoms, providing nursing interventions, medical treatment and health education [37], palliative care nurses provide direct patient care through a series of roles that include acting as a caregiver, counselor and psychologist, and therapeutic communicator.

Caregiver Nurses are the primary caregivers who spend most of their time with the patients. Whenever the patient cries out in pain, it is the nurse who responds immediately to ease the discomfort by providing either medical treatments, such as prescribed opioids without over-sedating the patient, or by educating the patient to manage pain using non-medical nursing interventions, such as relaxation therapies, distraction, massage and listening to the Quran. In the community, palliative nurses strive to understand the health issues from the standpoint of the patients and their families to provide culturally and religiously sensitive nursing care.

Counselor and psychologist Community palliative nurses provide emotional support to terminally ill cancer patients and their families by acting as a counselor, psychologist and caregiver [38]. Whenever dying patients express their feelings, the nurses guide them using an effective therapeutic communication approach to alleviate their sufferings and emotional burden.

Therapeutic communicator It is also the nurse's role to encourage and support the patients to make an informed decision about their care towards the final phase of their life [38]. This would be achieved by communicating significant health information to the patient appropriately and on time. Nurses' ethical communication of significant health information should be truthful and conveyed in a respectful, understandable and compassionate manner [36]. Moreover, it is expected of nurses to help their patients set realistic goals while providing genuine nursing care during the full period of their illness.

Indirect Patient Care

In addition to the direct patient care roles, palliative care nurses provide indirect patient care by acting as a case manager and an advocate for the patient.

Case manager Palliative care nurses provide indirect patient care by working in collaboration with a multidisciplinary team such as physicians, social workers, dietitians and physiotherapists, where the palliative care nurses coordinate and oversee the care provided for the patient [38]. As the primary care provider who is available around the clock and takes care of the patient, the nurses appear as gatekeepers to the services provided by other health-care providers. In the community, palliative care nurses coordinate care provided to the patient to maintain continuity of care and to provide optimal care to dying patients.

Advocator By profession, palliative care nurses are obligated to act as an advocate for the patient's rights and ensure that the care provided by the multidisciplinary team members meets patients' goals and preferences. Nurses spend more time with the patient than other health-care providers, and they establish a rapport with the patient and the family. Therefore, they are more aware of what the patient likes and dislikes, and they are more aware of the issues affecting patient care [36].

Clinical Training of Palliative Care in the Community

In the Middle East, clinical training of undergraduate nursing students in palliative care is still lacking [39]. The majority of nursing programs in the Middle East do not incorporate palliative care in their core curriculum, and they rarely examine the students in it. Only a few nursing programs have integrated palliative care into their curriculum. These include programs in Lebanon and Jordan [12]. Lebanon started incorporating palliative care into nursing programs in 2000. Jordan has a well-established interdisciplinary program for the provision of inpatient, outpatient and community palliative care [12].

Given the increase in the incidence of cancer across Middle Eastern countries, preparing nurses to provide quality palliative care is of priority. Many governments in the Middle East started recognising the importance of national palliative care services, such as in Saudi Arabia, Oman, Qatar and the United Arab Emirates [12]. For example, Saudi Arabia has a well-established inpatient palliative care unit at King Faisal Hospital, and it is well-recognised as a training centre in the region. Moreover, in the Sultanate of Oman, the Ministry of Health celebrated the graduation of the first group of palliative care nurses (360 nurses) in 2018. The graduated nurses attended a three-year palliative care nursing program at the national level. These nurses were trained to provide palliative care in various settings in Oman, including the community setting. The program was conducted under the umbrella of internationally recognised institutions, including the Middle East Cancer Consortium, the Oncology Nurses Society and the American Society of Clinical Oncology. This initiative started after a needs assessment in 2012 revealed the requirement to train a total of 360

Omani nurses in palliative cancer care to improve the QOL of cancer sufferers in the Sultanate. Since 2002, the palliative care services in Oman have been improving progressively, as evidenced by the provision of palliative nursing care in the National Oncology Centre [40].

Future Direction of Palliative Care in Nursing Curriculum

According to the World Health Organization, education is a priority for ensuring the effective implementation of cancer pain relief programs. It has, therefore, been recommended that training nurses and other health-care providers on palliative care generally and on cancer pain management specifically is essential to enable nurses to deliver a high standard of palliative care to terminally ill cancer patients.

To provide high standards of end-of-life care, nurses must be well-armed with essential knowledge and skills to provide effective palliative care. In addition, they must be well-trained to provide sympathetic and empathetic care to terminally ill cancer patients by working on their attitude and interpersonal competencies. These include effective communication skills, understanding the health issues from the patient's perspectives, an obligation to provide holistic and culturally sensitive care to the patient, and a focus on improving the patient's QOL while respecting the patient's beliefs, values and goals [38]. Therefore, integrating palliative care content into the nursing curriculum and considering interprofessional education of palliative care are urgent priorities. Also, emphasis on active learning strategies over passive strategies is essential to deliver palliative care education effectively. Furthermore, nursing students must be examined about their capabilities to provide palliative care; therefore, questions about palliative care should be included in the national nursing board exams. Nursing education should be designed in a way that prepares and trains nursing students to deliver the best evidenced-based palliative care practices.

Paediatric Palliative Care (PPC)

Palliative care is a care method directed toward patients with life-threatening illness with a main goal of improving their QOL. The same definition applies to children, but with more emphasis on integrating family-centred care, including family enabling and empowerment. Family enabling supports the family in caring for their chronically ill child with more independence, and family empowerment encourages the family to make sound decisions in matters related to their child's care [41].

Continuous family support and maximum utilisation of resources available in the community are essential in PPC. For effective PPC, a multidisciplinary team comprising physicians, nurses, social workers, child life specialists and psychology therapists should be involved in the care. It is important to note that the definition of children in the health-care settings of most Middle Eastern countries is limited to children under the age of 13 years because of cultural and religious considerations [42]. Children aged 13 years and older are transitioned to adult health-care settings and are managed by adult health-care teams.

PPC is highly needed in the Middle Eastern region. According to studied estimates, 20 to 120 out of 10,000 children worldwide need palliative care [43]. The rate of cancer among children aged 0 to 14 years in the Middle East is 11.4% [44]. Besides cancer, more than 35% of the total diseases in the Arab region were related to congenital malformations and chromosomal anomalies, which require PPC. These morbidities reached an alarming rate in the Middle East, which indicates a need for critical attention to palliative care in children.

Challenges to PPC

Children are a special group of people with needs that differ from those of adults, and so does their palliative care. However, palliative care in the Middle East is mainly directed toward adults, as no separate unit for PPC exists in the health-care settings of most countries in the Middle Eastern region [45]. Barriers to palliative care for children in the Middle East have been identified as a lack of policymakers' support, limited financial resources and inadequate provision of palliative care medication [46].

In addition, PPC poses challenges to health-care professionals themselves. There is a lack of professional training in both knowledge and coping mechanisms. PPC is not adequately emphasised in academic curriculum and causes added emotional distress. Sadness, feelings of failure and emotional detachment while caring for children who need palliative care have been reported [47].

Community-Based Paediatric Palliative Care (CBPPC)

Implementing PPC at home can be successful [48], particularly in the Middle Eastern region. People in the Middle East are overwhelmed by the family-centred culture and the social norms that undervalue the taking care of a terminally ill family member, especially children, by strangers. Parents of children with cancer in the Middle East have expressed needs such as wanting to know comprehensively about their child's health condition, to meet other parents with similar experiences and to receive adequate support from family, friends and health-care providers [49, 50].

CBPPC provides an opportunity for parents to take care of their terminally ill child at home. It is a cost-effective and holistic approach to care that is shown to improve children's QOL. Research findings indicate that CBPPC has remarkably reduced hospital utilisation and related costs and has significantly improved the health-related QOL among children with life-threatening illness and their families [51]. In addition, it has provided an opportunity for a home death to a majority of the families desiring it [52].

Palliative care is characterised by flexibility, and different models can be incorporated while providing palliative care, such as a consultative model, a few-personnel floating model and a telehealth model [53]. PPC centres in the Middle East, which suffers from limited human and financial resources and delivers care to a community that values a family-centred care approach, can benefit more from CBPPC. Collaboration with specialty clinics like the oncology clinic and the genetic clinic through consultation, sharing of human resources from community health centres and utilisation of technologies such as telehealth have the potential for successful CBPPC implementation in the Middle East.

Research and Professional Associations

Collaboration among Middle Eastern countries in palliative care for children's research and training has started recently. The Middle East Childhood Cancer Alliance has initiated a collaborative study to provide demographic and clinical data on children with acute lymphoblastic leukaemia (ALL) in the Middle East. The study was published in 2014 and provided comprehensive information on patient, laboratory and genetic characteristics; treatment protocol; response to induction therapy; and complications and toxicity among children with ALL [54]. In addition, the Paediatric Oncology East and Mediterranean (POEM) Group was established in 2013 to share experiences, initiate cooperative trials and develop common strategies. The group works toward care optimisation of paediatric oncology patients through needs assessment, robust registries, health-care provider training, guidelines, quality control, public awareness and strategic policy [55].

Research on Palliative Care in Arab Countries

Palliative care research has become a worldwide concern [56] and an important indicator of sustainable development goals [57]. With many people immigrating outside the Middle East in recent years, palliative care for the Arabic population must be investigated. Nevertheless, in Arab countries palliative care research is at its foundational stage [58, 59]. In this section, we provide an overview of the status of research in palliative care in Arab countries to assist researchers, funding institutions and policymakers in improving palliative care clinical advancements and outcomes. We conducted a systematic search in three databases (CINHAL, PubMed and Google Scholar) for each of the 22 Arab countries using the search terms *palliative care* and *end of life care*. Limits applied were academic articles and English language. The search was last updated on 30 July 2019. A total of 61 articles were located and reviewed.

Status of Palliative Care Research in Arab Countries

Scarcity of Literature

Each year, an estimated 40 million people require palliative care globally; 78% of them reside in low- and middle-income countries [60], such as Arab countries. However, our search results showed that the literature on palliative care research in this area is scarce, indicating that the Arabic population is understudied. This may be partially due to the unavailable palliative care services throughout this area [61, 62]. It may also be due to restricted controlled palliative care medicine, inaccessible palliative care services and lack of health professional training [60]. Of note, we found one study conducted in the Netherlands on Moroccans and Turks living there, which found inconsistent use of the available palliative care services among these Middle Eastern nationals [63]. This suggests that availability and access to palliative care may not be the only barriers to palliative care services and research.

The scant research output in this area may also be strongly linked to the low funding allotted for research in Arab countries generally and for palliative care research specifically. Numbers of published studies vary among the 22 Arab countries, as shown in Table 2. Lebanon has the highest number of palliative care publications (18 articles), followed by Jordan (13 article) and Morocco (seven articles). Eleven Arab countries have no palliative care publications. A good number of comparative studies between countries were published that were not included in the table but were used in our overall appraisal [59, 64–66]. A 2017 atlas of palliative care in the Middle East showed similar statistics to what we have presented here [61]. This indicates there is no significant increase in the number of published articles during the last two to three years. It is not surprising that most of these studies were published after 2010, indicating that palliative care research is fairly new.

Table 2 Number of published palliative care research articles by country

	Country	Number of published articles (excluding comparative studies)
1	Algeria	0
2	Bahrain	0
3	Comoros	0
4	Djibouti	0
5	Egypt	4
6	Iraq	0
7	Jordan	13
8	Kuwait	4
9	Lebanon	18
10	Libya	0
11	Mauritania	1
12	Morocco	7
13	Oman	1
14	Palestine	1
15	Qatar	4
16	Saudi Arabia	1
17	Somalia	0
18	Sudan	0
19	Syria	0
20	Tunisia	0
21	UAE	2
22	Yemen	0
	Total	**61**

Conceptual and Methodological Issues

Due to the increasing burden of non-communicable diseases and ageing populations, the field of palliative care continues to grow [67]. Many concepts and disease contexts related to palliative care need to be investigated, such as the concept of ageing and symptom management. Yet, almost all the studies conducted in Arab countries were focused on oncology palliative care only [64, 65, 68]. The focus of the published articles in the area of oncology palliative care was mostly on the perception of palliative care [69, 71], medication use [72] and symptoms [73, 74]. Other disease contexts that need palliative care were not studied, such as cardiovascular terminal illnesses (e.g. heart failure) and chronic obstructive pulmonary disease. A group of studies described the perception of physician nurses and nursing students' knowledge and attitude toward palliative care [39, 69, 70]. The timing of initiating palliative care was investigated by only one study [75]. Other important concepts have not been examined yet, such as ageing. No epidemiological studies have examined the number of people in need of palliative care. More importantly to note is that the concept of palliative care was not clearly defined in the studies and has been used interchangeably with the concept of end-of-life care [76]. Although both concepts are similar, it may create confusion that palliative care is only used in terminally ill patients versus in any condition that requires pain control and comfort measures.

From a methodological perspective, several issues were noticed across the appraised studies. Sample sizes were small in almost all studies, except for those conducted on students and healthcare professionals [69]. Nearly all studies reviewed were conducted on adult populations. Few studies were done on children [77–79]. In addition, we think that people living in rural areas have been overlooked in palliative care research in Arab countries. Moreover, studies were conducted in both inpatient and outpatient settings, but no studies have been conducted in community-based settings [14, 39, 80]. Further, most studies used quantitative approaches, except for a few that used qualitative approaches [63, 81]. All the quantitative studies used a prospective cross-sectional design.

Future Directions for Palliative Care Research

Palliative care research is as vital as palliative care service itself. Quality, rigorous research is needed to improve the lives of patients and families while advancing palliative care science. Proposed future areas of inquiry for researchers in palliative care may include advanced treatments (e.g. medications, other therapeutic interventions), epidemiology (e.g. underlying disease process, gender, age, multimorbidity, education of patients and families), self-care of patients, self-care of palliative care professionals, family caregiving and caregiver burden. More importantly, palliative care research should be directed to community-based studies, and special attention should be given to the difficult-to-reach populations, such as those in rural areas. Additionally, various research designs and approaches should be used to enhance the understanding of dynamics of palliative care. We recommend conducting more longitudinal studies to understand the effect of palliative care over time. Better representations of all age groups, gender and underlying diseases should be considered.

Funding institutions and policymakers may enhance research in palliative care by allocating funds, scholarships and fellowships. In addition, ensuring that quality data regarding palliative care are recorded in hospitals' electronic systems, such as the use of controlled substances, will enhance the accessibility of data for researchers to be used in studies and relevant scientific publications. Policymakers should also encourage cross-country and regional research collaboration to increase the understanding of palliative care through comparative studies. In addition, researchers worldwide should be supported and encouraged to examine how Arab immigrants use palliative services in the hosting non-Arab countries.

Conclusion

Community-based palliative care programs in Arab countries are underdeveloped and require a collective effort to overcome initial challenges. A limited amount of literature focusing on community-based palliative care programs in Arab countries has been published over the last 20 years. Accordingly, there is limited information describing the status of palliative care at community levels. Attention should now be directed toward optimising palliative care services by focusing on community-based program.

References

1. Fearon D, Kane H, Aliou ND, Sall A. Perceptions of palliative care in a lower middle-income Muslim country: A qualitative study of health care professionals, bereaved families and communities. Palliat Med. 2019;33(2):241–9.
2. Davidson PM, Phillips JL, Dennison-Himmelfarb C, Thompson SC, Luckett T, Currow DC. Providing palliative care for cardiovascular disease from a perspective of sociocultural diversity: a global view. Curr Opin Support Palliat Care. 2016;10(1):11–7.
3. Robinson S, Kissane DW, Brooker J, Burney S. A review of the construct of demoralization: History, definitions, and future directions for palliative care. Am J Hosp Palliat Med. 2016;33(1):93–101.
4. Seow H, Dhaliwal G, Fassbender K, Rangrej J, Brazil K, Fainsinger R. The effect of community-based specialist palliative care teams on place of care. J Palliat Med. 2016;19(1):16–21.
5. Youens D, Moorin R. The impact of community-based palliative care on utilization and cost of acute care hospital services in the last year of life. J Palliat Med. 2017;20(7):736–44.
6. Doumit M, Silbermann M, Fink RM, Mancuso MP, Brant J, Hajjar R, et al. Evaluating palliative care needs in Middle Eastern Countries. 2015.
7. al-Awamer A, Downar J. Developing a palliative care service model for Muslim Middle Eastern countries. Support Care Cancer. 2014;22(12):3253–62.
8. Silbermann M, Arnaout M, Daher M, Nestoros S, Pitsillides B, Charalambous H, et al. Palliative cancer care in Middle Eastern countries: accomplishments and challenges. Ann Oncol. 2012;23(suppl_3):15–28.
9. Nixon A. Palliative care in Saudi Arabia: a brief history. J Pain Palliat Care Pharmacother. 2004; 17(3–4):45–9.
10. Aljawi DM, Harford JB. Palliative care in the Muslim-majority countries: the need for more and better care. Contemporary and Innovative Practice in Palliative Care China. USA: InTech; 2012. p. 137–50.
11. Mendieta M, Buckingham RW. A review of palliative and hospice care in the context of Islam: dying with faith and family. J Palliat Med. 2017;20(11): 1284–90.
12. Zeinah GFA, Al-Kindi SG, Hassan AA. Middle East experience in palliative care. Am J Hosp Palliat Med. 2013;30(1):94–9.
13. Al-Zadjali M, Al Sinawi F, Al Touby S, Al Busaidi M, Al Jardani F. Palliative Care Nursing in Oman; Moving towards Palliative Care Nursing. J Palliat Care Med. 2015;5:40–4.
14. Shamieh O, Hui D. A comprehensive palliative care program at a tertiary cancer center in Jordan. Am J Hosp Palliat Med. 2015;32(2):238–42.
15. Gray AJ, Ezzat A, Volker S. Developing palliative care services for terminally ill patients in Saudi Arabia. Ann Saudi Med. 1995;15(4):370–7.
16. Meyers K, Kerr K, Cassel J. Up close: a field guide to community-based palliative care in California. Sacramento: California Health Care Foundation; 2014.
17. Brogaard T, Neergaard MA, Murray SA. Promoting palliative care in the community: a toolkit to improve and develop primary palliative care throughout Europe. Scand J Prim Health Care. 2016;34(1):3.
18. Seow H, Bainbridge D. A review of the essential components of quality palliative care in the home. J Palliat Med. 2018;21(S1):S–37-S-44.
19. Fallon M, Hanks G. ABC of palliative care. USA: Wiley; 2013.
20. Canada CoFPo. PALLIATIVE CARE priority topics for the assessment of competence: enhanced skills key features. Retrieved from https://www.cfpc.ca/uploadedFiles/Education/PC_KF_Final_ENG.pdf, 2017.
21. Webster R, Lacey J, Quine S. Palliative care: a public health priority in developing countries: Springer; 2007. p. 28(1), –39.
22. Ghaly M, Diamond RR, El-Akoum M, Hassan A. Palliative care and Islamic ethics. 2018.
23. Miller LL, Harvath TA, Ganzini L, Goy ER, Delorit MA, Jackson A. Attitudes and experiences of Oregon hospice nurses and social workers regarding assisted suicide. Palliat Med. 2004;18(8):685–91.
24. Al-Bahri A, Al-Moundhri M, Al-Mandhari Z, Al-Azri M. The role of patients' families in treatment decision-making among adult cancer patients in the Sultanate of Oman. Eur J Cancer Care. 2018;27(3):e12845.
25. Alzahrani AS, Alqahtani A, Alhazmi M, Gaafar R, Bajabir D, Alharbi IM, et al. Attitudes of cancer patients and their families toward disclosure of cancer diagnosis in Saudi Arabia: a Middle Eastern population example. Patient Prefer Adherence. 2018;12:1659.
26. Farhat F, Othman A, El Baba G, Kattan J. Revealing a cancer diagnosis to patients: attitudes of patients, families, friends, nurses, and physicians in Lebanon—results of a cross-sectional study. Curr Oncol. 2015;22(4):e264.
27. Obeidat R, Khrais HI. Jordanian physicians' attitudes toward disclosure of cancer information and patient participation in treatment decision-making. Asia Pac J Oncol Nurs. 2016;3(3):281.
28. Silbermann M, Hassan EA. Cultural perspectives in cancer care: impact of Islamic traditions and practices in Middle Eastern countries. J Pediatr Hematol Oncol. 2011;33:S81–S6.
29. Zirak M, Ghafourifard M, Mamaghani EA. Patients' dignity and its relationship with contextual variables: a cross-sectional study. J Caring Sci. 2017;6(1):49.

30. Ghaly M, Diamond RR, El-Akoum M, Hassan A. Palliative care and Islamic ethics. 2018:1–52.
31. Baharoon DA, Rahman HA, Fadhl SO. Publics' knowledge, attitudes and behavioral toward the use of solar energy in Yemen power sector. Renew Sust Energ Rev. 2016;60:498–515.
32. Sarafis P, Tsounis A, Malliarou M, Lahana E. Disclosing the truth: a dilemma between instilling hope and respecting patient autonomy in everyday clinical practice. Global J Health Sci. 2014;6(2):128.
33. Kassim PNJ, Alias F. Religious, ethical and legal considerations in end-of-life issues: fundamental requisites for medical decision making. J Relig Health. 2016;55(1):119–34.
34. Alwadaei S, Almoosawi B, Humaidan H, Dovey S. Waiting for a miracle or best medical practice? End-of-life medical ethical dilemmas in Bahrain. J Med Ethics. 2019;45(6):367–72.
35. Boucher NA, Siddiqui EA, Koenig HG. Supporting Muslim patients during advanced illness. Perm J. 2017;21:16.
36. Schroeder K, Lorenz K. Nursing and the future of palliative care. Asia Pac J Oncol Nurs. 2018;5(1):4.
37. Husaini A. The role of nurses in providing palliative care for dying cancer patients: a meta-ethnographic synthesis. BMJ Support Palliat Care. 2014;4(Suppl 1):A1–2.
38. Association AN. Call for action: Nurses lead and transform palliative care. https://www.nursingworld.org/~497158/globalassets/practiceandpolicy/health-policy/palliativecareprofessionalissuespanelcallforaction.pdf, 2017.
39. Al-Kindi SG, Zeinah GFA, Hassan AA. Palliative care knowledge and attitudes among oncology nurses in Qatar. Am J Hosp Palliat Med. 2014;31(5):469–74.
40. Daily M. Omanis graduate in three-year palliative care nursing program. https://muscatdaily.com/Archive/Oman/360-Omanis-graduate-in-three-year-palliative-care-nursing-program-5aqm: 2018.
41. Wilson D, Rodgers CC. Wong's essentials of pediatric nursing-e-book. Canada: Elsevier Health Sciences; 2016.
42. Abdwani R, Abdalla E, Al Abrawi S, Al-Zakwani I. Epidemiology of juvenile idiopathic arthritis in Oman. Pediatr Rheumatol Online J. 2015;13:33.
43. Connor SR, Downing J, Marston J. Estimating the Global Need for Palliative Care for Children: A Cross-sectional Analysis. J Pain Symptom Manag. 2017;53(2):171–7.
44. Steliarova-Foucher E, Colombet M, Ries LAG, Moreno F, Dolya A, Bray F, et al. International incidence of childhood cancer, 2001-10: a population-based registry study. Lancet Oncol. 2017;18(6):719–31.
45. Connor SR, Sepulveda Bermedo MC. Global atlas of palliative care at the end of life. 2018.
46. Mojen LK, Rassouli M, Eshghi P, Sari AA, Karimooi MH. Palliative Care for Children with Cancer in the Middle East: A Comparative Study. Indian J Palliat Care. 2017;23(4):379–86.
47. Verri ER, Santana Bitencourt NA, da Silva Oliveira JA, dos Santos Júnior R, Silva Marques H, Alves Porto M, et al. NURSING PROFESSIONALS: UNDERSTANDING ABOUT PEDIATRIC PALLIATIVE CARE. J Nurs UFPE/Revista de Enfermagem UFPE. 2019;13:1.
48. van der Geest IM, Bindels PJ, Pluijm SM, Michiels EM, van der Heide A, Pieters R, et al. Home-based palliative care for children with incurable cancer: long-term perspectives of and impact on general practitioners. J Pain Symptom Manag. 2017;53(3):578–87.
49. Doumit MA, Rahi AC, Saab R, Majdalani M. Spirituality among parents of children with cancer in a Middle Eastern country. Eur J Oncol Nurs. 2019;39:21–7.
50. Sasaki H, Bouesseau MC, Marston J, Mori R. A scoping review of palliative care for children in low- and middle-income countries. BMC Palliat Care. 2017;16(1):60.
51. Goldhagen J, Fafard M, Komatz K, Eason T, Livingood WC. Community-based pediatric palliative care for health related quality of life, hospital utilization and costs: lessons learned from a pilot study. BMC Palliat Care. 2016;15:73.
52. Chirico J, Donnelly JP, Gupton A, Cromwell P, Miller M, Dawson C, et al. Costs of Care and Location of Death in Community-Based Pediatric Palliative Care. J Palliat Med. 2019;22(5):517–21.
53. Brock KE, Snaman JM, Kaye EC, Bower KA, Weaver MS, Baker JN, et al. Models of Pediatric Palliative Oncology Outpatient Care-Benefits, Challenges, and Opportunities. J Oncol Pract. 2019;15(9): 476–87.
54. Al-Mulla NA, Chandra P, Khattab M, Madanat F, Vossough P, Torfa E, et al. Childhood acute lymphoblastic leukemia in the Middle East and neighboring countries: a prospective multi-institutional international collaborative study (CALLME1) by the Middle East Childhood Cancer Alliance (MECCA). Pediatr Blood Cancer. 2014;61(8): 1403–10.
55. Rodriguez-Galindo C, Friedrich P, Alcasabas P, Antillon F, Banavali S, Castillo L, et al. Toward the cure of all children with cancer through collaborative efforts: pediatric oncology as a global challenge. J Clin Oncol. 2015;33(27):3065.
56. Arias-Casais N, Garralda E, López-Fidalgo J, Lima L, Rhee JY, Pons-Izquierdo JJ, et al. Brief manual health indicators monitoring global palliative care development. 2019.
57. Ghebreyesus TA, Fore H, Birtanov Y, Jakab Z. Primary health care for the 21st century, universal health coverage, and the Sustainable Development Goals. Lancet. 2018;392(10156):1371–2.
58. Lynch T, Connor S, Clark D. Mapping levels of palliative care development: a global update. J Pain Symptom Manag. 2013;45(6):1094–106.
59. Silbermann M, et al. Evaluating palliative care needs in middle eastern countries. J Palliat Med. 2015;18(1):18.

60. Organization WH. Fact Sheet on Palliative Care. https://www.who.int/news-room/fact-sheets/detail/palliative-care: 2018.
61. Osman H RA, Garralda E, Rhee JY, Pons JJ, de Lima L, Tfayli A, Centeno C. Atlas of Palliative Care in the Eastern Mediterranean Region. Houston: IAHPC Press; 2017.
62. Pastrana T, Vallath N, Mastrojohn J, Namukwaya E, Kumar S, Radbruch L, et al. Disparities in the contribution of low- and middle-income countries to palliative care research. J Pain Symptom Manag. 2010;39(1):54–68.
63. de Graaff FM, Francke AL. Home care for terminally ill Turks and Moroccans and their families in the Netherlands: carers' experiences and factors influencing ease of access and use of services. Int J Nurs Stud. 2003;40(8):797–805.
64. Khatib O, Aljurf M. Cancer Prevention and Control in the Eastern Mediterranean Region: The Need for a Public Health Approach. Hematol Oncol Stem Cell Ther. 2008;1(1):44–52.
65. Silbermann M, Arnaout M, Daher M, Nestoros S, Pitsillides B, Charalambous H, et al. Palliative cancer care in Middle Eastern countries: accomplishments and challenges. Ann Oncol. 2012;23(suppl 3):15–28.
66. Zeinah GF, Al-Kindi SG, Hassan AA. Middle East experience in palliative care. Am J Hosp Palliat Care. 2013;30(1):94–9.
67. Fitch MI, Fliedner MC, O'Connor M. Nursing perspectives on palliative care 2015. Ann Palliat Med. 2015;4(3):150–5.
68. Hablas M. Palliative care in Egypt: the experience of the Gharbiah Cancer Society. Eur J Cancer. 2017;72:S161.
69. Al Qadire M. Knowledge of palliative care: An online survey. Nurse Educ Today. 2014;34(5):714–8.
70. Abu-El-Noor NI, Abu-El-Noor MK. Attitude of Palestinian nursing students toward caring for dying patients: A call for change in health education policy. J Holist Nurs. 2016;34(2):193–9.
71. Saad R, Huijer HAS, Noureddine S, Muwakkit S, Saab R, Abboud MR. Bereaved parental evaluation of the quality of a palliative care program in Lebanon. Pediatr Blood Cancer. 2011;57(2):310–6.
72. Wilby KJ, Mohamad AA, AlYafei SA. Evaluation of clinical pharmacy services offered for palliative care patients in Qatar. J Pain Palliat Care Pharmacother. 2014;28(3):212–5.
73. Qadire MA, Tubaishat A, Aljezawi MEM. Cancer pain in Jordan: prevalence and adequacy of treatment. Int J Palliat Nurs. 2013;19(3):125–30.
74. Alsirafy SA, El Mesidy SM, Abou-Elela EN, Elfaramawy YI. Pain prevalence in advanced cancer patients in Egypt. Eur J Palliat Care. 2010;17(6):303–5.
75. Bakouny Z, Assi T, El Rassy E, Daccache K, Kattan C, Tohme A, et al. Factors associated with the time to first palliative care consultation in Lebanese cancer patients. Support Care Cancer. 2019;27(4):1529–33.
76. Razeq NMA. End-of-life Decisions at Neonatal Intensive Care Units: Jordanian Nurses Attitudes and Viewpoints of Who, When, and How. J Pediatr Nurs. 2019;44:e36–44.
77. Mojen LK, Rassouli M, Eshghi P, Sari AA, Karimooi MH. Palliative care for children with cancer in the Middle East: A comparative study. Indian J Palliat Care. 2017;23(4):379.
78. Atout M, Hemingway P, Seymour J. The Practice of Mutual Protection in the Care of Children with Palliative Care Needs: A Multiple Qualitative Case Study Approach from Jordan. J Pediatr Nurs. 2019;45:e9–e18.
79. Atout M, Hemingway P, Seymour J. The experience of decision making in the care of children with palliative care needs: the experiences of Jordanian mothers. Compr Child Adolesc Nurs. 2017;40(4):240–56.
80. Shamieh O, Khamash O, Khraisat M, Jbouri O, Awni M, Al-Hawamdeh A, et al. Impact of outpatient palliative care (PC) on symptom burden in patients with advanced cancer at a tertiary cancer center in Jordan. Support Care Cancer. 2017;25(1):177–83.
81. de Graaff FM, Francke AL, van den Muijsenbergh ME, van der Geest S. Talking in triads: communication with Turkish and Moroccan immigrants in the palliative phase of cancer. J Clin Nurs. 2012;21(21–22):3143–52.

Part XXIII

Middle East: Lebanon

The Physician's Role in Running a Palliative Care Service in the Community: The Lebanon Experience

Ramzi R. Hajjar

Introduction and Background Construct

To best understand the role of physicians in providing palliative care for cancer patients in the community in Lebanon, it is helpful to briefly review the context in which palliative care is practiced. Demographics, case distribution, resource availability and conceptualization by the consumer (and provider) together determine the nature and ultimately effectiveness of this still fledgling specialty. The cultural milieu in which palliative care is practiced differs in many ways – as will be discussed – from Westernized countries on which our programs are structured and whose models of care we strive to emulate, befittingly or not.

Lebanon, like the rest of the world, has experienced a demographic shift over the past few decades that has profoundly impacted the practice of medicine and the delivery of healthcare. As the world population increased, life expectancy in developed and developing countries has also increased. Consequently, the absolute and relative number of older adults has grown at an unprecedented rate. This demographic shift will particularly be felt in Lebanon in the not-too-distant future, as the relatively young masses move up the population pyramid.

Lebanon is a diverse and heterogeneous country where politics, sectarianism, and party affiliation pervade most aspects of life, including the medical establishment. Microcosms within the tiny nation can differ widely in religious practices, economic privilege, and cultural norms, essentially discounting the "one size fits all" approach to care. The recent economic collapse has further eroded the ability of physicians to deliver effective and comprehensive medical care, and services deemed "non-essential" are first to fall victim to the struggling system. According to the World Bank, about 40% of Lebanese live in poverty. Healthcare services, which are increasingly being funded out-of-pocket, are beyond the reach of a rapidly increasing proportion of the population. It is imperative that healthcare providers working in this environment have a solid understanding of the elements that unite or separate different segments of the population, and are able to recognize and marginalize their own personal biases if meaningful end-of-life care is to be offered.

Imbedded within this diversity, however, are certain generalizable truths, not least of which are the inexorable progress toward old age, the family involvement in care of loved ones and the steady descent of large segments of the population into poverty even as healthcare costs escalate. Today, it is estimated that just under 10% of

R. R. Hajjar (✉)
Department of Internal Medicine, Geriatric Medicine Service, American University of Beirut Medical Center, Beirut, Lebanon
e-mail: rh110@aub.edu.lb

M. Silbermann (ed.), *Palliative Care for Chronic Cancer Patients in the Community*,
https://doi.org/10.1007/978-3-030-54526-0_32

the population is above the age of 65 years and 1.5% above the age of 85 years – a small proportion compared to Western Europe and the United States, but quite high regionally (Fig. 1). According to the World Health Organization (WHO), life expectancy lags only slightly behind that of developed countries, and currently stands at 75.1 years for men and 77.7 years for women [4]. It is projected that in 25 years, the number of Lebanese older than 65 will double, at which time one in five residents of this small Mediterranean country – with a current population of approximately six million – will be in the geriatric age group [1–3].

But with longevity comes chronic, costly, and serious illness, including many types of cancers, which the Lebanese healthcare system is ill-prepared to deal with. As elsewhere, aging is a major risk factor for many types of cancers and all-cause cancer incidence peaks at around age of 70 years (Fig. 2) [5, 6]. The number of new cases of cancer in Lebanon has increased steadily over the past decades, according to the National Cancer Registry of the Ministry of Health and the World Health Organization (WHO. In 2005, over 7400 new cases of cancer were reported in Lebanon, compared to 10,187 in 2010, and 12,238 in 2016 [6]. This worrisome trend is not entirely due to aging alone; expanded screening efforts and improved registration methods have likely contributed significantly. Nonetheless, the need for competent and effective end-of-life care in the community is immense and unmet [7].

Moreover, due to a high prevalence of cancer-promoting behavior (such as smoking) and apathy or aversion toward preventive care, many cancers present at an advanced stage when symptoms alert to the presence of disease and the only reasonable treatment option is palliative care [7, 8]. A comprehensive palliative care service clearly should not be restricted to terminal cancer patients, but in Lebanon referrals for end-of-life care are seldom generated from other services. In my experience at the American University of Beirut Medical Center, of 164 cases managed by both inpatient and outpatient care over the past 5 years, approximately 86% were above the age of 65 years and 74% were for management of terminal malignancies. This is in sharp

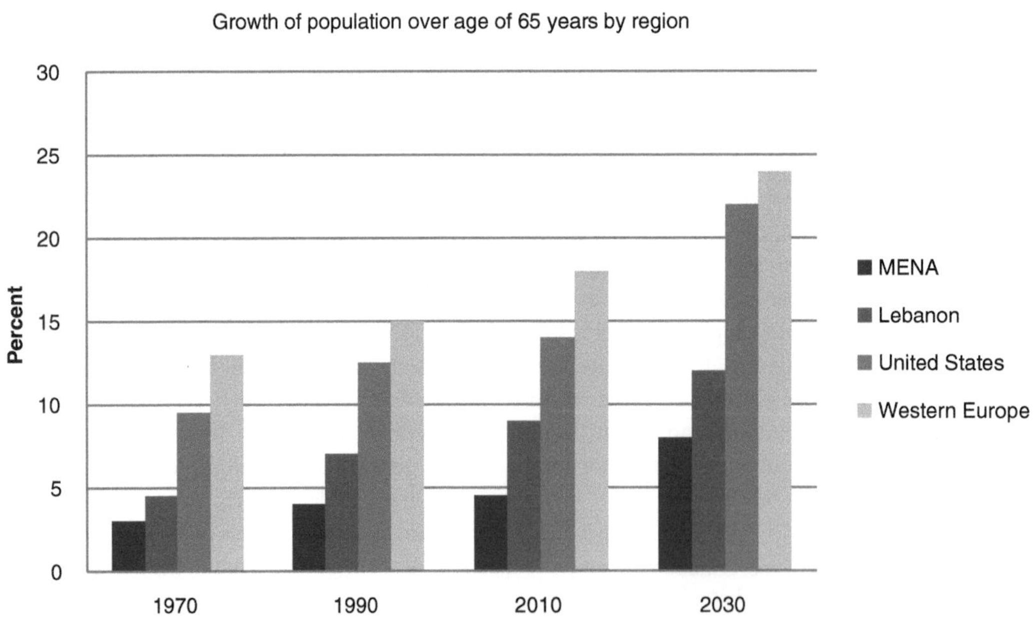

Fig. 1 Growth of population over age of 65 years by region [1–3, 25]. MENA Middle East and Northern Africa

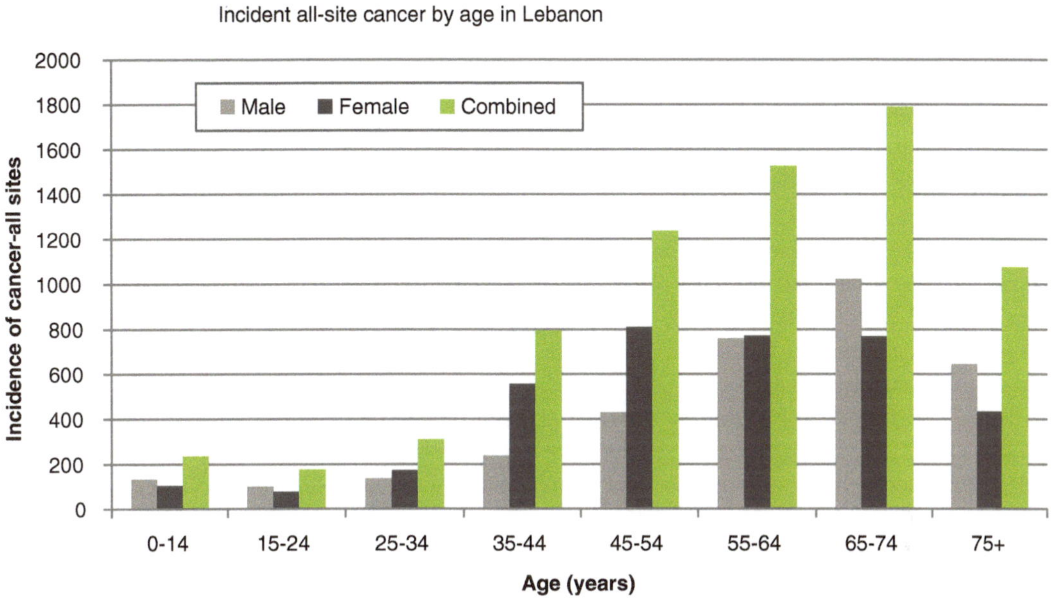

Fig. 2 Incident cancer cases in Lebanon by age. All-case cancer excludes non-melanoma skin cancer. (Source: National Cancer Registry (Ministry of Public Health, NCR))

contrast to the United States, where over two-thirds of hospice enrollees have non-malignant diagnoses, according to the Medicare Hospice Benefits report. Even so, by one estimate, less than 10% of patients with terminal malignancies benefited from palliative care services in Lebanon due to a deficiency of professionally trained providers, public awareness, and program availability and accessibility.

Seven medical schools currently exist in Lebanon. The abundance of well-trained physicians, however, are poorly distributed and clustered mainly in big cities, and large rural areas are deprived of specialty care. Despite being a tiny country, the crumbling infrastructure and choking traffic congestion resulting from decades of mismanagement prohibit willing providers from completing home care visits in an efficient and constructive manner. In addition, third-party payers do not cover home-based primary and specialty care. For these reasons, it is not cost effective for most providers to deliver care away from their clinic or hospital practice. Centralization of tertiary and specialty care means that many individuals requiring palliative care expertise will receive it late, if at all.

The cultural forces that affect acceptance and utilization of community palliative care services are many and have been reviewed elsewhere [9–11, 25]. Some healthcare professionals do not view symptom management as a goal in itself. Instead they continue to focus on curable interventions, even as these measures become futile. Home care, therefore, becomes paramount to dereliction of duties. Some might even view the dying process as a failure of modern medicine. Interestingly, many patients or their families harbor these same thoughts. Consequently, an inordinate number of patients with life-limiting illness spend extended periods in the hospital receiving tertiary care that does not necessarily alleviate symptoms or improve quality of life.

It is in this setting that physicians must carve out their role in the greater effort to assert themselves and the specialty of palliative care in the community at large. This unique construct offers both obstacles and opportunities. Done properly, and with the support of key stakeholders, the potential to build a culturally appropriate service from the ground up and integrate it into mainstream medicine is promising.

Role of the Physician in Community Palliative Care

When discussing the role of the physician in community-based palliative care programs for cancer patients, there are actually two issues that are being addressed: First, the role of the primary physician – the one making the referral – who knows the patient best and has most likely established rapport with him/her; second, the role of the palliative care specialist, who will oversee the end-of-life symptom management and transition to death. The former – the primary provider – may be a family physician, internist, specialist, or indeed the oncologist who diagnosed and managed early stages of the disease. The latter is the palliative care consultant and his/her team with expertise in managing the physical and mental distress experienced by a dying patient and their loved ones. When palliative care is delivered by a palliative care specialist working alongside the patient's general practitioner, it is referred to as "specialty palliative care". On the other hand, when it is delivered by practitioners not formally trained in palliative care, it is called "basic" or "primary palliative care". The degree of involvement of either physician can be quite broad, ranging from very limited participation to being the key administrator of care [12]. In Lebanon, many factors determine how these roles are carved out, and how physicians' roles evolve as the disease progresses. The primary care physician is generally viewed as being the professional best capable of providing comprehensive and continuous care. When the doctor/patient relationship is already established, issues of building trust and mutual understanding essential to the therapeutic relationship are already present. This allows the general practitioner to provide care to patients with life-limiting cancer in the context of an established relationship [13]. However, the connection between patients with cancer and their primary physician begins to dissolve as the disease progresses to an advanced stage, and is largely lost by the time the patient needs end-of-life care [14].

Historically, these two providers – the primary care provider and the palliative care specialist – have been studied and addressed independently, as though they comprise two separate aspects of the progression from disease management (curative care) to terminal care. It has long been known that optimal care requires the palliative care specialist be enlisted early in the course of the disease, as the primary care provider continues to take an active role throughout the journey. Such a cohesive approach is empirically known to lessen patient and family distress. However, a review of the literature shows that it was only at the turn of this century that the interaction and interdependence between these two key players began to be studied in an organized manner. Publications on interdisciplinary team dynamics in the home setting, and its effect on patients and their caregiver, have seen somewhat of a surge in the past 20 years, but many gaps remain, particularly in areas relating to cultural acceptance, community care models, and recruitment and training of personnel in regions of limited resources.

The three models of care that describe increasing interdependence among generalists and palliative care specialists are: sequential, parallel, and shared care. In the sequential model, care of the patient is virtually transferred in its entirety to the palliative care specialist after the terminal diagnosis is made. This can result in a disconnect and sense of abandonment during a vulnerable period. Patients with long-standing relations with their primary care provider have voiced concern that enrolling in palliative care with a "new doctor" means their trusted link to their general practitioner will be severed. This is not a misconception, unfortunately, as many physicians do not continue to follow their patients after referral to the palliative care specialist. Common reasons given by providers include role encroachment and inexperience in managing dying patients. While many patients do not wish – in fact, fear – losing their primary care provider, others welcome the expertise of the palliative physician and views him/her as best capable of meeting the needs as the goal of treatment shifts from curative to comfort care [14, 15]. These distinct views are mainly addressed by the parallel model of care.

In parallel care, the primary care provider continues to provide care and support to non-cancer medical problems (e.g., diabetes, heart failure, dementia) while the palliative specialist assumes the role of managing more complex symptoms and the dying process. There will undoubtedly be an overlap in the physicians' roles, and the efficacy of this model is in part determined by the involvement of each provider. The dynamics can get complicated. As mentioned above, primary care providers may have an aversion to managing dying patients in the community due to inexperience, lack of resources and accessibility, and their clinical workload may curb availability for community visits. Similarly, the palliative care specialist, particularly in Lebanon, may be viewed (rightfully or not) by patients and their families as being intrusive or callous. They may be perceived as less capable of communicating the overwhelming end-of-life events as effectively as the primary care provider who has a longer history with the patient and has established an emotional bond. Patients receiving palliative care in the community may find it easier to continue to view their primary provider as "their doctor" as the scarcity of palliative care specialists limits their ability to do home visits and often functions by team member proxy. Many factors determine how patients view each provider, and to whom they gravitate. In our experience with patients in Lebanon receiving palliative care in the community, physician availability was consistently ranked as one of the top determinants of who ultimately leads the care. At times of uncertainty and distress, the ability to consistently and reliably connect with a physician has, in itself, remarkable therapeutic power.

The shared model of care represents the highest level of involvement of both providers. It is generally accepted as the best approach to managing complex terminal patients, provided the elements necessary for a successful home care service are in place (which is not the case in Lebanon). The primary care provider is viewed as having an active role in discussing treatment alternatives, referring to the palliative care specialist and other services only when necessary. When appropriate, he/she will defer care to the palliative specialist as the leading expert in managing cancer symptoms, and jointly monitor effectiveness of interventions. Paramount to the success of the shared model of care is a functional interdisciplinary team that is conducted in an efficient and effective manner. Team challenges concerning role ambiguity, inadequate communication, interpersonal conflicts, remuneration, and work overload must be addressed and agreed upon at the onset. In an ideal community, public health programs should strive to achieve the shared model of care. This will require resources and is labor intensive. In reality, the type and model of care administered is determined by service availability, logistics, patient preference, and physician capability. Of these, the biggest obstacle, by far, is the availability of qualified palliative care providers, as will be discussed next.

Leveraging the Palliative Care Specialist for Community Care

In 2004, the Lebanese Ministry of Public Health introduced palliative care as a patient's right in the first article of the Law on "Patients' Rights and Informed Consent" [16]. At that time, human resources and expertise were the main obstacles in implementing the law as it was intended. The law was mainly driven by oncologists with a vision for their patients to die with dignity and without undue suffering. A few years earlier – in May 2000 – the Lebanese Pain and Palliative Care Initiative was launched under the auspices of the Lebanese Cancer Society [17, 18]. Members included physicians from various specialties, nurses, and other health professionals who work with terminal patients. The objectives of this initiative, among others, were to:

1. Promote the development of palliative care services and increase awareness of palliative care at academic, clinical, and social levels.
2. Promote the implementation of existing knowledge in palliative care and train professionals involved in the care of patients with incurable and advanced disease.
3. Consolidate the efforts of professionals from various disciplines who study and practice the

principles of palliative care (doctors, nurses, social workers, psychologists, volunteers, and others).
4. Address the ethical problems associated with the care of terminally ill patients, paying special attention to local cultural traditions and beliefs.
5. Strengthen home care agencies and social assistance programs.

According to the CIA World Fact Book, the death rate in Lebanon is 5.1/1000 population, or over 30,000 deaths per year [3]. With only five formally trained palliative care specialists currently in Lebanon, it has become clear that caring for patients with life-limiting cancer will not be delivered primarily by fellowship-trained palliative care practitioners. Our role is to help all those who deliver terminal care become more adept in the principles of hospice and comfort care. The shortage of certified palliative care providers in Lebanon is not unlike what is encountered in other developed and developing countries, only more severe. It was particularly apparent in the field of oncology after the 2017 Clinical Practice Guidelines of the American Society of Clinical Oncology strongly recommended that all patients with an advanced cancer diagnosis receive palliative care early in the course of the disease, along with active treatment [19]. As public awareness of this specialty grew in Lebanon, so did the demand… and the inadequate supply. To be certain, the void has been filled by many committed and qualified individuals from various specialties and disciplines. In fact, some aspects of palliative care (such as pain- and other symptom-management, discussion of code status and goals of care, and grief management) should be within the skill set of all clinicians taking care of seriously ill patients. Our duty as palliative care specialists is to facilitate the process by providing clinical pathways and algorithms to ensure that the quality of care meets standard guidelines. The dedication of those few clinicians who provide primary palliative care has sustained the momentum during this capacity-building phase. Despite their capable efforts, it is estimated that 5-10% of terminal cancer patients that need palliative care in Lebanon actually receive it [18, 20].

The previously described models of care are contingent on the presence of functional community palliative care programs that can assume care at some point in the disease progression. When such a service is not available, an alternative approach is necessary. The involvement of general practitioners as palliative care providers has been gaining momentum worldwide, and can potentially address the increasing shortage in Lebanon.

Therefore, by necessity (if not urgency), palliative care must be built into existing primary care systems in Lebanon by providing the tools to deliver quality palliative care to patients. This approach has been successfully developed (and replicated) in settings where it was integrated in existing primary care systems in the Western world [21]. Given adequate training, resources and access to specialist support, general practitioners should be capable of providing end-of-life care to most patients, with the palliative care specialist intervening in the most complex cases (Table 1).

A big step forward in establishing the specialty in Lebanon was reached on May 4, 2011 with the creation of the National Committee for Pain Relief and Palliative Care (NCPC) by the Ministry of Public Health (MPH – Decree no. 1/486) [22]. The NCPC was chaired by the Director of the MPH. It consolidated the efforts of professionals from various disciplines and institutions committed to advancing the principles of palliative care. The efforts undertaken by this multidisciplinary committee were divided into four broad categories with specific objectives:

1. Education:
   - Recommend a core curriculum for the training of healthcare professionals with an emphasis on knowledge, attitudes, and skill development.
   - Recommend specialization trajectories for physicians and nurses.
   - Institute the importance of continuing professional education in the field as a requirement for recertification and licensure.

Table 1 Some of the benefits and obstacles of obtaining home palliative care from a general practitioner (primary palliative care) versus fellowship-trained provider (specialty primary care) in Lebanon. The severe shortage of professionally trained palliative care clinicians means that most patients will receive end-of-life care from primary providers, if at all

Primary (basic) palliative care	Specialty palliative care
Benefits	
Established physician-patient trust and rapport already exists Continued management of preexisting and chronic conditions Decreased utilization of healthcare referrals and overall cost Clear and effective communication regarding the nature of the illness and possible trajectories towards inevitable death Referral to other specialties, including palliative care, when necessary	Expertise in managing refractory pain and pain syndromes Expertise in managing complex illnesses with multiple refractory symptoms Support of interdisiplinary team members Access to community resources Addresses all dimensions of physical, psychological, social, and spiritual suffering Prepares and educates patient/family of possible disease trajectory and imminent death Decreased utilization of healthcare resources and agressive interventions Help to facilitate events after death at home, or transfer to appropriate setting (hospital) when death is imminent.
Obstacles	
Inexperience in managing dying patients Time constraints (due to busy office/hospital workload) Patient/family loss of confidence in provider when disease progression is unanticipated or rapid	Shortage of specialty-trained providers Time constraints (due to overextension of limited human resource) Additional unreimbursed cost to patient Lack of provider availability – functions via team member proxy Fragmented care if communication with general practioner is suboptimal Role ambiguity and leadership conflict

- Develop strategies for public education and awareness in the field of palliative care.

2. Practice:
   - Develop national standards and competencies for pain relief and palliative care.
   - Implement strategies to engage professionals from different disciplines in the care process, such as the use of multidisciplinary care pathways.
   - Recommend models for service delivery such as home care and residential care and the use of palliative care teams in hospitals.
   - Develop mechanisms to empower the family and the patient to be actively involved in the care process, emphasizing the importance of family and patient-centered care.
3. Research:
   - Develop national research priorities for the field of pain relief and palliative care that target gaps in treatment, knowledge transfer, education, and policy.
   - To recommend research methods to address the gaps in information related to pain relief and palliative care in Lebanon.
4. Public Policy:
   - Promote legislation that ensures the availability and accessibility of opiates and the right to prescribe them.
   - Recommend strategies that will ensure the inclusion of interdisciplinary palliative care teams in the care process.
   - Develop models for cost allocation and reimbursement for pain relief and palliative care services.
   - Recommend the institution of pain relief and palliative care as integral parts of the healthcare system in Lebanon.

One obvious, but unstated, benefit of the ambitious goals outlined by the NCPC was to train general practitioners to implement the principles of palliative care, particularly in the community, where the need was dire. Training healthcare providers early in their career in essential skills such as communicating bad news, accepting the inevitability of death and dying, and reflecting on ethical implications of futile interventions bodes well for the future generation of providers. Each of the seven medical schools in Lebanon now include didactic sessions on end-of-life care in their core curriculum, but the quality and level of instruction remains inadequate despite having developed a national curriculum [23].

Evidence of the lack of training in previous years can be seen in the attitude of professionals toward the dying process. The inability, or refusal, of clinicians to discuss terminal issues with patients and their caregivers has become the prevailing medical culture. Most young physicians disengage in ambivalence and visible discomfort when faced with terminal patients for whom palliative care is the only reasonable approach. In a survey of 1205 practicing Lebanese nurses and physicians, only 19.1% of physicians reported routinely informing terminally ill patients about their diagnosis, although the majority of nurses and physicians (94% and 99%, respectively) believed that the terminal patient *should* be informed [18]. One-third of physicians (33%) said they do not inform patients of the diagnosis, and 37.7% said they would only do so if the family asked them to. This lack of communication creates a missed opportunity to initiate the palliative care process early and effectively. In another study of 126 medical students, three barriers to disclosing bad news were reported: fear of causing more distress to patients, family interference, and physician uncertainty [24]. Only 14% of students were given the opportunity to observe a senior physician disclose bad news to patients. To my knowledge, no students or residents are offered home visits as a routine part of their training. Most of their training continues to take place in tertiary care centers, and the pressing need for community support for older or terminal homebound patients is overlooked.

Founding members of the NCPC continue to actively promote the cause of palliative care in Lebanon, but the subcommittees have recently been dispersed due to the economic, political, and security situation on the ground, as well as the relocation of various members. The shortage of specialty-trained palliative care physicians is expected to grow. Currently there are no palliative care postgraduate training programs in Lebanon, and our dependence on well-trained generalists to address the need of community palliative care will persist in the foreseeable future. For many reasons, too few physicians-in-training are exposed to palliative care early and often enough to experience its rewards.

Conclusion

There is an urgent need to expand community palliative care services in Lebanon in order to provide person-centered compassionate care for patients with life-threatening cancer. Most terminal cancer patients have no access to palliative care, and they face needless suffering and isolation during the end-of-life progression. It is estimated that less than 10% of patients that could benefit from palliative care in Lebanon actually receive it, and palliative care currently remains mainly hospital-based. The social and family structure in Lebanon supports the expansion of palliative care into the community. Home-based care is facilitated by the presence and involvement of the extended family and affordable domestic caregivers. With limited resources and trained specialists, the integration of community palliative care service into existing primary care systems has been proposed as a bridging measure [13]. When the doctor/patient relationship has already been established, issues of building trust and mutual understanding, which are essential to the therapeutic relationship, are already present. This allows the general practitioner to provide palliative care in the context of an established relationship, while the palliative care specialist provides clinical guidelines and algorithms to ensure that current standards of practice are being met. Thus, the palliative care specialist plays the role of a custodian who promotes education, training, acceptance, and collaboration for the specialty. He/she should function as an advocate among policymakers at the government level to eliminate regulatory obstacles. Care for most community patients with terminal needs should be managed by primary providers, while the palliative care specialist manages the most complex cases with refractory symptoms. Primary palliative care providers should be given the tools to be able to carry out this role comfortably and competently. Most important among these tools are education and training. Leveraging the expertise of the palliative care specialist in this manner allows for the rapid expansion of palliative care for home-based patients during this capacity-building phase.

References

1. Center for Disease Control and Prevention; National Vital Statistic System. http://www.cdc.gov/nchs/nvss.htm. Accessed 17 Nov 2019.
2. United Nations., Department of Economic and Social Affairs, Population Division World population prospects 2019: highlights (ST/ESA/SER.A/423). 2019. Accessed 20 Feb 2020.
3. The World Factbook, Central Intelligence Agency. http://www.cia.gov/library/publications/the-world-fact-book. Accessed 17 Jan 2020.
4. World Health Organization. https://www.who.int/countries/lbn/en/. Accessed 20 Feb 2020.
5. Abu-Saad Huijer H, Saab M, Hajjar R. Palliative care for older adults: state of the art in Lebanon. Lebanese Med J. 2016;64(1):27–32.
6. Lebanese Ministry of Public Health, National Cancer Registry (NCR). https://www.moph.gov.lb/en/Pages/8/19526/national-cancer-registry. Accessed Dec 20 2019.
7. Hajjar RR, Atil T, Al-Mandhar Z, Oudrhiri M, Balducci L, Silbermann M. Prevalence of aging population in the Middle East and its implications on cancer incidence and care. Ann Oncol. 2013;232(Supplement 7):vii11–1124. https://doi.org/10.1093/annonc/mdt268.
8. Silbermann M, Arnaout M, Daher M, et al. Palliative cancer care in middle eastern countries: accomplishments and challenges. Ann Oncol. 2012;23(suppl 3):5–28. https://doi.org/10.1093/annonc/mds084.
9. Beernaert K, Van den Block L, Van Thienen K, Devroey D, Pardon K, Deliens L, Cohen J. Family physicians' role in palliative care throughout the care continuum: stakeholder perspectives. Fam Pract. 2015;32(6):694–700. https://doi.org/10.1039/fampra/cmv072.
10. Mouhawej MC, Maalouf-Haddad N, Tohmé A. Cultural challenges in imple-menting palliative services in Lebanon. Palliat Med Hosp Care Open J. 2017;SE(1):S15–8. https://doi.org/10.17140/PMH-COJ-SE-1-104.
11. Silbermann M, Fink RM, Min S-J, Mancuso MP, Brant J, Hajjar R, et al. Evaluating palliative care needs in middle eastern countries. J Palliat Med. 2015;18:1):1–8. https://doi.org/10.1089/jpm.2014.0194.
12. Ramanayake R, Dilanka G, Premasiri L. Palliative care; role of family physicians. J Family Med Prim Care. 2016;5:234–7. https://doi.org/10.4103/2249-4863.192356.
13. Murray SA, Osman H. Primary palliative care: the potential of primary care physicians as providers of palliative care in the community in the eastern Mediterranean region. East Mediterr Health J. 2012;18(2):178–83.
14. Norman A, Sisler J, Hack T, Harlos M. Family physicians and cancer care. Palliative care patients' perspective. Can Fam Physician. 2001;47:2009–16.
15. Ankuda CK, Patterson SM, Wingrove P, Bazemore AW. Regional variations in primary care involvement at the end of life. Ann Fam Med. 2017;15:63–7. https://doi.org/10.1370/afm.2002.
16. Lebanese Ministry of Public Health, Patient Rights and Informed Consent. Mibisterial Decree no. 574, Feb 11, 2004.
17. Daher M, Tabari H, Stjernsward J, et al. Lebanon: pain relief and palliative care. J Pain Symptom Manag. 2002;24:200–4. https://doi.org/10.1016/s0885-3924(02)00463-3.
18. Huijer H, Dimassi H. Palliative care in Lebanon: knowledge, attitudes and practices of physicians and nurses. Lebanese Med J. 2007;55:121–8.
19. Ferrell BR, Temel JS, Temin S, Smith TJ. Integration of palliative care into standard oncology care: American Society of Clinical Oncology Clinical Practice Guideline update. J Clin Oncol. 2017;35:96–112. https://doi.org/10.1200/JCO.2016.70.1474.
20. Daher M, Estephan E, Abu-Saad Huijer H, Naja Z. Implementation of palliative care in Lebanon; past, present, and future. Lebanese Med J. 2008;56:70–6.
21. Quill TE, Aberneethy AP. Generalist plus specialist palliative care--creating a more sustainable model. N Engl J Med. 2013;368(13):1173–5. https://doi.org/10.1056/NEJMp1215620.
22. Lebanese Ministry of Public Health, National Palliative Care Committee. Ministerial Decree no. 486, May 4, 2011.
23. Daher M, Doumit M, Hajjar R, Hamre R, Naifeh Khoury M, Tohme A. Integrating palliative care into healthcare education in Lebanon. Lebanese Med J. 2013;61(4):191–8.
24. Antoun J, Saab BR. A culturally sensitive audiovisual package to teach breaking bad news in a Lebanese setting. Med Teach. 2010;32(10):868–9.
25. Daher M, Hajjar R. Palliative care for cancer patients in Lebanon. In: Silbermann M, editor. Palliative care to the cancer patient, the Middle East as model to emerging countries. New York: Nova Sciences Publishers, Inc; 2014. p. 125–40.

Palliative Care in Lebanon: From Inception to Implementation

Myrna A. A. Doumit

Introduction

Lebanon is one of the world's smallest countries, with an area of 10,452 square kilometers. About four million people live in the country with over 80% living in urban areas. Since the end of the 15-year civil war in 1991, Lebanon has strived to reestablish its infrastructure. Over the same period, Lebanon's statistics have progressed, with life expectancy at birth rising to 74–77 years of age. Lebanon is undergoing an epidemiological transition, where diseases of affluence – diabetes, heart disease, cancer, high blood pressure – have noticeably augmented, while diseases of poverty – infectious and communicable diseases – are decreasing but have not yet disappeared [1].

Over the past century, the world experienced a demographic shift that has had a substantial influence on the delivery of health care. Improvements in health care have been accountable for the most significant years-of-life gains. In the twenty-first century, the world expectations of life and death are different from those a century ago [2]. As the world population has augmented, life expectancy in both developed and developing countries has also increased. With aging, older people are at high risk of developing complications from non-communicable diseases (NCDs).

In Lebanon, the number of people 65 years and older parallel those of the world. In 2015, Lebanon had the highest percentage of people aged 65 years and older (7.3%) in the Arab region and this number is projected to reach 12% by the year 2030 [3]. Subsequently, both the absolute and the relative number of older adults have increased at an unprecedented rate. This demographic shift will particularly be felt over the next few decades, as the relatively young population moves up the population pyramid and this change, as well, is expected to have its impact on the health care system [4].

Life expectancy in Lebanon lags only slightly behind that of developed countries, and currently stands at approximately 74 years for men and 77 years for women (as little as 50 years ago, it was 60 years). But with longevity comes chronic, costly, and serious illness, including many types of cancers, which the Lebanese health care system is ill-prepared to deal with. Aside from age-related degenerative disorders, aging is a major risk factor for many types of cancers. All-cause cancer incidence peaks at around age 70 [4].

The number of new cases of cancer in Lebanon has increased steadily over the past decade, according to the National Cancer Registry of the Ministry of Health and the World Health Organization (WHO). In 2004, almost 7200 new cases of cancer were reported in Lebanon,

M. A. A. Doumit (✉)
Alice Ramez Chagoury School of Nursing, Lebanese American University, Beirut, Lebanon
e-mail: Myrna.doumit@lau.edu.lb

M. Silbermann (ed.), *Palliative Care for Chronic Cancer Patients in the Community*,
https://doi.org/10.1007/978-3-030-54526-0_33

compared to over 9400 in the most recent report [5]. This worrisome trend is not entirely due to aging; expanded screening efforts and improved registration methods have likely contributed significantly. It is estimated that by 2030, the number of new cancer cases will approach 12,000.

The high burden of non-communicable diseases (NCDs) and the rapidly aging population in Lebanon makes palliative care (PC) an indispensable element of health services necessary to ease the suffering of patients. According to a report published in 2017, an estimated number of 15,000 patients need PC services each year. This number is expected to increase due to a number of factors such as the aging population and the rise in NCDs [6].

The World Health Organization (WHO) has defined palliative care as an approach that "improves the quality-of-life of patients and their families facing the problems associated with life-threatening illness, through the prevention and relief of suffering by means of early identification, impeccable assessment and treatment of pain and other problems, physical, psychosocial and spiritual" [7]. The WHO launched a public health model as well as a guideline to governments for the implementation of palliative care on the national level. This model was adopted by Lebanon. A major response to this initiative was the creation of the National Committee for pain relief and Palliative Care (NCPC) by the Ministry of Public Health (MPH – decree No 1/486).

Historical Background

Palliative care was first tackled in Lebanon in 1995 during a National Cancer Control Workshop with national health leaders and supported by the Ministry of Public Health and the WHO. This workshop was subsequently followed by another symposium in 1999 on palliative care and ethics which was organized by the Lebanese Cancer Society and sponsored by the WHO. Afterwards, in the year 2000, the Lebanese Pain and Palliative care initiative was launched and started under the auspices of the Lebanese Cancer Society. The team was multidisciplinary in nature and the purpose was to educate physicians and nurses about palliative care and to develop post-graduate training programs for physicians and nurses who wish to develop and introduce palliative care into medical and nursing curricula. After this workshop, nine fellows from different universities were chosen and sponsored for training in the United States to become EPEC (Education in Palliative and End-of-life Care) Trainers. Following this initiative, a 12-hour undergraduate curriculum and a continuing education program were developed for medical students; a continuing education program on pain and palliative care was also implemented for practicing nurses and courses on palliative care were implemented for nursing students.

In 2001, a symposium on pain and palliative care was organized and it yielded an increase in the number of patients receiving opioids; the morphine quota increased from 0.5 kg to 4.5 kg. National media was involved as well. The Ministry of Public Health introduced palliative care as a patient's right in the First Article of Law 574 (on patients' rights and informed consent) as a response to the Prague Charter [8] which states that: "Access to palliative care is a human right under the right to the highest attainable standard of physical and mental health". Another milestone was achieved in 2006 when the law 673 was amended by extending the duration of treatment outlined by a single prescription for opioids from 15 to 30 days [9]. In 2011, the Ministry of Public Health officially established the National Committee for pain relief and Palliative Care with the mandate of developing national plans for research, education, practice, and policy related to palliative care. In 2013, the Ministry of Public Health recognized palliative medicine as a new specialty [10].

National Need for Palliative Care

In Lebanon, the demand for PC services is expected to rise with the aging population and the high burden of NCDs. In 2015, Lebanon had the highest percentage of people aged 65 years and older (7.3%) in the Arab region and this number is projected to reach 12% by the year 2030 [3]. According to the national Pan Arab Project for Family Health (PAPFAM) survey, 75% of people aged 65 years and older reported suffering from at least one co-morbidity, where the leading causes of morbidity were hypertension (36.7%), heart disease (23.1%), and diabetes (21.4%) [3]. In addition, NCDs account for 91% of total deaths, with four types of NCDs accounting for the largest proportions of deaths: cardiovascular disease (47%), cancers (16%), chronic respiratory diseases (4%), and diabetes (5%) [1]. Moreover, children are less likely to receive PC [11]. A survey conducted among Lebanese nurses and physicians found that 98% of pediatric nurses and 100% of physicians reported the need for developing pediatric PC [12]. Furthermore, a study assessing the quality of pediatric PC for children with cancer in Lebanon found that management of distressing symptoms such as fatigue and difficulty sleeping was inadequate and focused mainly on treating symptoms such as pain and nausea [13]. Despite the latter, few patients who need PC receive the care they need. Furthermore, most PC services are provided in large cities and many patients cannot afford PC services [6]. Despite progress towards developing PC services in Lebanon, substantial challenges remain.

Integration of Palliative Care Services Within the Health Care System

Years 2011 and 2013, respectively, witnessed major steps towards the implementation of palliative care within the health care system in Lebanon by launching the National Committee for pain relief and Palliative Care (NCPC) and recognizing palliative care medicine as a new specialty.

The NCPC has defined for itself large-scale goals, and has merged the endeavors of professionals from different disciplines and institutions committed to enhancing principles of palliative care. The work undertaken by this multidisciplinary committee is divided into four large categories with explicit objectives:

1. Education:
   - Recommend a core curriculum for the training of health care professionals with an emphasis on knowledge, attitudes, and skill development.
   - Recommend specialization trajectories for physicians and nurses.
   - Institute the importance of continuing professional education in the field as a requirement for re-certification and licensure.
   - Develop strategies for public education and awareness in the field of palliative care.
2. Practice:
   - Develop national standards and competencies for pain relief and palliative care.
   - Implement strategies to engage professionals from different disciplines in the care process, such as the use of multidisciplinary care pathways.
   - Recommend models for provision of services such as home care, residential care, and the use of palliative care teams in hospitals.
   - Develop mechanisms to empower the family and the patient to be actively involved in the care process, emphasizing the importance of family and patient-centered care.
3. Research:
   - Develop national research priorities for the field of pain relief and palliative care that target gaps in treatment, knowledge transfer, education, and policy.
   - Recommend research methods addressing the gaps in information related to pain relief and palliative care in Lebanon.
4. Public Policy:
   - Promote legislation that ensures the availability, accessibility, and prescription rights of opiates.
   - Recommend strategies that will ensure the inclusion of interdisciplinary palliative care teams in the care process.
   - Develop models for cost allocation and reimbursement for pain relief and palliative care services.
   - Recommend the institution of pain relief and palliative care as integral parts of the health care system in Lebanon [14].

Unfortunately, the NCPC was not successful in implementing all the above recommendations. Despite significant strides, enormous challenges continue to defy the implementation of a holistic approach to palliative care. The primary concerns remain focused on funding, research, and public education.

Approaches and Barriers to Palliative Care

Education and PC in Lebanon

The National Committee for pain relief and Palliative Care took the initiative to advocate for integrating PC into nursing and medical curricula. Systemic reviews highlighted the advantage of including PC into health professionals' curricula at the undergraduate level [15–17]. Currently in Lebanon, 100% of nursing schools included PC as an entity but with different levels of emphasis and different core curricula. However, only 29% of the medical schools have integrated PC into their medical curriculum, at various levels. The national education subcommittee developed a modular curriculum for training undergraduate medical and nursing students. It recommended a one-credit course on palliative care (21-hour modular curriculum) be integrated into undergraduate training and be a requirement by all faculties of medicine and nursing in Lebanon. However, this core curriculum has not yet been officially adopted [18]. Unfortunately, the lack of education in palliative concepts currently translates into a lack of understanding of palliative care in clinicians' practices. Not all universities offer this concept with the same breadth and depth. Regrettably, this lack of minimal standardization is yielding to a discrepancy in the understanding and practice of the PC approach. One of the major barriers described in the Lebanese health system is the lack of communication skills to address end-of-life issues between health care workers and patients. There are a number of difficult conversations that doctors/nurses may need to have as a patient's disease progresses. Usually health care workers try to avoid discussing sensitive subjects with patients due to the controlling and dominant family system that still prevails; this could also be due to the lack of proper skills in communicating these sensitive issues. It is important that doctors/nurses become skilled in conversing with patients and their family members so that they can be more fully informed about the illness and make appropriate choices for their individual circumstances and preferences. Furthermore, doctors in Lebanon are reluctant to refer patients to palliative care services as they do not understand and/or believe in the discipline. Another barrier preventing physicians from handing over care to another doctor is that they are working under a system that is guided by a fee-for-service structure and therefore have concerns regarding the loss of income [19].

The NCPC has also recommended the inclusion of questions on pain management, palliative care, and end-of-life care in all official examinations tests of doctors and nurses. Moreover, it also recommended to tie continuous education as a precondition for licensure renewal. This step was recently adopted by the Order of Nurses, and nurses were able to issue a law that makes continuing education mandatory in order to practice medicine in Lebanon. Unfortunately, specialization trajectory in palliative care for nurses and physicians are still not developed enough to meet the country's needs. More emphasis is needed at the educational and practical levels.

Public education and awareness about palliative care was one of the main objectives for the NCPC. Unfortunately, this step was not properly pursued and the majority of people of Lebanon still do not fully understand the importance of palliative care for quality-of-life. In most cases, they relate the idea of palliative care to end-of-life, which delays the request for palliative care and is still not culturally accepted. This is an important aspect that needs close follow-up as supply of service is based on demand. As long as the people of Lebanon are not aware of the real meaning of PC and its impact on their quality of life, surely, they will not request it as a mode of care. Therefore, the main plan is to include education and use media to disseminate the reality regarding the importance and need to start palliative care the moment the individual is diagnosed with a chronic condition [20].

Palliative Care and Practice

(a) *At the hospital level*

The WHO strongly calls for the integration of PC in hospitals, especially those involved in treating cancer and chronic diseases. Hospital-based PC can improve patients' outcomes and symptom control, facilitate the discussion of patient's goals of care, reduce their length of stay, and promote transition of care to the community. In addition, hospital-based PC can help health professionals working in other fields to engage in and learn about PC. Hospital-based PC can be integrated in different ways: as an outpatient PC clinic; a PC consultation service for hospital inpatients; a PC day-care service; an inpatient PC unit; and as a PC outreach service [21]. Unfortunately, among the very few hospitals in Lebanon that were able to integrate palliative care into their system, many of them failed to continue. This letdown might be related to many factors, mainly financial, as most public and private insurance parties do not cover palliative care services. Lack of cooperation from physicians to refer patients to palliative care services may be due to a lack of understanding or belief in the discipline. They may also be concerned about losing their clients and, consequently, income. In addition, there is a lack of physicians specialized in PC.

Advanced care planning as an essential concept in the implementation of PC has not yet been introduced into the Lebanese culture. Patients are completely protected by family members. Decisions regarding treatment modalities are rarely taken by patients, especially when the condition is related to cancer. Usually family members are the decision-makers in such instances and patients willingly follow. Patient/family factors that present a barrier to palliative care include denial in patients/family that often hope or believe that the prognosis is better than what they are told; they may have an unrealistic expectation of the disease's response to treatment; lack of awareness. Misguided perceptions about PC among the Lebanese population is prevalent as well [22]. PC is associated with death and terminal diseases and is viewed as the last resort when all other treatment fails. The people of Lebanon, in general, closely relate palliative care to end-of-life.

(b) *At the primary health care level*

The first call to build the Primary Health Care (PHC) system in Lebanon dates back to 1977. Almost 20 years later, Lebanon held its first national conference on PHC. This was subsequently followed by the development of the first National Strategy for PHC in 1994. Two years later, a comprehensive assessment of health centers and dispensaries in Lebanon was conducted to identify those able to provide PHC services. Between 1977 and 1992, the health care system was busy responding to the emergency needs of the country due to the war status that prevailed during this period. Despite the continuous improvement in the PHC services provided across Lebanon, the concept of palliative care is still lacking in PHC due to health care workers' poor awareness and knowledge about PC and lack of the infrastructure needed for the implementation of this approach to care. The PHC system in Lebanon is not yet prepared to integrate the concept of PC into its services. This issue is related to lack of human and physical resources. The health care workers at the PHC do not have the educational preparation for providing PC. Special training sessions need to be planned and offered across the country's PHC system. Moreover, the physical structure and processes of the PHC are not helping as well. For example, there are no pain specialists nor psychological assessments for chronic care patients. It would be very helpful to have a comprehensive assessment of the services, reevaluating and restructuring the actual needs of the population of Lebanon and not simply to offer what we can based on our current human and physical resources.

Palliative Care at Patients' Home

There are currently two NGOs that provide palliative care at home for patients and do so free of charge. These two NGOs have played a major role in advocating for palliative care at the national level. They have also helped explain the concept of PC to patients and their families and raised physicians' awareness for the need to initiate PC at the time of diagnosis. One of the NGOs was more involved with capacity building; they organized local training workshops for people working in PC to enhance their knowledge and build their skills. There is still a lot that needed to be done at the community level since the two existing NGOs are not able to cover all regions of Lebanon, nor to respond to all needs, due to financial and human resources constraints [23–24].

In order to enhance the practice of PC in Lebanon, it is important to promote a multidisciplinary approach to care. This approach could be nurtured by promoting the interprofessional education among the different health care workers. This approach to education for health care workers started to thrive in Lebanon, but not to the extent of influencing a change to current health practices. Another recommendation is to develop national standards and competencies for pain and palliative care which must be followed by physicians and nurses. Moreover, empowering patients and families and teaching them about their rights to patient-centered care would enhance the social acceptance of palliative care.

The current NGOs which provide PC in Lebanon help seriously ill patients and their families with the objective to prevent and relieve suffering. They also try to maintain the best possible quality-of-life for patients despite the seriousness of their condition. Self-referrals and referrals from physicians are both acceptable for admission into the system, and an individualized interdisciplinary care schedule is planned. Home assessment visits are carried out by the PC nurse. Nurses practice in close collaboration with PC physicians who are part of the NGOs' team and with the patients' primary physician. The frequency of home visits is on an as-needed basis and it may vary throughout the course of the disease. The PC team is usually available around-the-clock for emergencies. Clinical psychologists and clinical pharmacists are also available. The main restriction for the two available NGOs is that they are only able to function within the capital and are not able to meet the needs of far-away patients, although at times they do travel to remote areas for consultations and do follow-ups by phone. It is significant to highlight that PC services in Lebanon are provided free of charge. The two NGOs depend on fundraising in order to maintain the services they provide.

Research and Palliative Care

Research in the field of palliative care in Lebanon is progressively developing; it remains, however, in its beginnings. Clinical approaches, overall, are still based on experience and trial and errors and necessitate to develop into evidence-based, emphasizing the importance of research in this field. Proper funding is required for palliative care research to develop and prosper. In order to improve palliative care research at the national level, multidisciplinary research groups must be developed; for this reason, it is important to train a good number of palliative care researchers and provide them with the support needed to work collaboratively [25].

Palliative Care and Public Policy

Public policy is the authority that governs the development and advancement of palliative care in Lebanon. The Ministry of Public Health, in collaboration with the private sector, promoted legislation to facilitate the implementation of palliative care in hospitals and in the community, affording the availability, accessibility, and prescription rights of opioids. It also developed and embraced a model for cost reimbursement, encouraging the provision of palliative care at home [26]. The Lebanese Ministry of Public Health took a milestone step in issuing the decree

1/447, which outlines criteria for the reimbursement of palliative care services. The decree defines coverage for both home and hospital-based programs and provides a plan for a reimbursement structure that can be used by the National Social Security Fund (NSSF) and private insurers.

Conclusion

For palliative care to thrive and grow it must be available, accessible, accepted, and provided with quality.

Palliative care should be sufficiently available in hospitals, primary health care centers, and homes. This includes health care professionals and other health care workers trained in PC and essential palliative care medicines being made available. It should be integrated into mainstream health care so that psychological support and symptom control can begin from the time of diagnosis.

Palliative care should be accessible to all people, regardless of their socioeconomic background, and should be provided along with bio-ethics, as there are often challenging decisions to be made regarding end-of-life care. Undoubtedly, the quality of care is a fundamental element and must be ensured through national standards.

Despite all its economic and political constraints, due to the strategic partnership between the private and public health sector, Lebanon is moving towards refining and enhancing the palliative care system already established in the country.

References

1. WHO noncommunicable diseases country profiles 2018. Geneva: World Health Organization; 2018. License: CC BY-NC-SA 3.0 IGO. Accessed 23 Dec 2019.
2. Rao JK, Anderson LA, Smith SM. End-of-life is a public health issue. Am J Prev Med. 2002;2393:215–20.
3. Mehio AS, Rizk A, Kronfol NM. Aging in Lebanon: perils and prospects. Le Journal Medical Libanais. Lebanese Med J. 2015;63(1):2–7.
4. Sibai A, Kronfol N. Country profile: older population in Lebanon: facts and prospects: Center for Studies on Aging A Publications; 2011. http://www.csa.org.lb/cms/assets/archives/2011/13%20country%20profile%20elderly%20population%20in%20lebanon%20facts%20and%20prospects%20english.pdf. Accessed 23 Dec 2019.
5. Ministry of Public Health website: www.moph.gov.lb. National Cancer Registry 2016; Accessed 23 Dec 2019.
6. Soueidan S, Osman H, El-Jardali F. K2P policy brief: integrating palliative care into the health system in Lebanon. Knowledge to Policy (K2P) Center, Beirut, Lebanon, July 2018 https://www.aub.edu.lb/k2p/Documents/K2P%20Policy%20Brief-%20Palliative%20Care-August%207%202018.pdf. Accessed 23 Dec 2019.
7. World Health Organization. WHO definition of palliative care. 2018. Retrieved from http://www.who.int/cancer/palliative/definition/en/.
8. Radbruch L, De Lima L, Lohmann D, Gwyther E, Payne S. The Prague Charter: urging governments to relieve suffering and ensure the right to palliative care. Palliat Med. 2013;27(2):101–2.
9. Daher M, Estephan E, Abu-Saad HH, Naja Z. Implementation of palliative care in Lebanon: past, present, and future. Le Journal Medical Libanais. Lebanese Med J. 2008;56(2):70–6.
10. Daher M, Doumit M. Palliative care in Lebanon: current practices, and perspectives for the future. New York: Palliative Care Vol 1, Nova Science Publishers, Inc; 2017. Chapter 21, p 307-316, isbn# 978-1-53612-084.
11. Osman H, Rihan A, Garralda E, Rhee JY, Pons JJ, de Lima L, et al. Atlas of palliative care in the eastern mediterranean region. Houston: IAHPC Press; 2017. http://dadun.unav.edu/handle/10171/43303; Accessed 23 Dec 2019.
12. Abu-Saad HH, Dimassi H. Palliative Care in Lebanon: knowledge, attitudes and practices of physicians and nurses. Le Journal Medical Libanais. Lebanese Med J. 2007;55(3):121–8.
13. Abu-Saad HH, Sagherian K, Tamim H, Naifeh MK, Abboud M. Quality of palliative care in children with cancer in Lebanon. Le Journal Medical Libanais. Lebanese Med J. 2013;61(4):228–36.
14. Daher M. Palliative Care in Lebanon: achievements and future. Human Health. 2012;20:14–7.
15. Ahmed N, Bestall JC, Ahmedzai SH, Payne SA, Clark D, Noble B. Systematic review of the problems and issues of accessing specialist palliative care by patients, carers and health and social care professionals. Palliat Med. 2004;18(6):525–42.
16. Centeno C, Rodriguez-Nunez A. The contribution of undergraduate palliative care education: does it influence the clinical patient's care? Curr Opin Support Palliat Care. 2015;9(4):375–91. https://doi.org/10.1097/SPC.0000000000000169.
17. Chung HO, Oczkowski SJW, Hanvey L, Mbuagbaw L, You JJ. Educational interventions to train

healthcare professionals in end-of-life communication: a systematic review and meta-analysis. BMC Med Educ. 2016;16(1):131. https://doi.org/10.1186/s12909-016-0653-x.
18. Osman H, Abboud M, El LZ, Ghusn H, Hanna J, Kanazi G. Setting practice standards for palliative care in Lebanon: recommendations of the subcommittee on practice - National Committee for pain control and palliative care. Le Journal Medical Libanais. Lebanese Med J. 2013;61(4):199–203.
19. Doumit M, Abu-Saad Huijer H. Lebanese cancer patients: communication and truth telling. Contemp Nurse. 2008;28:1–2.
20. Daher M, Doumit M, Hajjar R, Hamra R, Naifeh Khoury M, Tohmé A. Integrating palliative care into health education in Lebanon. Lebanese Med J. 2013;61(4):191–8. http://www.lebanesemedicaljournal.org/articles/61-4/review1.pdf.
21. World Health Organization. Planning and implementing palliative care services: a guide for programme managers. 2016. World Health Organization. https://apps.who.int/iris/handle/10665/250584.
22. Doumit M, Abu-Saad Huijer H, Kelley J. The lived experience of Lebanese oncology patients receiving palliative care. Eur J Oncol Nurs. 2007;11:309–19.
23. Balsam. The Lebanese Center for palliative care - annual report 2018. 2018. http://balsam-lb.org/wp-content/uploads/2018/04/Balsam-Annual-report-2018.pdf.
24. SANAD. SANAD annual report 2018. 2018. Retrieved from http://www.anadhospice.org/wp-content/uploads/SANAD-Annual-Report-2018.pdf.
25. Abu-Saad Huijer H, Deeb ME, Ghusn H, Karam GE, Zeineldine S. Palliative care research in Lebanon. J Med Liban. 2013;61(4):204–9.
26. Osman H. Lebanon's Ministry of Public Health issues decree on reimbursement for palliative care; An historic step toward more humane healthcare. 2019. https://www.executive-magazine.com/economics-policy/lebanons-ministry-of-public-health-issues-decree-on-reimbursement-for-palliative-care.

Part XXIV

Middle East: Palestine

Palliative Care for Palestinian Chronic Cancer Patients in the Community

Mohamad H. Khleif

Introduction

Millions of people around the world, principally in developing countries, endure great suffering and economic hardship due to life-threatening illnesses such as cancer. According to a WHO global perspective, the key feasible alternative to these urgent needs is to improve quality of life by developing an effective, low-cost approach for palliative care service of good quality and coverage. The best way to do so, in countries with strong family support and poor health infrastructure, is by home-based palliative care [1, 2]. So far in Palestine, palliative care services are not yet integrated within the Palestinian health-care system. Response-based actions are taken by health-care providers to control symptoms of patients with chronic diseases such as cancer, usually inside hospitals. In the community, the conditions are much worse, as still no community-based palliative care services are available.

In most cases, patients go from the hospital back to their homes and rely mainly on their family's help and care. Moreover, in most developing countries there are either very few community-based hospices for cancer patients or none at all, as is the case in Palestine. It is believed that this kind of situation cannot continue for too long a time since the sick patients, along with their families, very often cannot carry the load of both the physical and financial burden, as well as the emotional stress that is associated with chronic diseases such as cancer.

Cancer is one of the leading causes of death both worldwide [3], and in Palestine [4]. Approximately 70% of cancer deaths occur in low- and middle-income countries, and up to 50% of cancer deaths could be prevented by the implementation of evidence-based strategies for cancer prevention, early detection, and management [3]. In Palestine, cancer is the second leading cause of death, accounting for 15.4% (1863) of all deaths. In 2018, there were 3102 new cases reported in the West Bank of Palestine, with an incidence rate of 117.7 per 100,000 [4]. Most cases are diagnosed at the end stage of the disease [5, 6]; this late diagnosis makes it difficult to treat and resource cancer care, and results in poor health-related quality-of-life for cancer patients and a high financial burden on patients, their families, and the health-care system. One study measured the health-related quality-of-life of Palestinian cancer patients at as low as 42 points on a scale of 100 [5]. On the other hand, the cancer incidence in Middle Eastern countries is predicted to increase by 70% in the next 20 years - greater than any other region of the world [7]. Also, the high mortality rate is an indicator of late diagnoses of cancer and highlights the need for palliative care services for this

M. H. Khleif (✉)
AL-Sadeel Society for Palliative Care for Cancer and Chronic Diseases, Bethlehem, Palestine

M. Silbermann (ed.), *Palliative Care for Chronic Cancer Patients in the Community*,
https://doi.org/10.1007/978-3-030-54526-0_34

population. Literature discusses that the first point for estimating the need for palliative care is the number of deaths [8], especially as the reported overall survival rate in less-developed countries is 30% [9].

Additional resources are necessary in order to deal with advanced diseases, especially in the absence of integrated palliative care services within the health-care system. Costs were highest for those who died in chronic-care facilities and lowest for those who died in the community at home [10]. Home-based end-of-life hospice care has the potential to lessen the demand for acute hospital care, emergency department visits and admissions, as well as to increase patient satisfaction and number of home deaths [11, 12]. In several studies, home-based hospice palliative care was found to be cost-effective and reduced the need for other health services. Those receiving palliative care had health-care costs that were one-third lower [12]. A study in Israel found home hospice care during the last 2 months of life to be less costly than conventional care [13].

Subsequently, there is a significant need for palliative care services in the Middle East, including Palestine [14]. A survey of countries in the region showed that 86% of respondents wished to learn more about palliative care, whereas the question of how to finance such teams was one of the main concerns among the health-care professionals and administrators surveyed [9].

Current Situation

The rising financial burden of cancer care on health-care systems worldwide has led to the increased demand for evidence-based research to find ways to lower medical costs. 95% of stage four cancer patients in Palestine were undergoing expensive chemotherapy treatment, while their quality of life (QoL) was only 31% on a scale of 100 [5]. This shows the extremely deteriorated QoL of patients who are approaching the end of life, while maintaining expensive curative treatment modalities at hospitals, with no community backup, support, or care. A large proportion of the expenditure in Palestinian health care goes to expensive curative care outside the area [6], whereas a number of studies found that PC improves quality of life and lowers the costs of care to cancer patients and families [15, 16].

Nevertheless, most Middle Eastern cancer patients are not treated in the community. Home-based and hospice services must be sustained, as well as encouraging palliative care education [9]. This model of care is associated with additional benefits, such as increased patient and family satisfaction and choice, suggesting that cost alone may not be adequate to judge service delivery models [17].

There is a relatively low level of pain control, palliative care, staff training, and health facilities that care for cancer patients in Palestine. To the best of our knowledge, there are only three main centers for cancer care in the West Bank of Palestine, and only one non-governmental organization dedicated to palliative care. Unfortunately, there are no organized palliative care services in Palestine yet. As far as we know, there are no hospitals, community primary health centers, or home-based services available for cancer patients. In addition, there are no hospices or home hospice care available for such patients. Palliative care nursing is still underdeveloped in Palestine.

Even so, there are new initiatives to establish palliative care in the country. A non-governmental organization in Bethlehem, the AL-Sadeel Society for Palliative Care for cancer and chronic diseases, which was established in 2008, is the first palliative care society in the country. It focuses on spreading awareness about the importance of palliative care service and the need to integrate it within the health-care system. Its work includes follow-up on cancer and other chronic diseases at homes in the community on a small scale. This is done mainly by a small team of workers and based mainly on voluntary endeavors. One of their successful initiatives is the lending program of medical devices and equipment, which is trying to bridge the gap of the absence of such equipment provided by the governmental and private services. Some other programs are starting in the academic field either by integrating palliative care education within the curricula or by establishing stand-alone courses and programs on both undergraduate and postgraduate levels. One master program is expected to begin by the end of 2020 in Bethlehem, which will have a major focus on palliative care.

What Are the Difficulties?

Palliative care is not yet integrated within the national health-care system in Palestine [5, 14, 18]. The poorer QoL of cancer and chronic disease patients in the Palestinian community could be due to the deteriorating socio-economic and political situation in the country, as well as the lack of professional and specialized care to support those patients. Challenges include insufficient secured funds for organizations working in the field, weak governmental support, limited prioritization of palliative care by the policy makers, and absence of facilities for community-based palliative care and home care. Literature shows that the main problems in the region are shortage of funding or governmental support and lack of awareness among the public, as well as policy makers and professionals, concerning the need for such services [14].

Moreover, the national economy, strategic planning, health-care policy formulation, and the setting of national priorities are affected by the predominant geopolitical conditions, political, geographical, and administrative fragmentations of Palestine under occupation and barriers to movement; all these have damaging effects on the health-care system [6, 19], mainly in the community and on the most vulnerable people residing in areas remote from urban centers.

Community Involvement

Attitude toward end-of-life care and palliative care is somehow unclear due to the limited number of studies on the attitudes of the Palestinian communiity and population. Issues such as writing a will, choosing a health guardian, and peaceful death are not well-known, even amongst health-care professionals. There is an grave need for public awareness campaigns in the community and throughout the mass media. Topics should include the importance of palliative care for better quality-of-life for cancer and chronic disease patients and end-of-life care needs. Societal and religious figures of the community need to be involved in order to identify any cultural or religious barriers, which may not necessarily be in line with the concept of palliative care itself, but to education in palliative care [20]. However, some cultural thoughts are positive when it comes to death and dying. Death is somehow an acceptable event for many individuals, from a religious view, as it is the path to mortal life and happiness, as is the acceptance of associated pain or discomfort as a means to cleanse one's sins. Inside this debate, many patients would respond that they prefer to die at home, even though when the time comes, they and their families run to hospitals and die there, mainly as no services are available in the community to support these patients and families.

On the other hand, the community's and professionals' attitude toward the patients' perception of pain and their disbelief of the patients' complaint of pain hinders pain management in the community as well as in the hospitals. In many Middle Eastern countries, moderate to severe pain appears to be controlled using multimodal therapy, including the usage of nonsteroidal anti-inflammatory drugs and limited doses of injectable opioids [21]. In the Palestinian community structure, there is a culture of shame in admitting pain, especially in the masculine community, and the belief that bearing pain makes one stronger. The fear of addiction, fear of the limited available options, fear of complications, respiratory depression, fear of losing control, and the will to maintain the ability to communicate and be present with the people surrounding them, are some of the cultural barriers to better end-of-life care and pain management. Similar discussions can be found in literature, specific to the Middle Eastern region, debating the culture of taboo and the stigma of cancer and its pain, and citing that people consider and accept pain as part of the disease [20].

Furthermore, the community usually tries to help chronic disease patients and their families. The community provides good emotional and social support in the event of illness and loss. The society in Palestine, like other Arab countries, is collaborative in their support to individuals in need - emotionally, by giving them a sense of belonging, and even with financial assistance. Ultimately, these humanitarian endeavors are still limited and based on personal relationships and geographical boundaries; they cannot make up for the lack of community-organized palliative care services.

Community Professional Infrastructure

Palliative care (PC) is still a new theme in Palestine. As such, new palliative teams are advised to begin at the bedside, to show everyone what they can do, to be available, and also to educate other staff members [20]. There are a few palliative care nurses in Palestine who are officially trained and certified, through a combined oncology and palliative care diploma program. These efforts are still in the early stages and need a lot of support on both national and international levels. However, the AL-Sadeel Society for Palliative Care provides a palliative care consultative model through a team of palliative care nurses and two social workers specialized in palliative care. This is done mainly by telephone, as there is very limited access to the patients' homes. Approximately 200 patients were served by this team in 2018, according to the Society's registry. The author would like to add that the Society succeeded in acquiring a scholarship from the American National Cancer Institute for one doctor to be specialized in palliative care for oncology patients in Israel. This doctor is now practicing in East Jerusalem hospitals with limited access to Palestinian patients due to the restrictions on the freedom of movement by the Israeli authorities.

There are still no services such as hospices, geriatric homes, or home-nursing. There are, however, some unorganized and non official home care nursing services scattered throughout the centers of some urban areas, which are based on personal contact with patients undergoing hospitalization. There are two privately owned centers in the West Bank of Palestine that provide private home care nursing services for direct out-of-pocket payment [18].

A local study in the West Bank of Palestine showed that nurses had poor knowledge of palliative care [22]. Moreover, most health-care providers in Palestine who work in cancer units need training and education in providing patients with palliative care [23]. Palliative care requires competent practices which may be achieved through training programs, an essential part of standard cancer care. Of course, investments in human and logistic resources are needed [24].

What Can Be Done?

Based on the findings from a recent study by the author, the quality of life of Palestinian cancer patients is very poor, especially for those in the advanced stages. Palliative care was found to demonstrate improved outcomes of care and save costs for the health-care system. Long-term palliative care service and the persistent work of the palliative care team is essential for success. The adoption of such cost-effective strategies by policy makers would appear to be a wise use of public funds. The study recommends further research on a broader scale and longer follow-up periods to reinforce similar conclusions [25].

On the other hand, the incidence of cancer in the Middle East is predicted to double in the next 10 years, more than in any other region of the world [26]. The Worldwide Palliative Care Alliance recommends that palliative care be integrated into countries' health-care systems [27], as long as it is estimated that 80% of the adults requiring palliative care live in low- and middle-income countries [28]. Nevertheless, socio-cultural, ethical, and religious involvement are crucial to the palliative care initiation in the Middle East, due to the prevalence of religious observance and community structure [9].

Arguably, in order to develop palliative care teams in the Middle East, the most urgent task is to focus on the education of professionals [20]. Health professionals must be trained in palliative care, attend scientific workshops and conferences for professionals who are working in the field of cancer care, and palliative care education should be included within the curriculum of schools for health professions [18, 23, 29]. Cooperation and support from the Ministries of Health and Education, local cancer care centers, education bodies and international support are vital for success, extending to policy makers' involvement and priority-setting on both national and international levels.

Further recommendations include: providing support for patients with cancer and chronic diseases and to have palliative care and symptom-management facilities all over the country. Also, to ensure drug availability, especially adopting an essential drug list based on the international essential drug list for palliative care, to address the stigmatization of patients and, finally, to monitor systems for the proper practice and provision of oncology health services in the community and other health facilities. Regrettably, Middle Eastern countries still need governmental policies that recognize palliative care [30]. The successful example of the Al-Sadeel Society can serve as an inspiration for the initiation and adoption of palliative care models in Palestine.

Conclusion

There is a desperate need for integrating palliative care into the health-care and community-care systems in Palestine. The integration of cost-effective community-based palliative care services will provide a solution to the burden on the health-care system and patients at the same time. Efforts need to begin by integrating palliative care into the national health plans and health education, training providers of palliative care at different levels (including community health workers, nurses, and physicians) providing good home-based care and institutions providing home care, and valuing competent palliative care science and culture within the community and nation.

References

1. Sepulveda C, Marlin A, Yoshida T, Ullrich A. Palliative care: the World Health Organization's global perspective. J Pain Symptom Manag. 2002;24(2):91–6.
2. Stjernswärd J, Foley KM, Ferris FD. The public health strategy for palliative care. J Pain Symptom Manag. 2007;33(5):486–93.
3. WHO> Cancer. World Health Organization NCD Management Unit Cancer [Internet]. 2019. [cited 2018 Jan 27]. Available from: http://www.who.int/cancer/en/.
4. MOH. Health annual report Palestine 2018. Minist Heal PHIC, Heal Status, Palest 2018, July 2019 [Internet]. 2019.; Available from: https://site.moh.ps/Content/Books/fE4zsafxsjNVhJntidJnqnnEHUibMuC1NYu66TNEmoNUJ1ZxeRcCm3_Iei1j8d4YesYKxRyEhD6PZqdxzBa4z91pIhALGXoDGEhlEIPai9X9O.pdf.
5. Khleif MH, Imam AM. Quality of life for Palestinian patients with cancer in the absence of a palliative-care service: a triangulated study. Lancet [Internet]. 2013 [cited 2018 Jan 17];382:S23. Available from: http://www.sciencedirect.com/science/article/pii/S0140673613625957.
6. Husseini A, Abu-Rmeileh NME, Mikki N, Ramahi TM, Ghosh HA, Barghuthi N, et al. Cardiovascular diseases, diabetes mellitus, and cancer in the occupied Palestinian territory. Lancet (London, England). 2009;373(9668):1041–9.
7. Stewart BW, Wild CP. World cancer report 2014. World Heal Organ [Internet]. 2014:1–2. Available from: http://www.videnza.org/wp-content/uploads/World-Cancer-Report-2014.pdf.
8. Higginson I. Health care needs assessment: palliative care and terminal care. In: Stevens A, Raftery J, editors. Health care needs assessment. Oxford: Oxford Radcliffe Medical Press; 1997. p. 1–28.
9. Silbermann M, Fink RM, Min S-J, Mancuso MP, Brant J, Hajjar R, et al. Evaluating palliative care needs in middle eastern countries. J Palliat Med [Internet]. 2015;18(1):18–25. Available from: http://online.liebertpub.com/doi/abs/10.1089/jpm.2014.0194.
10. Walker H, Anderson M, Farahati F, Howell D, Librach SL, Husain A, et al. Resource use and costs of end-of-life/palliative care: Ontario adult cancer patients dying during 2002 and 2003. J Palliat Care. 2011;27(2):79–88.
11. Chitnis XA, Georghiou T, Steventon A, Bardsley MJ. Effect of a home-based end-of-life nursing service on hospital use at the end of life and place of death: a study using administrative data and matched controls. BMJ Support Palliat Care. 2013 Dec;3(4):422–30.
12. Brumley R, Enguidanos S, Jamison P, Seitz R, Morgenstern N, Saito S, et al. Increased satisfaction with care and lower costs: results of a randomized trial of in-home palliative care. J Am Geriatr Soc. 2007;55(7):993–1000.

13. Shnoor Y, Szlaifer M, Aoberman AS, Bentur N. The cost of home hospice care for terminal patients in Israel. Am J Hosp Palliat Med. 2007;24(4):284–90.
14. Bingley A, Clark D. A comparative review of palliative care development in six countries represented by the Middle East Cancer Consortium (MECC). J Pain Symptom Manag. 2009 Mar;37(3):287–96.
15. Smith S, Brick A, O'Hara S, Normand C. Evidence on the cost and cost-effectiveness of palliative care: a literature review. Palliat Med. 2014;28(2):130–50.
16. May P, Normand C, Morrison RS. Economic impact of hospital inpatient palliative care consultation: review of current evidence and directions for future research. J Palliat Med [Internet]. 2014;17(9):1054–63. Available from: http://online.liebertpub.com/doi/abs/10.1089/jpm.2013.0594.
17. Hodgson C. Cost-effectiveness of palliative care: a review of the literature [Internet]. 2012. Available from: http://www.hpcintegration.ca/media/36290/TWF-Economics-report-Eng-final-webmar7.pdf.
18. Khleif M, Dweib A. Palliative care initiative in a developing country: using Palestine as an example. In: Silbermann M, editor. Palliative care: perspectives, practices and impact on quality of life –global view. New York: Nova Science publishers; 2017. p. 345–54.
19. Physicians for Human Rights-Israel. Physicians for human rights-Israel [Internet]. Physicians for Human Rights-Israel. 2015. Available from: http://www.phr.org.il/phr.
20. Silbermann M, Arnaout M, Daher M, Nestoros S, Pitsillides B, Charalambous H, et al. Palliative cancer care in middle eastern countries: accomplishments and challenges. Ann Oncol J Eur Soc Med Oncol. 2012;23(Suppl 3):15–28.
21. Ben Arie E, Ali-Shtayeh M, Nejmi M, Schiff E, Hassan E, Mutafoglu K, et al. Integrative oncology in the Middle East: weaving traditional and complementary medicine in supportive care. Support Care Cancer. 2012;20:557–64.
22. Ayed A. The nurses ' knowledge and attitudes towards the palliative care. J Educ Pract. 2015;6(4):91–100.
23. Shawawra M, Khleif AD. Palliative care situation in Palestinian authority. J Pediatr Hematol Oncol. 2011;33(Suppl 1):S64–7.
24. Meier DE, Brawley OW. Palliative care and the quality of life. J Clin Oncol [Internet]. 2011;29(20):2750–2. Available from: http://www.ncbi.nlm.nih.gov/pmc/articles/PMC3139393/.
25. Khleif M. Economic and clinical impact of a consultative palliative care model for in-patients with cancer in Palestine. Unpublished thesis. Hebrew University of Jerusalem; 2019.
26. Boseley S. Global cancer surge fueled by alcohol, smoking, and obesity predicted by WHO. The Guardian [Internet] 2014 Feb 4.; Available from: https://www.theguardian.com/society/2014/feb/03/alcohol-sugar-smoking-fuel-cancer-surge.
27. Lancet T. Palliative care: a peaceful, humane global campaign is needed. Lancet [Internet]. 2014;383(9916):487. Available from: https://doi.org/10.1016/S0140-6736(14)60166-5.
28. Connor SR, Bermedo MCS. Global atlas of palliative care at the end of life [Internet]. Who. 2014. 111 p. Available from: http://www.who.int/cancer/publications/palliative-care-atlas/en/
29. Khleif M, Dweib A. Palliative care in Palestine. In: Silbermann M, editor. Palliative care to the cancer patient: the middle east as a model for emerging countries. New York: Nova Science publishers; 2014. p. 171–82.
30. Silbermann M. Availability of pain medication for patients in the middle east: status of the problem and the role of the Middle East Cancer consortium (MECC): implications for other regions. J Palliat Care Med. 2012;02(06):3.

Part XXV

Middle East: Turkey

Pediatric Palliative Care in the Community: The Turkish Experience

Rejin Kebudi and Fatma Betul Cakir

Introduction

PC is an approach that improves the QoL of patients and families facing problems associated with life-threatening illness, such as cancer, by prevention and treatment of symptoms and side effects of the disease, by means of early identification, assessment, and treatment of pain and other problems, physical, psychosocial, and spiritual. For a patient diagnosed with cancer, PC should begin at diagnosis and continue through treatment, follow-up care, and the end-of-life. PPC is the art and science of child-focused, family-oriented, relationship-centered medical care aimed at enhancing quality-of-life and minimizing suffering. Pain and symptom control, care coordination, and end-of-life care are important components of PPC.

Development of Palliative Care in Turkey

The health system reform in Turkey after 2002 (which coincided with the Health Transformation Program (HTP) that included universal health insurance coverage and easy health service access) has enabled all children to be admitted to tertiary health centers for diagnosis and treatment free of charge, totally reimbursed by the government [1–3]. In 2009, the TMH launched a national cancer control program including cancer registry, prevention, screening and early diagnosis, treatment, and PC. Turkey has accelerated the education programs on PC for health-care professionals since this project [4]. The establishment of PC in Turkey and in the region has also been supported by the Middle East Cancer Consortium (MECC) [5]. PC training programs organized in collaboration with the TMH and MECC between 2004 and 2014 were attended by a total of 434 people [6]. In 2014, the TMH published guidelines entitled "Directives for PC Services Implementation Procedures and Principles" to regulate the standards of PC units established in hospitals and revised them 1 year later [7, 8]. The directives highlighted the importance of teamwork, including psychological, social, and spiritual support to the patients, while integrating PC provision for the patient and the family. The role and necessity of integration of family physicians and home care teams to the PC units were also emphasized. In 2011, the majority of almost 40,000 patients who received home care had neurological disease (45%), cardiovascular disease (21%), and other chronic diseases; only 4% had cancer [3, 9]. Thus, most patients with cancer had not received home care. The number of patients

R. Kebudi (✉)
Pediatric Hematology-Oncology, Oncology Institute, Istanbul University & Istanbul Medical Faculty, Istanbul University, Istanbul, Turkey

F. B. Cakir
Bezmialem Vakif University Medical Faculty, Pediatric Hematology-Oncology, Istanbul, Turkey

M. Silbermann (ed.), *Palliative Care for Chronic Cancer Patients in the Community*,
https://doi.org/10.1007/978-3-030-54526-0_35

receiving home care increased to 760,645 in 2016; however, the number of cancer patients receiving home care was still inadequate [10]. After the new regulations for PC in 2015 [8], the number of PC units increased rapidly to 358 inpatient settings with a total of 4752 registered hospital beds in 81 cities by 2018 [10]. Although Turkey has reached about 50% of the PC beds as recommended by the European Association for Palliative Care for 1,000,000 inhabitants [10, 11], nearly all of them are hospital beds, since all these actively working PC units are inpatient units. There are only a few private outpatient hospices, but still no community hospice teams or specialized home PC teams designated for oncology or "hospital at home" organizations [10]. Although the number of PC units for adult patients increased rapidly after 2015, similar improvement did not occur in PPC. Only four PPC units have been recently established, and these inpatient hospital services take care of non-oncology PPC patients. Although acceptance of regulations for the implementation of PC services is encouraging, no formal national regulation for PPC exists.

The Current Status of Palliative Care Among Pediatric Oncology Patients in Turkey

Each year in Turkey, 2500–3000 new childhood cancer cases are expected [2, 9]. According to the Turkish Pediatric Oncology Group (TPOG) and Turkish Pediatric Hematology Society (TPHD) Registry initiated in 2002, about 2500–3000 new pediatric cancer cases are reported each year [2, 9]. In the previous decade, the majority of patients were diagnosed at quite advanced stages due to delay in diagnosis and late referral to oncology centers [9, 12]. However, in the current decade, there is a trend for earlier diagnosis of cancer due to improved awareness in the community, particularly among the health-care staff at primary level health-care settings. The health system reform in Turkey after 2002, which provided universal health insurance coverage and easy health service access, has enabled timely referral of all children to tertiary health centers for diagnosis and treatment, free of charge. The collaborative education program on "recognizing the signs and symptoms for early diagnosis of pediatric cancer and symptom management", organized by the TPOG and the TMH, has been afforded to primary physicians and nurses in many different cities and emphasizes pediatric and medical oncology topics in the medical school curriculum; this has also supported the improvement in the last decade [2, 9, 12].

In 2010, the first PPC unit was established in the Oncology Institute, Dokuz Eylul University Hospital in Izmir, by a dedicated team [13]. The unit actually served both adult and pediatric cancer patients. Although still no actively working PPC unit exists for children with cancer in Turkey, almost all pediatric hematologists and oncologists all over Turkey provide some form of PC at their inpatient or outpatient oncology clinics by way of consultations with the related disciplines [9]. Only a few university hospitals have dieticians, physiotherapists, and psychologists working full-time in the pediatric oncology units. In most centers, "consultations" are requested when necessary from psychologists, psychiatrists, dieticians, social workers, physiotherapists, algology units, or spiritual counselors who work at the hospitals or nearby hospitals. A collaborative training program has begun for spiritual counselors in Turkey [2, 9]. There are no professional art therapists employed in the pediatric oncology centers. An art therapist had worked voluntarily for over a year in two pediatric oncology centers, and her positive contribution to the children was immense [9, 14]. The primary physicians (the pediatric oncologists) and the oncology nurses working at the inpatient or outpatient services try to cover the role of the psychologist, social worker, and sometimes even the spiritual counselor in many centers; this may sometimes lead to a burn-out syndrome [15–17]. Nurses are in close contact with cancer patients at all stages of cancer, during treatment and at end-of-life, and they have more in-depth, day-to-day contact with the patient than the pediatric oncologist, which can be more proactive and innovative than the care efforts intended to maximize the health-related quality-of-life of children with cancer [2, 9, 15, 16]. In Turkey, there is no formal comprehensive PC curriculum in medical schools nor PC specialty/certification for physicians. PC continuing education for residents and doctors have improved. During the fellowship programs of medical or pediatric oncology specialties, there are few formal PC lectures in the curriculum. However, residents and fellows mostly learn PC while caring for these oncology patients during their hospitalization [2, 9]. A certification program for PC nursing was recently approved by the ministry of health [10]. Most nurses gain experience while working in the inpatient oncology clinic from more experienced nurses and pediatric oncologists/hematologists. PC training is increasing via an interdisciplinary care program in the inpatient clinics and via lectures and courses in national meetings. Oftentimes the relation between the health-care professionals and the children and their parents is very intimate or close. Good communication between the physicians and the parents promotes trust, from the time of diagnosis and throughout the continuing progressive stages of cancer; for terminal stage patients, this trust may even assist in their decision regarding where they choose to die [15, 16]. Most parents prefer to stay in the pediatric oncology ward in the hospital at the terminal stage, contrary to many countries in the Middle East [2, 9]. A few parents prefer home for the place of death.

The Current Status of Palliative Care Among Pediatric Non-Oncology Patients in Turkey

In 2015, the first PPC inpatient unit in Turkey was established in Bursa in the north-west part of Turkey. Bursa is a socioeconomically developed city. The other three inpatient PPC units were established in April 2017 in Erzurum, which is in the north-east part of Turkey, in May 2017 in Mersin, which is in the south of Turkey, and in December 2018 in Izmir, which is in the west of Turkey. All of them are located in government training and research hospitals. Each PPC units has seven to 20 beds and five to 10 nurses. In three PPC units, the chief physicians are pediatricians, and in the fourth is an anesthesiologist trained in intensive care. There is health staff on call for 24 hours/day, 7 days/week. The PPC units have no outpatient clinics for the periodic follow-up of the patients, except for the one in Mersin. The chief physician at this unit established a very well-organized outpatient clinic for the periodic follow-up of these chronic patients. Thus, acute problems that the families have to cope with could easily be solved during the outpatient clinic visits.

The primary aim of all these PPCs is to follow the children with permanent or progressive neuromotor disabilities with or without respiratory sequela, stabilize their medical condition, and prepare them for home care. The PPC staff is usually asked to treat children in the pediatric intensive care unit (ICU); however, patients from other departments of the same hospital, other hospitals, and from hospitals in other cities are also referred. The secondary aim of the PPC units is to educate mothers so that they can take care of their children who need complex health support measures such as BIPAP machines for home settings and to give psychosocial support to the patient and caregivers and to maintain a relatively good quality-of-life. There is no age limit for children; a neonate or an 18-year-old adolescent can be hospitalized as well at all PPC units. No PPC unit has cancer patient experience, except for the one in Bursa, where they followed one refractory acute leukemia patient who relapsed after an allogeneic bone marrow transplant and gave no response to salvage chemotherapies thereafter. The PPC team tried to support him and the parent palliatively at the terminal stage, but he died after a 15-day follow-up.

In the PPC units, in addition to the care of the patient by the primary physician and the nurses, consultations with psychiatrists, psychologists, physiotherapists, social workers, dieticians, spiritual counselors, and other relevant subdivisions/ departments throughout the hospital occur as needed. At every PPC unit, the physiotherapists and the psychologists visit the patients and the mothers every day if needed. Dieticians, social workers, and other staff members visit the patients once a week. At the PPC unit in Mersin, when a new patient is admitted to the unit, the psychologists, physiotherapists, and social workers are all introduced to the family, and they welcome the patient and the family.

Nurses have a very important role in all PPC units. They are at the core of the care for both the patient and the mother. They care for patient's medical problems and are also responsible for the education of the caregiver, which is usually the mother. All the nurses are well-trained and experienced in the intensive care of the patient, including eye/nose/mouth/anal and wound care, any catheter, nasogastric tube, tracheostomy or percutaneous endoscopic gastrostomy care, if present. They perform all the care and educate the mother or other caregiver and supervise them during all steps of the care. The nurses also support the physiotherapy exercises (particularly respiratory and mobilization physiotherapy) that the physiotherapist teaches the mothers to do. Although the nurses are not responsible for the psychosocial or spiritual well-being of the patients and the mothers, they witness and share all good and bad things that they experience throughout the day; thus, they are actually the first health-care staff that determine the need for a psychologist, a spiritual counsellor, or the social worker [15, 16]. In many PPC units or hospitals for children, volunteers from non-governmental organizations visit the patients and try to entertain them. The PPC unit in Izmir has recently published a palliative care book in Turkish (personal communication), and the same team established a one-day pediatric PC symposium that was held on 14 October 2019 in Izmir.

The mean duration of hospital stay in the PPC units range from 10 days to nearly 1 month, closely related to the time to provide the technical equipment that the children need at home and to educate the mothers to take care of their children at home. The cost of most of the equipment and the medication drugs are reimbursed by the government. At the PPC unit in Erzurum, however, the mean duration of hospital stay exceeds several months due to insufficient electricity infrastructure, particularly in small towns and villages within and around Erzurum. For example, a child that needs a ventilatory support system may not be discharged if continuous electricity is not available in their town. The low socioeconomic status of the patients is also another factor; the houses are small and the families are crowded with no extra suitable room for the patient at home. The municipalities, with the support of the social services of the government, try to improve the infrastructure of electricity at these rural areas and some non-governmental organizations support families financially.

Two other PPC units will be established in Ankara and in Kayseri in the upcoming months.

Multidisciplinary cancer treatment and other specialized care in Turkey are quite advanced in comparison to most countries in the region. Patients with cancer from the Middle East, Balkan or Turkish-speaking countries in the northeast of Turkey, such as Azerbaijan and Kazakhstan, come to Turkey for an accurate diagnosis and/or treatment. There are also refugees coming to Turkey from neighboring areas of conflict [2]. According to government estimates, since the onset of the civil war of Syria in March 2011, over four million Syrians have come to Turkey [18]. Since the beginning of the crisis in 2011, Disaster and Emergency Management Residency (AFAD), an organization activated for crisis circumstances, promoted ordinary daily life, regular education facilities, and health services [2, 19]. In April 2013, Turkey established its first asylum law, the "Law on Foreigners and International Protection" regulating all proceedings for refugees living in Turkey [2]. Refugees with cancer can be treated at tertiary government and university hospitals free of charge. The patients usually have very advanced stage diseases at diagnosis, and therefore have poor outcomes [20]. The refugee children with non-cancer chronic diseases are also allowed to receive PC support at these PPC units. However, the duration of their hospital stay maybe longer in the event of insufficient home facilities such as crowded rooms at small houses or longer time to obtain home-type ventilation machines.

Conclusion and Recommendations

Palliative care is an approach that improves the quality-of-life (QoL) of patients and families facing problems associated with life-threatening illness. PC should begin at diagnosis and continue through treatment, follow-up care, and the end-of-life. PPC is the art and science of child-focused, family-oriented, relationship-centered medical care aimed at enhancing quality-of-life and minimizing suffering. Pain and symptom control, care coordination, and end-of-life care are important components of PPC. Depending on the resources, PPC may be imbedded in the related clinic or may be in separate inpatient PPC units, inpatient, or outpatient children's hospice services; also, there should be dynamic local community or hospital-based specialized PPC home care teams for children with cancer. PPC providers should all respect traditional and cultural diversities. A national PPC network among PPC units would be very helpful, so that patients could be transferred when there is no available bed at a center. Guidelines for PPC should be prepared, the standard/minimal requirements of a PC unit should be established and future strategies should be planned. Inpatient PPC units and teams (acute) or inpatient pediatric hospices (chronic) should be established for the purpose of both acute problems of the patients that could be resolved in a limited time or for end-of-life care for the incurable cancer patients. All four PPC units now in Turkey take care of acute problems of the patients but sometimes are a place of death of the patients. Although there are local home care medical teams in the Ministry of Health, most of them are not experienced in PPC. PPC should be included in the national health policies, as well as the education of health-care workers, and public PC service provision should be seen as a priority. Scientific organizations and Societies for Pediatric Oncology, Pediatric Hematology, Pediatric Intensive Care, Perinatology, and other related disciplines should collaborate to improve PPC in the community. PPC should be included in the curriculum of both medical schools and nursing schools.

Acknowledgments We extend our thanks to Yelda Çufalı, MD, the chief of the Pediatric Palliative Care unit at Bursa Dörtçelik Training and Research Government Pediatric Hospital; Tuğba Güler, MD, and Nuri Alaçakır, MD; the chiefs of thePediatric Palliative Care unit at Regional Erzurum City Government Education and Research Hospital; Aydın Yücel, MD, the chief of the Pediatric Palliative Care unit at Mersin City Government Training and Research Hospital; and Nilgün Harputluoğlu, MD, the chief of the Pediatric Palliative Care unit at Behçet Uz Training and Research Government Pediatric Hospital for their valuable contribution.

References

1. Atun R, Aydın S, Chakraborty S, et al. Universal health coverage in Turkey: enhancement of equity. Lancet. 2013;382:65–99.
2. Kebudi R, Cakir FB. Cancer care in a country undergoing transition: Turkey, current challenges and trends for the future. In: Silbermann M, editor. Cancer care in countries and societies in transition. New York: Springer; 2016. p. 193–208.
3. Kebudi R, Cakir FB. Cultural challenges in implementing palliative services in Turkey. Palliat Med Hosp Care Open J. 2017;SE:S10–4.
4. Ozgul N, Gultekin M, Koc O, et al. Turkishcommunity-based palliative care model: a unique design. Ann Oncol. 2012;23(Suppl. 3):76–8.
5. Silbermann M, Arnaout M, Abdel Rahman Sayed H, et al. Pediatric palliative care in the Middle East. In: Knapp C, Madden V, Fowler-Kerry S, editors. Pediatric palliative care: global perspectives. Amterdam: Springer Science Business Media B.V; 2012. p. 127–59.
6. Hacıkamiloglu E, Utku ES, Cukurova Z, Keskinkilic B, Topcu I, Gultekin M, Silbermann M. Community palliative care in Turkey: a collaborative promoter to a new concept in the Middle East. J Public Health Manag Pract. 2016;22:81–8.
7. https://dosyamerkez.sağlık.gov.tr>4297.palyatif-bakim-yonergesi.doc. Last accessed on 10 Dec 2019.
8. https://www.saglikaktuel.com/d/file/palyatif-bakim-hizmetleri-yonergesi.pdf. Last accessed on 10 Dec 2019.
9. Kebudi R, Cakir FB, Gultekin M. Palliative care to the cancer patient in Turkey. In: Silbermann M, editor. Palliative care to the cancer patient: the Middle East as a model for emerging countries. New York: Nova; 2014.
10. Oguz GT, Silbermann M. International palliative care: update on Turkey's experience on developing community palliative care programs. J Fam Med. 2019;6(4):1172.
11. Radbruch L, Payne S, the Board of Directors of the EAPC. White paper on standards and norms for hospice and palliative care in Europe: part 2 recommendations from the European Association for Palliative Care. Eur J Palliat Care. 2010;17:22–33.

12. Kebudi R. Pediatric oncology in Turkey. J Pediatr Hematol Oncol. 2012;34:S12–4.
13. Mutafoglu K. Current palliative care practice in a university hospital. J Pediatr Hematol Oncol. 2010;32(suppl. 1):S36–8.
14. Kebudi R, Ozcan A. Understanding psychological states of children with cancer: art therapy as a communication tool. Psycho-Oncology. 2011., (abstract AA-3).;20(Supp):83.
15. Bar-Sela G, Schultz MJ, Elshamy K, et al. Training for awareness of one's own spirituality: a key factor in overcoming barriers to the provision of spiritual care to advanced cancer patients by doctors and nurses. Palliat Support Care. 2019;17(3):345–52.
16. Bar-Sela G, Schultz MJ, Elshamy K, et al. Human development index and its association with staff spiritual care provision: a Middle Eastern oncology study. Support Care Cancer. 2019;27(9):3601–10.
17. Alacacioglu A, Yavuzsen T, Dirioz M, Oztop I, Yilmaz U. Burnout in nurses and physicians working at an oncology department. Psycho-Oncology. 2009;18:543–8.
18. https://multeciler.org.tr/turkiyedeki-suriyeli-sayisi/.
19. Ben-Arye E, Bonucci M, Daher M, et al. Refugees in conflict: creating a bridge between traditional and conventional health belief models. Oncologist. 2018;23(6):693–6.
20. Kebudi R, Bayram I, Yagci-Kupeli B, et al. Refugee children with cancer in Turkey. Lancet Oncol. 2016;17:865–7.

The Role of the Community Nurse in Developing Palliative Care Services

Ayfer Aydin

Introduction

Chronic and non-infectious diseases have been steadily increasing around the world, resulting in an increasing demand for palliative care for patients with life-threatening conditions and the elderly population throughout the world. Each year, an estimated 40 million people are in need of palliative care, 78% of them live in low- and middle-income countries [1, 2]. Due to this increasing need for palliative care, the World Health Organization and the Worldwide Palliative Care Alliance proposed that palliative care can be provided in every locally available condition: at home, in hospitals, outpatient clinics and care centres, or wherever the patient is being cared for [1, 3–6].

Patients with life-threatening diseases suffer multiple physical discomforts, as well as a range of psychosocial and spiritual concerns [7–9]. With the progression of their diseases, the utilisation of health services by patients increases at the end-of-life stage [5, 6]. Studies show that the vast majority of patients prefer to spend their final days and die in their own homes. However, it is seen that patients are more likely to die in a hospital and not their homes. Furthermore, hospital deaths were determined to be in unpreferable conditions, suggesting a vital need for good community-based care. Providing palliative care in patients' home settings and their own habitat is the centre of many countries' health policies [4, 10].

Palliative Care in the Community

Developing palliative care services in primary care is essential for realising the expectations of dying people. Among the reasons for the need for palliative care in the community are the psychological stresses of coping with symptoms, dying in an unfamiliar environment among strangers, the burden of life-support, the shortage of available medical and disease-oriented care models, long hospital stays, the financial costs of medical care of a terminally ill patient and the lack of palliative care specialists in hospitals [11, 12].

Palliative care at home aims to increase the quality of life of the patient as much as possible by reducing the negative effects of the disease, relieving emerging problems with appropriate medical and nursing approaches, and ensuring that the patient's living conditions are affected as little as possible, thus allowing a comfortable death when the time comes [13]. The patients prefer to receive care at home rather than in a hospital setting [3, 10] because the home environment is more familiar, it allows the patient to maintain their normal life as much as possible and allows the family to be in charge.

A. Aydin (✉)
Koç University, School of Nursing, İstanbul, Turkey
e-mail: ayfer.aydin@deu.edu.tr

M. Silbermann (ed.), *Palliative Care for Chronic Cancer Patients in the Community*,
https://doi.org/10.1007/978-3-030-54526-0_36

Palliative care at home has many documented benefits [3, 8, 9, 13, 14]. These include the following:

- Reduced burden of symptoms on the patient and their family
- Increased patient and family compliance to care and treatment
- Improved recovery
- Improved patient and family satisfaction
- Reduced hospital, intensive care and emergency room stays
- Reduced hospitalisations
- Preserving family integrity
- Enabling the patient to live in their home setting
- Preventing the social isolation of the individual
- Providing the highest possible autonomy
- Allowing the patient to participate in family and social activities and hobbies
- Reduced risk of infection
- Allowing a more personal care
- Reduced stress for the patient and their family
- A lower short-term cost
- Uninterrupted health care from diagnosis to recovery
- Improved quality of life

The purpose of palliative care at home can vary depending on the needs of the patient and their family. The requirements and frequency of palliative care are subject to change as the needs of the patient and their family change, the disease progresses, and the required care gets more complex. The nature of the provided care will usually depend on the demands and expectations of the patient [10].

Community Palliative Care Team

Palliative care is a team effort. The palliative care team works together to meet the patient's physical, psychological, social, spiritual and cultural needs, and to help the families and carers. The members of the palliative care team may include physicians, nurses, allied health professionals, volunteers and carers. This team can provide continuous and coordinated supportive care in the community. The community nurse is a significant part of the palliative care team [15].

Community Nurse

The duties and the definition of a community nurse change according to the conditions and needs of each country. The literature indicates that nurses provide palliative care under different titles, such as a community nurse, public health nurse, home care nurse, the advanced practice registered nurse and district nurse [16–21]. Despite having different definitions and duties, we will use the term "community nurse" throughout this paper to include all of the above members of the nursing team.

Roles and Functions of the Community Nurse

Community nurses carry out significant roles and functions in a home care setting. The community nurse needs to plan systematic, integrated and effective care for the patient. In keeping with the nursing profession's principles, the nurses who work in this area focus on enhancing a person's quality of life, regardless of age, and on supporting family members and significant others. First of all, the community nurse must collect data regarding the patient and their family to determine the relevant problems, rank these problems in order of priority, plan and implement appropriate nursing interventions and evaluate the outcomes [22–24].

Assessment of the Palliative Care Patient

Data collection, the first stage of the nursing process, includes an assessment that aims to determine the care needs of the palliative care patient and their family [25]. It is important to determine the needs of the patient for palliative care at home for a successful outcome. For this purpose, the community nurse primarily needs to collect data and assess the patient.

The factors that should be evaluated during the assessment of the patient and their family in order to determine home care needs are as follows: the patient's ability to perform daily life activities (independence), disease-specific symptoms, nutritional status, cognitive functions and behaviours, communication, individual expectations and demands, changes in work and family life, understanding the disease, treatment and prognosis, and the ability to cope with the disease and its effects.

The community nurse should also evaluate the patient's carers to determine how the family perceives and defines the disease, whether they require information regarding the disease and their perception of the effects of the disease and treatments. The assessment of the family should also determine urgent priorities, the environment, family resources, family roles and relationships, family functions, social support systems, family expectations and demands and the impact of the disease on the family.

Another aspect of data collection is the evaluation of the home setting. It is important to make sure that the physical environment is adequate before the patient is brought home. The community nurse should determine the physical environment requirements to ensure safety and comfort for the patient's current and future care. It is important that the home environment is safe for nursing applications and adequate for safely storing the medical equipment. The community nurse also needs to determine and take the appropriate measures for bathroom and bedroom safety. All these considerations naturally involve the patient's resources of economic and social support [26, 27].

The data to be collected by the community nurse for the assessment of the patient and their family in the context of home care are presented in Table 1 [28].

Nursing Diagnosis

After data collection, the community nurse should evaluate the data and determine the needs of the patient and establish the nursing diagnosis. Among the most common nursing diagnoses in

Table 1 Assessment of patient

Medical history	The disease and its severity, stage and prognosis Previous medical conditions Treatment (previous and current) Other medical conditions Symptoms resulting from the disease and treatment Information needs regarding the disease and treatment The effects of the disease and treatment on daily life Emergency conditions
Recurring problems during the treatment process	Disease-related symptoms and problems; Pain Nausea and vomiting Diarrhea Constipation Mucositis Alopecia Dyspnea Itching Fatigue Level of consciousness Psychosocial problems Invasive interventions (e.g. port, catheter, ventilation)
Self-care	Carrying out daily activities (eating, drinking, bathing, etc.) Fulfilling family responsibilities (e.g. as a spouse or mother, shopping for groceries, maintaining the house) Need for counseling and support
Psychosocial assessment	Social relationships and support systems Fears (death, suffering, etc.) Coping behaviours Intellectual abilities (e.g. problem solving, educational status) Communication skills The patient's perception of the disease
Assessment of the carers	Health status of family members Relationship with the patient The family's ability to provide emotional and physical care Communication The family's knowledge of the disease and treatment The patient and their family's ability to cope with the disease Changes in domestic roles and lifestyle Sources of support The purpose and meaning of life, concerns about death

(continued)

Table 1 (continued)

Environment	Physical environment (temperature, lighting, sound, etc.) Physical security of the environment (bathroom, kitchen, stairs, etc.) Hygienic assessment Limitations to care (not having a telephone connection, etc.)
Financial status	Health insurance, solvency, sources of financial support

palliative care patients at home are pain, respiratory distress, fatigue, activity intolerance, impaired body image and social isolation [28].

Planning

The community nurse should determine the required interventions for the identified problems. The plan should include what needs to be done, how, and when, how to assess the patient, and how to include the family in the process. The patient and their family need to be a part of home care. The participation of the patients and their families has been shown to be positively correlated with their satisfaction with the care. The community nurse needs to be more careful when providing care for particular patients at home as they are more likely to have issues with home care due to their specific conditions.

Vulnerable Patients in Home Care

- Patients with complex or poorly treated conditions
- Patients with multiple symptoms and conditions
- Patients that undergo multiple and complex treatment procedures
- Patients that live alone
- Patients who are weak and/or elderly
- Patients with inadequate caregiver support
- Family disputes
- Patients that are confined to bed
- Patients without medical insurance

Nursing Interventions

The community nurse should apply and systematically evaluate the planned care. Community nursing applications need to be scientific and evidence-based, and compliant with the relevant legislation. Specific nursing interventions may vary depending on the patient's diagnosis, severity of the disease, frequency and severity of symptoms and the psychosocial status of the patient. Effective symptom management will ensure an increased quality of life and a peaceful death for the patient.

Evaluation

The community nurse must evaluate the patient's condition during home visits in order to provide the patient with solutions for problems that can be solved by nursing interventions. When the issue cannot be addressed in a home setting, the nurse is responsible for referring the patient to an institution where they can receive proper care.

All applications that are relevant to home care practices need to be documented. These records ensure the continuity and evaluation of the provided care and facilitate the communication between different members of the team. The roles and functions of community nurses who provide home care vary according to the factors mentioned above. A general summary of their functions are presented in Table 2 [29, 30].

Symptom Management

The community nurse should determine the problems of the palliative care patient with the nursing process, plan the required interventions for the determined symptoms and provide the necessary care [31–33]. The most common physical and psychosocial symptoms and nursing interventions for cancer PATIENTS that require palliative care at home are indicated below.

Table 2 The role and functions of the community nurse providing palliative home care

Initiate and maintain good communication with the patient and their family, using appropriate communication skills
Help patients and relatives access appropriate care and resources
Enable and support patients and their relatives to have a say in their care and to participate in decision making
Help the patient understand their own illness and the value of their life
Create a safe space for patients and their relatives
Explain to the patient and their family about their own responsibilities as a nurse and their role in the team
Accept that each patient and their family are unique
Respect the unique emotional reactions of the patient and their family
Respect the privacy of the patient and their family, and provide an adequate environment
Extensively evaluate each cancer patient and their family for an effective and acceptable plan, and provide the necessary support
Evaluate the cultural and religious values, emotions and behaviours of the patient and their family regarding death
Evaluate and try to fulfil the needs and expectations of the patient and their family
Encourage the patient and their family to express their fears, feelings and perceptions
Create a safe space for the patient and their family to talk about death
Enable the patient and their family to express their emotional and behavioural needs
Help the patient and their family understand the medical condition, and answer sensitive questions about death and grief
Provide continuous emotional support to the patient and their family
Help the patient and their family recognise their strengths
Be sensitive and respectful to the sexual needs of the dying patient
Plan care in collaboration with the patient and their family
Provide the patient and their family with information in a way that they can understand regarding;
Care options, available resources and services
Disease process and prognosis
Medication: effects, side effects, application
Treatment: purpose, benefits, side effects
Emergency conditions and complications: spinal cord compression, superior vena cava syndrome, cardiac tamponade, bleeding, seizures, hypercalcemia, opioid toxicity and delirium
Grieving: coping with grief, coping with the reaction of family members and the others
Death process: signs and symptoms of impending death, providing information regarding support of the patient in their final hours
Respect the patient's requests about complementary medicine and provide the necessary information
Evaluate the patient's pain and other symptoms, and help with management
Provide the patient and their family with the relevant phone numbers so that they can call and obtain information when necessary
Raise awareness regarding self-checking for symptoms at home
Provide the necessary information for accessing hospital and emergency services
Advise the patient and family about how and from whom to get help
Help maintain the patient's independence, creativity and control to increase their life satisfaction
Identify and aid the social support system of the patient and their family
Provide information to the patient and their family about the economic aspects of the disease and the available financial support
Provide the caregiving family members an opportunity to rest, if possible
Care During Death:
Inform family members about symptoms that suggest impending death
Evaluate the current treatment and discontinue unnecessary medication
Evaluate the religious and spiritual needs of the patient, family and carers
Provide the family and carers with appropriate written information
Help manage pain symptoms
Relieve breathing issues
Provide the necessary arrangements for the peaceful and dignified death of the patient
Enable the patient to be with relatives
Help the family realise any cultural or religious practices
Discuss the place of death with the patient and their family, and help with their decision
Help relieve the family's worries and fears
Grieving Process
Help meet the needs of the family
Support family members with home visits, if needed

Physical Symptoms

Pain; Pain is an unpleasant feeling arising from any part of the body, with or without an organic cause, that serves as a defense mechanism against physical damage and is commonly associated with past experiences. *Etiology*: Pain can occur due to many reasons. The etiology of pain can vary depending on its origin, cause and type. Acute pain is caused by prostaglandin, serotonin, histamine, bradykinin and substance P that are released as a result of sudden tissue damage, while chronic pain is caused by tumors and tumor-related structural changes, treatments, inactivity, inflammation, nerve pressure and decreased or hindered blood flow to an organ. *Signs and Symptoms*: Acute pain activates the sympathetic nervous system and causes physical symptoms such as paleness, sweating, increased pulse, high blood pressure, dilated pupils, tense skeletal muscles, rapid or superficial breathing and behavioural symptoms such as crying and holding the affected organ. Patients with chronic pain experience many difficulties in coping with the changes to their lifestyle. The pain can disrupt the patient's sleep patterns and quality, and they may experience sleep-related fatigue during the day. Chronic pain may negatively affect the patient's daily activities and self-care [26, 28, 34].

Nursing Interventions

- The patient is evaluated for pain [severity, frequency, type, duration, underlying cause)
- The pain is evaluated regarding its effect on the patient's life
- Other symptoms affecting pain are contained (fatigue, insomnia, etc.)
- Pharmacological treatment is provided as requested
- The patient and family are informed about pain management (effects of drugs, application, side effects)
- Non-pharmacological interventions are provided as requested to decrease pain (distraction, massaging, playing music, game therapy, hypnosis, acupuncture, exercise, etc.)

(a) *Fatigue*: It is an unpleasant subjective symptom that can prevent an individual from performing their regular functions at their normal capacity, ranging from slight burnout to an unbearable fatigue that affects their entire body. *Etiology*: The causes of fatigue include muscle weakness, accumulation of damaged cellular components, anemia, cancer pathology and treatment, fever, diarrhea, pain, nausea and vomiting, acute infections, electrolyte imbalances, nutritional disorders chemotherapy, radiotherapy, immunotherapy, side effects of some medications (corticosteroids, beta-blockers, etc.), disease-related anxiety, depression, social isolation and sleep disturbances. *Signs and Symptoms*: Fatigue can prevent the patient from performing daily living activities and self-care. It can impair concentration and decrease success and social interactions.

Nursing Interventions

- The patient is evaluated for fatigue (symptoms, severity, causes)
- Fatigue is evaluated regarding its effect on the patient's life
- Other symptoms affecting fatigue are contained (anemia, insomnia, pain, etc.)
- Laboratory findings are examined (electrolyte levels, transferrin levels, iron-binding capacity, folic acid level, B12 level, thyroid function tests, etc.)
- The patient and their family are asked about their knowledge of fatigue and relevant practices
- The environment is arranged to reduce the oxygen consumption of the patient
- The patient is provided with support for their daily activities
- The patient is encouraged to rest
- The patient is taught energy-saving approaches
- Fatigue-reducing alternative treatments are recommended (therapeutic touch, yoga, sleep hygiene, stress management, massage, regular exercise, reflexology)
- Assistance should be offered for housekeeping activities such as cleaning, meal preparation and related errands

- The importance of sleep hygiene should be emphasised
- The patient should be encouraged to participate in social activities that interest them

(b) *Loss of Appetite*: This is defined as decreased energy intake when compared with the energy requirement and the reduced desire to eat. *Etiology*: Anorexia can result from chemotherapy, other medication and changes in the ability to taste, as well as physical problems such as mucositis, stomatitis, nausea, vomiting, diarrhea, pain and difficulty swallowing. In addition, psychological factors such as anxiety, depression, fatigue, and insomnia associated with the disease can also contribute to anorexia. *Signs and Symptoms*: Reduced desire to eat, nausea and vomiting, weight loss, fatigue [26, 28, 34].

Nursing Interventions

- The nutritional status of the patient is evaluated
- Factors that cause inadequate fluid and nutrient intake are contained
- A nutritional program is prepared for the patient's disease and prognosis
- Meals are arranged to be small and frequent
- The patient is provided with high-protein and high-calorie foods
- Fatty and spicy foods are avoided to prevent nausea and vomiting
- Colorful and sightly food is preferred
- Antiemetic drugs are used before meals to prevent nausea and vomiting
- Enteral nutrition products are used as per the physician's instructions
- The patient's weight is monitored
- The patient is provided with oral care before and after meals
- The patient and their family are provided with nutrition education

(c) *Nausea and Vomiting*: Nausea is an uncomfortable feeling in the stomach, and vomiting is the expulsion of stomach contents as a result of the strong contraction of stomach muscles, often accompanied by nausea. *Etiology*: In the context of palliative care, nausea and vomiting may occur primarily due to the disease, but also from medical treatments, metastases, metabolic abnormalities, vestibular nerve stimulation, obstructions, increased intracranial pressure and anxiety. *Signs and Symptoms*: Patients with nausea and vomiting may experience gagging, anorexia, dehydration, electrolyte imbalance and malnutrition.

Nursing Interventions

- Nausea and vomiting are evaluated (type, form and severity)
- Other factors that cause nausea and vomiting are evaluated and contained
- The patient's nutrition is regulated (meal size, content, number, frequency and fluid intake)
- The diet of the patient is regulated
- Eating small amounts slowly
- Avoiding fatty, spicy, too hot and too cold foods
- Not consuming liquids while eating
- Arrangement of the environment (odour, image and sound, etc.)
- Ensuring proper oral hygiene
- The patient is taught nausea reducing methods
- The patient is provided with antiemetic medication as requested
- The patient's BMI and weight are monitored (weight loss of >10 kilos over 6 months)
- The patient is ensured to do relaxation and distraction exercises 30-60 minutes before a meal to reduce the stress caused by a meal and to increase the appetite

(d) *Constipation*: A defecation frequency of fewer than three times a week accompanied by a hard and painful stool lasting for more than two months. *Etiology*: The causes of constipation include drug treatments (aluminum- and calcium-containing antacids, anticholinergics, anticonvulsants, anti-emetics, antihypertensives, antispasmodics, barium sulfate-containing drugs, calcium and iron drugs, amine oxiadase inhibitors, opioids, tricyclic antidepressants), chemotherapy agents (vinca alkaloids, platinums, hormonal agents, taxanes), metabolic deficiencies (hypercalcemia, hyperglycemia, hypothyroidism), neurological deficiencies (sacral nerve infiltration, autonomic deficiencies, spinal cord compression and damage), intestinal obstruction (compression due to tumor growth, radiation fibrosis or scar tissue), low physical activity, immobility, poor muscle tone, various cognitive changes, sedation, depression, changes in bowel habits, history of laxative use, diet (insufficient fibre or fluid intake), nausea, fatigue, mucositis and anorexia. *Signs and Symptoms*: Decreased stool frequency, straining to defecate, hard and lumpy stool and difficulty defecating.

Nursing Interventions

- The patient's intestinal functions are evaluated daily
- The diet of the patient is regulated
- The patient is provided with plenty of liquid
- The patient is provided with natural foods such as prunes and prune juice
- The patient is provided with high-fibre foods
- The patient is to regularly take laxatives as ordered
- Rectal suppositories and enemas are avoided in patients with neutropenia or low platelet values
- The patient is encouraged to move as much as possible

(e) *Dyspnea*; This is defined as a subjectively difficult and uncomfortable breathing sensation. *Etiology*: The possible causes of dyspnea include anemia, anxiety, fears or claustrophobia, ascites, cerebral tumors, congenital heart disease, cystic fibrosis, hepatic or kidney failure, infection, metabolic and mechanical problems, pain, pleural effusion, left ventricular failure or pneumothorax, increased intracranial pressure and dysfunction of the respiratory muscles. *Signs and Symptoms*: Wheezing, retractions, nasal flaring, fatigue, fever, chills, headaches, the patient expressing increased number and depth of breathing, difficulty getting enough air, feeling short of breath and lack of air.

Nursing Interventions

- Breathing is evaluated (number, speed, rhythm and depth)
- The effect of dyspnea on the patient's life is evaluated
- Other symptoms affecting dyspnea are contained (fatigue, insomnia, etc.)
- The underlying causes of dyspnea are determined
- The patient is settled in a Fowler's or Semi-Fowler's position
- The patient is aided in moving while in bed and to change positions
- The patient is encouraged to do breathing and coughing exercises
- The patient is provided with adequate hydration
- Pulmonary aspiration, if necessary
- The patient is provided with oral care
- The patient is to avoid strenuous activities and exercises
- The patient is provided with support for their daily activities
- Providing a comfortable, calm and quiet environment and restricting visitors
- Providing oxygen therapy, if required
- Providing the adequate medication (mucolytics, bronchodilators, antibiotics, etc.)

(f) *Delirium*: Delirium is a disturbed state of mind that presents with impaired cognitive functions (primarily memory and perception), decreased or fluctuating unconsciousness, impaired attention and orientation, disorientedness, affective disorders, behavioural changes such as apathy and agitation and disturbances in the sleep-wake cycle. *Etiology*: Factors that can lead to delirium include infection, drugs and toxins, metabolic disorders, electrolyte disorders, kidney or liver failure, trauma, anemia, carbon monoxide poisoning, hypotension, heart failure, B12 or folic acid deficiency, hypertensive encephalopathy, circulatory shock and vasculitis. *Signs and Symptoms*: There are three clinical subtypes of delirium: hyperactive delirium, hypoactive delirium and mixed delirium. The clinical findings of delirium vary according to the type of delirium and the patient's age and developmental stage. "Hyperactive delirium" findings include excessive movement, talkativeness, psychomotor agitation, irritability, aimless navigation and disturbing behaviour. "Hypoactive delirium" findings include psychomotor slowing, sparse or slow speech, apathy, lethargy and sleepiness. In mixed delirium, it is possible to determine findings from both subtypes.

Nursing Interventions

- The patient is evaluated for delirium symptoms
- The patient is provided with symptomatic treatment
- Fluid and electrolyte balances are regulated
- The patient's nutritional status is evaluated
- The patient is treated in a quiet, tranquil and well-lit room at home
- It is recommended to place a familiar item next to the patient for grounding, such as a clock, a calendar or a photo

Psychosocial Symptoms

(a) *Anxiety*: Anxiety is intense internal distress, restlessness and a state of nervousness or unease that cannot be resolved. *Etiology*: The cause behind the development of anxiety may vary depending on the developmental stage of the patient and the severity of the disease. The potential causes include being subject to continuous procedures and hospitalisation, encountering a life-threatening disease, uncertainties concerning the disease and treatment, difficulties in keeping up with the changing social life and roles, inadequate pain and nausea control, difficulties adapting to the changing body image as a result of treatments, failed treatment response and learning about metastases. *Signs and Symptoms*: Restlessness, aggressive behaviours and bodily symptoms such as chest tightness, heart palpitations, difficulty breathing, shortness of breath, dry mouth, gastrointestinal complaints, tension in the whole body and insomnia.

Nursing Interventions

- Anxiety level is evaluated
- Causes of anxiety are determined
- The patient is encouraged to share their causes of anxiety
- The patient and their family are encouraged to express their thoughts and concerns about the disease and the treatment process
- The patient and their family are helped to bring out their strong sides
- The patient and their family are assessed in how much they know and how much they want to know about diagnosis, treatment, complications and prognosis
- The nurse creates an effective and safe communication space
- The nurse establishes a patient-nurse relationship based on trust
- Patients are encouraged to participate in the treatment and care process, while allowing visits from relatives and friends, if possible

(b) *Fear*: Fear is a sudden, emotional, undesirable behaviour and emotional response that occurs in the face of real or unreal danger. *Etiology*: Fear can root from the disease, hospitalisation, invasive procedures (injections, stitches), lack of information, uncertain prognosis, unfamiliar medical equipment, taking medication, bodily injuries and physical symptoms (pain, vomiting, etc.). *Signs and Symptoms*: Anxiety, sleep problems, crying, inability to be alone.

Nursing Interventions

- The patient's fears are determined
- The patient is encouraged to express their feelings by using age-appropriate communication methods
- The patient's routine is maintained
- The patient is allowed and encouraged to resume their routine activities
- The environment is adequately arranged
- The patient is encouraged to express their hospital-related fears
- The patient is taught relaxation techniques (slow rhythmic breathing, relaxation exercises, distraction methods, etc.)

(c) *Insomnia*: Difficulties in the onset, continuation, duration or quality of sleep despite suitable environments and conditions. *Etiology*: The causes of insomnia include many factors related to the patient, disease, treatment and environment, including the type, anatomical location and severity of the disease, chemotherapy, radiotherapy, hormonal therapy, nausea and vomiting, diarrhea, constipation, sweating, pain, dyspnea, fatigue, environmental factors such as noise and light and psychosocial causes such as anxiety, stress, and depression. *Signs and Symptoms*: Having difficulty falling asleep, having nightmares, impaired sleep quality and patterns, difficulty waking up, fatigue despite having slept, daytime sleepiness, fatigue due to changes in sleep, agitation.

Nursing Interventions

- The patient's sleep patterns are evaluated
- The nurse investigates the patient's normal sleep habits
- Causes of insomnia are determined, the effect of the treatment process on sleep is explained to the patient
- Other symptoms affecting insomnia are contained
- The patient is informed about effective interventions to prevent insomnia
- Drinking warm milk before bedtime
- Massaging
- Music
- Progressive muscle relaxation exercises
- A warm shower before bed
- Pharmacological treatment as prescribed by a physician, if necessary
- Arranging the environment
- Reducing loud noises, creating a quiet environment
- Reducing alarm sounds
- Adjusting the lights as desired by the patient
- Medical processes are in a way that will minimise the number of times that the patient needs to be woken during sleep (e.g. combining nighttime medications with measuring vital signs)
- The patient is helped to comply with their bedtime routines (e.g. watching TV for 10–15 minutes before sleep if the patient finds it relaxing)
- Methods of relaxation are recommended such as massage, yoga, contemplation, progressive muscle relaxation, breathing techniques and aromatherapy

Support for Family Members

The responsibilities of family members have recently become more significant and complex in the context of home care. Palliative care at home has evolved from a simple to a more complex modality of care that often requires advanced skills such as opioid treatment and symptom management. The exact nature of the responsibilities of family members in providing palliative care at home depends on the patient's physical and psychosocial needs and the dynamics of the relationship between the carer and the patient. The family member that is responsible for providing palliative care at home may also have other responsibilities such as caring for other family members.

The nurse should be in continuous communication with family members. They must evaluate the family members' roles and responsibilities in palliative care and their relationship with the patient. They are responsible for providing information that is pertinent to the care of the patient. Family members can also experience physical and psychosocial problems. Thus, it is essential to allow them to express their own problems as well. The nurse should plan the necessary interventions after determining the problems experienced by the family members. The nurse should evaluate the physical and psychological burden on the family and provide the necessary support. It is also the nurse's responsibility to identify the causes of stress in the family and provide coping methods. The nurse should provide family members with the necessary training and counseling services regarding patient care.

References

1. Worldwide palliative care alliance: global atlas of palliative care at the end of life. 2014. http://www.who.int/nmh/Global_Atlas_of_Palliative_Care.pdf. Accessed 29 Feb 2020.
2. Etkind SN, Bone AE, Gomes B, Lovell N, Evans CJ, Higginson IJ, et al. How many people will need palliative care in 2040? Past trends, future projections and implications for services. BMC Med. 2017;15(1):102.
3. Chiang JK, Kao YH. Impact of home hospice care on patients with advanced lung cancer: a longitudinal population-based study in Taiwan. J Palliat Med. 2016;19(4):380–6.
4. Stjernswärd J. Palliative care: the public health strategy. J Public Health Policy. 2007;28(1):42–55.
5. Murray SA, Firth A, Schneider N, Van den Eynden B, Gomez-Batiste X, Brogaard T, Villanueva T, Abela J, Eychmuller S, Mitchell G, Downing J. Promoting palliative care in the community: production of the primary palliative care toolkit by the European Association of Palliative Care Taskforce in primary palliative care. Palliat Med. 2015;29(2):101–11.
6. Mitchell G. Rapidly increasing end-of-life care needs: a timely warning. BMC Med. 2017;15(1):126.
7. Burge F, Lawson B, Johnston G, Asada Y, McIntyre PF, Flowerdew G. Preferred and actual location of death: what factors enable a preferred home death? J Palliat Med. 2015;18(12):1054–9.
8. Peters L, Sellick K. Quality of life of cancer patients receiving inpatient and home-based palliative care. J Adv Nurs. 2006;53(5):524–33.
9. Lai XB, Chen LQ, Chen SH, Xia HO. An examination of home-based end-of-life care for cancer patients: a qualitative study. BMC Palliat Care. 2019;18(1):1–1.
10. Thomas K. Out-of-hours palliative care in the community. Continuing care for the dying at home. London: Macmillan Cancer Relief; 2001.
11. De Lima L, Pastrana T. Opportunities for palliative care in public health. Annu Rev Public Health. 2016;37:357–74.
12. European Association of Palliative Care (EAPC) task force in primary palliative care.
13. Wiencek C, Coyne P. Palliative delivery models. Seminars in Oncology Nursing. 2014;30(4):227–33.
14. Appelin G, Brobäck G, Berterö C. A comprehensive picture of palliative care at home from the people involved. Eur J Oncol Nurs. 2005;9(4): 315–24.
15. Dunne K, Sullivan K, Kernohan G. Palliative care for patients with cancer: district nurses' experiences. J Adv Nurs. 2005;50(4):372–80.
16. King N, Melvin J, Ashby J, Firth J. Community palliative care: role perception. Br J Community Nurs. 2010;15(2):91–8.
17. Austin L, Luker K, Caress A, Hallett C. Palliative care: community nurses' perceptions of quality. BMJ Quality & Safety. 2000;9(3):151–8.
18. Luker KA, Wilson K, Pateman B, Beaver K. The role of district nursing: perspectives of cancer patients and their carers before and after hospital discharge. Eur J Cancer Care. 2003;12(4):308–16.
19. Fitzgerald GP, Naugle MA, Wolf JP. The palliative advanced practice registered nurse in the home setting. Adv Pract Palliat Nurs. 2016;25:180.
20. Sekse RJ, Hunskår I, Ellingsen S. The nurse's role in palliative care: a qualitative meta-synthesis. J Clin Nurs. 2018;27(1–2):e21–38.
21. Maybin J, Charles A, Honeyman M. Understanding quality in district nursing services. London: Kings Fund; 2016.
22. McKenzie H, Boughton M, Hayes L, Forsyth S, Davies M, Underwood E, McVey P. A sense of security for cancer patients at home: the role of community nurses. Health Soc Care Community. 2007;15(4):352–9.
23. Walshe C, Luker KA. District nurses' role in palliative care provision: a realist review. Int J Nurs Stud. 2010;47(9):1167–83.
24. Canadian Nurses Association. Joint position statement: the palliative approach to care and the role of the nurse. Available from: www. cna-aiic. ca/~/media/cna/page-content/pdf-en/the-palliativeapproach-to-care-and-the-role-of-the-nurse_e. pdf. 2015.
25. Kuebler KK, Lynn J, Von Rohen J. Perspectives in palliative care. Seminars in Oncology Nursing. 2005;21(1):2–10.
26. Ferrell BR, Coyle N, Paice J, editors. Oxford textbook of palliative nursing. New York: Oxford University Press; 2015.
27. Dahlin C, Coyne P, Ferrell BR, editors. Advanced practice palliative nursing. New York: Oxford University Press; 2016.
28. Bookbinder M, McHugh ME. Symptom management in palliative care and end of life care. Nurs Clin. 2010;45(3):271–327.
29. Palliative Caring at Home. Information for those caring for a person with advanced and terminal illness. Western Australia Edition – January 2012 www.palliativecarewa.asn.au. Accessed 6 Mar 2017.
30. Carter L. Delivering palliative care in the community: community nurses' experiences and perceptions of their role. Unpublished masters thesis. University of Nottingham; 2008.
31. End of Life Nursing Education Consortium (ELNEC) APRN curriculum. www.aacn.nche.edu/elnec. Erişim Tarihi 9 February 2018.
32. Milone-Nuzzo P, Ercolano E, McCorkle R. Home care and hospice care. In: Oxford textbook of palliative nursing. New York: Oxford University Press; 2015.
33. NCCN clinical practice guidelines in oncology 2008. http://www.nccn.org/professionals/physician_gls/PDF/occult.pdf.
34. North of England Cancer Network (NECN) 2012. Palliative and end of life care guidelines for cancer and non-cancer patients. https://southtees.nhs.uk/content/uploads/NECN-palliative-care-guidelines.pdf.

Caring for the Cancer Patient in the Community: In Mind, Body and Spirit

Gonca Tuncel-Oguz

Introduction

Cancer is the second leading cause of death worldwide, accounting to an estimated 9.6 million deaths in 2018. Although it is one of the major health challenges in many countries, more than 70% of all cancer deaths occur in low- and middle-income populations, where resources available for prevention, diagnosis and treatment of cancer are limited or nonexistent [1]. In 2030, 12 million people are expected to lose their lives due to cancer [2]. Advances in cancer screening and detection techniques, remarkable improvements in antineoplastic and supportive care treatments result in more than 65% of patients diagnosed with cancer living five years, and often more, beyond their diagnosis [3]. Along with the rising global cancer rates and progress in survival, many cancer survivors have to cope with the accumulating symptom burden, deterioration of function and other concerns inherent to slowly progressive, life-limiting disease [4].

Palliative care is an approach to patient/family/caregiver-centred health care that focuses on optimal management of distressing symptoms while incorporating psychosocial and spiritual care according to their needs, values, beliefs and cultures. The goal of palliative care is to anticipate, prevent and reduce suffering and to support the best possible quality of life for the patient/family/caregiver, regardless of the stage of the disease or the need for other therapies [5]. For cancer patients, combined standard oncology care and palliative care should be considered early in the course of illness for any patient with metastatic cancer and/or high symptom burden [6]. It should be delivered concurrently with disease-directed, life-prolonging therapies and should facilitate patient autonomy, access to information and choice.

In the last years, there has been a strong tendency for new community-based palliative care models to meet the needs of the growing population of patients living with cancer who are well enough to be in home-like settings, yet experience the very real burden of advanced and progressive illness [4]. The World Health Organization (WHO) recommends that all countries adopt a national palliative care policy as a human right, providing different resources and settings, including home-based care [7]. Besides, studies show that most of the patients with advanced cancer want to be cared for or spend their last days at home [8, 9]. A good palliative care program encompassing interventions at all levels of care, with a particular focus on primary health-care services and home-based care, could eventually result in a reduction in hospitalisation, use of health-care resources and costs while

G. Tuncel-Oguz (✉)
Palliative Care Clinic, Department of Anesthesiology, Dr. A.Y. Ankara Oncology Education & Research Hospital, University of Health Sciences, Ankara, Turkey

M. Silbermann (ed.), *Palliative Care for Chronic Cancer Patients in the Community*, https://doi.org/10.1007/978-3-030-54526-0_37

improving the symptom burden and satisfaction of the patient and caregivers [10, 11]. Given the projected increases in the number of cancer survivors and intensified focus of health-care professionals on community-based palliative care, the palliative care needs of cancer patients living in the community should be comprehensively addressed.

Palliative Care Needs of Patients with Advanced Cancer Living in the Community

Cancer patients often experience multiple symptoms simultaneously, which may be difficult to manage from the time of diagnosis and throughout the treatment or terminal phase of the illness [12]. The individuals living and receiving care in the community have to confront the psychological, social, emotional and spiritual issues related to advanced cancer, as well as burdensome cancer-related symptoms, in a context other than an inpatient cancer centre [4]. For advanced illness, continuity of care throughout the disease trajectory and across different settings in the health-care system is mandatory. Therefore, an expanded community and home-based palliative care with input from specialist physicians enabling the management of complex pain and other symptoms at home can be beneficial.

In a recent study, it has been shown that patients referred to community-based palliative care experience multiple and often severe symptoms that have been insufficiently addressed [4]. Nearly all (95%) patients with cancer had at least one reported symptom, and two-thirds (67%) reported three or more symptoms. Fatigue, anorexia and pain were the first three symptoms and the others followed. A review of interventions prescribed before referral to palliative care demonstrated that a substantial proportion of patients were not receiving treatments aimed at addressing their symptom concerns. For example, most of the patients reporting moderate/severe constipation and depression were not being treated, although the treatments are available and familiar. It was found that there is a clear need for a better discussion of advance care planning and goals. Worries about the future, flagging hope and social needs have been identified as the most burdensome issues facing patients with cancer [13]. Riolfi et al. have conducted a study to assess the effectiveness of appropriate palliative home care services in reducing hospital admissions, and to identify factors predicting the likelihood of patients treated at home being hospitalised [11]. Irrespective of age, gender and type of tumor, patients taken into care by the palliative home care team were more likely to die at home, have fewer hospitalisations and spent fewer days in hospital in the last two months of their lives. The patients with hematological cancers and hepatocellular carcinoma were more likely to be hospitalised and certain symptoms, such as dyspnea and delirium, were determined as predictives of hospitalisation.

Providing palliative care at home preserves the dignity of terminally-ill patients and allows them to spend their last days with loved ones at their homes. A growing body of evidence from both population and patient surveys shows that the majority of cancer patients would prefer to die in their own home [14]. Concerning the efficiency of palliative care services, it was demonstrated that changing the focus of care-providing policy from the hospital to the home reduces health-care costs by reducing hospital admissions and the length of hospital stays [15]. Alonso-Babarro et al. found that, when an appropriate palliative home care team was available, there were fewer deaths in hospital and a drop in the overall hospitalisation rates for patients in the last two months of their lives [16]. Gomes and Higginson reviewed numerous studies from around the world, analysing the factors affecting the place where terminally ill cancer patients die [17]. They found consistent evidence of the influence of several factors on the place of death, six of which were strongly associated with death at home. Those were determined as patients' functional status, their preferences, the availability of home care and its intensity, living with relatives and extended family support. Other studies have found that around 75% of respondents desire to experience their last phase of life at home [14].

However, this is linked to the presence of a strong social and family network; the percentage of younger, single or widowed patients preferring to die at home seems to be well below that percentage. Although patients with advanced illness who are near the end-of-life report wanting to be cared for and die at home, most of them also contradictorily referred to the emergency departments (EDs) in the last weeks or days of life [18]. People with cancer frequently present with exacerbation of existing problems and new symptoms, complications of treatments or difficulties with the care and support systems. The distress of family members while managing the end-of-life symptoms may also contribute to the increase in admissions [18, 19]. In a French study, the most frequent reasons for ED admissions were generalised weakness, social isolation and end-of-life care for home-hospitalised palliative care patients. They also report in their study that half of the transfers to EDs were potentially avoidable for terminally-ill patients in home care [20]. Mercadante et al. showed that, in a population of patients with advanced cancer, most of the problems could be solved just by phone explanations or by a simple medical visit at home [21]. The results of the studies emphasised the fact that many dying people are admitted to hospital for terminal care because of inadequate support in the community.

The diagnosis of a patient with cancer involves both the patient and his/her family members in processes of care and in making medical decisions. Caregivers often play a critical role in providing care to patients in the home-hospice setting and are often responsible for performing health-care activities such as administering medications when patients are unable to. They usually undertake the complex process of managing cancer pain, which is reported to be one of the most frequent and distressing symptoms, reaching a rate of 90% at the terminal phase of the disease [22, 23]. Pain management is usually a challenging aspect of the caregivers' role as it is an ongoing issue for family caregivers due to the variability in severity and types of pain [23]. Poorly managed pain results in frustration not only for patients but also for family caregivers. Caring for a patient in advanced stages of disease poses severe challenges to the caregivers' personal life, including the spiritual aspects. Spirituality is an essential part of health care that is defined in the context of religion and culture and affects the individual's perception of illness and health [24]. Studies have shown that high levels of spirituality are associated with high levels of development and transcendence and a good understanding of the meaning and purpose of life; therefore, it plays a significant role in improving the overall satisfaction and the quality of life in both patients with cancer and their caregivers [25]. Patients with advanced cancer and family caregivers have a wide range of unmet needs; patients report psychological and physical unmet needs while caregivers identify emotional management as being the most difficult [26]. The concepts of presence, in the sense of availability and home visits, and competence, in the sense of effective symptom control and skillful communication, have been identified as crucial for both patients and family caregivers to feel a sense of security [27]. Psychosocial care must be provided, including attention to the psychological, emotional, social and financial well-being of both the patients and the family members while, at the same time, respecting their autonomy.

Current Status of Community Palliative Care in Turkey and Barriers to Implementation

In Turkey, cancer was reported to be the leading cause of death (20%) after cardiovascular diseases. According to the most recent results of the Turkish Ministry of Health, cancer incidence was 210.2 per 100,000 people, which means that each year approximately 163,500 patients had a new diagnosis of cancer or, in other words, 450 patients in each day [28]. The high rate of cancer as a chronic illness necessitates the integration of palliative care into comprehensive oncology care early in the disease trajectory for there to be an improvement in the quality of life for both patients and caregivers.

The awareness of palliative care began in the 1990s and has disseminated very slowly through the years in Turkey. It gained acceleration with the Health Transformation Program (HTP) in 2003, which emphasised the protection of the individual's as well as the communities' health. "Good quality and sustainable health service accessible to everyone" was its central theme [29]. In 2009, the Turkish Ministry of Health launched a five-year National Cancer Control Program which included: Central Registry, Prevention, Screening and Early Diagnosis, Treatment and Palliative Care. Among these, palliative care was the weakest part of current cancer control activities in Turkey. The Pallia-Turk project followed in 2010, which was focused on two main topics: (a) opioid availability and (b) implementation of a community-based palliative care model [30]. Guidelines entitled 'Directives for Palliative Care Services Implementation Procedures and Principles' were published by the Ministry of Health in October 2014 and revised in July 2015 [31]. This directive highlighted the importance of teamwork, psychological, social and spiritual support and integrated provision of palliative care. Palliative care services were to be provided in palliative care centres at inpatient care facilities and by family physicians and home care teams outside the hospitals. According to the directives, palliative care services could be offered to people living in nursing homes by implementing a palliative care protocol with the inpatient care facilities and by obtaining approval from the Directorate. The palliative care centres were also made responsible for regulating the necessary coordination with family physicians and home care teams to ensure the continuity of care after discharge. The most recent results from the Turkish Ministry of Health show that the country has reached 5481 palliative care beds in 410 health-care facilities throughout 81 cities. All of the beds are localised in inpatient care units and, unfortunately, there are still no designs for hospices, community hospice teams, home palliative care teams or 'hospital at home' organisations in Turkey.

Global cancer rates have been increasing with an associated rise in the number of cancer survivors living in the community with symptoms and disabilities as a result of their disease and/or treatment. Palliative care becomes the primary focus of care when disease-directed, life-prolonging therapies are no longer effective, appropriate or desired [5]. Most of the patients prefer to be cared for in their own homes until the time of death. Home-based care aims to provide symptom control and quality of life while integrating the family members into the process. In Turkey, the directive 'Regulation on the provision of home care services' was first announced in 2005. Home care teams provide health care and follow-up on the patients in line with their medical needs, including rehabilitation, physiotherapy and psychological treatment in their own environment where they live with their families. The patients or families may apply through a central phone number and an appointment is made with the home care team serving that region. After the interview, the necessary interventions and follow-up of care starts. The teams are available only during working hours and cannot help with emergency situations. The existing home care teams are not specialised in palliative care but are expected to provide such care. Although cancer patients can also apply for home care services, statistics show that only a small percentage of advanced cancer patients received home care. Most of the served population were patients with neurologic or cardiovascular diseases [32]. The integration of palliative care and home care services is well-defined in the directives of the Health Ministry, but regional networks, the transition of care and effective coordination are not standardised in the country. Some of the palliative centres try to visit their patients regularly after they are discharged from the inpatient unit. The other palliative care teams work as consultative clinics and visit patients at home after having received consultation from home care teams, especially in cases of symptom control, specific pain or transitioning to inpatient palliative care centres. Nevertheless, many cancer patients and their families feel desperate in the community, waiting for physical, psychosocial and spiritual support.

Nurses play an essential role in various settings for the care of cancer patients, both in the community and in hospitals. They are the major components of the multidisciplinary palliative care teams and their presence is mandatory in home care services. In a study examining the roles, satisfaction and adequacy of home health-care nurses on the provison of palliative home care, the nurses specified significant deficiencies regarding home care, such as personnel shortages, lack of funding and policies, poor access to end-of-life or hospice services and decreased community awareness of what services are available. Respondents identified lack of time, funding and concerns about staff relief coverages as the primary obstacles to palliative care education [33]. Several similar problems also hinder good-quality home palliative care in Turkey, educational barriers being the most important one.

Palliative care in the community is an emerging concept in Turkey, as well as palliative care itself. Most health-care providers find themselves unable to appropriately recognise and palliate the symptoms related to cancer or its treatment, especially pain. Treating an advanced cancer patient with multiple disabling symptoms and suffering in pain is very frustrating for the home care teams. Opiophobia, which is still very common among the health-care providers, patients and families, contributes to the undertreatment of cancer pain. Turkey is one of the countries with statistical evidence of inadequate morphine consumption per capita. In 2010, the adequacy of opioid analgesic consumption was only 7% – based on a per capita consumption of 14.31 mg morphine equivalents [34]. Moreover, opiophobia, lack of education and a burdensome regulatory system for prescribing opioids prevent many physicians in the community from prescribing opioids, even when palliative care teams or oncologists have previously prescribed them. Patients surviving at home must visit inpatient palliative care centres several times in order to get their prescriptions for opioid drugs. Philosophy and principles of palliative care are not yet included in curricula for medical and nursing faculties in Turkey. After the palliative care directives by the Health Ministry, several workshops, symposiums and conferences were organised to improve the quality of palliative care skills, and were attended by health-care professionals from different disciplines, including family physicians and home care teams. A certification program of palliative care nursing was approved and started country-wide, aimed to cover all nurses working in palliative care units. A workshop about ‘Pain Management in Palliative Care’ was organised with the participation of many experts and a national guideline was published in 2016. Despite the evidence of its benefits and ongoing training programs, palliative care is often underutilised or initiated late in the course of cancer treatment, as it is in many countries. There is a growing number of people diagnosed with cancer as a chronic illness in the community. Common triggers for referral to community-based palliative care, such as diagnosis of metastatic disease, poor expected prognosis or decline in performance status may transform early involvement palliative care into comprehensive care. One important issue that home care teams cited about advanced cancer patients is that most of them were not satisfactorily informed about the incurable nature of their disease. Although their primary oncologist gave information to the patient and family, there is a tendency to withhold the diagnosis of cancer from the patient for fear that disclosing the prognosis might be damaging. The discussion surrounding death and dying can be emotionally challenging, and avoiding entire discussions regarding goals of care and end-of-life presents obstacles for the home-based palliative care team. Sometimes the expectations of patients/families vs. the services provided by home care teams cannot coincide.

Psychosocial care involves attention to the psychological, emotional, social and financial well-being of patients and family members. Members of palliative home care teams usually need to assess and treat psychological symptoms such as anxiety, depression and delirium just as carefully as physical symptoms. Community support is often offered to bereaved family members and encourages spirituality while facing the loss associated with dying and bereavement. Under the present circumstances in Turkey, it is not easy for the home care teams to provide a holistic approach and to address the psychological and spiritual needs of the patients and families. The ideal multidisciplinary team, which would include nurses, doctors, psychologists/counselors, social workers and trained volunteers or community health workers, is often incomplete in-home care teams; therefore, the physicians and, primarily, the nurses carry the responsibility. They feel under-trained for such skills and do not have enough time or staff available. They may avoid administering simple intravenous infusions, or other invasive procedures that can be performed at home, due to uncertainty about ethical or legal regulations.

Support for family caregivers is a core aspect of palliative care provision. Besides physical and psychological morbidity, they are often financially disadvantaged and frequently become socially isolated. In fact, family caregivers make a significant and under-recognised economic contribution to health care [35]. The Turkish government, along with the collaboration of various ministries, executes several programs to solve reimbursement and financial constraints. The patients are supported in terms of medical devices and materials used at home, such as oxygen concentrators, diapers, suctions, etc. A care allowance is paid to the caregivers when verification of the patients' disability and/or chronic life-limiting disease is confirmed by an expert physician. In order to be eligible for this payment, the ratio of disability must be over 50% and the family must have a low monthly income. Unfortunately, most family members do not learn of this opportunity until it is too late in the disease trajectory, when there is not enough time to complete the legal procedures necessary in order to benefit before the patient's death. This issue also reflects on the role of social workers who are the essential components of the multidisciplinary team of comprehensive cancer care.

Future Perspectives

The WHO defines home care as the provision of health services by formal and informal caregivers in the home in order to promote, restore and maintain a person's maximum level of comfort, function, and health, including care towards a dignified death. Understanding the palliative care needs of community-based patients in the advanced stages of cancer represents a first step toward the development of delivery models that integrate care across settings, and that coordinate community oncologists and palliative care providers to meet identified needs of this population. There is a lack of information regarding home-based palliative care, and more studies in this area (descriptive/observational, etc.) are needed.

National health systems are responsible for including palliative care in the continuum of care for people with chronic life-limiting health problems and developing national policies and plans following the principles of universal health coverage [36]. The service delivery model must take into account the country's social and health system context. In Turkey, setting up a palliative home care service by integrating palliative home care into existing home care services will be beneficial. Although the country has a social policy supporting the patients and families in many aspects of health-care coverage, reimbursement and other financial procedures must be improved and regulations must be facilitated. Beyond the provision of care, the networks should determine consensually defined goals and quality standards. The use of uniform outcome measurements, especially patient-reported outcomes, and incorporation into routine clinical practice are promoted to evaluate the services given in different settings. Up-to-date training and research activities based on scientific evidence should be organised and supervised, covering all health-care professionals. Previously mentioned barriers such as lack of sufficient time, financial problems and the shortage of available substitute human resources while attending the training courses should also be considered.

Cancer patients may require support from different levels of palliative care services during the course of their illness. Home care is one of the desirable palliative care models empowering the patient and family in providing the necessary care [37]. It is crucial to develop uniform criteria for admission and discharge and a functional referral pathway at all levels of care.

Conclusion

As the advances in new detection and treatment methods of cancer proceed, the number of advanced cancer patients living with multiple unaddressed symptoms in the community increase. Early palliative care interventions in comprehensive cancer care of patients have been shown to provide better symptom control, reduce hospital re-admissions and costs and facilitate transitions through different settings.

The World Health Assembly, the decision-making body of WHO, has resolved that palliative care is an ethical responsibility of health systems and integration of palliative care into public health-care systems is essential for the achievement of the sustainable development goal on universal health coverage. The demand for the delivery of multi-professional palliative care at home is increasing with examples of improvement in the physical, psychosocial and spiritual burden of cancer survivors and caregivers. However, many high-quality studies regarding the outcomes of home palliative care and the effectiveness of organisations are needed for the best evidence.

References

1. Cancer control, knowledge into action, WHO guide for effective programmes. Palliat Care. 2007.
2. Sutcliffe SB. Cancer Control: life and death in an unequal world. Curr Oncol. 2012;19(1):12–5.
3. Australian Institute of Health, Welfare. Cancer survival and prevalence in Australia: period estimates from 1982 to 2010. Asia Pac J Clin Oncol. 2013;9:29–39.
4. Kamal AH, Bull J, Kavalieratos D, Taylor DH Jr, Downey W, Abernethy AP. Palliative care needs of patients with cancer living in the community. Oncol Pract. 2011;7(6):382–8.
5. National Comprehensive Cancer Network Guidelines, Version 1. Palliat Care. 2019.
6. Smith TJ, Temin S, Alesi ER, Abernethy AP, Balboni TA, Basch EM, et al. American Society of Clinical Oncology provisional clinical opinion: the integration of palliative care into standard oncology care. J Clin Oncol. 2012;30:880–7.
7. Gwyther L, Brennan F, Harding R. Advancing palliative care as a human right. J Pain Symptom Manag. 2009;38(5):767–74.
8. Beccaro M, Costantini M, Giorgi Rossi P, ISDOC Study Group, et al. Actual and preferred place of death of cancer patients. Results from the Italian survey of the dying of cancer (ISDOC). J Epidemiol Community Health. 2006;60(5):412–6.
9. Gomes B, Higginson IJ, Calanzani N, et al. Preferences for place of death if faced with advanced cancer: a population survey in England, Flanders, Germany, Italy, the Netherlands, Portugal and Spain. Ann Oncol. 2012;23(8):2006–15.
10. Brumley R, Enguidanos S, Jamison P, et al. Increased satisfaction with care and lower costs: results of a randomized trial of in-home palliative care. J Am Geriatr Soc. 2007;55:993.
11. Riolfi M, Buja A, Zanardo C, Marangon CF, Manno P, Baldo V. Effectiveness of palliative home-care services in reducing hospital admissions and determinants of hospitalization for terminally ill patients followed up by a palliative home-care team: a retrospective cohort study. Palliat Med. 2014;28: 403–11.
12. Dodd MJ, Miaskowski C, Paul SM. Symptom clusters and their effect on the functional status of patients with cancer. Oncol Nurs Forum. 2001;28:465–70.
13. Baile WF, Palmer JL, Bruera E, et al. Assessment of palliative care cancer patients' most important concerns. Support Care Cancer. 2011;19:475–81.
14. Radbruch L. Payne S and the Board of Directors of the EAPC. White paper on standards and norms for hospice and palliative care in Europe: part 2 recommendations from the European association for palliative care. Eur J Palliative Care. 2010;17(1):22–33.
15. Lukas L, Foltz C, Paxton H. Hospital outcomes for a home-based palliative medicine consulting service. J Palliat Med. 2013;16:179–84.
16. Alonso-Babarro A, Astray-Mochales J, Dominguez-Berjon F, et al. The association between in-patient death, utilization of hospital resources and availability of palliative home care for cancer patients. Palliat Med. 2013;27(1):68–75.
17. Gomes B, Higginson IJ. Factors influencing death at home in terminally ill patients with cancer: a systematic review. BMJ. 2006;332(7540):515–21.
18. Barbera L, Taylor C, Dudgeon D. Why do patients with cancer visit the emergency department near the end of life? CMAJ. 2010;182(6):563–8.
19. van der Meer DM, Weiland TJ, Philip J, et al. Presentation patterns and outcomes of patients with cancer accessing care in emergency departments in Victoria, Australia. Support Care Cancer. 2016;24(3):1251–60.
20. Cornillon P, Loiseau S, Aublet-Cuvelier B, Guastella V. Reasons for transferral to emergency departments of terminally ill patients – a French descriptive and retrospective study. BMC Palliat Care. 2016;21(1):87.
21. Mercadante S, Porzio G, Valle A, et al. Home Care Italy Group (HOCAI). Emergencies in patients with advanced cancer followed at home. J Pain Symptom Manag. 2012;44(2):295–300.

22. Lobchuk MM, Vorauer JD. Family caregiver perspective-taking and accuracy in estimating cancer patient experiences. Soc Sci Med. 2003;57:2370–84.
23. Vallerand AH, Collins-Bohler D, Templin T, Hasenau SM. Knowledge of and barriers to pain management in caregivers of cancer patients receiving home care. Cancer Nurs. 2007;30:31–7.
24. Singh DKM, Ajinkya S. Spirituality and religion in modern medicine. Indian J Psychol Med. 2012;34:399.
25. Glajchen M. The emerging role and needs of family caregivers in cancer care. J Support Oncol. 2003;2:145–55.
26. Klarare A, Rasmussen BH, Fossum B, Hansson J, Fürst CJ, Lundh Hagelin C. Actions helping expressed or anticipated needs: Patients with advanced cancer and their family caregivers' experiences of specialist palliative home care teams. Eur J Cancer Care. 2018;27(6):e12948.
27. Sarmento VP, Gysels M, Higginson IJ, Gomes B. Home palliative care works: but how? A meta-ethnography of the experiences of patients and family caregivers. BMJ Support Palliat Care. 2017;7:1–14.
28. Republic of Turkey Ministry of Health, Turkey cancer statistics. 2014.
29. Turkey Health Transformation Program Assessment Report (2003–2011). (2012). Republic of Turkey Ministry of Health, Ankara.
30. Ozgul N, Koç O, Gultekin M, et al. Opioids for cancer pain: availability, accessibility and regulatory barriers in Turkey and Pallia-Turk project. J Pediatr Hematol Oncol. 2011;33(Suppl 1):S29–32.
31. Directives for Palliative Care Services Implementation Procedures and Principles. (2018). http:/dosyamerkez.saglik.gov.tr/Eklenti/2817.palyatif.bakim.hizmetleri.yonergesi pdf.pdf.
32. Aslan Ş, Uyar S, Güzel Ş. Home health care services practice in Turkey. J Soc Res Manag. 2018;1:45–56.
33. Brant JM, Fink RM, Thompson C, et al. Global survey of the roles, satisfaction, and barriers of home health care nurses on the provision of palliative care. J Palliat Med. 2019;22(8):945–60.
34. Duthey B, Scholten W. Adequacy of opioid analgesic consumption at country, global, and regional levels in 2010,its relationship with development level, and changes compared with 2006. J Pain Symptom Manag. 2014;47:283–97.
35. Hudson P, Payne S. Family caregivers and palliative care: current status and agenda for the future. J Palliat Med. 2011;14(7):864–9.
36. Planning and implementing palliative care services: a guide for programme managers. World Health Organization; 2016.
37. Farahani AS, Rassouli M, Mojen LK, et al. The feasibility of home palliative care for cancer patients: the perspective of Iranian nurses. Int J Cancer Manag. 2018;11(8):e80114.

Part XXVI

Middle East: Yemen

Prevalence and Management of Cancer Pain in Developing Countries

Gamal Abdul Hamid

Introduction

A developing country, additionally referred to as the least-developed country or an underdeveloped country with low income, is a nation with a retrogressive mechanical base and a low human advancement record contrasted with different nations [1]. This categorization does not really reflect the advancement status of the global regions such as: South Asia and Sub-Saharan Africa, North Africa and the Middle East, Europe and Central Asia, the Caribbean and Latin America, and East Asia and the Pacific [2]. In 2015, the worldwide recorded cancer cases were 17.5 million, and death due to cancer diseases reached approximately 8.7 million cases [3, 4]. Cancer pain ranges from moderate to severe and is considered to be one of most common diseases in low- and middle-income countries. Most of the patients reach the hospital in late advanced stages and when treatment options are limited.

The World Health Organization (WHO) showed that cancer occurs mainly in developing countries, primarily in Africa, Asia, and South and Central America [3]. Throughout the years, the burden of cancer has moved to low-income countries that, as of now, represent about 57% of cases and 65% of cancer deaths worldwide. In developing countries with low income, stomach and liver cancer among males and cervix cancer among females are the main causes of cancer mortality [4]. Poor survival rates due to late-stage diagnosis and the absence of access to convenient treatment were common in patients registered in developing countries [5].

The prevalence of cancer in developing countries has markedly increased with a parallel increase of cancer globally [6]. More than 85% of countries throughout the world have low incomes and suffer from the burden of global cancer [7]. Africa, Asia, and Latin America make up more than 50% of all cancer patients [8] and statistically indicate a high death rate of more than 50% in Asia alone [8].

Cancer is one of the leading causes of high death rates worldwide [9]. Although cancer is one of the chronic diseases that can be prevented and treated, in 2018, statistics reported the deaths of nearly 9.6 million people, and indicated a high incidence of cancer diseases for more than 18 million new cases, most of which occurred in developing countries [10–12]. Despite the differences in the spread of cancer types, cancer has a negative effect on all societies. While the overall cancer burden in high-income societies is still considered high, low-income societies are also overcoming this issue. Developing countries are experiencing a marked lifestyle change similar to that of developed countries, and this exposes them to high cancer rates, particularly colon and

G. A. Hamid (✉)
Clinical Laboratory and Hematology Faculty of Medicine, University of Aden, Aden, Yemen

M. Silbermann (ed.), *Palliative Care for Chronic Cancer Patients in the Community*,
https://doi.org/10.1007/978-3-030-54526-0_38

prostate cancer in men and breast and uterine cancer in women [12]. The high incidence of cancer in developing countries is a greater burden for chronic, non-communicable diseases than for infectious diseases. The great similarity of high mortality rates in chronic diseases in the past two decades, particularly cancer, has exceeded infectious disease mortality rates on all continents, except Africa [13].

Despite the various causes of cancer, age and tobacco, diet, and infectious agents are considered factors for global cancer trends. Certain types of cancer, such as prostate, colon, and breast cancer, are related to Western lifestyle in the more developed and less developed countries [14].

Prevalence of Pain

Cancer incidence clearly differs between developed and developing countries in introducing tobacco controls and programs to prevent infectious diseases. Programs for early detection and the introduction of modern diagnostic methods and targeted treatments are also being introduced in developed countries, which lead to a reduction in cancer incidence as well as a high recovery rate and a low death rate that has not occurred in less developed countries.

The global cancer burden, higher rates of cancers and prevention methods, high recovery rates and cancer prevention resulting from epidemiological data, and the role of economic and political factors highlighted and challenged the fundamental differences in cancer burden in developing countries to introduce programs to mitigate the potential impact of current and future cancer control.

Pain suffering is one of the most common, difficult, and frightening symptoms in cancer patients [15–18]. At the time of cancer diagnosis, more than 30% of patients complain of pain and, when their disease progressed, 85% of patients experience pain. In addition, it is suggested that 25–35% of cancer patients require treatment and, with the progression of the disease, more than 75% of the patients suffer pain. The symptoms of pain vary and are unique. However, there are some generalizations regarding specific types of cancer and the associated intensity of pain (Table 1) [19].

Table 1 Causes of moderate to severe cancer pain

Type of cancer	Prevalence %
Oral	80–90
Bone	80–90
Genitourinary male	70–80
Genitourinary female	65–75
Breast	50–55
Bronchus	40–50
Lymphoma	20–25

Pain is one of the most complex symptoms due to its cognitive, behavioral, sensory, and emotional components [20], and more than 50% of cancer patients suffer pain; patients in developing countries show an increased number of pain cases, as most cases are diagnosed at late stages [18], 25% of cancer patients suffer from acute pain, while more than 50% of cancer patients suffer from moderate to severe pain [17, 21]. More than 75% of all cancer patients complain of pain and require pain treatment interventions.

The recommendations in the WHO's guidelines are divided into a three-level ladder approach for methods of pain management with regard to drugs, including the use of opioids. The purpose of this ladder is to make pain relievers readily available to all cancer patients with advanced stages and to access effective medications at reasonable prices or even free of charge (Fig. 1) [22]. These guidelines are universally acceptable and appropriate for all cancer patients [23]. According to clinically-proven clinical guidelines, the prevalence of cancer pain is about 39% in the USA, 40% in Europe [24], 42.1% in Latin America [25, 26], 52% in Asia [27–29], 70% in the Middle East [30–32], and 61.6% in Africa [33, 34].

Not undergoing treatment for pain or not being regularized to treat pain has a negative impact on mental and physical health and lifestyle, causes severe suffering, and impacts the functional activity of cancer patients [16, 20, 25]. Repercussions from pain suffering include an effect on movement and daily activity, disturbance in entertainment, sleeping hours, and professional and social life [16, 17, 35–37]. Also, the

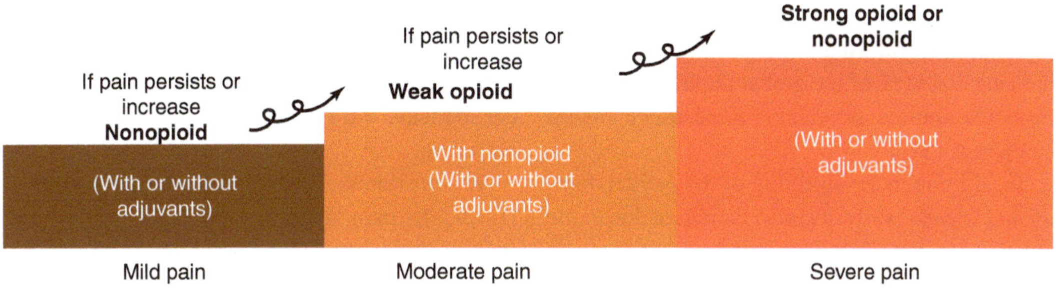

Fig. 1 WHO analgesic ladder. (Modified from the World Health Organization [22])

severity and duration of pain reflects quality of life (QoL) [16].

In cases of acute pain, the patient may lose his/her appetite, refrain from taking pain medications, or have suicidal thoughts [38]. In this case, the patient's health deteriorates, and despite the rules and principles of international pain relief agreed upon by the World Health Organization [39] treatment is, in practice, weak and underserved in developing countries [40–42]. A comparison was performed between the consumption of and the need for opioid analgesics at country, regional, and global levels and showed improvement in the treatment of pain in developed countries [43, 44]. Cultural, legislative, and regulatory barriers to health care are major obstacles and adversely affect pain management [20].

Opioid treatment and health care are not readily available or easily accessible [45]. Physicians face obstacles and challenges at many levels when it comes to opioid acquisition [46]. The poor training of health-care professionals and lack of patient awareness worsens the health situation, as it leads to an increased negative impact on the patient's QoL [45–47].

The increasing suffering of cancer patients is linked to the lack of professional training for doctors and nurses, administrative bureaucracy, and the lack of financial resources for purchasing opioids and chemical and palliative drugs to relieve pain [48, 49]. In addition, factors such as poverty and illiteracy increase suffering.

The prevalence of pain experienced in advanced-stage cancer patients is 70–80% when not being treated and factors such as weak strategic prevention, illiteracy, and low income exacerbates the patients' condition in the late stages of the disease [48]. The persistent suffering from discomfort and its accompanying symptoms reduces the patients' quality of life and places a burden on the family's economic and general health that, in turn, has a negative impact on the patient's ability to tolerate treatment [48–50].

Palliative Care of Pain

The increasing incidence of cancer in developing and developed countries, as well as the high rate of aging globally, presents the urgent need to raise the level of palliative care. Despite the importance of palliative care, it is difficult to gauge the need for it using current research methodologies [51, 52]. According to the World Health Organization, the response to suffering, which includes professionals in the psychological, physical, spiritual, legal, and social fields, requires professional availability in a number of specializations in the field of health care [53, 54].

Despite the burden of population density, India and China have witnessed a significant improvement in the development of palliative care services and have integrated them into their health-care strategy systems. This is considered a major advancement in reaching both curative medicine and the pain relief associated with limited economic and social situations [55].

The low rate of early diagnosis and the registration of 75–80% of patients in late stages reflects the weakness of cancer prevention services in developing countries. Palliative care often works to relieve pain symptoms, and health-care services that have no benefit in improving quality of life or longevity are less important, especially in the final stages of the disease. Estimated World Health Organization statistics indicate that 80% of the global population suffers from the limited provision of adequate opioid analgesics [51].

In addition to the suffering of the patient, family and friends' suffering also increases due to the patient not receiving appropriate treatment to relieve the pain. Therefore, in order to help patients, there must be strong pain management to prevent this suffering.

Palliative care is considered to be one of the most important resources that are not given adequate attention and use in developed countries. At the same time, it is considered to be a resource that is unavailable or limited in developing countries. Most cancer cases in developing countries are diagnosed in advanced late stages, and the limited treatment options, if available at all, are necessary in these countries. According to the guidelines of the World Health Organization, palliative care is the fourth major option for controlling pain in developing countries. Improving the quality of life of patients and their families is one of the priorities of palliative care, with a comprehensive methodology for psychological, physical, and cultural aspects [56].

Unfortunately, 80% of cancer patients in developing countries do not have access to palliative care and this number will surely rise in the coming years; this is an indication of how serious the consequences are for patients with low incomes, and requires urgent intervention from the local governorates of these countries to improve palliative care services [56].

Due to the governmental ban of opioids by some countries and the scarcity of their availability in the market, there is an urgent need to provide morphine and opioid derivatives to suffering cancer patients in order to reduce the severe pain associated with the disease and its treatments [57].

Opioid Availability in Developing Countries

Adequate treatment of pain is considered by professional health organizations to be one of the most important human rights [58, 59]. In accordance with strict legal regulations governing the optimal and legitimate use of opioid analgesics, it is necessary to dispense these analgesics to cancer patients who need them to alleviate their suffering.

In most low- and middle-income countries (LMICs), pain medications are limited and require strict procedures and laws, negatively affecting patients' lives. The availability of opioid analgesics is often a special problem, presented in Table 2, Analgesic medications listed in the WHO's Model List of Essential Medicines (WHO's MLEM) [60].

According to the requirements of the Global Opioid Policy Initiative (GOPI), the opioid formulations that are available for the treatment of cancer patients in developing countries are: morphine injection (Minj), codeine, morphine immediate release (MIR), fentanyl transdermal (FTD), oxycodone immediate release, and methadone per oral (MPO) [42].

Morphine and codeine are the most common pain medications available in most countries. The

Table 2 Analgesic medications listed in the WHO's MLEM

Opioid analgesics	Form of Administration
Morphine	Injection, oral liquid, tablet
Codeine	Tablet
Non-opioids and non-steroidal anti-inflammatory medications	
Ibuprofen	Tablet
Aspirin	Tablet, suppository
Paracetamol	Tablet, oral liquid, suppository,
Medicines used in mood disorders	
Amitriptyline	Tablet
Anticonvulsants, anti-epileptics	
Sodium valproate	Tablet, oral liquid
Carbamazepine	Tablet, oral liquid
Local anesthetics	
Lidocaine	Injection
Lidocaine with adrenaline	Injection
Bupivacaine	Injection
General anesthetics	
Nitrous oxide	Inhalation
Ketamine	Injection

Philippines, China, Malaysia, Israel, Qatar, and Saudi Arabia have all seven formulations available; in Algeria, Morocco, and Iran about six opioid formulations; five formulations are available in Hong Kong, Japan, Vietnam, South Korea, and Thailand; while four formulations are available in Egypt, Lebanon, Yemen, and Palestine. Oral MIR formulation is not available in Cambodia, Kazakhstan, Afghanistan, Bhutan, Bangladesh, and Laos [61].

Other countries such as Bangladesh, Afghanistan, Myanmar, and Bhutan have access to only three formulations: codeine, MPO, and Minj.

Access to FTD was achieved in many countries, despite the lack of morphine tablets, which are at a lower cost, and the availability of FTD, which is expensive. Many countries provide these drugs free of charge to all cancer patients and some countries require paying 25% of the treatment cost as a community contribution; however, in some countries such as the Philippines, Cambodia, Nepal, Laos, Bangladesh, and Indonesia, the patient is forced to pay all the costs of treatment [62].

Barriers to Palliative Care

Despite support for cancer treatment programs, there are still gaps between the palliative care service offered and patients' need for care. Eliminating obstacles and filling the gaps is a major global necessity that needs greater attention from the parties that care for cancer patients. Since most cancer patients in many developing countries have been diagnosed at the late advanced-stages of the disease, palliative care and pain therapy are the best realistic treatment options. The barriers to the health-care system that interfere with the adequate management of pain on a large scale is considered a problem for health-care professionals [50].

Unfortunately, priority is not given to pain management or individual patient care by either global or governmental organizations. At the global level, the lack of governmental attention was reflected in the World Health Organization's poor level of interest in pain management and its focus on communicable disease control.

One of the main challenges in providing pain relief treatment is the significant absence in cultural programs regarding the awareness of assessment and management of pain through the already available medications. Also, there is a lack of interest on the part of medical institutes and colleges in improving nursing curricula and medical colleges regarding cancer pain management. In some areas, palliative care services are provided according to international standards; however, patients in many developing countries in Asia and Africa and, in particular, the countries of the Middle East and Asia, resort to traditional treatment such as herbs. In many cases, when there are gaps between the level of pain and the provision of treatment, patients must endure the pain and live with it. Palliative care policies' guidance for health-care systems in most developing countries is necessary and gaps and weaknesses are well-covered in the literature. Also, there is a decrease in the number of palliative care teams in most countries. The absence of chemotherapy and supportive treatment for cancer patients along with the limited quantities of opioids to treat cancer pain has had a negative impact on patients' lives. The burden of travelling to search for opioids and the lack of financial resources for patients to purchase these drugs are factors that negatively affect them [63].

The rate of opioid consumption is an indicator of palliative care services in any country. The availability of opioids in the region does not necessarily reflect the availability of opioids to patients.

Opioid Availability and Legislation

Developing countries are making great efforts to overcome difficulties in the provision and availability of essential medicines to all patients. All countries have standards and regulations for prescribing morphine after it has been approved by the supervising authorities in the Ministry of Health and to ensure that treatment reaches the oncology centers easily. Although some medications are almost always available to patients in some countries, a few countries such as Yemen, Cambodia, Afghanistan, Myanmar, and Bangladesh require that opioids be administered only with special permission. This requires the registration of all patients attending outpatient clinics, inpatient clinics, and departments of chemotherapy in countries such as Pakistan, the Philippines, Afghanistan, Kazakhstan, and Bangladesh [62]. However, some countries such as Vietnam and China have compulsory registration for outpatients.

Most countries have regulatory and administrative restrictions for prescriptions. While some (Pakistan, the Philippines, Cambodia, China, Mongolia, Laos, Myanmar and Thailand) have restrictive access to these prescription forms, in a few countries such as Cambodia, Mongolia, Pakistan, and the Philippines, the prescription requires payment [64].

The regulations for licensing physicians and pharmacists to prescribe the opioids vary from one country to another in the developing countries. The pharmacists in Afghanistan are allowed to give prescriptions in emergency situations and in conditions of acute pain, during official holidays and evening shifts. Pakistan, Malaysia, and Indonesia have permitted doctors to be approved by phone or fax [42].

There are differences in the rules and guidelines for prescribing opioids in the Middle East region according to each country's regulations [65, 66]. "Opioid phobia" is one of the daily problems in the region that lead to insufficient pain and symptom management. When comparing countries in the Middle East region, we note that Cyprus and Israel have educational programs for doctors, pharmacists, and other health professionals in the optimal use of opioids in palliative care [67, 68].

Turkey's experience has been unique in developing a continuous awareness training program for government leaders, doctors, nurses, and the public. It is a pioneering endeavor that can be applied in other countries. Jordan, along with the World Health Organization, has been remarkable in developing and improving prescription regulations for opioids and developing the field of rehabilitation and training for doctors and pharmacists. Cyprus and Israel are the largest consumers of opioids, as they are among the most educated and have opioid education programs that distinguish their specialized palliative care services. Lebanon, Libya, Palestine, Syria, and Yemen have no restrictions on inpatients, but in other countries patients may require a permit to receive opioid treatment.

The most common opioids available and registered for palliative care are codeine, morphine, and pethidine (meperidine). More than 20 years ago, the International Narcotics Control Board (INCB) recorded a perception that assumed interest in using proprietary opioids in the treatment of pain in all cancer cases, which included palliative care, the most expensive form of treatment. In recent years, doctors tend to prefer prescribing fentanyl treatment, especially in the form of skin patches.

Opioid Availability and Cost

Most countries cover the cost of opioids and dispense them free of charge to all cancer patients, and some countries cover 75% of the cost of treatment and the patient bears 25% of the cost of opioid analgesics. In Afghanistan, Lebanon, Morocco, and Syria, patients bear the full cost of medicines. Iraq, Lebanon, Libya, Afghanistan, and Palestine have ceased to supply controlled-release procedures of injectable morphine. Oxycodone, methadone, and fentanyl are not regularly available in most countries [69]. Suffering from cancer pain remains one of the most significant global problems, especially in developing countries. The suffering of the patients must be given greater attention and the practice of patient care should consider all of the social, psychological, spiritual, and cultural aspects of the individual; the pain should be evaluated in a comprehensive and continuous manner, and pain management must be given greater attention, with a comprehensive approach.

Raising the level of awareness for cancer and its consequences, along with cancer treatment programs relating to the spread of cancer pain, is of urgency and one of the most important criteria for improving health care. The responsible institutions are committed to developing programs to educate medical personnel and patients on how to use and recognize painkillers, and governments are working to provide effective drugs according to the basic list agreed upon with the World Health Organization. Studies and statistics from the United States of America, Canada, and the United Kingdom indicate that palliative care programs for cancer-related diseases play an important role in reducing the costs of health-care programs [70].

Future plans throughout developing countries include comprehensive strategies that are beneficial for improvement in other regions and countries around the world. In developing and low-income countries, the basic guidelines for palliative care providers to negotiate with governments of developing countries to develop palliative care are as follows:

1. Develop a comprehensive strategy that supports the integration of palliative care and pain treatment programs in the health-care system, in addition to incorporating the palliative care program into the heath plan to monitor the national cancer program
2. Create and develop safe financing
3. Recognize the right of patients to appropriate assessment and management of pain
4. Determine and ensure staff competency in pain assessment and management, and address pain assessment and management in the orientation of all new staff
5. Establish policies and procedures that support the appropriate prescription and ordering of effective pain medications
6. Educate patients and their families about effective pain management
7. Examine adequate supply methods to secure opioid and other essential materials and medications for palliative care programs
8. Establish training programs for all cadres of health professionals on highly trained analgesics care
9. Coordinate with universities to adopt a palliative care program as a medical specialty, and to consider it as part of basic education programs for the medical and nursing curricula
10. Support programs for developing elderly care and home medical services for centers of health-care systems.

References

1. Sullivan A, Sheffrin SM. Economics: principles in action. Upper saddle river. New Jersey: Pearson Prentice Hall; 2003. p. 471.
2. Soyannwo OA. Cancer pain management for developing countries. IASP. 2009;17:1.
3. Fitzmaurice C, Allen C, Barber R, et al. Global, regional, and national cancer incidence, mortality, years of life lost, years lived with disability, and disability-adjusted life years for 32 cancer groups, 1990 to 2015: a systematic analysis for the global burden of disease study. JAMA Oncol. 2017;3:524e48.
4. Bray F, Ferlay J, Soerjomataram I, Siegel RL, Torre LA, Jemal A. Global cancer statistics 2018: GLOBOCAN estimates of incidence and mortality worldwide for 36 cancers in 185 countries. CA Cancer J Clin. 2018;68:394–424. https://doi.org/10.3322/caac.21492. Available online at cacancerjournal.com.
5. Jemal A, Bray F, Center MM, Ferlay J, Ward E, Forman D. Global cancer statistics. CA Cancer J Clin. 2011;61:69–90.
6. Islam SMS, Purnat TD, Phuong NTA, Mwingira U, Schacht K, Fröschl G. Non-Communicable Diseases (NCDs) in developing countries: a symposium report. Glob Health. 2014;10:81.
7. Mishra A, Meherotra R. Head and neck cancer: global burden and regional trends in India. Asian Pac J Cancer Prev. 2014;15(2):537–50.
8. Shah SC, Kayamba V, Peek RM, Heimburger D. Cancer control in low- and middle-income countries: is it time to consider screening? J Global Oncol. 2019;5:1–8. https://doi.org/10.1200/JGO.18.00200.
9. Ovayolu O, Ovayolu N, Aytaç S, Serçe S, Sevinc A. Pain in cancer patients: pain assessment by patients and family caregivers and problems experienced by caregivers. Support Care Cancer. 2015;23(7):1857–64. https://doi.org/10.1007/s00520-014-2540-5.
10. Sener SF, Grey N. The global burden of cancer. J Surg Oncol. 2005;92:1–3.

11. Salminen E, Izewska J, Andreo P. IAEA's role in the global management of cancer-focus on upgrading radiotherapy services. Acta Oncol. 2005;44:816–24.
12. World Health Organization. Global cancer rates could increase by 50% to 15 million by 2020 (April 3, 2003). [On-line]. http://www.who.int/mediacentre/news/releases/2003/pr27/en/ (January 10, 2020, date last accessed).
13. Beaglehole R, Yach D. Globalisation and the prevention and control of noncommunicable disease: the neglected chronic diseases of adults. Lancet. 2003;362:903–8.
14. Stewart BW, Kleihues P. International agency for research on cancer. World cancer report. Lyon: IARC Press; 2003.
15. Liang SY, Ding SA, Wu WW, Liu CY, Lin CC. Opioid-taking self-efficacy affects the quality of life of Taiwanese patients with cancer pain. Support Care Cancer. 2015;23(7):2113–20.
16. Deng D, Fu L, Zhao YX, et al. The relationship between cancer pain and quality of life in patients newly admitted to Wuhan Hospice Center of China. Am J Hosp Palliat Care. 2012;29(1):53–9.
17. He QH, Liu QL, Li Z, Li KZ, Xie YG. Impact of epidural analgesia on quality of life and pain in advanced cancer patients. Pain Manag Nurs. 2015;16(3):307–13.
18. Hong SH, Roh SY, Kim SY, et al. Change in cancer pain management in Korea between 2001 and 2006: results of two nationwide surveys. J Pain Symptom Manag. 2011;41(1):93–103.
19. Toth JA. Concepts in cancer pain management. US Pharm. 2009;34(11):3–12.
20. Ovayolu N, Ovayolu Ö, Serçe S, Tuna D, Pirbudak Çöçelli L, Sevinç A. Pain and quality of life in Turkish cancer patients. Nurs Health Sci. 2013;15(4):437–43. https://doi.org/10.1111/nhs.12047.
21. Breivik H, Cherny N, Collett B, et al. Cancer-related pain: a pan-European survey of prevalence, treatment, and patient attitudes. Ann Oncol. 2009;20(8):1420–33.
22. Gamal Abdul Hamid, Gunida Algneid, Nasser Baom, Shatha Yassin. Prevalence and management of Pain in Yemeni patients with Cancer; NCRI Cancer Conferences book 2014, Presentation page 29 https://www.researchgate.net/publication/341549392_Prevalence_and_management_of_Pain_in_Yemeni_patients_with_Cancer.
23. Zech DFJ, Grond S, Lynch J, Hertel D, Lehmann KA. Validation of World Health Organization Guidelines for cancer pain relief: a 10-year prospective study. Pain. 1995;63(1):65–76.
24. Javier FO, Irawan C, Mansor MB, Sriraj W, Tan KH, Thinh DHQ. Cancer pain management insights and reality in Southeast Asia: expert perspectives from six countries. J Glob Oncol. 2016;2(4):235–43.
25. Nogueira RTE, de Moraes Viera EB, Sousa LHA, Garcia JBS. Difficult situation in cancer pain: breakthrough pain. Revista Dor. 2014;15(1):41–7.
26. Pracucho EM, Lopes LR, Zanatto RM, et al. Profile of patients with gastrointestinal stromal tumors (GIST). Arq Bras Cir Dig. 2015;28(2):124–7.
27. Rau KM, Chen JS, Wu HB, et al. The impact of pain control on physical and psychiatric functions of cancer patients: a nation-wide survey in Taiwan. Jpn J Clin Oncol. 2015;45(11):1042–9.
28. Yang P, Sun L-Q, Lu Q, Pang D, Ding Y. Quality of life in cancer patients with pain in Beijing. Chin J Cancer Res. 2012;24(1):60–6.
29. Kim JY, Jang WY, Hur MH, et al. Prevalence and management of pain by different age groups of Korean cancer patients. Am J Hosp Palliat Care. 2013;30(4):393–8.
30. Al Qadire M, Tubaishat A, Aljezawi MM. Cancer pain in Jordan: prevalence and adequacy of treatment. Int J Palliat Nurs. 2013;19(3):125–30.
31. Halawi R, Aldin ES, Baydoun A, et al. Physical symptom profile for adult cancer inpatients at a Lebanese cancer unit. Eur J Intern Med. 2012;23(8):e185–9.
32. Hamid GA, Saeed NM, Ba-Ashen Y, Ba-Kubirah R. Colorectal carcinoma at Al-Gamhouria Teaching Hospital, Aden, Yemen. Gulf J Oncolog. 2012;11(11):16–9.
33. Beck SL, Falkson G. Prevalence and management of cancer pain in South Africa. Pain. 2001;94(1):75–84.
34. Harding R, Selman L, Agupio G, et al. The prevalence and burden of symptoms amongst cancer patients attending palliative care in two African countries. Eur J Cancer. 2011;47(1):51–6.
35. Kim YS, Do H, Lee JW, et al. Patient reporting pain intensity immediately after surgery can be associated with underlying depression in women with breast cancer. Psychooncology. 2016;25(3):308–15.
36. Bushenell MC, Ceko M, Low LA. Cognitive and emotional control of pain and its disruption in chronic pain. Nat Rev Neurosci. 2013;14(7):502–11. https://doi.org/10.1038/nrn3516.
37. Oliveira KG, von Zeidler SV, PodestJ JR, et al. Influence of pain severity on the quality of life in patients with head and neck cancer before antineoplastic therapy. BMC Cancer. 2014;14(1):39.
38. O'Mahony S, Goulet J, Kornblith A, et al. Desire for hastened death, cancer pain and depression: report of a longitudinal observational study. J Pain Symptom Manag. 2005;29(5):446–57.
39. Jadad AR, Browman GP. The WHO analgesic ladder for cancer pain management. JAMA. 1995;274(23):1870–3.
40. Fairchild A. Under-treatment of cancer pain. Curr Opin Support Palliat Care. 2010;4(1):11–5.
41. Deandrea S, Montanari M, Moja L, Apolone G. Prevalence of under treatment in cancer pain. A review of published literature. Ann Oncol. 2008;19(12):1985–91.
42. Cleary J, Radbruch L, Torode J, Cherny NI. Formulary availability and regulatory barriers to accessibility of opioids for cancer pain in Asia: a report from the Global Opioid Policy Initiative (GOPI). Ann Oncol. 2013;24(Suppl 11):xi24–32.
43. Lynch T, Connor S, Clark D. Mapping levels of palliative care development: a global update. J Pain Symptom Manag. 2013;45(6):1094–106.

44. Seya MJ, Gelders SF, Achara OU, Milani B, Scholten WK. A first comparison between the consumption of and the need for opioid analgesics at country, regional, and global levels. J Pain Palliat Care Pharmacother. 2011;25(1):6–18.
45. Foley KM, Wagner JL, Joranson DE, Gelband H. [database on the Internet]. Pain control for people with cancer and AIDS. In: Jamison DT, Breman JG, Measham AR, editors. Disease control priorities in developing countries [Internet]. 2nd ed. Washington, DC: World Bank; 2006. [cited February 20, 2017]. Available from: http://www.ncbi.nlm.nih.gov/books/NBK11800/. Accessed 9 Oct 2018.
46. Lebaron V, Beck SL, Maurer M, Black F, Palat G. An ethnographic study of barriers to cancer pain management and opioid availability in India. Oncologist. 2014;19(5):515–22.
47. Li YX, Yu JQ, Tang L, et al. Cancer pain management at home: voice from an underdeveloped region of China. Cancer Nurs. 2013;36(4):326–34.
48. Gehdoo RP. Cancer pain management. Indian J Anaesth. 2006;50:375–90.
49. McCarberg BH, Nicholson BD, Todd KH, Palmer T, Penles L. The impact of pain on quality of life and the unmet needs of pain management: results from pain sufferers and physicians participating in an internet survey. Am J Ther. 2008;15:312–20.
50. Paice JA, Ferrell B. The management of cancer pain. CA Cancer J Clin. 2011;61:157–82.
51. Connor S, Sepulveda C. Global atlas of palliative care at the end-of-life 2014. Available from: http://www.thewpca.org/resources/global-atlas-of-palliative-care/. [Last accessed 24 Aug 2016].
52. Callaway M, Foley KM, De Lima L, Connor SR, Dix O, Lynch T, et al. Funding for palliative care programs in developing countries. J Pain Symptom Manag. 2007;33:509–13.
53. Gwythere L, Krakauer E. WPCA policy statement on defining palliative care 2011. Available from: http://www.thewpca.org/resources/?WPCA%20policy%20defining%20palliative%20care. [Last accessed 13 Apr 2014].
54. Sepúlveda C, Marlin A, Yoshida T, Ullrich A. Palliative care: the World Health Organization's global perspective. J Pain Symp Manag. 2002;24(2):91–6. https://doi.org/10.1016/s0885-3924(02)00440-2.
55. Rajagopol MR, Twycross R. Providing palliative care in resource-poor countries. In: Hanks G, Cherny NI, Christakis NA, Fallon M, Kaasa S, Porteno RK, editors. Oxford textbook of palliative medicine. 4th ed. Oxford: Oxford University Press; 2010. p. 23–31.
56. WHO: Palliative care. http://www.who.int/mediacentre/factsheets/fs402/en.
57. Human Rights Watch: Unbearable pain: India's obligation to ensure palliative care. https://www.hrw.org/report/2009/10/28/unbearable-pain/indias-obligationensure-palliative-care.
58. Radbruch L, Payne S, de Lima L, Lohmann D. The Lisbon challenge: acknowledging palliative care as a human right. J Palliat Med. 2013;16:301–4.
59. Méndez JE. Report of the Special Rapporteur on torture and other cruel, in human or degrading treatment or punishment. United Nations General Assembly, Contract No: A/HRC/22/53; 2013.
60. World Health Organization. WHO model lists of essential medicines. Available from: http://www.who.int/medicines/publications/essentialmedicines/en/. Accessed 19 Jan 2018.
61. WHO webpage on the Internet; Availability of narcotic drugs for medical use; Available on https://www.incb.org/incb/en/narcotic-drugs/Availability/availability.html. Accessed 11 Mar 2020.
62. Saini S, Bhatnagar S. Cancer pain management in developing countries. Indian J Palliat Care. 2016;22(4):373–7. https://doi.org/10.4103/0973-1075.191742.
63. Grant M, Elk R, Ferrell B, Morrison RS, Von Gunten CF. Current status of palliative care-clinical implementation, education, and research. CA Cancer J Clin. 2009;59:327–35.
64. Bosnjak S, Maurer MA, Ryan KM, Leon MX, Adiye GM. Improving the availability and accessibility of opioids for the treatment of pain: the international pain policy fellowship. Support Care Cancer. 2011;19:1239–47. https://doi.org/10.1007/s00520-011-1200-2.
65. AlBahrani BJ, Mehdi I. The need for regulatory reforms in the use of opioids for pain management and palliative care in the Middle East. Gulf J Oncolog. 2018;1(27):52–9.
66. Silbermann M. Opioids in middle eastern populations. Asian Pac J Cancer Prev. 2010;11(Suppl 1):1–5.
67. Sapir R, Catane R, Strauss-Liviatan N, Cherny NI. Cancer pain: knowledge and attitudes of physicians in Israel. J Pain Symptom Manag. 1999;17:266e272.
68. Kakas J, Pitsillides B. Managing cancer pain at home: the experience of Cyprus. Available at http://www.whocancerpain.wisc.edu/eng/10_2/cyprus.html. Accessed 29 June 2005.
69. Cleary J, Silbermann M, Scholten W, Radbruch L, Torode L, et al. Formulary availability and regulatory barriers to accessibility of opioids for cancer pain in the Middle East: a report from the Global Opioid Policy Initiative (GOPI). Ann Oncol. 2013;24(Supplement 11):xi51–9. https://doi.org/10.1093/annonc/mdt503.
70. TWF. Cost-effectiveness of palliative care. Available from: http://hpcintegration.ca/media/24434/TWF-Economics-report-Final.pdf.

Prevalence and Management of Cancer Pain in Developing Countries

Part XXVII

Central Asia: Afghanistan

Palliative Care: The Care That Is Rarely Practiced in Health System of Afghanistan

Maihan Abdullah, Najia Niazi, and Musa Pakteen

Afghanistan is a landlocked country in South-Central Asia surrounded by six countries [1]. It was estimated in 2018 that the population was more than 37 million [2], of which three quarters live in rural areas. The average size of a family in Afghanistan is 7.7 people. Even though more than 75% of the nation's labor force is employed, about 80% of jobs are categorized as vulnerable and only 20% are deemed as decent employment. Approximately 45% of the jobs are in the agricultural sector and only 18% are in the area of manufacturing. According to a recent survey, more than half of Afghans live below the national poverty line. While the literacy rate among Afghans aged 15–24 is nearly 55%, the adult literacy rate is only 35%, one of the lowest in the world. In Afghanistan, women of childbearing age have, on average, 5.3 children. The life expectancy at birth for women is 67 years and for men 64. Nearly half of the Afghan population is under the age of 15, and only 3% are 65 and older, making Afghanistan one of the youngest nations on earth [3, 4].

The responsibility for the Afghans' health primarily falls on the Ministry of Public Health (MoPH). The health system in Afghanistan has considerably improved since the fall of the Taliban in 2002 [5]. With the support of international donors in 2003, the MoPH established the Basic Package of Health Services (BPHS), contracting out primary healthcare services in rural areas to non-governmental organizations (NGOs). In 2005, the Essential Package of Health Services (EPHS) was prepared outsourcing secondary health services in Provincial and Regional Hospitals to NGOs. Out of 34 provinces, 31 are contracted out to NGOs while health services in the remaining three provinces are managed by MoPH itself. In addition, tertiary healthcare services which are mainly located in the capital city, Kabul, are managed by the MoPH. Currently, 93% of people are within two hours distance from a public clinic through any means of transportation [6–8].

The Current Health Expenditure (CHE) in 2017 was approximately USD 2.4 billion, accounting for 12% of the gross domestic product (GDP), which is higher than other low- and middle-income countries (LMICs) such as India, Pakistan, Egypt, Nepal, and Tajikistan. Of the USD 2.4 billion, USD 1.8 billion (75.5%) was out-of-pocket expenditures paid by households, USD 470 million (19.4%) was funded by international donors, and only USD 123 million (5.1%) was paid by the Afghan government. More than half of the household out-of-pocket expenses was spent on medical goods and medicine, 34.6% on diagnostic services, and 10% on outpatient ser-

M. Abdullah (✉)
National Cancer Control Program, Ministry of Public Health, Kabul, Afghanistan

N. Niazi · M. Pakteen
The Cancer Center at Jumhuriat Hospital, National Cancer Control Program, Ministry of Public Health, Kabul, Afghanistan

M. Silbermann (ed.), *Palliative Care for Chronic Cancer Patients in the Community*,
https://doi.org/10.1007/978-3-030-54526-0_39

vices. According to the above statistics, household out-of-pocket spending pushed almost 14% of people into poverty [9, 10].

Considering that infant, child, and maternal mortality rates in Afghanistan have been one of the highest in the world, it is not surprising that international donors and the government have prioritized these conditions since 2003 [8]. According to the Afghanistan Mortality Survey conducted in 2010, however, the leading causes of death among Afghan men and women are were non-communicable diseases (35%) and infections (30%), whereas perinatal conditions account for 13%. Maternal conditions represent only 5% of total deaths in Afghanistan. Cancer accounts for 6% of all deaths [1].

Based on International Agency for Research on Cancer (IARC) estimates, in 2018 about 20,000 Afghans suffered from different types of cancer (9150 male and 10,300 female). In the same year, almost 15,000 Afghans died of cancer. However, these figures are conservative, and it is assumed that between 30,000 and 40,000 Afghans live with cancer. The leading cancers in Afghanistan are that of breast, stomach, lip and oral cavity, esophagus, lung, and blood, respectively [11].

Until 2016, there was not a single bed dedicated for oncology patients in the Afghanistan health system; however, hematologic oncology patients were admitted to the hematology departments in Jamhuriat Hospital and the Indira Gandhi Institute of Child Health (IGICH), which were already established. As a result of two years of advocacy efforts for cancer control by known social and political figures, the Cancer Diagnosis and Treatment Project was established in 2016 within the Ministry of Public Health. The Cancer Diagnosis and Treatment Project was promoted to the National Cancer Control Program (NCCP) in January 2017.

The first and only Cancer Center in Afghanistan was established in Jumhuriat Hospital (located in downtown Kabul) in late 2016, with a 10-bed day care unit and 20-bed inpatient unit. At the moment, the oncology ward has a 20-bed day care, a 20-bed surgical, and a 40-bed medical oncology unit with a staff of about 100 in total. On average, 100 patients visit the outpatient department every day. As of 2019, it was estimated that nearly 50,000 visits were paid to the ward. In addition, the NCCP established a 15-bed medical oncology ward in Herat and Balkh, which are the regional capitals in the west and in the north of Afghanistan, respectively. Moreover, breast cancer diagnostic centers were established in Kabul and Herat provinces. Unfortunately, radiotherapy is not available in Afghanistan [12, 13].

As the Cancer Center in Jumhuriat Hospital and the oncology wards in the two provinces are recently established, the public and some healthcare providers are not aware of the oncology services. Patients suffering from symptoms of cancer usually seek care at district, provincial, regional, and national hospitals. Data from the Kabul Cancer Registry clearly show that of 8000 cancer cases, most patients were diagnosed at late stages. The most common presenting symptoms are pain, constipation/obstipation, nausea/vomiting, dysphagia, dyspnea, odor, especially in breast cancer and sarcoma of bone, stomatitis, anxiety and depression, and ulcer/bed sores. In addition to pain and other physical problems, cancer patients and their family members face psychological, social, and spiritual distress.

Due to the relatively low incidence of cancer and young population, Afghanistan is in the category of countries where the percentage of adults in need of palliative care for cancer at the end of life is the lowest; however, when it comes to the need for pediatric palliative care for cancer, Afghanistan ranks among the countries with the highest percentages [14]. Even though the Worldwide Palliative Care Alliance (WPCA) has reported that Afghanistan does not have hospice-palliative care services [15], a home-based palliative care project called Hamdardi was established by a non-profit organization, Silk Road Development, back in 2010. This nurse-run project provides hospice care in the Dasht-e-Barchi neighborhood, which is located in western Kabul. The nurses provide psychological, social, and emotional support as well as pain management with nonsteroidal anti-inflammatory drugs (NSAIDs) and tramadol [16].

In view of the fact that 60–70% of patients are diagnosed at advanced stages, most of them need palliative treatment. The most common complaint in these patients is pain, ranging from mild to severe, depending on the type of cancer and treatment as well as on personal characteristics. The most commonly used analgesic for moderate pain is diclofenac sodium injection 25 mg/ml (3 ml). If pain persists, the second choice of most physicians in Afghanistan is tramadol HCL 75 mg plus paracetamol 650 mg per oral ingestion tablet. Subsequently, if pain continues or increases, physicians usually prescribe tramadol HCL 100 mg injections. These pain medications are administered at almost all levels of public health facilities as well as at individual practices and private hospitals.

If pain is not controlled through the above-stated measures, patients are referred to provincial, regional, or national public hospitals. At these hospitals, patients are assessed for pain and paracetamol, NSAIDs, and tramadol, pentazocine, or nalbuphine are prescribed parentally in different combinations. Generally, when pain is not relieved through enteral analgesics or few doses of parenteral analgesics, patients are referred to public health facilities for parenteral analgesics, especially opioids. Morphine injection, usually available in public and private hospitals, is rarely used for pain management, particularly for cancer-related pain.

In Afghanistan, regulation of opioid drugs and other pharmaceuticals is the responsibility of the National Medicine and Healthcare Products Regulatory Authority (NMHRA). The NMHRA also develops and reviews the Essential Medicine List (EML), National Licensed Medicine List (NLML), and National Formulary [17]. EML is implemented in public health facilities including the BPHS, EPHS, National Hospitals, and in all other national programs, while the NLML is used in the private health sector. The medicines in NLML can be manufactured in the country as well as imported. The opioid analgesics in the NLML are fentanyl, morphine (HCL and sulfate), nalbuphine, codeine, pentazocine, pethidine, and tramadol. Methadone is also present in NLML but under the "drugs used in addictive disorders" category, whereas codeine is listed under the "Expectorants, excl. combinations with cough suppressants" category.

Of these opioids, only morphine, pethidine, and tramadol are present in the EML. Public health facilities can merely procure and administer medicines that are included in the EML while methadone can only be used in addiction rehabilitation centers, mostly run by the MoPH. In Afghanistan, tramadol and methadone are available in oral ingestion and injection forms but morphine, nalbuphine, and fentanyl are available only in injectable form. In addition, codeine is available in oral ingestion as well as in syrup form [18–20].

Although the MoPH has allowed the import and sale of a few opioids, the uses of those medicines are limited at all levels of health facilities both in public and private sectors. Morphine, recommended by World Health Organization (WHO) and the International Association for Hospice and Palliative Care (IAHPC) [21, 22], is used for pain management of acute cardiovascular conditions and sometimes in orthopedic cases. In addition, morphine is used at the Indira Gandhi Institute of Child Health. It is noteworthy that the use of opioids at the French Medical Institute of Children (FMIC), the Cure International Hospital of Kabul, and in hospitals run by the International Committee of the Red Cross (ICRC), Médecins Sans Frontières (MSF), and the Emergency is different from the rest of the country; however, they generally do not provide services to cancer patients. The barriers to the use of opioids in palliative care are due to the systems, clinicians, and patients.

System-Related Barriers

Many essential analgesics, especially opioids, are not listed in the NLML and thus the import is illegal.

- Few opioids can be procured and used by public health facilities, even at tertiary levels.
- The import processes of opioids are time-consuming, complicated, and bureaucratic.
- The supply of opioids on the market is insufficient and some formulations are not available at all.

- Opioids are not available in many pharmacies.
- The expiration dates of opioids on the market are usually short.
- There is no national guideline or protocol for pain management in health facilities.

Clinician-Related Barriers

- Clinicians usually do not have sufficient skills to assess pain.
- Clinicians often do not possess adequate knowledge of pain management.
- Clinicians typically do not take pain seriously and do not prioritize it.
- Clinicians fear side effects.
- Clinicians are unwilling to prescribe opioids.

Patient-Related Barriers

- Communication problems between patients and healthcare providers exist at all levels of health facilities. In Afghanistan's traditional and religious society, especially in rural areas, most female patients communicate with male providers through their male caregivers.
- In order to please the clinician, patients tend to tolerate the pain and do not make it obvious.
- If patients' pain is not relieved, they frequently change hospitals and doctors [23].

Even more than pain, dysphagia and dyspnea are bothersome and inconvenient for patients and their family members. In almost all cases of dysphagia, physicians at provincial and regional levels do not provide care and refer the patients to Kabul. Those who are willing and can afford to get to Kabul can only receive palliative treatment in a few hospitals. If patients can tolerate it, endoscopic metal stenting, gastrostomy, or jejunostomy is performed. On the other hand, other symptoms such as nausea and vomiting, anorexia, bed sores, diarrhea, constipation, and stomatitis are treated at all levels with the medicines recommended in the Essential Package (EP) of Palliative Care; however, pressure-reducing mattresses are not available. Patients with sarcoma of the bone, oral cavity, and advanced breast cancer present with malodor. This is not only discomforting for patients and their family members but also for healthcare providers and other patients. Sometimes a debridement or toilet mastectomy is performed, but otherwise not much is done for such patients.

In the only Cancer Center in Afghanistan located in Jumhuriat Hospital, 60–70% of the treatment is palliative. Most surgical palliative procedures are performed at provincial, regional, and national public hospitals as well as in most private hospitals. Nerve block procedures for pain relief is not available in Afghanistan. NCCP could not find a single surgeon or anesthesiologist in the public or private sector to block the nerve of an advanced breast cancer patient who had unbearable neck and shoulder pain. Palliative chemotherapy is performed at some private hospitals in Kabul, at the Cancer Center in Jumhuriat Hospital, as well as at the newly established oncology wards in Herat and Balkh provinces. Those who require palliative radiation are referred to neighboring countries.

Along with pain and other physical symptoms, cancer patients suffer from psychological, social, and spiritual distress. The term "cancer" sounds devastating and there are many factors that contribute to this notion; most patients and their families believe cancer is not curable. In addition, those who believe cancer can be treated, do not trust the doctors in Afghanistan. Therefore, patients go to other countries for treatment, mainly Pakistan, India, and Iran. Most patients sell their homes, livestock, farmland, vehicles, and jewelry, and even borrow money to afford the journey and treatment. Despite enduring the many problems and expense of going abroad, at the end of the day, their palliative care is done in Afghanistan.

Sameera sold her daughter in order to afford treatment to get well for the rest of her family. Later, when she started feeling better, she regretted selling her daughter. She tried to get her daughter back by paying through any means but the family did not agree to return the daughter to her mother.

In Afghanistan, a "Mullah", or traditional and spiritual healer, also plays an active role in the treatment of terminally ill patients. We often hear that a traditional healer in a rural district has prepared a medicine that can cure cancer. In 2018, a 16-year old boy from Ghazni province approached the MoPH claiming that a medicine he prepared can cure cancer. Recently, a traditional healer posted some videos on Facebook which show that he has prepared a cancer medicine which has cured some patients. A friend of mine, who is a doctor himself, and has a doctor and a pharmacist in his family, drove four hours to buy that medicine for his father. His father had been receiving palliative chemotherapy due to advanced stomach cancer. Depending on the level of belief, educational level, and financial status, most patients go to a traditional or spiritual healer at some point during their illness.

Afghanistan is one of the most religious countries in the world and the majority of the people believe in faith healing. Patients or their caregivers travel long distances to find a Mullah with the hope of being cured. Many patients report the physical and/or mental efficacy of faith healing following unsuccessful medical treatment inside or outside the country. A Mullah in Ghorband district of Parwan province, who is a cancer survivor himself, provides faith healing to many cancer patients. He claims that he heals patients with the help of Jinns (spirits). Anosha, who has breast cancer for the past four years, told her psychologist that one of her relatives gifted a car to this Mullah after being successfully treated. Anosha now also goes to this Mullah and finds the treatment effective.

Many patients report that a Mullah does not provide treatment for monetary gains. In fact, he treats patients solely because of the gift he has for treating them. Many patients have reported positive effects while some have reported otherwise. In such cases, religious beliefs of these people may overrule everything they witness or experience. Most Muslims strongly believe,

> Our Lord, Allah, has command over everything and he has taken the responsibility of three things: provides food to His people, choses the life partners for His people, and gives death to His People.

Therefore, based on the above belief, if a patient dies, their families go through all five stages of grief more easily. We have witnessed family members reporting that it was Allah's will and neither they nor we could do anything to help the patient. These statements are based on the following verse of the Quran:

> Indeed we belong to Allah, and indeed to him we will return.

Furthermore, many people in Afghanistan consider cancer to be a curse. Many patients die due to the rejection they feel and encounter everywhere in society, especially in their own homes. People believe cancer is a communicable and incurable disease, and even eating together with a cancer patient is no less than a disaster for them. Additionally, many female patients have been left by their husbands when they come to know that their wives have cancer.

> Bibi Zulaikha was an orphan girl brought up by her aunt. When she grew up she got married and had five children. As soon as the husband discovered that she had cancer, he left her and got married to another woman during the course of her treatment. When Bibi Zulaikha received a donation of about $300 from her cousins, who live outside of Afghanistan, the husband took that money and spent it on his new wife. Bibi Zuleikha, like many other patients, was left without any money. Even though the Cancer Center in Jumhuriat Hospital managed to raise some funds for her treatment, the mental stress exacerbated her illness. At last, news of Bibi Zulaikha's death was received by the Cancer Center.

Cancer patients develop psychological and emotional problems when they experience bullying, sometimes even by their close family members. This may lead to low self-esteem, poor self-image, an inferiority complex, or poor body image due to deformities that may appear with the progression of illness. Even though there are families that have a very good understanding of how to deal with such patients, most families, particularly those who are less educated and poor, have problems coping with terminally ill patients.

> Zainab was a breast cancer patient with five children, the youngest being one year old. Her husband was unemployed. She was receiving palliative chemotherapy along with psychosocial therapy at

the Cancer Center. She was telling her psychologist that she was at the end stage of her life and she would soon die. Her children would be left behind without anyone to take care of them. She said she could not serve herself nor her family. Her sister-in-law would tell her that God had seen her sins and that is why He cursed her with cancer. She would curse herself and wished to die sooner. Close to her death, when she was receiving supportive treatment at home, she wished to see her psychotherapist; however, even her last wish was not fulfilled. The psychotherapist received a phone call from Zainab's mother that she was no longer in this world.

Suicidal thoughts while going through cancer, especially during the palliative stages, are exceedingly common. In Afghanistan, dozens of problems are found to contribute to such thoughts among cancer patients; poverty or a low socioeconomic situation are probably the biggest factors. In addition, the failure to recognize psychological disorders and the value of psychosocial support, the stigma surrounding receipt of mental health support, the presence of generalized fears, mood disturbances, low self-esteem, and poor self-image each play an important role in giving up on life. Some other personal problems include unemployment, disturbed sexual relations, self-neglect, distressing interpersonal relationships, anger outbursts, poor parenting, and communication gaps. Some social issues include the failure of families to resolve long-term conflicts in patients' lives, forced marriages (particularly at a young age), gender inequality, being the only earning member of the family, indecisiveness about initiating treatment, and isolation and a limited social circle. In addition to all the above problems, side effects and complications of treatment, especially deformity and loss of hair, contribute to suicidal thoughts.

At the end stages, many take their ill family member to a hospital rather than letting them stay at home even when these patients can continue the necessary supportive treatment at home. There are several reasons why end-of-life patients are taken to the hospital; one of the main reasons is the families' fear of denigration from relatives – that the family did not spend enough money or value the patient enough, and let the patient die at home; sometimes, families try their best and wish to spend more money if there is a chance of saving the patient; at other times, due to lack of caregivers at home or the overburden on one caregiver, the patient is taken to a health-care facility.

Challenges to Palliative Care

Even though some palliative care services are provided to cancer patients at end-of-life and at different levels of health facilities, the idea of palliative care is quite new in Afghanistan. The barriers to establishing and implementing palliative care in Afghanistan can generally be categorized into one of three areas: the lack of government commitment, lack of education, and lack of medicine.

Lack of Government Commitment

Considering the fact that the MoPH subsidizes only 5% of the country's health expenditure, it is extremely difficult to convince the leadership to prioritize cancer in general and palliative care in particular. It was only five years ago that the MoPH agreed to provide limited cancer care services in the country. Currently, people wait for weeks to receive their curative or palliative chemotherapy at the Cancer Center in Jumhuriat Hospital because of the limited number of beds. Therefore, the Cancer Center cannot admit most patients that require palliative care services who are referred from across the country. Since 2018, NCCP has been advocating for funding from the Ministry of Finance to establish a small palliative care unit at the Cancer Center.

Lack of Education

Palliative care is not taught in medical schools nor during residency programs. The Mental Health Department at the MoPH has trained hundreds of psychosocial counselors through its one-year program; however, they are not trained in palliative care. There is currently only one clinical psychologist who provides psychosocial counselling to cancer patients. To the best of our knowledge, there are no doctors, nurses, pharmacists, or psychosocial counsellors trained in palliative care in Afghanistan.

Lack of Medicine

Based on the NLML and EML, there are very few drugs that may be procured and administered by public health facilities. As a result, many cheap, effective, safe, and conveniently-administered medicines and their different formulations are not available on the market. For example, controlled and immediate-release oral morphine listed in the Essential Package of Palliative Care are not available in Afghanistan.

Recommendations for Implementing Palliative Care

Since the establishment of the Cancer Diagnosis and Treatment Project in 2016 and NCCP in 2017, a number of initiatives have been taken. One of the most important achievements was the inclusion of 34 chemo-drugs in the NLML. In addition, palliative care interventions were included in the new health system package, the Integrated Package of Essential Health Services for Afghanistan. (IPHS). Besides, considering its limited resources, the Cancer Center has provided palliative care services to hundreds of cancer patients. For the first time, the WHO's pain management ladder approach is implemented at the Cancer Center. As most cancer patients are diagnosed at advanced stages, palliative care services need to be fully integrated in the healthcare system and implemented. In order to do so, the following interventions are needed.

- To include palliative care in the National Health Policy and Strategy
- To integrate palliative care into BPHS, EPHS, and hospitals at the national level
- To allocate a budget for the implementation of palliative care
- To develop pain management guidelines and SOPs
- To provide palliative care training to existing healthcare providers, especially to nurses, midwives, psychosocial counsellors, and community health workers (CHWs) around the country
- To educate people about palliative care
- To include more analgesics, especially opioids, in the NLML and EML
- To allocate special funding for training healthcare providers in palliative care outside the country [23–25]

References

1. Afghanistan Mortality Survey. 2010. Demographic health program. https://dhsprogram.com/pubs/pdf/fr248/fr248.pdf. Accessed 24 Jan 2020.
2. The World Bank. Afghanistan. https://data.worldbank.org/country/afghanistan. Accessed 21 Jan 2020.
3. Afghanistan Living Conditions Survey, 2016–17. National statistics and information authority, Kabul. https://www.nsia.gov.af:8080/wp-content/uploads/2019/04/ALCS-2016-17-Analysis-report-.pdf. Accessed 23 Jan 2020.
4. Afghanistan Development Update. 2018. The World Bank. http://documents.worldbank.org/curated/en/985851533222840038/Afghanistan-development-update. Accessed 23 Jan 2020.
5. National Health Strategy 2016–2017. Ministry of Public Health. http://old.moph.gov.af/en/page/579. Accessed 25 Jan 2020.
6. Afghanistan Health Survey. 2018. Royal Tropical Institute, Amsterdam. https://www.kit.nl/wp-content/uploads/2019/07/AHS-2018-report-FINAL-15-4-2019.pdf. Accessed 25 Jan 2020.
7. Afghanistan Demographic and Health Survey. 2015. Demographic health program. https://dhsprogram.com/pubs/pdf/FR323/FR323.pdf. Accessed 24 January 2020.
8. Afghanistan Services Provision Assessment. 2018. Demographic Health Program. https://www.dhsprogram.com/pubs/pdf/SPA31/SPA31.pdf. Accessed 27 Jan 2020.
9. Health Financing Policy 2012–2020. 2012. Ministry of Public Health. http://old.moph.gov.af/Content/files/ Health%20Financing % 20Policy%202012-2020.pdf. Accessed 25 Jan 2020.
10. Afghanistan National Health Accounts with Disease Accounts, 2017. Ministry of Public Health, Kabul. https://moph.gov.af/sites/default/files/2019-09/Afghanistan% 20National %20Health%20Accounts%

202017Final%20% 28Annexes%29%2024-8-2019% 20-min.pdf. Accessed 23 Jan 2020.
11. International Agency for Research on Cancer. 2018. https://gco.iarc.fr/today/data/factsheets/populations/4-afghanistan-fact-sheets.pdf. Accessed on 29 Jan 2020.
12. National Cancer Control Program. 2019. Ministry of public health. https://moph.gov.af/index.php/en/national-cancer-control-program-nccp. Accessed 15 Feb 2020.
13. National Cancer Control Program Afghanistan. 2020. Union for international cancer control. https://www.uicc.org/membership/national-cancer-control-program-afghanistan. Accessed 16 Jan 2020.
14. Stephen RC, Maria C, Sharon B, David C, James C, Dennis F, et al. Global atlas of palliative care at the end of life. World Health Organization. 2014. https://www.who.int/nmh/Global_Atlas_of_Palliative_Care.pdf. Accessed 30 Jan 2020.
15. Thomas L, Stephen C, David C. Mapping levels of palliative care development: a global update. J Pain Symptom Manag. 2013;45(6):1094–106. https://doi.org/10.1016/j.jpainsymman.2012.05.011.
16. Alaina dalton. Hamdardi development of a hospice program in Afghanistan. A pilot project. Slideplayer. 2011. https://slideplayer.com/slide/10342478/ Accessed 2 Feb 2020.
17. National Medicines and Healthcare Products Regulatory Authority. 2019. https://nmhra.gov.af/. Accessed 16 Feb 2020.
18. National Licensed Medicines List of Afghanistan. 2014. [Updated 2018]. General directorate of pharmaceutical affairs. http://gdpa.gov.af/Content/Media/Documents/AfghanistanLML_online 20150127122015117234l1553325325.pdf. Accessed 25 Jan 2020.
19. National Essential Medicines List of Afghanistan. 2014. World Health Organization. https://apps.who.int/medicinedocs/documents/s21737en /s21737en.pdf. Accessed 25 Jan 2020.
20. Afghanistan National Medicine Policy 2014–2019. 2014. General Directorate of Pharmaceutical Affairs. http://gdpa.gov.af/Content/Media/Documents/NMP_E_2014_20193010201473846558553325325.pdf. Accessed 25 Jan 2020.
21. Eric LK, Xiaoxiao K, Stéphane V, Hector A, Afsan B, Oscar M, et al. Palliative care and pain control. Disease control priorities: improving health and reducing poverty. National Center for Biotechnology Information. 2018. https://www.ncbi.nlm.nih.gov/books/NBK525289/pdf/Bookshelf_NBK525289.pdf. Accessed 27 Jan 2020.
22. World Health Organization Model List of Essential Medicines. 2019. https://apps.who.int/iris/bitstream/handle/10665/325771/WHO-MVP-EMP-IAU-2019.06-eng.pdf. Accessed 30 Jan 2020.
23. James C, Hellen G, Judith W. Cancer pain relief. Disease control priorities. 2018. http://dcp-3.org/sites/default/files/chapters/DCP3 %20CancerCh%209.pdf. Accessed 27 Jan 2020.
24. Anderson RE, Grant L. What is the value of palliative care provision in low-resource settings? Br Med J. 2016;2(1) https://doi.org/10.1136/bmjgh-2016-000139.
25. Henry D. Palliative care: what approaches are suitable in developing countries? Br J Haematol. 2011;154(6):728–35. https://doi.org/10.1111/j.1365-2141.2011.08764.x.

Part XXVIII

Central Asia: Armenia

Palliative Care for Cancer Patients in Armenia: A Silent Pain

Narine Movsesyan, Nune Karapetyan, Gevorg Tamamyan, and Jemma Arakelyan

Geography and the Sociodemographic Situation

The Republic of Armenia (RA) is located in South Caucasus. The RA borders with Georgia, Iran, Turkey, and Azerbaijan [1]. The total population of the country is 2.97 million. There is a slight female predominance: the gender ratio is 0.89 (53% female, 43% male) [2, 3].

From the beginning of RA's independency (in 1991), there was a number of obstacles to the country's development, including war, natural disasters, and the global financial crisis. In 1990, the gross domestic product (GDP) was US$ 2.26 billion. There has been remarkable progress in the economy since the end of 2018 when the new parliamentary government was formed after the Velvet Revolution. Currently, Armenia is considered to be an upper-middle-income country, and the GDP was expected to reach US$ 13.673 billion dollars in 2019; the gross national income (GNI) per capita was US$ 4680 in 2019 [4, 5].

During the years of the Soviet Union, Armenia's health-care system had a centralized, tertiary care-oriented structure; the state funding for health-care services were decided by the higher governing bodies. Patients were not informed regarding the available health-care options, such as choosing their physicians, and the hospitals were not prepared to compete and adapt to the changing demands of the market. After the independence of the Republic of Armenia in 1991, the health-care system faced a number of challenges, including war, earthquakes, and a socio-economic crisis. In parallel with the above-mentioned challenges, the health-care system experienced a number of reforms. Nowadays, public, primary and secondary health-care facilities are administered by the Ministry of Health (MoH) of RA and local governance bodies, such as municipalities. Along with public health-care facilities, there are a number of private ones. Health care is paid for by state and local budgets, medical insurance and out-of-pocket payments, including co-payments [7]. However, the majority of health-care services provided are not subsidized and are covered by the patients themselves. There is, however, a list of people with certain social and health conditions

N. Movsesyan
Department of Anesthesiology and Intensive Care, Yerevan State Medical University, Yerevan, Armenia

N. Karapetyan · J. Arakelyan (✉)
Department of Oncology, Yerevan State Medical University, Yerevan, Armenia

Chemotherapy Department of Adult Solid Tumors, Hematology Center after Prof. R. Yeolyan, Yerevan, Armenia

G. Tamamyan
The Pediatric Cancer and Blood Disorders Center of Armenia, Hematology Center after Prof. R. Yeolyan, Yerevan, Armenia

Department of Pediatric Hematology and Oncology, Yerevan State Medical University, Yerevan, Armenia

M. Silbermann (ed.), *Palliative Care for Chronic Cancer Patients in the Community*,
https://doi.org/10.1007/978-3-030-54526-0_40

whose health expenses are partially or fully funded by the state budget, known as the Basic Benefits Package (BBP). The BBP utilizes public funds to cover maternity, emergency, primary, pediatric, and oncological health-care services; the socially vulnerable population also receives health-care services under the BBP. Some of these services are fully covered, while others are partially covered (as with the treatment of oncological diseases) or require a co-payment. Most palliative care is not covered by the BBP [6–8].

Cancer in Armenia: Epidemiological Overview

Each year, approximately 18.1 million new cancer cases and more than 9.6 million cancer-related deaths are reported worldwide. 70% of these deaths resulted from malignant tumors and occur in low- and middle-income countries [9, 10].

It is estimated that the number of cancer cases will increase by 63% by 2040, which will pose additional burdens on health systems and require additional measures to improve the effectiveness of patient care [11].

Trends in Morbidity, Prevalence, and Mortality of NCDs in the Republic of Armenia (RA)

In recent years, the incidence of cancer reported among the RA population has somewhat stabilized. For example, in 2014 the number of first-time tumors diagnosed was 8365, and in 2017 it was 8389 (males 50.3%), increasing by only 0.02%. At the same time, in 2017 the number of registered cases increased by 14% (compared to 2008) and by 63% (compared to 1998) [12]. This could be attributable to the improvements in diagnostics, quality, and accessibility of health-care services and better registration, but could also be due to the increase in absolute numbers, meaning more people get cancer because of the aging population and increase in risk factors [19].

One of the leading identified risk factors for cancer is tobacco use [13–15]. In Armenia, GLOBOCAN 2018 reported that the mortality and morbidity rate of lung cancer, specifically, were 20% and 15.6%, respectively. According to the WHO Global Health Observatory data repository, in Armenia in 2018, the age standardized prevalence of smokers aged 15 years and older was 26.8%, meaning 52.1% of males and 1.5% of females were current smokers [16]. At the same time, the STEPS (Noncommunicable Disease Risk Factor *Survey*, part of the STEPwise approach to surveillance) project survey indicated that the number of males and females exposed to second-hand smoking at home and indoor workplaces are 56.4% and 26.6% of the population, respectively [17].

Among the other risk factors, infections are considered responsible for 15% of new cancer cases in the world. In Armenia, infections contribute to 12.2% of cancer cases [18]. Human papillomavirus infection, hepatitis B and C viruses, the Epstein-Barr virus, and others increase the risk of cancer. Also, alcohol abuse, malnutrition, ultraviolet radiation, obesity, sedentary lifestyle, etc. contribute to cancer development [13].

About 90% of all deaths in Armenia are attributable to noncommunicable diseases (NCDs) and the probability of premature mortality (up to the age of 70) caused by NCDs accounts for 22% [20].

Over the last five years, the analysis of cancer mortality rates has shown positive dynamics (Tables 1 and 2) [12].

Cancer Types

In 2018, the five most common cancer types sited in Armenia were lung (1375 cases), breast (1054 cases), colorectal (990 cases), prostate (636 cases), and stomach (586 cases) [21].

Table 1 Mortality structure of the RA population by causes of death [12]

Cause of death	2013	2014	2015	2016	2017	2018	Dynamics
CSD (cause-specific death)	12,960	13,268	12,817	13,571	15,106	14,209	897
Malignant tumors	5589	5685	6069	5662	5550	5199	↓351
Respiratory diseases	1645	1862	2126	2148	1644	1978	↓334
Diabetes mellitus	1305	1191	1276	1171	809	579	↓230

Table 2 Mortality dynamics of malignant tumors in Armenia, 2013–2018 [12]

		2013		2014		2015		2016		2017		2018	
№	RA Marz	I.[a]	N[b]	I.	N	I.	N	I.	N	I.	N	I.	N
1	RA, Total	1849	5589	1886	5685	202	6069	1892	5662	186.3	5550	175.1	5199
2	Yerevan	2109	2242	2053	2196	2129	2283	1886	2027	183.5	1976	1768	1909
3	Aragatsotn	1379	181	1555	205	1769	231	1656	215	186.2	238	1964	248
4	Ararat	1972	511	1575	410	1757	456	1596	413	149.2	385	1240	319
5	Armavir	1408	374	1434	383	1552	414	1476	393	155.4	412	1294	342
6	Gegharkunik	1116	261	1203	281	1463	340	1605	271	155.1	357	1624	372
7	Lori	2342	545	2629	603	2799	634	2561	571	267.8	587	2597	562
8	Kotayk	183	467	1855	473	219	557	2183	553	204.2	515	1848	465
9	Shirak	1998	498	2102	520	2263	554	2148	518	222.9	529	2061	483
10	Syunik	172	243	229	322	2125	297	2213	308	201.9	280	1587	219
11	Vayots Dzor	1712	89	1802	93	2114	108	1465	74	150.1	75	1643	81
12	Tavush	1391	178	1566	199	1546	195	176	220	158.1	196	1619	199

[a]Per 100,000 population
[b]Absolute numbers

Predictive Assessment of Disease

In 2016, it was reported that 10.97% of the RA population was age 65 years and older, and in 2018 this increased to 11.25%, or 98,000 more people [22], bringing Armenia to the top of the list of aging societies. The UN Population Fund forecasts indicate that Armenia will soon break that threshold, predicting that by 2050, those over 65 will make up more than 22% of the population [23, 24].

Currently in Armenia, the rate of cancer morbidity is high, and is expected to increase. It is predicted that the number of incidents of malignant neoplasms will reach 9915 in 2025, compared to the baseline of 8835 cases in 2018 [25]. Various factors contribute to these tendencies, including increasing demographic indicators. At the same time, there is a high prevalence of various risk factors responsible for the increased cancer morbidity and mortality rates, such as high body mass index, poor diet, lack of physical activity, tobacco use, and alcohol abuse.

Diagnostic Phase

The increased probability of longer survival rates for patients with malignant tumors is largely due to the greater number of options for early detection. It is concerning that in 2017 in Armenia, only 44.7% of all types of malignant tumors were diagnosed at Phases I and II, and 56.3% were diagnosed at Phases III and IV (Table 3). Furthermore, 68% of tracheal, bronchial, and lung cancers, 66% of stomach cancers, and 44% of colorectal and prostate cancers were detected at stage IV. Early detection of cervical cancer is also low. There has been positive progress in the early diagnosis of breast and bladder cancers, where 74% and 66% were found in stages I–II, respectively [12].

Considering the high prevalence of noncommunicable diseases and its increasing tendency in Armenia, a large number of patients suffering from pain, disabilities, etc., need qualified palliative care.

Palliative Care: General Principles and Epidemiology

According to the World Health Organization (WHO), "Palliative care is an approach that improves the quality of life of patients and their families facing the problems associated with life-threatening illness, through the prevention and relief of suffering by means of early identification and impeccable assessment and treatment of pain and other problems, physical, psychosocial and spiritual [26]". In addition to the foregoing, it should also be noted that the WHO has recognized palliative care as an integral component of health care that should be accessible to those in need and in urgent situations, including those with limited resources [27].

One of the key components of palliative care is pain management. Globally, about 80% of patients

Table 3 Stage of detection for most common malignant tumors, 2018

	Stage					
	I–II		III		IV	
Tumor type	*n*	%	*n*	%	*n*	%
Breast	751	73.6	66	6.5	204	20
Colon	14	35.6	124	30.8	135	33.6
Trachea, bronchi, lungs	119	18.6	106	16.6	414	64.8
Prostate	73	33	52	24	95	44
Cervix	68	38	101	43	45	19
Uterus	138	55	31	16	57	29
Ovary	41	37	57	35	46	28
Stomach	92	17	57	17	221	66
Bladder	239	67	31	10	70	23

with malignant tumors and AIDS, and 67% of patients with cardiovascular and chronic obstructive pulmonary diseases suffer from chronic pain at the late stages of the disease [28]. In 2011, WHO estimated that annually, 5.5 million late-stage cancer patients and 1 million patients with end-stage HIV/AIDS worldwide experience moderate to severe pain but have no access to adequate pain treatment [27]. Sixty to 80% of patients with malignant tumors suffer from chronic pain. In the case of advanced cancer, the number of patients with chronic pain reaches 45–100%, with 20–40% of the patients not controlling the pain. Moderate to severe pain has a profound effect on the quality of life, so permanent pain has a number of physical, psychological, and social consequences. It can reduce a person's mobility and result in loss of strength, weaken the immune system, and limit the ability to eat, concentrate, sleep, and interact with others [29].

Palliative Care in Armenia

After the collapse of the Soviet Union, the health-care system in Armenia was devastated. The main reason was the centralized structure of health-care system that required huge funding that cannot be afforded by a state budget at that time. During that period, palliative care was performed on a voluntary basis by certain individuals.

In 1993, given the impact of pain on a person's health and quality of life, the Single Convention on opioids has been implemented. The convention states that "the medical use of narcotic drugs continues to be indispensable for the relief of pain and suffering and that adequate provision must be made to ensure the availability of narcotic drugs for such purposes" [30].

In 2009–2010, to highlight the role and purpose of palliative care in Armenia, Stephen R. Connor, an international palliative care consultant, conducted a study on "Palliative Care Needs Assessment in Armenia", under the patronage of the Open Society Foundation. It was found that 18,000 people need palliative care annually. The research was followed by the implementation of palliative care in the country. Progress has been made due to the joint advocacy of international and local NGOs and local sectoral health-care providers. However, the study revealed that the lack of palliative care and accessibility to painkillers are still prevalent throughout the country [6, 31].

At the beginning of the 2010s, there were major legislative improvements in the field of palliative medicine. On August 15, 2012, the Government of Armenia signed the Palliative Care Concept Paper and its Action Plan [32]. On December 11, 2014, the Ministry of Health approved the "Clinical Guidelines for Prescribing Medicines and Psychotropic Drugs for Palliative Care and Services."

After the legislative changes from 2011 to 2014, within the framework of the Global Fund's "Health System Strengthening" grant program for four medical institutions of the Republic of Armenia: the National Center of Oncology of the RA MoH; the Heratsi Hospital Complex of Yerevan State Medical University; the Vanadzor Hospital Complex in Lori Marz; and the Ararat Medical Center in Ararat Marz, palliative care experimental programs were carried out in combination with home care, outpatient and inpatient services when needed. These programs were instructed to perform need assessments in terms of staff, expenditures, etc., for the full implementation of palliative care in Armenia. The information collected was then incorporated into a number of legislative regulations.

In 2012, a 10-bed palliative care department was established at the National Center of Oncology, but the provided services were not in high demand and the unit was soon dissolved. The low demand was due to, among other reasons, the fact that the palliative care provided in the unit was not included in the Basic Benefit Package (BBP) and was funded based on out-of-pocket payments.

In 2017, a state program for palliative medical care and the development of corresponding services was implemented; it intended to establish and introduce mechanisms for the provision of palliative medical care in inpatient and outpatient services. It also planned to improve legislation, develop clinical guidelines on palliative care, and to include this branch of medicine into postgraduate studies as well as other higher education programs.

Currently, the Ministry of Health (MoH) of the RA has launched a pilot project in which mobile palliative care will be delivered in two primary health-care facilities in Yerevan. The service is covered by the BBP. In 2020, the MoH plans to establish inpatient units/hospices at hospitals licensed to provide palliative care.

Another initiative aiming to address pediatric cancer palliative care has been carried out by the City of Smile Charitable Foundation and Hematology Center after Prof. R.H.Yeolyan. A five-bed, state-of-the-art pediatric palliative care clinic is currently under construction at the Hematology Center, where the only Pediatric Cancer and Blood Disorders Center of Armenia is located, and it is expected to begin operating in June 2020. The design and implementation of this program was corroborated by world-known experts from St. Jude Children's Research Hospital (SJCRH, USA). These specialists who will be running the clinic are involved in palliative care improvement programs within the framework of Eurasian Alliance for Pediatric Oncology, under the umbrella of SJCRH.

The overwhelming majority of the financial resources directed to implement palliative care programs have been funded by international organizations. Hence, the portion of the total budget envisaged for the health sector must be reviewed and funds should be allocated to provide palliative care services within existing resources.

Despite the fact that the use of drugs for pain relief is not prohibited in Armenia by either domestic legislation or international regulations, the analysis of responses to inquiries and real-life cases have revealed inadequate pain management among patients in Armenia who need palliative care.

Availability of Drugs: Morphine Need Assessment in RA

The use of opioid analgesics, especially morphine, in palliative care for pain control is extremely low in Armenia. In 2010, the morphine-equivalent Adequacy Consumption Measure (ACM) per capita was found to be 0.88 mg., while the actual need of the morphine equivalents in the country was 305.56 mg [33].

One of the conditions for providing access to pain control within the framework of palliative care is the compatibility of the medications available with the WHO Model List of Essential Medicines. The opioid analgesics included in this list are as follows [34]:

- Codeine phosphate
- Fentanyl patch
- Morphine hydrochloride or morphine sulphate for injections, pills, intravenous solutions and granules, oral solution
- Methadone

Most of the opioid analgesics (morphine for injection, and oral, methadone) intended for pain relief and palliative care were approved by the RA MoH in 2018 and are fully in line with the WHO Model List of Essential Medicines [35].

According to the opioid prescription regulations, the drugs are discharged without a commission. The prescription for drugs containing narcotics and psychotropic substances must be written by the treating physician (regardless of specialty), and then endorsed by the director of the medical institution. The prescription for the dose and quantity approved by the physician is valid for 10 days. Legislation has been approved for the assessment and management guidelines for patients' pain within palliative care and services, by which the health-care provider can determine what type of medication and dosage should be assigned to the patient. However, even after these changes, health-care providers often do not prescribe narcotic painkillers and avoid prescribing large doses [36].

Education and Training of the Medical Staff

The provision of palliative care depends on many factors, including financial capabilities, staffing, and more.

Palliative care in Armenia is much more advanced than in many countries of the former Soviet Union, as, in 2017, numerous legislative regulations were put into place to strengthen and facilitate the implementation of palliative care. However, there are some obstacles that have led to the delay in the widespread introduction of palliative care such as the lack of awareness and education of the staff.

In 2017, the only postgraduate program for nurses and physicians specializing in palliative care was in Yerevan State Medical University (YSMU). The duration of the program was four months for physicians and three months for nurses. There is currently only one course on palliative medicine in YSMU, which was introduced in 2017 for primary care fellows and taught during the second year of clinical residency. Only 10 second-year interns specializing in family medicine passed this course.

Programs for specialized and advanced training of graduate students were developed at YSMU. Between 2016 and 2018, a total of 29 nurses attended the one- and two-week training courses. In addition, from 2010 to 2017, a number of NGOs, with assistance from the Open Society Foundation of RA, provided one- and two-week trainings courses to primary care physicians [31].

According to local experts, there currently 20 doctors and 20 nurses specialized in the field of palliative medicine in Armenia, but only a few of them actually practice palliative care.

Currently, there are no educational programs on palliative care in Armenia. Principally, in countries where palliative medicine is an integral part of health care, there is a three-tiered educational approach: palliative care is first taught at university, then as a postgraduate training program, and thereafter, those physicians who wish to specialize in palliative care attend subspecialty courses [37].

Gaps in Palliative Care in Armenia

For most societies and health-care providers, palliative care is generally viewed as an abstract idea or service, separate from public life; however, the social component is a large part of palliative care.

Over the years, adapting and improving procedures to facilitate access to pain relievers in medical institutions has been hampered due to various factors: among them are a lack of guidelines for the use of narcotic substances for medical purposes, supervisory actions of the police and fear of the medical staff, low awareness of patients and their families about drug use for medical purposes, as well as the shortage of trained doctors.

The country does not have an adequate amount of specialists or integrated sub-specialty projects, nor the general vision for how palliative care should be integrated into the medical field or society, and no work is being carried out to rectify this matter.

Legislative and policy reforms for palliative care in the RA were introduced in 2008. However, they have not been sufficient to ensure availability and accessibility of the service. Even if all the necessary legislative changes are made and the relevant medical institutions are licensed to provide palliative care services, it will still not be possible to ensure full palliative care as long as there are no specialists with proper specialized education. The problem lies in that the professionals involved in the palliative care team are the primary source of information for the patients. Lack of awareness and education among healthcare personnel results in misconception among patients and their family members about the different components of palliative care. It is believed that only terminally ill patients receive this care. Therefore, it is extremely important to include well-trained, knowledgeable professionals in the team. Also, it is necessary to provide regular training opportunities for all team members [38].

A number of NGOs performed field visits and face-to-face interviews to assess the palliative care provided in Armenia. The results showed that majority of patients are in need of palliative care and do not receive services that meet the WHO standards, including proper pain relief [38]. The reason for this disparity is the fact that measures aimed to ensure patients' access to opioid analgesics are in constant competition with the policy of combating drug trafficking [36]. There are few countries in the world that have managed to maintain a balance between proper patient pain and drug control. Most countries prefer restrictive policies for opioid analgesics utilization and maintain strict oversight. For this reason, in the most former Soviet Union countries, patients are deprived of the opportunity to live without pain [39, 40]. Conversely, there are countries where the liberalization and excessive prevalence of opioid painkillers have caused problems such as deaths due to opioid overdose and physician-mediated drug dependence, mainly related to unnecessary prescriptions [41].

Therefore, palliative care may be fully introduced if the role of health-care policymakers and authorities responsible for carrying these out – the Ministry of Health, police officers dealing with drug trafficking, as well as inpatient and outpatient (including mobile) palliative care providers, are fulfilled properly and harmoniously, and the actions of one interested party do not limit the responsibilities and regular activities of the other.

References

1. About Armenia – Geography – The Government of the Republic of Armenia [Internet]. [cited 2020 Jan 22]. Available from: https://www.gov.am/en/geography/.
2. About Armenia – Demographics – The Government of the Republic of Armenia [Internet]. [cited 2020 Jan 22]. Available from: https://www.gov.am/en/demographics/.
3. Armenia Demographics 2020 (Population, Age, Sex, Trends) – Worldometer [Internet]. [cited 2020 Jan 22]. Available from: https://www.worldometers.info/demographics/armenia-demographics/#age-structure.
4. Data for Armenia, Upper- middle-income|Data [Internet]. [cited 2020 Jan 22]. Available from: https://data.worldbank.org/?locations=AM-XT.
5. Armenia Overview [Internet]. [cited 2020 Jan 22]. Available from: https://www.worldbank.org/en/country/armenia/overview#1.
6. Richardson E. Health systems in transition. Vol. 15, Armenia health system review. 2013. [cited 2020 Jan 22]. Available from: http://www.euro.who.int/_data/assets/pdf_file/0008/234935/HiT-Armenia.pdf?ua=1.
7. Report National Health Accounts of Armenia – 2017 [Internet]. [cited 2020 Jan 22]. Available from: https://nih.am/assets/pdf/atvk/9a41bb8fb3968df4046c1466e4404fa0.pdf.
8. Rouselle F. Lavado, Susanna Hayrapetyan, and Samvel Kharazyan. Universal Health Coverage Study Series No. 27 Expansion of the Benefits Package: The Experience of Armenia [Internet]. [cited 2020 Jan 22]. Available from: http://documents.worldbank.org/curated/en/615741516195329170/pdf/Expansion-of-the-benefits-package-the-experience-of-Armenia.pdf.
9. PRESS RELEASE N° 263 [Internet]. 2018 [cited 2020 Jan 22]. Available from: https://www.who.int/cancer/PRGlobocanFinal.pdf.
10. Cancer [Internet]. [cited 2020 Jan 22]. Available from: https://www.who.int/news-room/fact-sheets/detail/cancer.
11. Cancer Tomorrow [Internet]. [cited 2020 Jan 22]. Available from: https://gco.iarc.fr/tomorrow/home.
12. Statistics – Ministry of Health of the Republic of Armenia. [cited 2020 Jan 22].
13. Jacob L, Freyn M, Kalder M, Dinas K, Kostev K. Impact of tobacco smoking on the risk of developing 25 different cancers in the UK: a retrospective study of 422,010 patients followed for up to 30 years [Internet]. [cited 2020 Jan 22]. Available from: www.oncotarget.com.
14. O'Keeffe LM, Taylor G, Huxley RR, Mitchell P, Woodward M, Peters SAE. Smoking as a risk factor for lung cancer in women and men: a systematic review and meta-analysis. BMJ Open. 2018;8(10):e021611.
15. Taylor R, Gumming R, Woodward A, Black M. Passive smoking and lung cancer: A cumulative meta-analysis. Aust N Z J Public Health. 2001;25(3):203–11.
16. GHO|By category|SDG Target 3.a|Tobacco control – Data by country [Internet]. [cited 2020 Feb 9]. Available from: https://apps.who.int/gho/data/node.main.SDG3A?lang=en.
17. Andreasyan D, Bazarchyan A, Torosyan A, Sargsyan S. Prevalence of tobacco smoking in Armenia, STEPs survey. Tob Induc Dis. 2018;16(3)
18. Infection|The Cancer Atlas [Internet]. [cited 2020 Jan 22]. Available from: https://canceratlas.cancer.org/risk-factors/infection/.
19. Shah SC, Kayamba V, Peek RM, Heimburger D. Cancer control in low- and middle-income countries: is it time to consider screening? J Glob Oncol. 2019;5:1–8.
20. UN in Armenia: News: Launch of the Armenia Noncommunicable Diseases (NCDs) Investment Case report [Internet]. [cited 2020 Jan 22]. Available from: https://www.un.am/en/news/860.
21. Armenia Source: Globocan 2018. [Internet]. [cited 2020 Jan 22]. Available from: https://gco.iarc.fr/today/data/factsheets/populations/51-armenia-fact-sheets.pdf.
22. Population ages 65 and above (% of total population) – Armenia|Data [Internet]. [cited 2020 Jan 22]. Available from: https://data.worldbank.org/indicator/SP.POP.65UP.TO.ZS?locations=AM.
23. Ada. FINAL EVALUATION REPORT [Internet]. 2016 [cited 2020 Jan 22]. Available from: https://www.unfpa.org/sites/default/files/Armenia_CPE_report_2016-2020.pdf.
24. World Population Ageing [highlights]. [Internet]. [cited 2020 Jan 22]. Available from: https://www.

un.org/en/development/desa/population/publications/pdf/ageing/WPA2017_Highlights.pdf.
25. Cancer Tomorrow [Internet]. [cited 2020 Jan 22]. Available from: https://gco.iarc.fr/tomorrow/graphic-isotype?type=1&population=900&mode=population&sex=0&cancer=39&age_group=value&apc_male=0&apc_female=0.
26. WHO|WHO Definition of Palliative Care [Internet]. [cited 2020 Jan 22]. Available from: https://www.who.int/cancer/palliative/definition/en/.
27. Strengthening of palliative care as a component of integrated treatment throughout the life course Report by the Secretariat [Internet]. [cited 2020 Jan 22]. Available from: https://apps.who.int/gb/ebwha/pdf_files/EB134/B134_28-en.pdf.
28. Palliative Care [Internet]. [cited 2020 Jan 22]. Available from: https://www.who.int/news-room/fact-sheets/detail/palliative-care.
29. Brennan F, Carr DB, Cousins M. Pain management: a fundamental human right. Anesthesia Analgesia. 2007;105:205–21.
30. United Convention on Drugs of 1961, Compliance to Protocol 1972, Amendments to United Convention on Drugs of 1961 [Internet]. [cited 2020 Jan 22]. Available from: https://www.arlis.am/DocumentView.aspx?DocID=76214.
31. Papikyan A, Connor SR, Amiryan D. Development of palliative care in Armenia. J Pain Symptom Manage. 2018;55:S19–24. https://doi.org/10.1016/j.jpainsymman.2017.02.023.
32. Executive Summary of the Government Session of the Republic of Armenia on Approval of the Concept of Palliative Care and Assistance of Palliative Care. [Internet]. [cited 2020 Jan 22]. Available from: https://www.arlis.am/DocumentView.aspx?DocID=77569.
33. Beatrice Duthey B, Scholten W. Adequacy of Opioid Analgesic Consumption at Country, Global, and Regional Levels in 2010, Its Relationship with Development Level, and Changes Compared With 2006 Journal of Pain and Symptom Management 1. J Pain Symptom Manage [Internet]. 2013 [cited 2020 Jan 22]; Available from: https://www.esmo.org/content/download/34220/681134/file/Journal_of_pain_&_symptom_management_Scholten2013.pdf.
34. WHO Model List of Essential Medicines [Internet]. 2017 [cited 2020 Jan 22]. Available from: http://www.who.int/medicines/publications/essentialmedicines/en/.
35. Drugs [Internet]. [cited 2020 Aug 17]. Available from: http://pharm.cals.am/pharm/drug_images/index.php.
36. Barros De Luca G, Zopunyan V, Burke-Shyne N, Papikyan A, Amiryan D. Palliative care and human rights in patient care: an Armenia case study. [Internet]. [cited 2020 Jan 22]. Available from: https://publichealthreviews.biomedcentral.com/track/pdf/10.1186/s40985-017-0062-7.
37. Education in Palliative Care: Building a Culture of Learning – Google Books [Internet]. [cited 2020 Jan 22]. Available from: https://books.google.am/books?id=a4iHZxK_F7IC&pg=PA50&lpg=PA50&dq=palliative+care+three+tiered+education&source=bl&ots=uVIKIzfY0S&sig=ACfU3U2Qo8i0e4nTn7AHLA4MwsWJNExHlA&hl=ru&sa=X&ved=2ahUKEwjDj5iktZTnAhUBwsQBHWpzAAwQ6AEwCnoECAgQAQ#v=onepage&q=palliative care three tiered education&f=false.
38. Cancer and the Struggle for Palliative Care in Armenia|HRW [Internet]. [cited 2020 Jan 22]. Available from: https://www.hrw.org/report/2015/07/14/all-i-can-do-is-cry/cancer-and-struggle-palliative-care-armenia.
39. Clark F. Russia's war on drugs leaves patients without pain relief. Lancet. 2015;386:231–2.
40. Lohman D, Schleifer R, Amon JJ. Access to pain treatment as a human right [Internet]. 2010 [cited 2020 Jan 22]. Available from: http://www.biomedcentral.com/1741-7015/8/8.
41. Opioid Overdose Crisis|National Institute on Drug Abuse (NIDA) [Internet]. [cited 2020 Jan 22]. Available from: https://www.drugabuse.gov/drugs-abuse/opioids/opioid-overdose-crisis.

Part XXIX

Central Asia: Kazakhstan

Mobile Teams in Kazakhstan: Improving Cancer Patients' Access to Palliative Care

Gulnara Kunirova, Dilyara Kaidarova,
and Tolganai Ansatbayeva

Introduction

Cancer is the second leading cause of premature death in Kazakhstan with the incidence rates increasing by approximately 1–1.5% annually. In 2018, cancer claimed 14,369 lives of Kazakhstan citizens, at the rate of approximately 39 people a day; 32,228 new cases of the disease were registered. The total number of patients receiving cancer care by the end of 2018 was 181,202. Within the last 25 years, the overall cancer death rates have dropped by 29% due to significant improvements in prevention and early detection. However, the percentage of late stage diagnosis remains relatively high at 37–40% [2].

Even though most cancers are not immediately fatal, many patients experience months to years of life-limiting illness with a relatively brief period of decline prior to death, when they will need palliative care at a certain point.

Since the early 2000s, in-patient hospice services in the country have been available to provide nursing care and symptom management only to a limited number of cancer patients approaching end of life. Located very sporadically across the country, without being justified by any statistical data, they served only the needs of locally residing citizens. Long distances between province centers (where the majority of health-care facilities are located) and rural districts (some may be as far away as 600 kilometers), added to the inequality of access to hospice care. The number of hospice beds did not change much within two decades, with only one new hospice, opened in Taraz in 2017.

To address the urgent deficit of palliative beds, 208 new beds were deployed during the last 5 to 6 years in 13 out of 17 regional cancer centers under the overpassed National Cancer Care Development Plan for 2012–2016 [3]. Unintentionally, the inclusion of palliative care into the clinical practice of oncology centers highlighted the difference between end-of-life care provided in hospices and earlier palliative care provided in specialized cancer treatment facilities. It became more obvious that patients should not have to choose between treatment with curative intent or comfort care, and there is a need for both, in varying degrees, throughout the course of cancer, whether the eventual

G. Kunirova (✉)
Kazakhstan Association for Palliative Care (KAPC), Together Against Cancer Foundation, International Association for Hospice and Palliative Care (IAHPC), Almaty, Republic of Kazakhstan

D. Kaidarova
Kazakh Institute of Oncology and Radiology, Kazakhstan Association of Oncologists, National Academy of Sciences, Almaty, Republic of Kazakhstan

T. Ansatbayeva
Almaty Oncology Center, Kazakh Institute of Oncology and Radiology, Almaty, Republic of Kazakhstan

M. Silbermann (ed.), *Palliative Care for Chronic Cancer Patients in the Community*,
https://doi.org/10.1007/978-3-030-54526-0_41

outcome is long-term survival or death [3]. While hospices provide care for people from the point at which they can no longer receive any specialist anticancer treatment to the end of their lives, palliative care wards in cancer clinics provide symptomatic and pain treatment to patients still receiving chemotherapy or radiation therapy aimed at cure [4].

As of today, the total number of palliative care beds available for cancer patients is 354, including hospices (146 beds) and special wards in cancer clinics (208 beds). However, the estimated need in in-patient palliative care for cancer patients is about 810 beds. This estimation is based upon the National Standard of Organization of Palliative Care, which provides for 30 in-patient palliative beds to be established per 400,000 of population [5], and the assumption that 60% of patients in need of palliative care in Kazakhstan are those with cancer.

Concurrently with the opening of in-patient palliative care wards in oncology centers, various nongovernmental organizations in different parts of the country started their home-based services for those patients who were no longer receiving in-patient specialist care and had no access to hospice facilities. Although only few of them have proven their financial and institutional sustainability, their contribution to the development of outpatient palliative care services in Kazakhstan was outstanding. In fact, they set a new model of holistic multidisciplinary in-home palliative care to patients, proving to the government that it is economically efficient, socially beneficial, and humane.

As an example, the Almaty Mobile Team was launched in December of 2013 in Kazakhstan's biggest city of 1,777,000 people. During the first 2 years, it functioned as a pilot project, funded by the Open Society Foundation, but later the service became part of the Almaty Oncology Center. Due to the continuing support of the Together Against Cancer Foundation, today, families of cancer patients are able to use functional beds, oxygen concentrators, wheelchairs, walking frames, gel mattresses preventing bed sores, folding bathtubs, etc., for free. The Foundation also provides methodological assistance to newly opening mobile teams across the country and conducts training courses for palliative care specialists. To date, over 7000 home visits were made by the Almaty Mobile Team, and each year the number of visits almost doubled due to better awareness among medical community and public as well as improvement of referral procedures.

A "Good Care" Case

At 09:15 a.m. the hotline operator of the Almaty Mobile Team received a request from a district oncologist. Each primary care oncologist can place a formalized request for Mobile Team visit through a WhatsApp group or by email. Family carers can also make their requests through a hotline telephone number. The operator collects and processes requests. Depending on the urgent need of the family, at first visit the doctor can be accompanied by a nurse and/or a psychologist and/or a social worker. Although the Mobile Team is not an emergency ambulance but a visiting service, some calls require urgent reaction (Fig. 1).

T. was a 59-year-old driver with a Stage 3 Pancoast tumor (a rare form of lung cancer) with bone metastasis. He looked exhausted after 19 cycles of chemotherapy. He was still receiving bisphosphonates and targeted therapy, but his condition had significantly deteriorating in the last three days. At the time of first visit, he had multiple complaints: breathlessness even at rest, anxiety, lack of appetite due to nausea, sleep disorder, irritability, anxiety, constipation, and

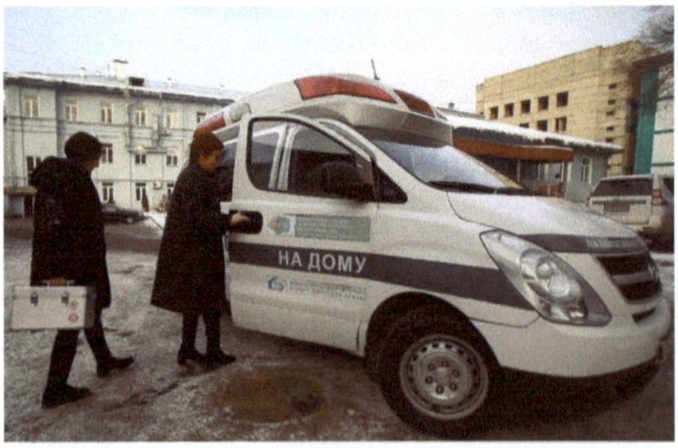

Fig. 1 A local bank sponsored the purchase of a car for the Almaty Mobile Team

fatigue. On top of all, his pain score was 9/10 and was characterized as excruciating, persistent, multiple, irradiating, burning, and intensifying with movement. Tramadol, a weak opioid used for treatment of moderate pain given by the physician of the district primary care clinic to which T. was assigned, had no effect.

The doctor was supported by the psychologist at her first visit, and while the doctor talked to the patient, conducted physical examination, provided necessary care, and administered medication to ease pain and breathlessness, the psychologist worked with the wife and children. She assessed the psychosocial needs of the family and answered their questions. Through the 45-minute visit, one could notice the change in the physical and emotional condition of the patient. The family was left with new medication prescriptions and corrected dosage of previously prescribed painkillers, instructions concerning care, and necessary telephone numbers for emergency calls. For the first time in many weeks, the patient gave a weak smile and waved goodbye to his saviors (Fig. 2).

During the next 7 days, the patient was visited by the nurse, who made her assessment of the patient's care needs, administered his daily treatment prescribed by the doctor, taught the family caregivers how to keep the patient clean and provide better care and how to administer medications and help him with everyday procedures.

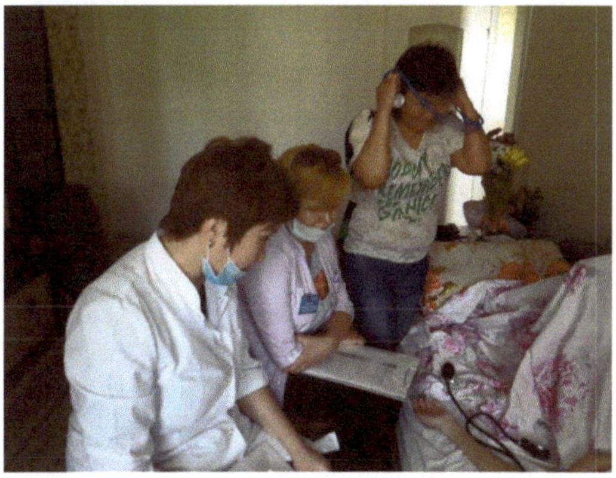

Fig. 2 Physician, psychologist, and nurse visiting the patient in Almaty

On the third day from the first visit, the nurse reported improvement of the quality of life of the patient. He was now able to sleep at night; he started to eat food and his respiratory condition improved. His pain scores had dropped from 8–9 to 3–4.

The next visit of the doctor took place 2 weeks later: the pain therapy scheme was corrected and other symptoms, like lymphedema and urinary difficulties, were addressed. The family also asked for the support of the social worker and the psychologist.

When T.'s pain and breathlessness worsened again after 5 weeks, he was switched to morphine. Adjuvants and oxygen therapy were added. A portable oxygen concentrator, a special mattress to prevent the bedsores and diapers were provided for free by the Together Against Cancer Foundation.

The patient was under the patronage of the Mobile Team for 8.5 weeks, during which the doctor visited him six times, the nurse 20 times, the psychologist five times, and the social worker two times. All team members were available for consultations at certain hours.

T. passed away on Sunday. His wife wrote a little note: "Dear Doctor Tolganai, last night my husband passed away. There was no pain, he wasn't suffocating, his heart just failed. Thank you for being with us during this difficult time. There is no way we could get through it without your team. What you do is priceless."

A "Bad Care" Case

Around the same time, in the small town of Shemonaikha, 1270 kilometers away from Almaty (equivalent to the driving distance between Paris and Madrid), a man was suffering from severe pain. B. was a 57-year-old electrical engineer recently diagnosed with late stage thyroid cancer. He was discharged home from the oncology center, where he received chemotherapy, with a metastasis in his lungs and progressive tumor intoxication.

Shemonaikha is the center of a rural district with a population of only 44,350 people. There is a Central District Hospital, which includes a local network of small primary care facilities, but the closest palliative care ward is located 110 kilometers away, in the city of Ust-Kamenogorsk.

In order to support his family, B. had to work in spite of his rapidly deteriorating health condition. “When things got worse, we could neither get proper help at home, nor have him admitted to the central hospital. There is no oncologist in our hospital or in the local outpatient clinic. A nurse from the outpatient clinic visited us several times to help with care. But every time he was in pain, we’d have to call the ambulance.” Searching for help, B.’s sister found the number of the Kazakhstan Palliative Care Association on the Internet. She had several telephone consultations with the Almaty doctors and received psychological support, but at some point B.’s breathlessness became worse and the family decided to take B. to the palliative care ward in the Ust-Kamenogorsk oncology center. Winters are harsh in Eastern Kazakhstan and the trip was not very easy for the family. Worst of all, the clinic ran out of some drugs, so the relatives had to buy some medicines in the nearby pharmacy. After B. received oxygen and medication, he let his sister go back home. The next day she had to take this long trip once again to spend time with her brother, who died in her arms 30 minutes after she arrived.

Light at the End of the Tunnel

Despite the disparity in access to palliative care and multiple challenges to its overall development, the best way to describe the current status of palliative care in Kazakhstan would be with an analogy showing the light at the end of the tunnel.

From being nonexistent only 20 years ago, palliative care in Kazakhstan is now moving slowly, but straightforwardly, toward integration into the mainstream health-care system.

There are several reasons for optimism on the global and national scale.

In 2014, the global resolution on palliative care (WHA67.19) called upon the WHO Member States to improve access to palliative care as a core component of health systems, with an emphasis on primary health care and community/home-based care. In the WHO Global Action Plan for the Prevention and Control of Noncommunicable Diseases 2013–2020, palliative care was clearly recognized as part of the comprehensive services required for noncommunicable diseases. High-quality palliative care is an explicit element of the WHO Framework on integrated people-centered services, approved at the 69th World Health Assembly in 2016 [6].

Palliative care and pain relief are essential elements of universal health coverage (UHC) and a special focus is made on equity for all populations, particularly the poorest and most marginalized, who should be able to access the health-care services that they require [7].

The Lancet Commission on Palliative Care and Pain Relief assessing global palliative care needs was released in October 2017 with the aim of quantifying the heavy burden of serious health-related suffering (SHS), identifying an essential package of palliative care medicines and measuring the unmet need for the use of opioids [8].

On October 25, 2018, the Declaration of Astana was approved by the Heads of State and Ministers of Health during the historical Global Conference on Primary Healthcare held in the Kazakhstan capital, Astana (recently renamed to Nur-Sultan). For the first time in history, palliative care was mentioned in the context of universal coverage and primary health care. The Declaration includes the following two references to palliative care: (1) “Promotive, preventive, curative, rehabilitative services and palliative care must be accessible to all”; and (2) under the heading “Build sustainable primary health care” the declaration states: “We will prioritize disease prevention and health promotion and will aim to meet all people’s health needs across the life course through comprehensive preventive, promotive, curative, rehabilitative services and palliative care.” Thus, The Astana Declaration explicitly calls for countries to integrate palliative care into primary health care [9] (Fig. 3).

In the 2014 edition of the Global Atlas of Palliative Care at the End of Life, Kazakhstan ranked as a Group 3A country but, according to

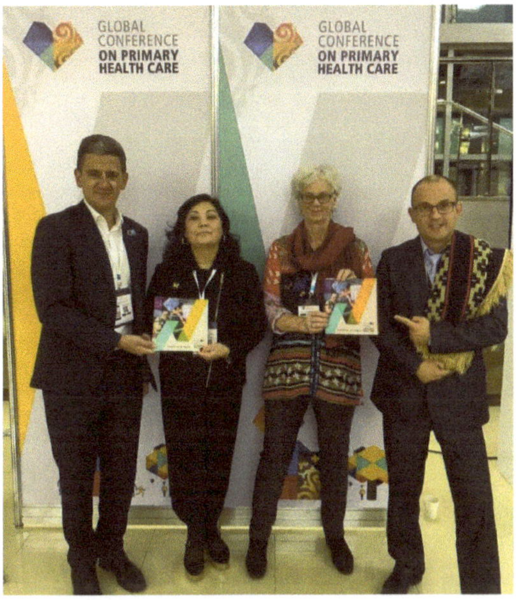

Fig. 3 The IAHPC delegation at the 2019 Global Conference on Primary Healthcare in Astana, Kazakhstan

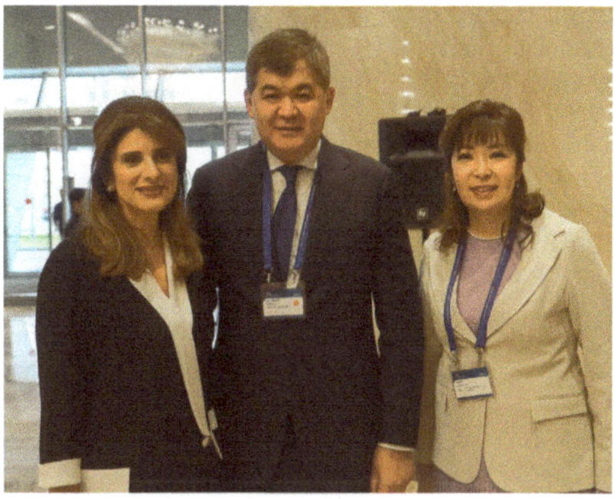

Fig. 4 The UICC President, H.R.H. Princess Dina Mired, Minister of Health, Dr. Yelzhan Birtanov, Director of KazIOR, Acad. Dilyara Kaidarova on the opening of the 2019 World Cancer Leaders' Summit in Nur-Sultan, Kazakhstan

Stephen Connor, Executive Director of the Worldwide Hospice Palliative Care Alliance (WHPCA), Kazakhstan has risen to a 4A group in the new edition of the Atlas that will be published later in 2020. The 4A group refers to countries where hospice and palliative care services are at the preliminary stage of integration into mainstream service provision. This group of countries is characterized by: the development of a critical mass of palliative care activism in a number of locations; a variety of palliative care providers and types of services; awareness of palliative care on the part of health professionals and local communities; the availability of morphine and some other strong pain-relieving medicines; limited impact of palliative care upon policy; the provision of a substantial number of training and education initiatives by a range of organizations; and interest in the concept of a national palliative care association [10].

This progress was made due to tireless efforts of a group of highly committed individuals and organizations, especially those united under the umbrella of the Kazakhstan Association for Palliative Care (KAPC), which serves as the main driving force of changes in the legislation, methodology, education and training, institutional development, clinical practices, and attitudes of the public to hospice and palliative care (Fig. 4). KAPC was created with the intention to combine efforts of local champions, from Members of Parliament to volunteers, international experts, partner organizations like the Open Society Foundation, IAHPC, WHPCA, EAPC, UICC, ASCO, NIH/NCI, MECC, and many others, to speed up the development of palliative care in Kazakhstan [11].

On the national level, a major change in the health-care system is taking place right now with the transition to insurance medicine and a number of other important developments.

The Mandatory Social Health Insurance (MSHI) system was launched on January 1, 2020, under which all citizens and permanent residents of Kazakhstan will have access to two packages of medical care: the state-guaranteed basic package and the health insurance fund package. Palliative care is included in the so-called guaranteed package of medical assistance, which means that it will remain free-of-charge for defined categories of patients irrespective of their status within the insurance system [12].

The growing attention of the oncologists to the problems of incurable cancer patients was demonstrated during the 2019 World Cancer

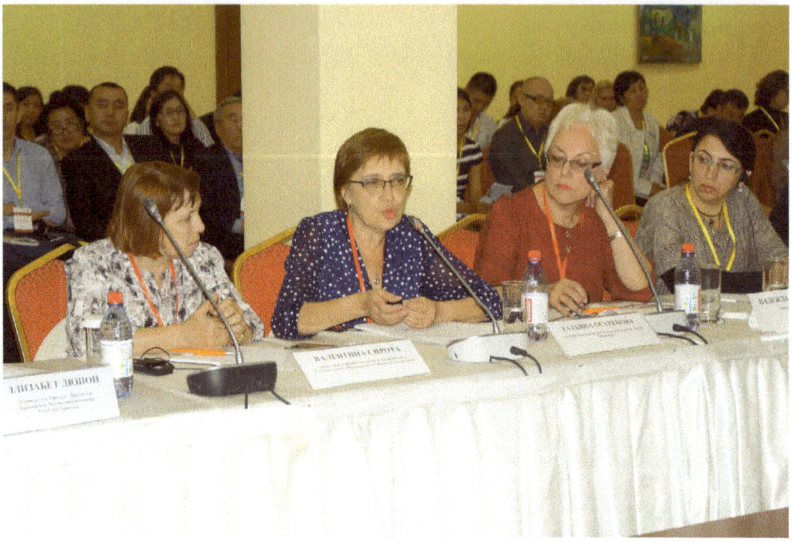

Fig. 5 Palliative care champions from KAPC speaking at the International Round Table on access to opioids "Stop My Pain" in Nur-Sultan

Leader's Summit, hosted by the Kazakh Institute of Oncology and Radiology (KazIOR) in Kazakhstan's capital, Nur-Sultan, from October 15 to 17; 350 global influencers and leaders in cancer control and public health from 82 countries and from across governments, UN agencies, academia, nonprofit organizations, and private sectors considered the ways in which cancer detection, treatment, and care can contribute to the achievement of Universal Health Coverage [13] (Fig. 5).

The Comprehensive Cancer Control Plan for 2018–2022 devotes a special section to the integration of palliative care into cancer care practices. It includes measures aimed at the introduction of mobile teams for incurable patients; training physicians, nurses, psychologists, and social workers; estimation of tariffs for palliative care services; and development of guidelines for service providers and cooperation with NGOs [3].

A broader perspective on future developments of palliative care in the short-term was presented in the Roadmap for the Improvement of Palliative Care in the Republic of Kazakhstan for 2019–2020, developed and approved by the Ministry of Health of the Republic of Kazakhstan in collaboration with the Kazakh Association for Palliative Care, oncologists, and international experts. The document provides for further amendment of the legislation and regulations, review of clinical protocols, analysis of the current resources, including human capacity, activities of NGOs, training of regional trainers, raising awareness, etc. The Roadmap contains goals that are achievable in a 2-year period, but these are only initial steps on the way to full integration of palliative care in the health-care system [14].

Advantages and Barriers to the Development of Home-Based Palliative Care in Kazakhstan

It would not be an exaggeration to say that the achievement of mutual understanding and the focus on cooperation between all stakeholders was the main breakthrough of recent years. However, we are still facing a lot of challenges, ranging from important political decisions to the everyday delivery of palliative care to patients at all levels of care: primary, secondary, and tertiary.

Home-based palliative care is needed for people with various chronic and life-limiting health problems – not only cancer, but many other conditions such as advanced cardiac, renal, and respiratory diseases, HIV/AIDS, and chronic neurological disorders.

Based on the work of the Lancet Commission on Global Access to Palliative Care, the total number of patients in need of palliative care in 2015 was estimated at 134,190 patients with serious, life-threatening conditions. Over 55,000 of them were patients with cancer. At this point of time, in-home palliative care is only available to cancer patients in Kazakhstan.

The development of mobile teams contributes to the progress of integrating cancer treatment, primary medical care, and palliative care services that are administratively separated. It also opens opportunities for patients to get broader access to consultations with oncology specialists, diagnostic facilities, and minor surgeries.

The WHO Guide for Program Managers on Planning and Implementing Palliative Care Services points at a number of advantages of home-based palliative care in many situations. Many patients feel more comfortable in their home than in a health-care setting. In a country like Kazakhstan, where several generations of a family tend to stay together, this is particularly true. A home-based service means that family members are integrated into the process, which, in turn, means that the patient has better access to care. A home-based approach provides advice and support to family members to help them as caregivers, and the home-care team is able to facilitate referral to additional services. While the home-based care helps the family maintain privacy and confidentiality, at the same time it helps to increase community awareness about palliative care. Local mass media, especially social media, contributes a lot to the promotion and dissemination of information about available palliative care services and the feedback stimulates providers to make improvements to patient care [15].

Immediate-release oral morphine was registered in the country over a year ago, thanks to the local producer VivaPharm, but difficulties with supply and distribution still occur at year end and beginning. Besides, physicians are poorly informed about the availability of such a drug and primary medical organizations do not order oral morphine, habitually using injection forms. Slow-release fentanyl patches are available, but again, more training is required for health professionals to properly prescribe and administer these medicines.

The following are barriers that exist in the health-care system and stand in the way of many people receiving high-quality palliative care where and when they needed it most:

- Inadequate training in pain and symptom management, as well as other palliative care skills, among health-care professionals dedicated by medical organizations to provide in-home care
- Lack of material and technical preparedness of medical organizations for home care
- Insufficient guidelines for the provision of assistance to palliative cancer patients
- Regulatory restrictions, for example, the mobile team is prohibited from carrying strong analgesics (opioids have to be prescribed only by the district primary care clinic and obtained in a designated pharmacy)
- Insufficient use of instruments and indicators to assess the quality of care provided
- Low remuneration for palliative care employees working with a high load of psycho-emotional stress
- Prevalence of paternalistic versus patient-centered attitudes in modern health care
- Underestimation of the benefits brought by the multidisciplinary palliative care team as part of medical organizations (time and budget saving, relieving social tension, providing continuity of care, improving statistics, supporting positive image of medical organizations, etc.)

Conclusion

No matter how much funding, effort, and resources are invested, the most reliable indicator of the level of palliative care development in the country will be the patients' satisfaction with the quality of care.

The results of a survey we conducted among 88 recipients of in-home palliative care in Almaty, aimed at studying satisfaction, showed: satisfaction among our patients (15.9%), their family carers (36.4%), and both (47.7%).

Without going into details of this survey, it was revealed that 100% of the respondents at the time of the first visit were in need of medical assistance for relief of pain and other symptoms, organization of care and training of relatives in nursing skills, providing psychological support to the patient and family members and social support to the family. Only 13.63% of all recipients reported that they needed spiritual support.

88.6% reported a general improvement in their condition as a result of the mobile team's interventions; 9.1% reported no improvement, and 2.3% reported a deterioration in their condition. 84.1% of respondents scored professional competence of team members as excellent (5/5), 11.4% as good (4/5), and 4.5% as satisfactory (3/5).

The majority of patients (79.5%) said that they prefer to receive palliative care at home if the support of mobile team is provided, while 20.5% wished to receive in-patient hospice care.

The general level of satisfaction with the performance of the mobile team, on a scale from 1 to 5, was as follows: "5" (84.1%), "4" (11.4%), and "3" (4.5%).

Despite the fact that this survey was modest in scope, it provided additional evidence that in-home palliative care significantly increases patient satisfaction while reducing the need of more expensive medical services at the end of life, such as hospice facilities.

With more evidence in place, local champions will be better armed to advocate for broadening access to palliative care through the introduction of home-based services.

References

1. Kaidarova D. Cancer control plan for 2018–2022. 2018. Retrieved from https://onco.Kz/news/razrabotan-proekt-kompleksnogo-plana-po-borbe-s-onkologicheskimi-zabolevaniyami-na-2018-2022-gody/.
2. CancerRegister.n.d..Retrievedfromhttps://www.ezdrav.kz/61-elektronnyj-registr-onkologicheskikh-bolnykh.
3. Order of the Minister of Health of the Republic of Kazakhstan, November 14, 2013. No. 657 On Approval of the Standards for Providing Palliative Care in the Republic of Kazakhstan. Available from http://www.rcrz.kz. Accessed June 2015.
4. Institute of Medicine (US) and National Research Council (US) National Cancer Policy Board. In: Foley KM, Gelband H, editors. Improving palliative care for cancer. Washington, DC: National Academies Press (US); 2001. From: https://www.ncbi.nlm.nih.gov/books/NBK223534/.
5. On Approval of the Standard for Organization of Palliative Care to the Population of the Republic of Kazakhstan. Decree of the Minister of Health of the Republic of Kazakhstan #657, dated November 14, 2013. From: https://tengrinews.kz/zakon/pravitelstvo_respubliki_kazahstan_premer_ministr_rk/zdravoohranenie/id-V1300008956/.
6. Planning and implementing palliative care services: a guide for program managers/ISBN: 978-92-4-156541-7 (NLM classification: QV 250) © World Health Organization, 2016 https://apps.who.int/iris/bitstream/handle/10665/250584/9789241565417-eng.pdf.
7. Morris C. Universal health coverage and palliative care. London: Worldwide Hospice Palliative Care Alliance; 2014.
8. Knaul FM, Farmer PE, Krakauer EL, De Lima L, Bhadelia A, Kwete XJ, Arreola-Ornelas H, Gómez-Dantés O, Rodriguez NM, Alleyne GA, Connor SR. Alleviating the access abyss in palliative care and pain relief – an imperative of universal health coverage: The Lancet Commission report. Lancet. 2017;391:10128.
9. WHO Declaration of Astana. October 2018, www.who.int/primary-health/conference-phc/declaration. November 20, 2018. On Declaration of Alma-Ata International Conference on Primary Health Care, Alma-Ata, USSR, September 6–12, 1978. www.who.int/publications/almaata_declaration_en.pdf?ua=1 (Last accessed November 20, 2018). 3. Knaul FM, Farmer PE, Krakauer El, et al.; on behalf of the Lancet Commission on Palliative Care and Pain Relief Study Group.
10. Global Atlas of Palliative Care at the End of Life. Edited by Stephen R. Connor, PhD, Senior Fellow to the Worldwide Palliative Care Alliance (WPCA), Maria Cecilia Sepulveda Bermedo, MD, Senior Adviser Cancer Control, Chronic Diseases Prevention and Management, Chronic Diseases and Health Promotion, World Health Organization Worldwide Hospice Palliative Care Alliance 2014. ISBN: 978-0-9928277-0-0.
11. Kazakh Association of Palliative Care //http://www.palliative.kz/.
12. Ministry of Health Care of the Republic of Kazakhstan n.d. Retrieved from http://dsm.gov.kz/ru/kategorii/gobmp-i-osms.
13. World Cancer Leader's Summit n.d. Retrieved from https://www.uicc.org/what-we-do/convening/world-cancer-leaders-summit/2019-world-cancer-leaders-summit
14. Order of the Ministry of Health of the Republic of Kazakhstan No. 30 dated 31· January 2019. On Approval of the Roadmap for the Improvement of Palliative Care in the Republic of Kazakhstan for 2019–2020.
15. World Health Organization. Planning and implementing palliative care services: a guide for programme managers. World Health Organization 2016. https://apps.who.int/iris/handle/10665/250584

Part XXX

South Asia: Pakistan

Provision of Palliative Care for Oncological Patients in Pakistan: A Review of Challenges and Current Practices

Muhammad Atif Waqar,
Nasreen Muhammad Saleem,
and Muhammad Shamvil Ashraf

Introduction

Pakistan is the sixth most populated country in the world with more than 200 million people, with approximately 37% of the population above 60 years of age and an average life expectancy of 66 and 67 years in males and females, respectively [1]. It is predominantly an Islamic country. It is ranked 186th out of 189 countries in the matter of total expenditure on health as a percentage of the gross domestic product (GDP), with 45% of the population living below the poverty line. Cancer has emerged as a major health issue within Pakistan. Although oncological services in the country have progressed over the past few decades and is now better rooted for curative oncology, preventive oncology and palliative care services are still poorly developed [2].

Palliative medicine in Pakistan is a fairly new discipline with only handful of institutions providing specialized services to those in need [3]. The remaining burden of palliation has been shared by oncologists, internists, and family physicians of the country with little or no training in palliative medicine. This results in enormous unmet needs of palliative care for those suffering with life-limiting illnesses. This chapter aims to examine the current state of palliative medicine in Pakistan with a review of challenges, existing services and models, resources, and future prospects.

M. A. Waqar (✉) · N. M. Saleem
Section of Palliative Medicine, Department of Oncology, The Aga Khan University Hospital, Karachi, Pakistan
e-mail: atif.waqar@aku.edu; nasreen.salim@aku.edu

M. S. Ashraf
Indus Health Network and Consultant Pediatric Oncology, The Indus Hospital, Karachi, Pakistan

Current Palliative Care Landscape in Pakistan

The International Observatory at the End of Life Care (IOELC) published a survey of palliative care facilities around the world and have observed a "least favorable ratio" of patients served by palliative care facilities in Pakistan as only one service was identified for a population of 157,935,000 [4]. The Worldwide Hospice Palliative Care Alliance (WHPCA) published a global atlas of palliative care development in each country around the world and, in their assessment, they observed that <1% of Pakistan's population has access to specialty palliative care services [5]. The WHPCA records that in 2012, more than 350,000 people needed pain relief for

M. Silbermann (ed.), *Palliative Care for Chronic Cancer Patients in the Community*,
https://doi.org/10.1007/978-3-030-54526-0_42

palliation in Pakistan, but only about 300 of those patients received any – likely due to the lack of specialty palliative care services, poor access, and overtly stringent regulations on opioid procurement and dispensing. The Global Cancer Observatory noted that there are approximately 173,937 new cases of cancer diagnosed in Pakistan each year [6]. Most of these cancer patients present at very advanced stages of the disease, where cure of the malignancy becomes impossible and control of the disease is the primary goal. Simultaneously, it is estimated that there are 118,422 deaths each year from cancer in Pakistan. In terms of pediatric cancers alone, it is estimated that approximately 8000 children under the age of 18 are diagnosed with cancer each year in Pakistan [7]. Unfortunately, less than 50% of these patients are actually diagnosed and treated correctly. This results in over 70% of pediatric cancer patients presenting at very advanced stages of the malignancy. With an estimated 57.2% mortality rate from cancer in the first year after diagnosis, these are all patients who are in dire need of and would benefit from palliative care in the last year of their life.

Health Care Systems/Infrastructure

Pakistan's Public Health Care System (PPHCS) was established in 1979. Pakistan's health care system is three-tiered; it begins with Basic Health Units, Rural Health Units, and Dispensaries in Tier 1, Tier 2 comprises the District Health Quarters Hospitals (Secondary Care) throughout the nation, and Tier 3 consists of Tertiary Care Hospitals in major urban cities [8]. However, access to care in the PPHCS is extremely challenging: long waiting periods, ineffective health care providers, and often defunct health care systems have become the bane of the average patient in the nation; more than 45% of the health budget is directed toward curable diseases at the tertiary care level; and 86.8% of the total expenditure on health care is out-of-pocket costs that patients must endure. Many then turn to the private health care services in the nation out of desperation. Unfortunately, the private health care services are an unorganized system varying from well-equipped tertiary care hospitals to a local general practitioner with a medicine counter providing care to patients in need. Pakistan's Medical and Dental Council (PMDC), responsible for regulating hospitals affiliated with medical colleges, was dissolved in late 2019 due to corruption; therefore, the PMDC's affairs are currently being run by the newly constituted Pakistan Medical Commission (PMC) under direct Presidential Ordinance.

Challenges to Developing Palliative Care in Pakistan

Community and Society-Based Challenges

The median survival rate of patients has increased in Pakistan owing to advances in medicine, better screening modalities, and improved access to health care. However, the nation is very ill-equipped to handle the tsunami of patients who will be transitioning into the geriatric age group in the coming decades. Additionally, the household dynamics have also changed over the course of the past three decades – youths have immigrated abroad seeking better opportunities for employment leaving behind aging parents who will require long-term care. The lack of assisted living facilities, nursing homes, and institutionalized long-term care facilities is creating an unprecedented problem for an aging population with multimorbidity and life-limiting conditions but with limited resources.

Joint family systems are still prevalent in much of Pakistan, with many extended families living together in a single household. While this lends support to caregivers in the form of added helping hands and relieves caregiver stress and burn-out, it also leads to many unique challenges. Family members each exhibit varying degrees of understanding and acceptance at terminal stages of the disease process, leading to difference of opinions in terms of the extent of aggressive medical management that is provided for patients with terminal stages of cancer. A shift in the place of death has occurred in recent times with the medicalization of death, and more patients are dying in institutional settings rather than at home.

Health Care and Institutional-Based Challenges

Given the dearth of cancer care services and long waiting periods in the PPHCS, many cancer patients seek care in the private sector. Antineoplastic treatments tend to generate significant revenue to institutions and private practice oncologists; there is little incentive for them to de-escalate such treatments even in the face of unfavorable prognosis and refractory diseases. Pharmaceutical companies continue to pour large sums of money into this very lucrative branch of medicine, often luring cancer care providers to industry- sponsored events and promises of fringe benefits if their brand of antineoplastic treatments is increasingly prescribed. Patients are still thought of as commodities, and referring patients to palliative care providers is often associated with loss of business and revenue. The concept of co-managing a patient amongst health care providers is still a relatively alien concept; often such providers tend to hold onto their patients until the end, despite the increasing burden of distressing symptoms and their inability to address them effectively.

Health care facilities are focused on revenue generation rather than cost savings. Given the fee for service models, there is a greater incentive for them to keep patients in the intensive care units on artificial life support and mechanical ventilation. Palliative care teams are thought to be counterproductive to this philosophy and investment in areas of improving quality of end-of-life care is often ignored. Since most health care expenditures are ultimately out-of-pocket costs for patients, a visit to the palliative care provider is often thought to lead to additional financial burden, with many electing not to invest any additional funds and to forgo seeing the palliative care team, especially as a cure is no longer an option.

With the exception of a select few tertiary care hospitals that have developed specialty palliative care services, most hospitals even in the urban settings do not possess a palliative care service or mechanism to provide good end-of-life care. There are currently no home-based hospice services in the nation. Free-standing hospice facilities are also very scarce and are often run by either faith-based charitable organizations or non-governmental entities. The services provided at these centers often mimic a shelter home with a focus on residential care for the desolate rather than symptom management and end-of-life care.

Required medications that provide palliation are also not readily available to relieve complex cancer-related pain. Opioids are very stringently regulated by at least four different regulatory bodies, each requiring separate licenses to stock and dispense opiates. Each federally designated cancer hospital will receive an annual quota of opiates based upon their consumption in the preceding year; once these medications are depleted there are no alternatives available and health care providers have to use suboptimal, inferior non-opiate analgesics to relieve pain. Currently, morphine (oral extended release and injectable) is the only available opiate to prescribe in these cancer centers. The opioid consumption per capita in Pakistan is 0.05, much below the median consumption in the region which is 3.27. The lack of technical knowledge on opiate prescribing on the part of health care providers as well as fears associated with opiate use also results in inadequate opiate use [9].

Professional Education, Training, and Workforce-Based Challenges

There is a shortage of trained palliative care clinicians and allied health workforces in Pakistan. Since there are no national palliative care polices, the specialty of palliative medicine is still not recognized by the leading medical education regulatory bodies. The PMDC does not require that palliative care or end-of-life care be taught as part of the mandatory undergraduate medical curriculum. Similarly, the College of Physicians and Surgeons (CPSP) who are tasked with regulating post graduate education and training do not recognize palliative medicine as a separate training specialty nor do they require dedicated experience for oncologists in training during their residency and fellowship. The Higher Education Commission (HEC) has taken a similar stand and does not mandate that palliative care be taught as a core curriculum in undergraduate and post graduate nursing education. Education for allied disciplines in palliative medicine is virtually non-existent. Sporadic workshops and brief courses have been offered by some hospitals and universities in Pakistan's major cities over the past few years. Public awareness campaigns and educational sessions for caregivers and support groups are also very minimal. There are no national palliative care associations or groups in Pakistan at present.

Development of Palliative Care and Existing Models in Pakistan

On an institutional level, palliative care is being offered as a specialty multidisciplinary service in five tertiary care hospitals in Pakistan. These include the Aga Khan University Hospital (AKUH) and the Indus Hospital (TIH) in Karachi, Shaukat Khanum Memorial Cancer Hospital and Research Center (SKMCHRC) in their sites at Lahore and Peshawar, and Shifa International Hospital (SIH) in Islamabad. All the aforementioned hospitals offer inpatient palliative care consultations as well as outpatient palliative care clinic services. At present, only AKUH and SKMCHRC have dedicated palliative care units where patients can be admitted for intractable symptom management or end-of -life care. TIH is the only charity-based tertiary care hospital that provides completely free pediatric palliative care services to all patients in need. Additionally, only AKUH has an established network of Home-Based Palliative Care services comprised of a multidisciplinary team that offers comprehensive palliative care visits and around-the-clock, end-of-life care services at home.

There are currently three free-standing hospice centers in the city of Karachi that have been providing end-of-life care free of charge to the desolate, terminally ill cancer patients of Karachi. Bait Ul Sukoon Hospice in Karachi was founded a decade ago with the vision to provide residential hospice care for underprivileged terminal cancer patients. However, a number of cancer patients with better prognoses and salvageable disease processes prompted a change in philosophy and the institution has since evolved into a cost-free Cancer Hospital for the underprivileged with a hospice that provides inpatient end-of-life care.

Al-Mehrab Tibi Imdad is another hospice for underprivileged cancer patients where they receive residential end-of-life care. Patients and their families are provided living quarters and housing while they undergo palliative treatments at the hospice. However, due to its complete dependence on donations and charity, the facility is understaffed and many of the beds remain unoccupied. Rahat Kada Hospice came into existence in 1991 due to philanthropic efforts and charitable donations and provides community-based hospice services. It has since morphed into a 100-bed hospice and is now part of the Medical Aid Foundation that also provides cost-free cancer treatment to underprivileged patients of Karachi.

The Way Forward (Future Prospects, Innovations, Opportunities)

Technology-Based Solutions

Advancements in technology have benefited health care globally by increasing access and reducing costs [10]. Telemedicine can prove to be promising for the people with life-limiting illnesses, especially for those living in remote areas of Pakistan. Success of e-health interventions by Sehat Kahani, an entrepreneurial initiative empowering female health care providers to offer teleconsultations for underserved communities, serves as a model that can be replicated with modifications for on-going management of palliative patients residing at far distances from the tertiary care facilities [11]. This will enable them to spend last days of life close to their loved ones without fear of poor symptom control and unnecessary suffering.

Similarly, now with more than 74 million people in Pakistan having access to 3G/4G internet services, mobile health apps are gaining popularity [12]. Although the standardization of palliative care solutions is arguably the base of the discipline and requires an individualized care plan, some basic solutions and options can be incorporated into accessible health apps for patients and their caregivers. This can additionally contribute in reducing the burden of the already stretched and over-worked health workforce in Pakistan.

Another model that has been practiced in one of the only tertiary care hospitals in Pakistan, having all essential service components of palliative medicine, is Aga Khan University, which aids in reducing emergency visits for palliative patients. It is a WhatsApp-based helpline service for patients and families already utilizing outpatient palliative medicine services from the hospital. This enables families to seek immediate consultation for the changing symptoms and clinical condition of patients. It has a number of advantages over a telephonic helpline, including the ease of sharing pictures of wounds, vitals and sugar monitoring records, laboratory reports and, if needed, videos and recording of symptoms the family is unable to explain. Such services need more standardization and consideration for confidentiality and privacy issues before further expansion.

Integration with Primary Care Providers

Primary care physicians are the first point of contact in communities where a large number of patients have palliative needs. Despite this high burden of expectations, general practitioners find it challenging to deal with terminally ill patients. They report the strong need for training and capacity-building to effectively manage palliative patients in the community [13].

Although Pakistan has a three-tiered health care system, the integration of these systems is negligible, which leads to a major disconnect between family physicians and specialists [14]. Family physicians have the potential to bridge the gap among primary, secondary, and tertiary health care systems in Pakistan [15].

Empowering general practitioners with capacity-building training for coping with terminally ill patients in the community and integrating them with the specialists of palliative medicine in tertiary care hospitals by proper referral systems, can improve the prospect of palliative medicine in Pakistan. The initial steps are already in place in a tertiary care hospital in Pakistan, where palliative medicine training and clinical rotation is a mandatory part of PGME Family Medicine. This has shown a positive impact on family practitioners' confidence and palliative patients' satisfaction in the community.

Universal Health Care Coverage

Financial burden is one of the major factors that inhibit people with chronic cancer to seek palliative care in the country [2]. With Pakistan being one of the LMIC, it still has an inadequate health care infrastructure that struggles to provide equitable access of quality health care to the masses [14].

Pakistan categorized Universal Health Coverage (UHC) among the top priorities of the 17 Sustainable Development Goals (SDG) to be achieved by the year 2030 [16, 17]. Palliative care as part of UHC will gain resources at the national level. This, in turn, has the potential to overcome financial barriers to accessing palliative services. It is also promising for the development of health care systems and providing skilled human resources that can deliver quality palliative services to currently underserved populations in the country.

Volunteer-Based Home Hospice Care

Pakistan has a rich and deeply rooted culture of volunteerism in the country. The enormous spirit to help those in need is reflected at both individual and institutional levels, sharing the burden of the State. The practice of community service has carried through generations in some of the smaller communities of Pakistan, where people from all age groups participate in some form of voluntary work. These communities have fairly well-structured institutional systems that provide services in the areas of health, educational, economic, and social development [18].

The notion of engaging volunteers to support family caregivers of palliative patients for home-based care can prove to be an effective strategy for strengthening palliative care services provided to chronic cancer patients in Pakistan. One such model is being tested by the Aga Khan Health Board for Pakistan, a Jamati institution of Pakistan's Ismaili community which has trained volunteer nurses, doctors, and social workers as master trainers who work toward capacity-building of family caregivers of patients with life-limiting chronic illnesses. The Training of Trainers (ToT) model is aimed at developing community-owned resources across Pakistan that will help in the multifaceted care of palliative patients. Although results of these efforts will take some time to be evaluated, this springs a solid ground for other such volunteer-based models to overcome the inequalities of palliative care in Pakistan.

National Health Policy for Palliative Care

Since its inception, Pakistan has been struggling with numerous obstacles in establishing a quality health care system. One of them is formulating a nationwide health policy. This has had the worst effect on the discipline of palliative medicine where the lack of well-coordinated infrastructure, trained human resources, and the provision of essential drugs of comfort, i.e., opioids, have failed to receive their due attention.

To overcome the challenge, in 2016, Pakistan formed the National Health Vision (NHV) 2016–2025. WHO is extending its full support in the strategic planning, monitoring, and capacity-building for the success of this vision. The primary focus of NHV is to provide equitable access to essential quality health care by protecting the vulnerable population financially and creating responsive and robust health care systems [19]. The Sehat Sahulat program, benefiting more than 6.3 million families, mostly in underserved parts of Pakistan, is one of the remarkable outcomes of NHV 2025 [20].

As the National Health Vision 2025 further unfolds in coming years, it must have concrete strategies, such as the inclusion of oncological and palliative care services in micro-insurance schemes like Sehat Sahulat. These policies can have practical implications only with the presence of an expert body for palliative care at the national level within the government that can advocate for essential, evidence-based, and cost-effective solutions for the country.

AKHSP: Integration

The Aga Khan Health Service, Pakistan (AKHS,P) is a non-profit, community-based organization working within the umbrella of the Aga Khan Development Network. It shares the State's burden by being one of the largest non-profit private health care systems providing primary- and secondary-level health care services across the country, especially in the most challenging northern belt of Pakistan [21].

Working with the unique challenges of mountainous rural areas of Pakistan has enabled the organization to try and test innovative strategies. They have successfully established e-health programs in two major hub towns, Gilgit city in Gilgit Baltistan and Booni in Chitral, with technical support from Aga Khan University (AKU), one of the esteemed and internationally recognized universities of AKDN.

The future plan is to establish a partnership with AKU for palliative medicine telemedicine consultations via e-health programs of AKHS,P. The pre-requisite intervention is to train and empower the on-ground medical staff on the basics of palliative medicine. This will improve access to palliative medicine services for the underserved population of northern Pakistan.

Dedicated Institute of Palliative Care

Scarcity of trained human resources and an absence of structured educational programs on palliative medicine for physicians, nurses, and allied health professionals present excessive challenges in promoting palliative care services in Pakistan. Although institute level fellowship programs and short training courses at the Aga Khan University & Shaukat Khanam Memorial Cancer Hospital and Research Centre are trying to address the urgent needs, in the long run this gulf can only be filled by a dedicated national level institution that has both public and private representation.

A specialized academic institute of palliative medicine focusing on academics and research will be able to consolidate the patchy efforts of various institutions at a national level, and provide innovative and contextual solutions for the unmet needs of quality palliative care services in Pakistan. This has been realized at the Institute for Palliative Care that is under construction in Lahore, the first dedicated 100-bed hospital to cater to cancer patients in need of palliative care. Upon completion, the hospital will have a 10-bed emergency room for palliative care emergencies, telemedicine rooms to provide care for cancer patients living in remote areas of Pakistan, and teaching and conference rooms to provide advanced training and education in the realm of palliative care.

Conclusion

Although palliative medicine in Pakistan is currently complex and challenging, there is still a promising future. Access to opioids and health care financing are the urgent issues that need to be addressed by the State. Multilayered integrated solutions are needed to strengthen material and human resources that can alleviate suffering for chronic cancer patients in Pakistan. The distinctive and diversified culture and society, if dealt with sensitively, can serve as a source to advance palliative care in the country. Geographical challenges will be overcome by technological innovations in the near future. Collaboration between different stakeholders at the national level can be instrumental in creating lasting solutions for palliative care in Pakistan.

References

1. WHO country profile – Pakistan. Retrieved from https://www.who.int/countries/pak/en/.
2. Shad A, Ashraf MS, Hafeez H. Development of palliative-care services in a developing country: Pakistan. J Pediat Hematol Oncol. 2011;33(1):S62–3.
3. Punjwani R, Khatoon A, Dias JM, Kurji ZA, Siddiqui DF, Bana S, Baig-Ansari N. Palliative care in nursing – where are we in Pakistan? J Palliat Care Med. 2015;5:002.
4. Clark D, Wright M. The international observatory on end of life care: a global view of palliative care development. J Pain Symptom Manag. 2007;33(5): 542–6.
5. WHO global atlas on palliative care at the end of life. 2014. Retrieved from http://www.thewhpca.org/resources/global-atlas-on-end-of-life-care.
6. Globocan 2018 – WHO. Pakistan global cancer observatory. Retrieved from https://gco.iarc.fr/today/data/factsheets/populations/586-pakistan-fact-sheets.pdf/.
7. Ashraf MS. Pediatric oncology in Pakistan. J Pediat Hematol Oncol. 2012;34(Suppl 1):S23–5. https://doi.org/10.1097/MPH.0b013e318249abf9. PubMed PMID: 22357147.
8. Khan RI. Palliative care in Pakistan. Indian J Med Ethics. 2017;2(1):37–42. PubMed PMID: 27867144.
9. Atlas of palliative care in the eastern mediterranean region. 2017. Retrieved from http://www.thewhpca.org/resources/item/atlas-of-palliative-care-in-the-emro-region.
10. Kvedar J, Coye MJ, Everett W. Connected health: a review of technologies and strategies to improve patient care with telemedicine and telehealth. Health Aff. 2014;33(2):194–9.
11. Sehat Kahani. 2020. Retrieved on https://www.sehatkahani.com/.
12. Pakistan telecommunication authority. 2019. Retrieved on https://www.pta.gov.pk/en/telecom-indicators/.
13. Wakefield MA, Beilby J, Ashby MA. General practitioners and palliative care. Palliat Med. 1993;7(2):117–26.
14. Hassan A, Mahmood K, Bukhsh HA. Healthcare system of Pakistan. Int J Adv Res Publ. 2017;1(4):170–3.
15. Zuberi RW. Family medicine: a brief review of its history and concepts and its relevance to Pakistan. J Pakistan Med Assoc. 1993;43(5):102.
16. National initiative of sustainable development goals 2030. 3. Good health & well-being. Retrieved from https://www.sdgpakistan.pk/web/goals/goal3/.
17. Universal health coverage partnership, country profile: Pakistan. Retrieved from https://uhcpartnership.net/country-profile/pakistan/.
18. Deneb Sumbul. The good samaritans: volunteerism in Pakistan 2016. Retrieved from https://newslinemagazine.com/magazine/good-samaritans-volunteerism-pakistan/.
19. National Health Vision (NHV) Pakistan – 2016–2025. Retrieved from http://www.nationalplanningcycles.org/sites/default/files/planning_cycle_repository/pak-

istan/national_health_vision_2016-25_30-08-2016.pdf/.
20. Sehat sahulat program Pakistan. Retrieved from https://www.pmhealthprogram.gov.pk/.
21. Aga khan health service, Pakistan – company profile. Retrieved from https://www.akdn.org/aga-khan-health-service-pakistan-0/.

Part XXXI

South Asia: India

Collaborative Programmes Between Government and Civil Society: Scope, Challenges and Models

Suresh Kumar, Libby Sallnow, and Heather Richardson

Introduction

The past four decades have witnessed a growing interest around the world in the ways in which public involvement in governance may be enhanced [1]. This has been particularly true in health care since the Alma-Ata Declaration of 1978. Governance is the process of decision-making and the participatory nature of the process is considered to be one of the features of good governance [2]. International agencies such as the World Bank have been strong advocates of community participation in development projects [3]. The World Health Organisation has been particularly vocal on the role of community participation in health care since the 1978 Alma-Ata Declaration [4]. At the same time, questions have been raised about what exactly civil society is and to what degree is it legitimised to act on behalf of the public [5].

S. Kumar (✉)
Institute of Palliative Medicine, WHO Collaborating Center for Community Participation in Palliative Care and Long Term Care, Kozhikode, Kerala, India

L. Sallnow
Central and North West London NHS Foundation Trust & St Christopher's Hospice, London, UK
e-mail: libby.sallnow@nhs.net

H. Richardson
St Christopher's Hospice, London, UK
e-mail: H.Richardson@stchristophers.org.uk

Civil Society and Participation

The term 'civil society' is often used without clearly defining what it meant. Related terms such as community participation/community mobilisation are also often defined imprecisely, used in a multitude of differing contexts and not measured or monitored systematically. It has been pointed out that participation can range from 'tokenistic', with no meaningful impact, to assuming control over the decision making process. The aim of community participation is to build support networks in a pro-active way within communities [6]. Historically, the early notions of civil society meant the public domain, including the state, the market and the church, but not the private domain [7]. But later, this concept began to emphasise the distinction between the official realm of the state and the grassroots activities of the general public. Civil society also differentiates between the market and the world of ordinary people. The concept was meant to include not only various autonomous associations, cooperatives, social movements, mutual aid and other informal groups, but also families and informal personal networks [8]. Currently, however, according to the libertarian notion, civil society is synonymous with the private market sector. Society as a whole is perceived in terms of a two-celled model, that is, comprising the state and the civil or private domain. On the other hand, according to the communitarian perspective, civil society is synonymous with community [9].

M. Silbermann (ed.), *Palliative Care for Chronic Cancer Patients in the Community*,
https://doi.org/10.1007/978-3-030-54526-0_43

Civil society is not monolithic. A possible dynamic relationship can exist between the state, which can exercise coercive force in its interventions, and a civil society where freedom is exercised and experienced and a range of possibilities are offered. The range of participation can be as different as that of a government-organised non-governmental organisations (GONGO) aiming to further the government's political interests to civil society triggering political transformations, as in Eastern Europe [10, 11].

Collaboration Between Civil Society and the State

The Cambridge English Dictionary defines collaboration as the 'act of working together with other people or organizations to create or achieve something' [12].

Three forms of interaction between the state and non-governmental organisations within civil society have been described. There are groups which detach themselves from the state system and develop parallel health, political and economic systems. This can be termed the 'exit option'. Other groups are seen to engage the state in dialogue for the purpose of addressing inefficiencies, corruption, and bad policies, and to ensure that the state meets minimum obligations to its citizens – activities under what can be called the 'voice option'. The third form of interaction, termed 'straddling', describes those groups that oscillate between the 'exit option' and the 'voice option' according to the circumstances [13]. Within these three categories, what we call 'collaboration' comes under the exit or straddling options.

Broadly, from the government's point of view, there can be two approaches to collaboration between civil society and the state. The first one is what can be called a 'utilitarian approach' to civil society participation. Participation here is seen as a means to achieve something the government wants. The government invites civil society to participate in a pre-set task in order to legitimate interests and to 'use' local resources to offset costs. The second approach, which can be called the 'empowerment approach', sees participation as 'a set of empowering practices seeking to achieve a re-balancing of power structures while developing the conscientization and citizenship of socially excluded communities.' The two approaches, although both can be described as collaborative initiatives, are based on different philosophies and politics [14]. The ideal arrangement would be one in which the government and civil society work together with the same objectives, agreeing on and sharing the same strategy, complementing each other. Whatever the approach, the effectiveness of civil society organisations in these collaborative ventures derives from their flexibility in adapting to local contexts and addressing diverse and interrelated needs, a quality not usually characteristic of government projects and procedures. This quality is all the more relevant in the case of state–civil society collaboration in the development and delivery of palliative care services which require a great deal of individualisation and flexibility.

The interface between civil society and the state in such collaborative ventures has been widely discussed. Concerns have also been expressed about the relationship between the government and civil society sometimes being 'too close for comfort' [15]. For example, there is an argument that contracting NGOs to provide health services may improve the equity, efficiency and quality of services in underserved areas, a concept very much in line with the World Bank's notion of 'participation' [16, 17]. But many people have pointed out the risk of civil society organisations collaborating in this manner with the government and losing their social justice or community development perspectives and getting co-opted as little more than service providers [18].

The context in which collaboration takes place is also understood to determine the outcome. A paper analysing studies from Taiwan, Kerala, Mexico, post-Communist Russia and Ceará (in Brazil), concludes that the 'synergies' which are a prerequisite for positive developmental outcomes are best achieved when political competition compels policymakers to make services available and even accept alliances with communities [19]. This is significant, as there is evidence to show that policy change is determined by the ways in which state and societal actors are constituted, become politically significant and interact across the public-private divide [20].

Another issue which is often raised, particularly in situations where civil society contributes voluntary manpower in health care, is that of the balance between professional and lay expertise. The question of whether it is safe, cost-effective and consistent with equitable outcomes to transfer power away from health experts has been raised frequently [21].

State–Civil Society Interactions in Palliative Care

Interactions between civil society and the government regarding the issue of palliative care are spread out over a wide spectrum, beginning with advocacy/lobbying, and moving on to collaboration in policymaking/development of services/education and training and outsourcing components of services. Many CSOs have multiple layers of interaction with the government.

International non-governmental organisations in palliative care are primarily active in the area of advocacy. The United Nations recently hosted a hearing in New York in April 2019 as part of the preparatory process for the UN General Assembly's high-level meeting on universal health coverage. The Worldwide Hospice Palliative Care Alliance (WHPCA), International Children's Palliative Care Network (ICPCN), African Palliative Care Association (APCA) and Kenya Hospices and Palliative Care Association (KEHPCA) from the palliative care community were represented. These organisations argued through prepared statements about why Universal Health Coverage should not neglect those with the highest health needs, specifically those requiring palliative care services [22].

As a rule, the first attempts at developing palliative care services in most countries were through civil society initiatives. Governments then began to take notice, either due to advocacy programmes by these civil society organisations, international NGOs or international agencies such as the World Health Organisation.

The history of the palliative care movement was rooted in the care of patients with advanced cancer by civil society initiatives [23]. Faith-based hospices existed in Europe and in Pondicherry, India (a French colony at that time), much before the establishment of modern hospices [24]. Most of these early initiatives were led by faith-based organisations. In the United Kingdom, St. Christopher's Hospice was the first modern hospice, which opened its doors in 1967 and, with its focus on both patient care and research, became a major stimulus for hospices and hospital-based palliative care services [25]. Faith-based organisations initiating palliative care services was seen later in many regions. For example, the first faith-based palliative care organisation in Thailand opened in 1992 at Pharbat Numpu temple in the Lop Puri province. Care was provided by Buddhist monks and volunteers [26]. Churches continue to play an indirect role in the delivery of palliative care services by the state. It has been observed that 'dying and end-of-life care has, to a great extent, been moved out of hospitals and back into the local community, and renewed attention is given to dying and spiritual care issues' with the result that local churches play a role in palliative care [27].

The situation in the United Kingdom evolved significantly after 1967. Charitable hospices today in the UK raise their funding through a combination of support from their local communities, such as fundraising and statutory funding – from the National Health Service and local authorities, although there have been complaints that the National Health Service's contribution for many hospices have not increased in proportion to rising expenses [28].

The nature of collaboration with civil society organisations in the field of palliative care (or the lack of collaboration) varies from country to country and from region to region within countries. Financial support for programmes is a major issue. Contributions from multiple sources, although a positive development, are often grossly inadequate to deliver the services needed across a population. A series of examples from different regions are discussed below.

Europe

The history of palliative care in Europe demonstrates regular attempts by civil society organisations, both national and regional, to engage the government. Some examples follow.

A civil society organisation to promote palliative care in Europe was first formed in 1988 when the European Association for Palliative Care (EAPC), supported by the Floriani Foundation, came into being [29]. Since then, policy issues relating to end-of-life care in Europe have been raised by both non-governmental and intergovernmental organisations. Exhortatory declarations were made at palliative care conferences calling for government action on palliative care at the national level [30]. The European Federation of Older Persons (EURAG), a non-governmental organisation representing the interests of older persons in Europe, with 152 member organisations in 33 countries, launched a campaign in 2004 to make palliative care a priority topic on the European health agenda [31].

Germany shows two separate tracks, called hospice care and palliative care. German hospice care developed as a civil society movement and, from the beginning, volunteers played an active role. Palliative care, on the other hand, was led by a few pioneer physicians and started independently from hospices. The clear distinction between professionally-run health care palliative care units and civil society-led inpatient hospices continues. Over the last two decades, these two areas of care have moved further into the regular health care service with government interventions. One implication of this collaboration with the government is that volunteer services are becoming increasingly subjected to regulations. This also means that there is an increasing amount of competition and economic pressure on both streams [32].

Russia's first hospice was founded in St. Petersburg in 1990 as a charity, but with the support of the city's board of health. Later, in many other cities, hospices were founded by charitable organisations. A major development was the securing of funding for these hospices by local government. Running parallel to these initiatives from civil society, the Ministry of Health established the Moscow Centre for Palliative Care with its focus on the development of palliative care services in hospitals in Russia [33].

The initial attempts to develop palliative care initiatives in Eastern Europe were all made by civil society organisations. The first service in the region was a volunteer hospice service which began in 1976 in Krakow, Poland [34]. Most of them, with the exception of the first, started in the 1990s and early 2000s. Throughout the last decade, Romania has shown rapid progress in public policy, education, training and the establishment of palliative care services. The lead institution for palliative care in Romania is Hospice Casa Sperantei in Brasov, which was established in collaboration with overseas partners and run by a civil society organisation. It is now a resource centre for palliative care development in Eastern Europe, offering training programmes for countries in the Balkan region and Commonwealth of Independent States countries [35].

Africa

Palliative care in Africa is mostly civil society organisation-driven and to a large extent dependent on external donors and funds [36]. One notable exception is Uganda, where the government has dedicated part of its national budget specifically to palliative care development [37].

Uganda has a rich presence of civil society organisations in palliative care. The first national organisation (Hospice Uganda) was formed in 1993. Advocacy by civil society organisations, governmental collaboration and lobbying led to palliative care being recognised as an essential service in the Ugandan National Health Policy Plan and Strategy. These advocacy efforts have been supported by several national and global non-governmental organisations [38]. Oral morphine is locally reconstituted and distributed through a collaborative partnership between the Ugandan government and Hospice Africa Uganda [39]. Hospice Africa Uganda also involves community volunteer workers who advocate for palliative care in the community and help to destigmatise death and dying [40]. There are still limitations, primarily due to gaps in the collaborative model. A recent joint report by civil society organisations pointed out that a lack of government ownership of the programmes and the lack of a legal and policy framework has resulted in patchy coverage [41].

Kenya has shown an evolution from predominantly charity-based palliative care services to one in which the government has started taking interest. Until 2010, palliative care provision in Kenya was mainly supported by non-governmental organisations and managed by independent hospices and mission hospitals. In 2010, Kenya's Director of Medical Services mandated that 10 public hospitals integrate palliative care into service provision [42]. A partnership between Kenya Hospices and Palliative Care Association and Kenya's Ministry of Health played a major role in this palliative care service expansion. Financial support for the project came from the Diana Princess of Wales Memorial Fund and the True Colors Trust [43]. Mentorship and funding to integrate palliative care into nursing and undergraduate medical curricula in Kenya was also provided by the Diana Princess of Wales Memorial Fund [44].

Pacific Region

Fiji, in the Pacific, has a dynamic interaction between national and international non-governmental organisations and the government in the field of palliative care. Unlike most other countries, the initial attempt was made by the government. In 2008, the Government of Fiji decided to establish the first palliative care service in the country in the form of an eight-bedded hospice at Tamavua Rehabilitation Hospital. The old building designated for the unit was cleaned and prepared by local organisations and then renovated and equipped with the help of funds sourced from donors. The Fiji Cancer Society, a civil society organisation formed in 1997, was responsible for this project [45].

The Ministry recently appointed a palliative care nurse in the Central Division. The Fijian Cancer Society provides a car and driver to support this nurse for conducting home visits. Many other agencies, local and international, are involved in the development of palliative care programmes in Fiji. In 2016, the International Atomic Energy Agency also supported a capacity-building workshop in Fiji [46].

Asia

Several models of collaboration between the state and civil society have emerged in Asia. Three are discussed below.

Mongolia has a very successful programme and is an example of good collaboration between the civil society organisation and the government. Mongolia began developing palliative care in 2000 with the creation of the civil society organisation, 'Mongolian Palliative Care Society'. Advocacy activities involving international players resulted in palliative care being included in Mongolia's Health Law, Health Insurance Law, Social Welfare Law, National Cancer Control Program and the National Program for Non-Communicable Diseases. The country has also recently approved Palliative Care Standards and Pain Management Guidelines. Palliative care education is included in the undergraduate and postgraduate curriculum in all medical universities. In 2014, a paediatric palliative care in-patient unit was established with five beds. Essential drugs for palliative care including opioids have been available since 2015 [47].

Telangana in India shows a different model, with the government outsourcing the running of palliative care services in districts to a civil society organisation. The government allots funds to the pain relief and palliative care society and the civil society organisation which is responsible for selecting and training the staff and the day-to-day management of palliative care centres. The non-governmental organisation also enlists the support of local volunteers to supplement the paid manpower [48].

Kerala in India is unique in that it has seen direct involvement of political parties in palliative care. Palliative care in Kerala began in 1993 as a civil society organisation-run service, linked to a government medical college. The programme had a small outpatient service and a basic home care service and was managed with support from the local community in the form of donations and voluntary work. Seven years later a programme named Neighbourhood Network in Palliative Care was launched to expand the programme and to encourage better participation from the community. The community groups formed were encouraged to take responsibility for developing palliative care initiatives in the locality. Approximately 50 such local palliative care initiatives developed over the next eight years. By that time, the local government in Kerala had also begun taking an interest in the programme. Palliative home care units were soon established by over 1000 local government institutions in the region, guided by a Pain and Palliative Care Policy by the State Government of Kerala. Two decades after the initial attempts for a deeper involvement of the community, Kerala now has about 1100 palliative care units linked to local government institutions and more than 450 units run by local community groups. Over 300 of these civil society projects developed spontaneously over the last decade, 'uninvited' and not as part of the original system. New community groups in palliative care continue to form regularly. All 1550 local initiatives are organisationally and financially independent from each other and new players continue to enter. A recent entry into the palliative care scene is the largest political party in Kerala, the Communist Party of India (known as CPM). CPM formally decided to train their cadre, working with existing groups in the community and setting up new groups in villages where there were none. The Party has linked palliative care with other social and political activities with the suggestion that participation in palliative care is a political responsibility of citizens [49, 50].

Volunteering

Volunteer work is one of several kinds of productive activities and is defined as 'unpaid work provided to parties to whom the worker owes no contractual, familial or friendship obligations'. It adds use value to goods and services [51]. Volunteering by individuals is a major means through which civil society contributes to palliative care services. Volunteer work in palliative care can be informal or formal. Formal volunteering is usually carried out in the context of an organisation. Informal volunteering (e.g. helping friends, neighbours, and family members living outside the household, etc.) is more private and is not organised. Obligations often have a more powerful influence on informal assistance than they do on formal volunteer work. There is an argument that formal volunteer work, being public, would have different roots than the more private form of informal volunteering. Social ties contribute more to informal volunteering than to formal volunteering [52].

Informal voluntary work in palliative care comes under the general category of 'helping a patient or family'. Formal voluntary work is collective endeavour taken up as part of an agreed project for common good. Collective work has an advantage in terms of the sustainability of voluntary action by an individual as it is strongly dependent on similar action by other individuals in the community. Such resources for collective action in the community are collectively termed 'social capital', meaning the social ties, including friendship networks and organisational memberships that supply information, foster trust, make contacts, provide support, set guidelines and create obligations. This promotes volunteer work by fostering norms of generalised reciprocity, encouraging people to trust each other and amplifying reputations [53]. It has been observed that the benefits for patients and families include emotional support, companionship and practical assistance (e.g. respite or breaks from caregiving). Volunteering in hospice palliative care also provides many benefits for the volunteers, including being able to make a difference in the lives of others, personal growth and greater appreciation of what is really important in life [54]. Attrition among formal volunteers is a relatively understudied but an important area of study [55].

Conclusion

Participation of civil society in governance is a regularly recurring theme in development discourses. Different models of interaction between civil society and the state exist. The roles and relative positions of the government and civil society in decision-making and implementation vary enormously in these projects. These different models are based on radically different ideologies and philosophies.

Civil society plays a prominent role in the initiation and running of palliative care services in many countries. Flexibility in adapting to local contexts and addressing diverse and interrelated needs makes civil society organisations an effective player in the delivery of palliative care services, which require a great deal of individualisation and flexibility.

Civil society organisations also played key roles in the initiation and development of palliative care services in most countries. Governments entered the scene later either due to advocacy programmes by these civil society organisations, international NGOs or international agencies such as the World Health Organisation. Interactions in the area of palliative care between civil society and the government are spread out over a wide spectrum, starting with advocacy/lobbying, moving on to collaborating in policy-making/development of services/education and training. Civil society organisations are found to follow the 'exit', 'voice' and 'straddling' options in their interactions with governments. There is no uniform pattern of collaboration and many civil society organisations have multiple layers of interaction with the government.

References

1. Fung A, Wright EO. Deepening democracy: innovations in empowered local governance. Polit Soc. 2001;29(1):5–41.
2. What is good governance? – United Nations ESCAP. Available at https://www.unescap.org/sites/default/files/good-governance.pdf. Accessed 13 Mar 2020.
3. Paul S. Community participation in development projects. In: World Bank discussion papers, vol. 6. Washington: The World bank; 1987. Available at http://documents.worldbank.org/curated/en/850911468766244486/pdf/multi-page.pdf. Accessed 13 Mar 2020.
4. Haldane V, Chuah FLH, Srivastava A, Singh SR, Koh GCH, Seng CK, et al. Community participation in health services development, implementation, and evaluation: a systematic review of empowerment, health, community, and process outcomes. PLoS One. 2019;14(5):e0216112. https://doi.org/10.1371/journal.pone.0216112.
5. Kotzian P, Steffek J. Legitimacy and activities of civil society organizations, Working Papers 156, University of Bremen, Collaborative Research Center 597: Transformations of the State 2011.
6. Kellehear A. Third-wave public health? Compassion, community, and end-of-life care. Int J Appl Psychoanal Studies. 2004;1(4):313–23.
7. Ehrenberg J. Civil society: the critical history of an idea. New York, NY: NYU Press; 1999.
8. Bush Zetterberg K. Det civila samhället i socialstaten [The Civil Society in a Welfare State]. Stockholm: City University Press; 1996.
9. Hanberger A. Policy and program evaluation, civil society, and democracy. Am J Eval. 2001;22(2):211–28.
10. Hasmath, et al. Conceptualizing government-organized non-governmental organizations. J Civ Soc. 2019;15(3):267–84.
11. Brannan T. From antipolitics to anti-politics: what became of east European civil society. 2003 Working Paper 41, London School of Economics and Political Science, London.
12. https://dictionary.cambridge.org/dictionary/english/collaboration.
13. Nyangg'oro JE. NGOs, civil society and the State in Africa: in search of relevance. In: Tandon R, editor. Civil society, the State and African development in the 1990s. Nairobi: Central Graphics Services; 1993.
14. Morgan LM. Community participation in health: perpetual allure, persistent challenge. Health Policy Plan. 2001;16(3):221–30.
15. Hulme D, Edwards M. NGOs, states and donors: too close for comfort? London: Macmillan; 1997.
16. La Forgia M, Cerezo C. Is the perfect the enemy of the good? A case study on large-scale contracting for basic health services in rural Guatemala. In: La Forgia G, editor. Health system innovations in Central America: lessons and impact of new approaches. Washington, DC: World Bank; 2005.
17. Cammack P. What the World Bank means by poverty reduction, and why it matters. New Political Economy. 2004;9(2):189–211.
18. Gideon J. 'Consultation' or co-option? A case study from the Chilean health sector. Prog Dev Stud. 2005;5(3):169–81.
19. Evans P. Government action, social capital and development: reviewing the evidence on synergy. World Dev. 1996;24(6):1119–32.
20. Houtzager P. Introduction: from polycentrism to the polity. In: Houtzager P, Moore M, editors. Changing paths: international development and the new politics of inclusion. Ann Arbor: University of Michigan Press; 2003. p. 1–13.
21. Florin D, Dixon J. Public involvement in health care. Br Med J. 2004;328:159–61.

22. http://www.thewhpca.org/latest-news/item/un-civil-society-interactive-hearing-statements-on-palliative-care.
23. Abrams R, Jameson G, Poehlman M, Snyder S. Terminal care in cancer — a study of two hundred patients attending Boston clinics. N Engl J Med. 1945;232:719.
24. Zaman S, Inbadas H, Whitelaw A, Clark D. Common or multiple futures for end of life care around the world? Ideas from the 'waiting room of history'. Soc Sci Med. 2017;172:72.
25. National Council for Palliative Care. The distinctive characteristics of cancer. London: The National Council for Palliative Care; 2006.
26. Wright M, Hamzah E, Phungrassami T, Bausa-Claudio A. Hospice and palliative care in Southeast Asia: a review of developments and challenges in Malaysia, Thailand and the Philippines. 1st ed. New York: Oxford University Press; 2010.
27. Grassman EJ, Whitaker A. End of life and dimensions of civil society: the Church of Sweden in a new geography of death. Mortality. 2007;12(3):261–80. https://doi.org/10.1080/13576270701430635.
28. Hospice UK 'Rising costs and precarious "Jenga-like" funding model undermining capacity of hospices to meet demand for care' 5/07/rising-costs-and-precarious-jenga-like-funding-model-undermining-capacity-of-hospices-to-meet-demand-for-care.
29. Blumhuber H, Kaasa S, De Conno F. The European Association for Palliative Care. J Pain and Symptom Manage. 2002;24:124–7.
30. Barcelona declaration on palliative care. Eur J Pall Care 1995;3:15. Poznan declaration. Eur J Pall Care 1998;6:61–5.
31. www.eurag-europe.org/palliativ-en.htm.
32. Hesse M, Radbruch L. Volunteering in hospice and palliative care in Germany. In: Scott R, Howlett S, editors. The changing face of volunteering in hospice and palliative care. Oxford: Oxford Scholarship Online; 2018.
33. Novikov G. The integration of palliative care into the health system of the Russian Federation. In: Wright M, editor. Sharing the vision: hospice and palliative care collaboration in Russia. A report of the international seminar, held 5 May 2004 at Hospice House. London: Help the Hospices; 2004.
34. Clark D, Centeno C. Palliative care in Europe: an. https://doi.org/10.7861/clinmedicine.6-2-197.
35. Mosoiu D, Ryan KM, Joranson DE, Garthwaite JP. Reform of drug control policy for palliative care in Romania. Lancet. 2006;367:2110.
36. Clark D, Wright M, Hunt J, Lynch T. Hospice and palliative care development in Africa: a multi-method review of services and experiences. J Pain Symptom Manag. 2007;33:698–710.
37. Murray S, for the economist intelligence unit. The 2015 quality of death index. In: Line D, editor. Ranking palliative care across the world. 2015. https://www.eiuperspectives.economist.com/sites/default/files/2015%20EIU%20Quality%20of%20Death%20Index%20Oct%2029%20FINAL.pdf. Accessed 24 Feb 2020.
38. Harding R, Higginson IJ. Palliative care in sub-Saharan Africa. Lancet. 2005;365:1971–7.
39. Republic of Uganda Ministry of Health. National palliative care policy. Uganda: Ministry of Health Kampala; 2015.
40. Hannon B, Zimmermann C, Knaul FM, et al. Provision of palliative care in low- and middle-income countries: overcoming obstacles for effective treatment delivery. J Clin Oncol. 2016;34:62–8.
41. Joint civil society report on palliative care in Uganda 2016. Available at prdoc.ohchr.org. Accessed 14 Mar 2020.
42. Republic of Kenya Ministry of Health: National palliative care guidelines. http://kehpca.org/wp-content/uploads/National-Palliative-Care-Guidelines-02.10.pdf.
43. Kenyan hospitals introducing palliative care. Science Africa. 2011;18:1–2.
44. Rawlinson F, Gwyther L, Kiyange F, et al. The current situation in education and training of healthcare professionals across Africa to optimise the delivery of palliative care for cancer patients. Ecancermedicalscience. 2014;8:492.
45. http://www.health.gov.fj/wp-content/uploads/2018/03/Annual-Report-2008.pdf.
46. Spratt J Palliative Care in the Pacific: initial research 2019 DevPolicy Blog. https://devpolicy.org/publications/reports/Palliative-Care-in-the-Pacific-initial-research.pdf.
47. Davaasuren O, Frank D. Ferris palliative care development in Mongolia. J Pain Symptom Manage. 2018;55(2 Supplement):S59–66.
48. Civil Society News, Hyderabad https://www.civilsocietyonline.com/interviews/we-have-set-up-palliative-care-centres-in-8-districts/.
49. Kumar S. Models of delivering palliative and end-of-life care in India. Support Palliat Care. 2013;7(2):216–22.
50. Kumar S. Community participation in palliative care: reflections from the ground. Progress in Palliative Care. 2020;28(1):83–8. https://doi.org/10.1080/09699260.2019.1706272.
51. Tilly C, Tilly C. Capitalist work and labor markets. In: Smelser N, Swedberg R, editors. Handbook of economic sociology. Princeton: Princeton University Press; 1994. p. 283–313.
52. Wilson J, Musick MA. Who cares? Toward an integrated theory of volunteer work. Am Sociol Rev. 1997;62(5):694–713.
53. Putnam R. Bowling alone: America's declining social capital. J Democr. 1995;6:65–78.
54. Claxton-Oldfield S. Hospice palliative care volunteers: the benefits for patients, family caregivers, and the volunteers. Palliat Supportive Care. 2015;13(3):809–13. https://doi.org/10.1017/S1478951514000674.
55. de Vries DH, Pool R. The influence of community health resources on effectiveness and sustainability of community and lay health worker programs in lower-income countries: a systematic review. PLoS One. 2017;12:e0170217.

The Role of the Palliative Care Team in Keeping Paediatric Oncology Patients at Home

Mary Ann Muckaden

Introduction

Cancers in children are the most curable along its varying spectrum. However, at first presentation to the hospital, they have a plethora of sometimes severe symptoms. These need urgent attention, along with the management of the cancer. Oncologists tend to focus on the treatment of cancer, while palliative care specialists offer holistic care for the individual. It is logical therefore that the American Society of Clinical Oncology, along with Oncologists and most other cancer organizations, recommends early integration of palliative care, along with oncology care, for all cancer patients with high-risk disease or high-symptom burden, which are based on robust clinical evidence [1, 2].

WHO Definition of Palliative Care for Children [3]

Palliative care for children represents a special, albeit closely related field, to adult palliative care. WHO's definition of palliative care is applicable for children suffering from cancer and other paediatric chronic disorders, and their families.

- Palliative care for children is the active total care of the child's body, mind and spirit, and involves giving support to the family.
- It begins when an illness is diagnosed and continues regardless of whether or not a child receives disease directed treatment.
- Health providers must evaluate and alleviate a child's physical, psychological and social distress.
- Effective palliative care requires a broad multidisciplinary approach that includes the family and makes use of available community resources; it can be successfully implemented even if resources are limited.
- It can be provided in tertiary care facilities, in community health centres and even in children's homes.

Most paediatric palliative care centres all over the world incorporate the above principles when working alongside the oncologists to provide optimal care. The same is true in India, where, at the Tata Memorial Centre and a few other cancer centres, trained PPC specialists join the tumour boards for 5 years, where management decisions are jointly taken for every individual child. The combined care allows proper symptomatic treatment, along with cancer-directed therapy, choices to reducing intensity when burdens outweigh therapy benefits and ultimately a take-over of the case when cancer-directed treatment is stopped. This allows good rapport building between child,

M. A. Muckaden (✉)
Department of Palliative Medicine, Tata Memorial Center, Mumbai, India

M. Silbermann (ed.), *Palliative Care for Chronic Cancer Patients in the Community*,
https://doi.org/10.1007/978-3-030-54526-0_44

family and PPC teams. Care of the child in areas other than the hospital can also be discussed when the family feels assured that all decisions are individual, shared and in the best interest of the child. This concept is well elucidated in a review paper by Baker et al. [4] and is the standard practice in the majority of PPC centres.

Home Care: An Integral Component of Palliative Care

Initial treatment plans are formatted at the hospital; the child may even be admitted. However, when the therapy enters the less intense maintenance phase, a hospital environment is not overly conducive to the best quality of care for the child due to ever crowding and the presence of hospital resistant infections, especially in-between multiple hospital admissions. The aim of this chapter, therefore, is to discuss an alternative to this place of care. Home care teams should be utilized whenever needed, and should be part of the care team from initiation of the treatment trajectory; the child would be symptomatic due to the disease process.

Home is the castle for child and family; they are more in control of their own lives in their familiar surroundings. Child is assured a comfortable and safe environment. Whether child is undergoing maintenance therapy, relapse metronomic therapy or best supportive care, continuity of care is planned and provided by the treating paediatrician, nurses, family members and often the community. Medicinal and nursing interventions appropriate at home, adequate nutrition, psychological care, social support and spiritual care are part of palliative home care.

Often the circumstances under which the family is existing are not clear. Home care comprehensive assessment includes home itself – cleanliness, ventilation, status of surroundings, presence of helpful neighbours, panchayat, NGOs in vicinity, any other sources of support, etc.

Care includes simple solutions to improve the hygiene and ventilation of the home and the surroundings. The number of people in the home at any one point in time may have to be discussed and arranged to prevent infections and be conducive to rest; yet not an empty home which would lead to depression and loneliness. An optimum environment is one allowing the child to rest, as well as play.

In Asia, and maybe other parts of the world, cancer is still a social stigma. It takes a lot of convincing of parents of the child's peers that the child's cancer is not contagious, and his peers can come and play, as long as they do not have any active infection.

Cooking facilities for the family need to be assessed and solutions arranged. An appetizing aroma for the rest could induce nausea in the sick child. Can cooking be done somewhere else? Or be restricted to certain time of the day while the child is enjoying the ventilation outside the home.

Most of the care of physical symptoms, discussed below, can be adapted at home. Oral medications, rarely even the sub-cutaneous route, is taught to the primary caregivers. Follow-up is provided on the helpline. This would in turn reduce the need for hospital visits, which would in turn reduce the exposure to infections and fatigue. These experiences are echoed in a study conducted in Germany, [5] where the provision of home care to children was done by the Pediatric Oncology Departments in 39% of children. The same paper describes the experience at Great Ormond Street Hospital in London. Authors conclude the necessity of incorporation of palliative care including home care into the care of children with cancer. Across the Atlantic, similar discussion is available in the review paper by Baker et al. [4] from St Jude's Cancer Hospital.

Indian experience, including ours, has shown home care integration to be very fruitful in keeping hospital visits and hospitalization to an optimum level. This in turn improves the quality of life for the child and makes care more doable for the family. Neighbours and social groups help whenever they can. Counselling and social interventions are arranged regularly. The helpline is a constant resource for families to reach out to the doctor or nurse for advice.

Common Symptoms and their Management

Some common symptoms of advanced cancer and their management are discussed here; with a special emphasis on management at home.

Common symptoms commonly found in patients with advanced cancer, as discussed by Wolfe et al. [6] and Torres et al. [7] are pain (48%), nausea (50%), fatigue (46%), lack of appetite (43.7%), drowsiness (39%) and irritability (37%).

The most frequent psychological symptoms were difficulty sleeping (21.1%), worrying (18.3%), feeling sad (18.3%) and feeling nervous (16.9%) [6, 7].

Social issues depend on region from where the family hails. Common findings in India and Tata Memorial Hospital are as follows:

1. Majority of patients come from low socio-economic strata; therapy has taken a toll on often meagre resources
2. Levels of education are often low, or child and siblings have dropped out for economic reasons
3. Lack of availability of oncologist/paediatrician/local general practitioners; especially in rural areas to make home visits

Spiritual issues – In a Prospective Cohort study by Kamper et al. [8], a Spiritual Quality of Life Questionnaire was developed to understand how children deal with their advanced cancer. When asked about what they do to get close to God when they are sick, many children said that they pray to God, while others go to church, read spiritual books or perform other spiritual acts.

Management

Pain – Assessment and management of pain has been described elsewhere in this book. For advanced cancer, especially for children residing at home, there is adequate evidence of the use of the WHO two-step analgesic ladder (2012) for the management of pain. The first step includes paracetamol and ibuprofen, when a nonsteroidal anti-inflammatory drug (NSAID) is needed. Step 2 – Oral morphine is very safe and easy to administer and titrate; it is started by the oncologist/palliative care physician and continued at home, under the close supervision of the home care nurses and doctors. No doctor should avoid the use of oral morphine just because the patient is being discharged home. Patients are more at ease in their familiar surroundings, and the helpline is a source for any queries to be addressed, including stopping, if the side effects become severe. Fentanyl patches are easily administered at home. The use of a patient-controlled analgesia (PCA) devices to administer opioids in children has been described in a systematic review by Nijland L. et al. [9], where the benefits were seen for young children and those who were cognitively impaired, although not specifically reported in a home setting.

In India, although there is a big issue with morphine availability, most children are administered pain medication safely at home.

Fatigue, loss of appetite, cachexia syndrome – Fatigue, occurring within the context of an advancing cancer, is much more difficult to treat. It is often reported as part of a syndrome encompassing anorexia, cachexia and fatigue. Ulrich [10, 11] has enumerated causes of fatigue as physical, psychosocial and due to sleep disturbances. Some physical causes are untreated symptoms like pain, nausea/vomiting or drugs used in treatment of these symptoms, e.g. opioids.

Management

Like any symptom, possible reversal of the direct cause is the first dictum, along with exercise and psychotherapy, as the cornerstone of therapy. Parents, as well as the child, are educated about providing small frequent meals, using a variety of foods, sometimes cold, to stimulate appetite, thus reducing fatigue. In India, not being able to feed a child causes distress. Parents are taught that there are other ways to care.

Drugs, e.g. methylphenidate and modafinil, have a limited role. Useful drugs in adults like Medroxyprogesterone acetate and steroids have not been adequately tested in children and should be used with caution. The latter are part of many chemotherapy regimens, and are being used by our team with some benefits, short term, although more for management of anorexia than fatigue. All these measures are very easily managed at home and should be encouraged as part of routine care.

Irritability and lack of sleep are probably inter-related. Sleep disturbances can be relieved by non-drug measures like sleep hygiene and simple anti-anxiolytic drugs. Irritability could be a symptom of early delirium, the most common cause being metabolic disorders. Early delirium is best treated by haloperidol (Table 1), raised intra cranial tension if suspected as a cause should be confirmed and treated with low dose steroids.

Management of Other Common Physical Symptoms

Some other common symptoms, which occur with advancing cancer, and common medications prescribed are listed in Table 1. They can be safely used at home.

Table 1 Adapted from Levine et al. [1]

Symptom	Medication	Common pediatric dose (<60 kg)	Max daily dose
Constipation	Lactulose (can be diluted in water, juices, milk)	<12 years 7.5 mL orally/day, may be repeated after 2 hours	60 mL/day
		>12years 15–30 mL orally/day, may be repeated after 2 hours	
	Polyethylene glycol (mix in 4-8 oz liquid)	1/2 to 1 packet (17 gms) orally every day up to TID	3 packets per day
	Docusate/senna (Senna-S)	2–<6 years: ½ tab daily	1 tab BID
		6–<12 years: 1 tab daily	2 tabs BID
		≥12 years: 2 tabs daily	4 tabs BID
Nausea	Ondansetron	0.15 mg/kg/dose orally or IV every 6–8 hours	8 mg/dose
	Promethazine	>2 years: 0.25 mg/kg/dose orally or IV every 6–8 hours	1 mg/kg/24 hours
	Scopolamine (transdermal)	8–15 kg: ½ patch every 3 days	1 patch every 3 days
		>15 kg: 1 patch every 3 days	
Secretions	Hyoscyamine	2–12 years: 0.0625–0.125 mg/dose orally or SL every 4 hours	2–12 years: 0.75 mg/24 hours
			>12 years: 1.5 mg/24 hours
		>12 years: 0.125–0.25 mg/dose orally or SL every 4 hours	
	Glycopyrrolate	0.04–0.1 mg/kg/dose orally every 4–8 hours	1–2 mg/dose or 8 mg/day
Agitation/ delirium	Haloperidol	0.01–0.02 mg/kg/dose orally, SL, or PR every 8–12 hours	0.15 mg/kg/day
Agitation/ seizures	Lorazepam[b]	0.05 mg/kg/dose orally, SL (preferred for seizure), or PR every 4–6 hours	2 mg/dose
Pruritus	Diphenhydramine[b]	0.5–1.0 mg/kg/dose orally every 6–8 hours	5 mg/kg/24 hours or 400 mg/24 hours
	Hydroxyzine	0.5–1 mg/kg/dose orally every 6–8 hours	4 mg/kg/24 hours

Table 1 (continued)

Symptom	Medication	Common pediatric dose (<60 kg)	Max daily dose
Nausea/ inflammation	Dexamethasone	2.5–10 mg/m^2/day in divided doses every 6–12 hours	20 mg/dose
Pain	Acetaminophen (mild pain)	10–15 mg/kg/dose orally every 4–6 hours	75 mg/kg/24 hours
	Ibuprofen (mind pain)	5–10 mg/kg/dose orally every 6–8 hours	40 mg/kg/24 hours
	Oxycodone (moderate pain)	0.1 mg/kg/dose orally every 4 hours	Patient dependent
		Sustained release formulation available for daily to TID dosing	
	Morphine (moderate pain)	0.3 mg/kg/dose orally, SL, or PR every 3–4 hours	Patient dependent
		0.1 mg/kg/dose IV every 2–4 hours	
		Sustained release formulation available for daily to TID dosing	
	Gabapentin (adjunct for neuropathic pain)	Initially 5–10 mg/kg per day divided TID, increase dose every 3 days	70 mg/kg/24 hours or 3600 mg/24 hours
	Amitriphyline (adjunct for neuropathic pain)	0.1 mg/kg orally at bedtime, increase by doubling dose every 3–5 days	1 mg/kg/24 hours

Severe pain	Recommended infusion starting doses			
Opioid	Infusion/hour[a]	Boost dose[a]	Interval between boosts	Max
Morphine	0.02 mg/kg/hr	0.02 mg/kg	15 minutes	NA, titrate to effect
Hydromorphone	0.004 mg/kg/hr	0.004 mg/kg	15 minutes	NA, titrate to effect
Fentanyl	0.05 mcg/kg/hr	0.5 mcg/kg	10 minutes	NA, titrate to effect

Abbreviations: *BID* twice daily, *IV* intravenous, *NA* not applicable, *PCA* patient-controlled analgesia, *PR* per rectum, *SL* sublingual, *TID* three times daily

[a]May consider boosts only for the opioid-naïve patient for the initial 12–24 hours

[b]Both lorazepam and diphenhydramine may also be used to help manage nausea

Psycho-Social Care

At home, psychological support for the child, siblings and parents (extended as well) will continue, as was being offered in hospital settings, as a continuum. Often, the child cannot express anticipatory grief and fear of the future, even death, with their loved ones. Trained counsellors visit the homes regularly, either alone or with the rest of the team. They facilitate good communication between members of the family, which is easier in the home environment. Coping strategies are also based upon cultural needs and should be individualized; strategies suggested by Baker et al., which are applicable across the globe.

Social care involves rectifying any of the home issues enumerated above. Referrals to available NGOs for any financial, schooling or other community issues are arranged. Social workers are also trained for counselling and can take on the role of the counsellors when required.

Spiritual Care

Spiritual resources, including relationships with pastoral care staff and clergy, may provide additional spiritual support for a child with cancer at the end-of-life [12]. In countries like India where so many religions co-exist, the palliative care team members provide the spiritual care. Dealing with the spiritual suffering of a parent, often with an only child diagnosed with advancing cancer, needs immense spiritual strength on the part of the professional. This develops over time. At Tata

Memorial Centre, for over 20 years, trained volunteer counsellors have been teaching children and their parents coping strategies, under the watchful guidance of us doctors. Active and non-judgmental listening is the cornerstone. As with counselling, solutions emerge from ventilation, and leave the person at least in control of the situation, with an enhanced ability to cope.

End-of-Life Care

Not all cancers in children are curable. A certain percentage will ultimately enter the end-of-life phase and need terminal care. During this period, a coordinated multidisciplinary effort is crucial in working with the patient and family to address their specific needs. Open, honest, thoughtful and caring communication at this time can provide emotional comfort in a situation filled with uncertainty and fear.

The parents are frightened at the prospect of the patient dying at home and may choose the familiarity and security of the hospital; the child may also express a preference about where he or she likes to be, even if not explicitly referring to death [13]. All these factors must be considered – identifying the patient's and family's preferences may help to determine referral to hospice care, the desired location of death, the avoidance to referral to intensive care unit, the adoption of "do not resuscitate" order and plans for funeral arrangements.

In our hospital, if the ward is the choice for End-of-Life Care (EoLC), a corner of the ward is more preferable than the ICU. Family members are allowed around the bed, doctors and nurses ensure comfort care. No resuscitation is the norm in our hospital, as a policy.

At home, EoLC is anticipated and arranged between palliative care teams and local paediatrician and nurses. Symptoms are managed as enumerated above. The local physician/paediatrician is of immense benefit, a prior arrangement will facilitate the death certificate.

Two difficult symptoms to be managed are pain and respiratory distress. Pain guidelines have been enumerated above. It needs to be emphasized that a terribly ill child still feels pain and the dosage of drug should be not be reduced but titrated as per the pain score. The oral route may not be as convenient, the existing central line or a device for sub-cutaneous bolus or infusion are very well tolerated.

For respiratory distress, the reversible causes should be considered, keeping in mind the EoLC situation, where comfort care is paramount. Although blood transfusions may not be warranted for a low Hb, a draining of a large quantity of ascitic or pleural fluid may reduce symptoms. Antibiotics are not warranted but round-the-clock antipyretics will provide adequate comfort. Usually, bronchodilators and steroids will not help. The judicious use of low dose morphine, which reduces perception of breathlessness and respiratory drive, will provide a reduction in the distress caused by the dyspnoea. Ideal starting dose is 0.2 mg/kg every 4 hours orally or buccal. Keeping the room cool and moist, with oxygen only when medically indicated, will provide comfort. A propped-up position with adequate ventilation and a fan breeze on the face, are other useful techniques. The addition of low-dose benzodiazepines like lorazepam and rarely midazolam will lessen anxiety. Judicious use of glycopyrrolate or hyoscine hydrobromide can reduce secretions when the child cannot cough. They should be used with caution, as secretions may become excessively dry. It is to be kept in mind that the death rattle is more distressing to parents than the child itself.

There is sufficient evidence today to concede that all patients, even very young children, know they are dying and that they are able to discern the exceptional distress among family and caregivers around them when death becomes imminent [14, 15]. The same tenets of counselling and communication apply here also. This gives the child courage and comfort as they live in the present and are not too concerned about the future [16].

At the Tata Memorial Hospital where we have practiced paediatric palliative care for over 20 years, our experience has allowed the majority of the children dying of incurable cancer to die at home. This has been possible with the palliative home care team working closely with the doctors and nurses in the community, even in the rural areas. Although some parents do panic and reach the hospital at the end-of-life, these have been few. Most parents have been extremely grateful when asked about the same during the bereavement visits/phone calls.

Bereavement Support

Research and clinical experience have shown that grieving for the parents and siblings can take many different paths, over many years; to incorporate the loss and yet continue with their lives. Most families seem to be able to integrate their feelings and thoughts about the loss experience, with the demands of daily life – they often find the necessary internal and external resources to cope on their own. It is our experience and that of many other services, that bereaved parents may, at some point, find it helpful to share their experiences with other bereaved families through supervised support group meetings.

However, there would be a certain percentage of families who would experience abnormal grieving, manifesting symptoms of major depression and generalized anxiety disorder; and would benefit from appropriate and timely professional help [17]. For siblings, the most common immediate or long-term effects include poor school performance, depression, severe separation anxiety, distress and fear for their own health. The roles of the grief counsellor/palliative care teams include regular contact over several months, with the caveat to call in additional professional help whenever required.

Care for Carers

Anticipatory prevention of compassion fatigue and burn-out among care providers is essential. This happens more commonly when dealing with children. As with primary caregivers, ventilation is useful for the team members. It is important to facilitate opportunities for open discussions during and after challenging cases, along with ample opportunities for stress busting activities.

At our hospital over 20 years, we have experienced only two professionals who developed burn-out while working with children.

Conclusion

Integrating palliative care with the paediatric oncology, to deliver optimum holistic care to a child with advanced cancer and their family, has been a very rewarding experience. It has led to optimum anti-cancer therapy, home care to a large percentage of children, even at the end-of-life, thus achieving a dignified death at a place of their choice and bereavement care for the family. It should be integrated early in the trajectory of the child's cancer journey for maximal benefit.

References

1. Levine D, Lam C, Cunningham M, Remke S, Chrastek J, Klick J, Macauley R, Baker J. Best practices for pediatric palliative cancer care: a primer for clinical providers. J Support Oncol. 2013; https://doi.org/10.12788/j.suponc.0012.
2. Weaver MS, Heinze KE, Kelly KP, Wiener L, Casey RL, Bell CJ, Wolfe J, Garee AM, Watson A, Hinds PS. Palliative care as a standard of care in pediatric oncology. Pediatr Blood Cancer. 2015; https://doi.org/10.1002/pbc.25695.
3. WHO. WHO definition of palliative care for children: WHO; 1998.
4. Baker JN, Hinds PS, Spunt SL, Barfield RC, Allen C, Powell BC, Anderson LH, Kane JR. Integration of palliative care practices into the ongoing care of children with cancer: individualized care planning and coordination. Pediatr Clin N Am. 2008;55:223–50.
5. Friedrichsdorf SJ, Menke A, Brun S, Wamsler C, Zernikow B. Status quo of palliative care in pediatric oncology – a nationwide survey in Germany. J Pain Symptom Manag. 2005; https://doi.org/10.1016/j.jpainsymman.2004.05.004.
6. Wolfe J, Orellana L, Ullrich C, Cook EF, Kang TI, Rosenberg A, Geyer R, Feudtner C, Dussel V. Symptoms and distress in children with advanced cancer: prospective patient-reported outcomes from the PediQUEST study. J Clin Oncol. 2015; https://doi.org/10.1200/JCO.2014.59.1222.
7. Torres V, Nunes MDR, Silva-Rodrigues FM, Bravo L, Adlard K, Secola R, Fernandes AM, Nascimento LC, Jacob E. Frequency, severity, and distress associated with physical and psychosocial symptoms

at home in children and adolescents with cancer. J Pediatr Heal Care. 2019; https://doi.org/10.1016/j.pedhc.2018.11.007.
8. Kamper RL, Van Cleve L, Savedra M. Children with advanced cancer: responses to a spiritual quality of life interview. J Spec Pediatr Nurs. 2010; https://doi.org/10.1111/j.1744-6155.2010.00253.x.
9. Nijland L, Schmidt P, Frosch M, Wager J, Hübner-Möhler B, Drake R, Zernikow B. Subcutaneous or intravenous opioid administration by patient-controlled analgesia in cancer pain: a systematic literature review. Support Care Cancer. 2019; https://doi.org/10.1007/s00520-018-4368-x.
10. Ullrich CK, Dussel V, Hilden JM, Sheaffer JW, Moore CL, Berde CB, Wolfe J. Fatigue in children with cancer at the end of life. J Pain Symptom Manag. 2010; https://doi.org/10.1016/j.jpainsymman.2010.02.020.
11. Ullrich CK, Mayer OH. Assessment and management of fatigue and dyspnea in pediatric palliative care. Pediatr Clin N Am. 2007; https://doi.org/10.1016/j.pcl.2007.07.006.
12. Hart D, Schneider D. Spiritual care for children with cancer. Semin Oncol Nurs. 1997; https://doi.org/10.1016/S0749-2081(97)80023-X.
13. Friedrichsdorf SJ, Collins JJ. Management of non-pain symptoms in pediatric palliative care. Med Princ Pract. 2007; https://doi.org/10.1159/000104540.
14. Liben S, Papadatou D, Wolfe J. Paediatric palliative care: challenges and emerging ideas. Lancet. 2008; https://doi.org/10.1016/S0140-6736(07)61203-3.
15. Epelman CL. End-of-life management in pediatric cancer. Curr Oncol Rep. 2012; https://doi.org/10.1007/s11912-012-0218-z.
16. Kreicbergs U, Valdimarsdóttir U, Onelöv E, Henter JI, Steineck G. Talking about death with children who have severe malignant disease. N Engl J Med. 2004; https://doi.org/10.1056/NEJMoa040366.
17. Breyer J, Sanfeliz A, Cieurzo CE, et al. Loss and grief. In: Brown RT, editor. Comprehensive handbook of childhood cancer and sickle cell disease. New York: Oxford University Press; 2006. p. 358–80.

Part XXXII

South Asia: Indonesia

Experiences in Extending Palliative Care to Neuro-Oncology Patients in Indonesia

Tiara Aninditha, Henry R. Sofyan, Feranindhya Agiananda, and Jonathan Odilo

The Importance of Palliative Care in Neuro-Oncology

Neuro-oncology cases have devastating consequences for patients and family. Tumor of the CNS could deteriorate patient's clinical symptoms rapidly more than other systemic malignancy due to the disability caused by involvement of brain area that regulate motoric and executive functions which lead to the decline of QoL.

The neurological symptoms in brain tumors are unique from one patient to another, related to location and size of the tumor. For example, frontal lobe tumor could induce apraxia, loss of motivation, and psychiatric symptoms that prevent patients from performing daily activities. Furthermore, the tumor mass could shift the brain and cause cerebral edema and brain herniation that can cause death [1–3].

Despite the development of therapeutics modality had increased survival of cancer, mortality caused by CNS tumor remains high. While the incidence of primary brain tumor is low, the incidence of brain metastasis of systemic cancer outnumbers primary brain tumor by three to ten times [4].

The curative treatments for CNS tumor remain limited and the life expectancy of patients are relatively short because of the involvement of eloquent and vital structure of the CNS. With the high number of morbidity and mortality, CNS caused physical and psychological distress to patients and their families. A research done by Sitorus et al. [5] showed that there were 68.6% brain tumor patients who suffer from psychological distress. The distress is mainly caused by physical distress and emotional distress. This distress should be addressed on palliative care as part of comprehensive management.

Therefore, the palliative care in neuro-oncology must begin from the time of diagnosis to the end-of-life phase. The approach of palliative treatment is more emphasized in neuro-oncology than other medical oncology due to higher morbidity and mortality [1–3].

Palliative care in developing countries is a challenge. Aside from health care professionals and regulations, the challenge came from patient's family. The patients who come from lower income

T. Aninditha (✉)
Department of Neurology Cipto Mangunkusumo General Hospital, Faculty of Medicine Universitas Indonesia, Jakarta, Indonesia

H. R. Sofyan
Department of Neurology Cipto Mangunkusumo General Hospital, Faculty of Medicine Universitas Indonesia, Jakarta, Indonesia

Arva Paramaniaga, Jakarta, Indonesia

F. Agiananda
Department of Psychiatry, Awal Bros West Hospital, Jakarta, Indonesia

J. Odilo
Universitas Indonesia Hospital, Faculty of Medicine Universitas Indonesia, Jakarta, Indonesia

M. Silbermann (ed.), *Palliative Care for Chronic Cancer Patients in the Community*,
https://doi.org/10.1007/978-3-030-54526-0_45

family are hard to be appointed. Meanwhile, a patient's family with low education background is hard to be trained. The appointed caregivers cannot recognize the symptoms and needs of patients; the drugs and health care provider facility for palliative care are poorly distributed [6].

Palliative Care in Neuro-Oncology Patients

The aim of palliative care in neuro-oncology is to alleviate symptoms in patients and to preserve QoL. Neurologists mostly handle the clinical symptoms caused by CNS tumor and its complications, but it actually involves multidisciplinary medical specialties capable of managing oncology patients.

Varied symptoms suffered by patients increased the difficulty of palliative care in neuro-oncology. The symptoms that should be addressed by a physician and must be informed to the family that takes care of the patients are listed as follows.

Impaired Consciousness

Impaired consciousness is common in brain tumor patients as manifestations of increased intracranial pressure (ICP). Tumor mass could directly compress the center of consciousness in brain. Cerebral edema produced as the consequences of blood brain barrier (BBB) disruption could also compress the brain. Thus, decrease of consciousness is inevitable. Comelli et al. stated that 25% of patients with brain tumor presented with decrease of consciousness in emergency department (ED) [7]. The condition worsened in the last day of life. In the end-of-life phase, 82% of patients had decreased consciousness in the last week of life [8]. The transient loss of consciousness in patients with long-standing disease could be an indication to start end-of-life care.

Patients with impaired consciousness usually receive intravenous (IV) dexamethasone in emergency department (ED). However, the administration of dexamethasone is debatable since it is futile to give IV dexamethasone to brain tumor patients with refractory cerebral edema. This caused patients' caregiver to admit patients with end-of-life phase to ED repeatedly. The administration of IV dexamethasone should be considered carefully in these patients.

Headache

Almost half of CNS tumor patients would suffer headache in their life. It is mostly due to peritumoral edema which increased the ICP, even after patients have had therapy. In Indonesia, the resource is mostly given to patients who are expected to be cured, thus making it difficult to perform palliative surgery. Instead, pharmacology therapy is resorted to.

Headache occurred at any time during clinical course of brain tumor, and the most irritating symptom compared to other symptoms. Common analgesic could not relieve the headache, and steroid is usually administered. Administration of common analgesic is a common mistake among caregivers. Patients should be educated by a physician to adjust their activity to decrease the headache. Re-evaluation of tumor should be done if there is a suspicion of progressivity.

Seizure

Seizure is a disabling symptom because it inflicts fear to the caregiver and makes patients uncomfortable. Late onset seizure or recurrent seizure could indicate progressive disease, and it could be a burden toward patients. Klein et al. found that seizure in LGG patients lower the physical functioning, limit daily role, vitality, and social functioning [9]. Each uncontrolled seizure could deteriorate the clinical status of patients; therefore, it needs adequate treatment in palliative care.

The main choice of antiepileptic in patients is levetiracetam because of its high efficacy in controlling seizures and low interaction with other drugs. Other antiepileptics such as topiramate or lamotrigine could be used but will need a longer duration of therapy to control seizure [10]. Unfortunately, the choices of antiepileptic in Indonesia are limited. Some hospitals only provide phenytoin or valproic acid. The interaction of phenytoin and dexamethasone to alleviate brain edema is challenging. Phenytoin would lowered the dexamethasone effect, resulting inincreasing dose of dexamethasone to attain equivalent response. This limitation is challenging in controlling seizures in brain tumor.

Swallowing and Nutrition Problem

Swallowing impairment greatly increased in brain tumor patients compared to other tumors. Park et al. found that 72.5% of patients with brain tumor had swallowing problem [11]. Dysphagia in patients could reduce nutritional intake, liquid, and drugs, let alone the increased risk of pulmonary inhalation of solid/liquid mass [12]. This could increase the risk of malnutrition and reducing QoL, especially in brain metastases patients.

Malnutrition in primary brain tumors remains unnoticed. The associated symptoms are nausea, vomiting, headache, dysphagia, fatigue, and weight losses. Malnutrition could cause direct consequences such as infections, decreased functional status, and prolonged recovery from surgery. Thus, the nutritional assessment of brain tumor patients should be done at the time of diagnosis.

In Indonesia, patients usually live with extended family. The patients' nutrition are easily taken care of because the other family members generally cook for the patients. However, nutrition monitoring is still inadequate in Indonesia considering the need of nutrition is different in every phase of disease course.

Motor Deficits

Motoric deficits cause significant disability on patients and greatly burden caregivers compared to other tumors. This prevents patients to perform daily activities, causes distress, and lowers the QoL. Moreover, this deficit is sometimes irreversible due to sequelae after treatment. Long-term steroid use could also cause myopathy in proximal muscle and produce generalized weakness [13]. Ijzeman-Korevaar et al., in a systematic review, shown that 44.2% patients presented with motor deficits in end-of-life phase [14]. Thus, compared to other types of cancers, the motor deficits have more impact on QoL compared to other advanced cancers [13].

Until now, the best choice to preserve motor function in patients is through physical rehabilitation. This therapy is difficult to be performed in home care due to insurance coverage and regulation. Patient's family members are taught simple movement to prevent further complications and to mobilize patient. In cooperative patients, patients are taught to maximize the intact body function to adapt to physical disability.

Cognitive Dysfunction

Cognitive dysfunction is common in brain tumor patients (up to 68.9% in primary brain tumor [15] and as high as 80% in brain metastasis [16]). A systematic review by Ijzerman-Korevaar et al. showed that 36% of patients with glioma presented with cognitive dysfunction in diagnosis and increased to 44.3% at the end-of-life phase [14]. The cognitive domain ranged from executive and attention, memory, language, visuospatial, and psychomotor speed [15]. Even the treatment modality such as surgery, chemotherapy, radiotherapy, and supportive treatment (antiepileptic, steroid) could induce cognitive dysfunction.

Cognitive dysfunction could be rooted from tumor or sequelae of and after treatment. Cognitive preserving drugs (donepezil or memantine) could be given to patients who underwent curative modality. Unfortunately, these drugs are not suitable for patients with partial therapy. These drugs are expensive and not covered by insurance. Therefore, the importance of curative treatment is emphasized to prevent cognitive dysfunction. This is a challenging matter in Indonesia because patients come with tumor of unresectable size due to delayed diagnosis.

Psychiatric Changes

Brain tumor patients tend to have a range of psychiatric symptoms because of the tumor itself, the disability caused by the tumor and the difficulty to restore the symptoms, and overall problems encountered in the course of the disease. Depression found in 25–44% of patients with primary brain tumor [17] can be associated on women, less educated subjects, lower tumor grade, and in frontal area [18]. Arnold et al. shown that anxiety found on 48% of brain tumor patients is predominantly on women and lower grade tumor. Psychosis could also be found in 22% of patients with pituitary gland and temporal lobe tumors [17].

In several Academy Health Center (AHC), psychiatrists are involved at the beginning of the diagnosis and treatment of brain tumor patients, even giving medical support, until patients are ready for home care to prevent further distress. Unfortunately, this service is not yet widely implemented and difficult to follow-up. The peer group communication and social worker psychological support are only available in the big cities. Furthermore, psychological distress is not the main reason caregivers bring patients to hospital which complicate the symptoms.

Adaptation of Palliative Guidelines in Indonesia

In Indonesia, the policy of palliative care has been made. A minister regulation No. 812/Menkes/SK/VII/2007 was issued to assure that palliative care is established as part of healthcare in Indonesia [19]. In 2015, the national guideline for palliative cancer program was already composed. The program emphasized on establishing palliative care by integrating healthcare facilities, provision of human resources and infrastructure, and increasing accessibility of palliative care on oncology patients [20]. The implementation of palliative care in Indonesia is still in developing phase. There are many limitations challenging the implementation of palliative care. The total number of specialist physicians in Indonesia is low compared to population, let alone the physician specialized in palliative care. This condition is worsened by the maldistribution of physicians in Indonesia.

Despite limitations of palliative health care professionals in Indonesia, every personnel involved in neuro-oncology palliative team has an expertise to take care of the patients. The tumor board which decides whether patients must be subjected to palliative treatment or not is composed of neurologist, neurosurgeon, hematology oncology internist, radiotherapist, medical rehabilitation therapist, psychiatrist, medical nutrition specialist, and other specialist as patients need. In Indonesia, Cipto Mangunkusumo General Hospital and National Cancer Center Dharmais Hospital are the top referral hospitals which give comprehensive care for neuro-oncology patients, among other government and private hospitals in the big cities.

The palliative patients decision algorithm (Fig. 1) is started as early as the patients are admitted to the hospital. Patients were screened with Palliative Score (Table 1); if the score is equal or greater than 4, they should be consulted at the palliative division. All patients will be discussed in tumor board meetings to have comprehensive assessment for medical inpatient care, palliative care, and to prepare home care. Before going home, the patient's caregiver will be educated on how to take care of the patients, his/her nutritional needs, including psychiatric, rehabilitation, and any symptoms or condition that need special attention. Soon as the patient is discharged, home care could be started.

Admission of palliative care is different and unstandardized among specialists. No curative treatment is given to patients. By principle, only symptomatic treatments are given by many physicians. Because of this principle, further diagnosis is not done in patients. Meanwhile, in neuro-oncology case, diagnosis determines the need for palliative care. The difference in perception caused palliative care in neuro-oncology to lack multidisciplinary approach. Many physicians in Indonesia perceive that palliative care equals to hospice care, resulting in inadequacy of treatment given to patients and the rate of readmission of patients is high.

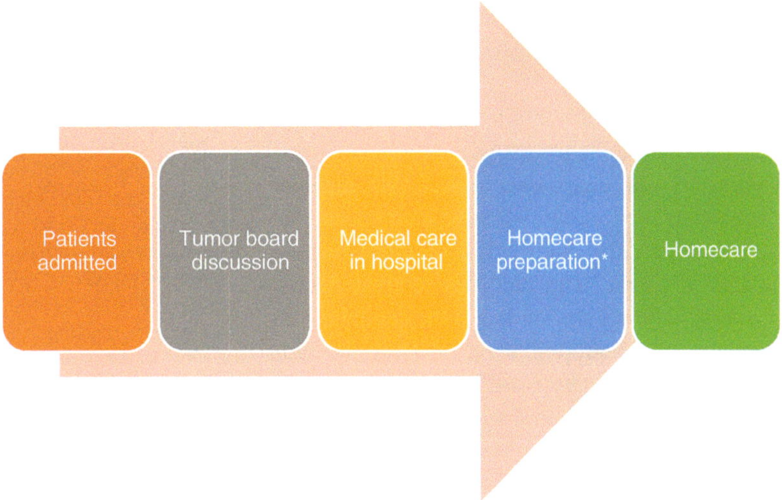

Fig. 1 Palliative patient decision algorithm. *Home care preparation consisted of family meeting, family education, nutritional education, physiotherapy, and psychiatry counseling. In home care, case manager and social worker help patient's family

Table 1 Palliative score in Cipto Mangunkusumo General Hospital

Baseline disease (score 2 for every item present)	
1. Metastatic or recurrent cancer	
2. COPD	
3. Stroke (with functional preservation <50%)	
4. Chronic kidney disease	
5. Late stage heart disease (congestive heart failure (CHF), coronary artery disease, cardiomyopathy with left ventricular ejection fraction (LVEF) <25%)	
6. HIV/AIDS	
7. Other severe congenital disorder	
Comorbidity (score 1 for every item present)	
1. Chronic liver disease	
2. Moderate kidney disorder	
3. Moderate COPD	
4. CHF	
5. Another disease or complications	
Eastern Cooperative Oncology Group (ECOG) performance status	
ECOG scale	Score
0	0
1	0
2	1
3	2
4	3
Other criteria (score 1 for every item present)	
1. No curative treatment planned	
2. Decided not to continue therapy	
3. Uncontrolled pain >24 hours	
4. Uncontrolled symptoms (e.g., nausea and vomiting)	
5. Psychosocial and spiritual condition	
6. Emergency department admission >1 time/month for the same diagnosis	
7. Diagnosed with same problem >1 time/month	
8. Hospital admission without meaningful clinical treatment	
9. ICU admission without meaningful clinical treatment	

Home care in Indonesia is made possible by referral back system of the Indonesian National Health System where patients are referred back to Primary Health Center (PHC) after treatment in hospital. The main problems of palliative care after hospital treatment are lack of hospice care, social worker, and case manager of patients at post-hospital treatment. The available service is centralized in metropolitan and capital city, and done by an NGO. There is no standardized care, and not all patients need the treatment covered by the said service. The culture of Indonesian people from marginal areas is to spend the rest of their lives in the home without the aid of health care professionals.

Although a regulation of palliative care is already established, hospice and home care regulations in oncology patients were lacking. The health care professionals are not protected by the law while caring for oncology patients. There is no standard of care set by the policymakers and standardized outcome to be achieved. Thus, home care is only performed by certain health care institution, mainly in central referral in every province.

Financing is one of the problems faced in palliative care in Indonesia. Palliative care is taking a significant amount of cost needed in health care. Many patients in Indonesia could not afford the care for oncology patients. The national health insurance provided by Indonesian government only has limited and without home care coverage. Many patients depend on external financing such as non-governmental organization (NGO).

Indonesia has only limited resources given to palliative care in neuro-oncology patients. There were only 20 neuro-oncologists, 90 medical oncologists, and a few palliative care specialists in Indonesia. The distribution of those professionals is sparse. The facilities to treat neuro-oncology patients are limited in the capital of the provinces and metropolitan cities. Thus, the education of hospice care is difficult, due to fear of patients going back home without palliative care facility.

Although it seems pessimistic, an effort to enforce palliative care services for patients has already started in Indonesia. In many AHC and referral hospitals, tumor board meetings have already been set up. Hopefully in the near future, palliative care services in Indonesia could fulfill the needs of palliative patients and families so that their quality of life will be better.

References

1. Mummudi N, Jalali R. Palliative care and quality of life in neuro-oncology. F1000Prime Rep. 2014;6
2. Borasio GD, Bausewein C, Lorenzl S, Voltz R, Wasner M. Palliative care in neuro-oncology. In: Tonn J-C, Reardon DA, Rutka JT, Westhpal M, editors. Oncology of CNS tumors. Berlin: Springer-Verlag; 2010.
3. Burnet NG, Bulusu VR, Jefferies SJ. Management of primary brain tumours. In: Booth S, Bruera E, editors. Palliative care consultations: primary and metastatic brain tumours. New York: Oxford University Press; 2004.
4. Soffietti R, Franchino F, Ruda R. Brain metastasis as complication of systemic cancers. In: Schiff D, Arrilaga I, Wen PY, editors. Cancer neurology in clinical practice: neurological complications of cancer and its treatment. 3rd ed. USA: Springer; 2018.
5. Sitorus JJR, Agiananda F, Anninditha T, Wiguna T, Lukman PR. Distres in brain tumor patients and its related factors. Neurona. 2017;34(2):91–6.
6. Higginson IJ, Evans CJ. What is the evidence that palliative care teams improve outcome for cancer patients and their families? Cancer J. 2010;16(5):423–35.
7. Comelli G, Lippi G, Campana V, Servadei F, Cervellin G. Clinical presentation and epidemiology of brain tumors firstly diagnosed in adults in the emergency department: a 10-year, single center prospective study. Ann Transl Med. 2017;5(13):269.
8. Faithfull S, Cook K, Lucas C. Palliative care of patients with a primary malignant brain tumour: case review of service use and support provided. Palliat Med. 2005;19:545–50.
9. Klein M, Engelberts NHJ, van der Ploeg HM, Trenite DGAK, Aaronson NK, Taphoorn MJB, et al. Epilepsy in low-grade gliomas: the impact on cognitive function and quality of life. Ann Neurol. 2003;54(4):514–20.
10. Thomas AA, Carver A. Essential competencies in palliative medicine for neuro-oncologists. Neurooncol Pract. 2015;2(3):151–7.
11. Parks DH, Chun MH, Lee SJ, Song YB. Comparison of swallowing functions between brain tumor and stroke patients. Ann Rehabil Med. 2013;37(5):633–41.
12. Pace A, Di Lorenzo C, Guariglia L, Jandolo B, Carapella CM, Pompili A. End of life issues in brain tumor patients. J Neuro-Oncol. 2009;91:39–43.
13. Amidei C, Kushner DS. Clinical implications of motor deficits related to brain tumors. Neurooncology Pract. 2015;2(4):179–84.
14. Ijzeman-Korevaar M, Snijders TJ, de Graeff A, Teunissen SCCM, de Vos FYF. Prevalence of symptoms in glioma patients throughout the disease trajectory: a systematic review. J Neuro-Oncol. 2018;140:485–96.
15. van Kessel E, Baumfalk AE, van Zandvoort MJE, Robe PA, Snijders TJ. Tumor-related neurocognitive dysfunction in patients with diffuse glioma: a systematic review of neurocognitive functioning prior antitumor treatment. J Neuro-Oncol. 2017;134:9–18.
16. Gertsnecker A, Nabors LB, Meneses K, Fiveash JB, Marson DC, Cutter G, et al. Cognition in patients with newly diagnosed brain metastasis: profiles and implications. J Neuro-Oncol. 2014;120:179–85.
17. Madhusoodanan S, Ting MB, Farah T, Ugur U. Psychiatric aspects of brain tumor: a review. World J Psychiatr. 2015;5(3):273–85.
18. Arnold SD, Forman LM, Brigidi BD, Carter KE, Schweitzer HA, Quinn HE, et al. Evaluation and characterization of generalized anxiety and depression in patients with primary brain tumors. Neuro-Oncology. 2008;10(2):171–81.
19. Palliative Care Policy. 2007 Jul 19; 812/Menkes/SK/VII/2007.
20. Ministry of Health Republic of Indonesia. National Guidelines of Cancer Palliative Program. Jakarta: Indonesia; 2015.

Establishment of Home-Based Pediatric Palliative Care: The Indonesian Experience

Lynna Chandra and Ying Pin Toh

Background

Rachel House was established in 2006 to provide palliative care for children living with life-threatening illnesses, in particular, cancer and HIV. At that time, palliative care was not widely known [1–3], with the development of the local palliative care policy only in 2007 by the Ministry of Health of Indonesia [1, 3]. Indonesia is part of Southeast Asia and one of the most populated countries in the world [1].

The initial intent when Rachel House was set up was to build a 60-bed inpatient facility. The decision was subsequently made to convert the service to follow a home-based palliative care model, responding to the needs and demands of the children and the families Rachel House was meant to serve, many of whom were from marginalized communities.

The added challenge was that the home care model was new to the Indonesian healthcare system and, at the time, there were few community services serving the poor. Patients were discharged from hospitals with minimal support in the community setting. The only available avenue, when crisis hit, was for patients to be rushed back to the hospital, if finances permitted.

L. Chandra (✉)
Rachel House (Yayasan Rumah Rachel), Jakarta, Indonesia

International Children's Palliative Care Network, Assagay, South Africa
e-mail: lynna@rachel-house.org

Y. P. Toh
Rachel House (Yayasan Rumah Rachel), Jakarta, Indonesia

Asia Pacific Hospice Network, Singapore, Singapore

Hospice or Home Care

The experience of Eka,[1] a 12-year-old boy diagnosed with acute myeloid leukaemia, influenced the decision to switch from a hospice to a home care model for the delivery of community palliative care. Eka was referred to Rachel House in the early part of our journey, having been discharged from the hospital after enduring months of treatment that, unfortunately, did not curb the progression of the disease. He was referred to Rachel House's inpatient service with a large wound at the perineum that bled profusely. Despite his difficulties, Eka strongly desired to go home and flatly refused further institutional care. He cited friends and home-cooked meals as the two overriding factors for this decision - even when going home meant sleeping on a thin mattress on the dirt floor in the living room of a house that measured no larger than 3 m × 3 m. During the six weeks of journeying with Eka, the Rachel House

[1]Name has been changed to protect the privacy of the child.

M. Silbermann (ed.), *Palliative Care for Chronic Cancer Patients in the Community*,
https://doi.org/10.1007/978-3-030-54526-0_46

team organized a movie screening in his home, where Eka lay on his mattress surrounded by his friends, enjoying the camaraderie! This story demonstrates the child's hunger for the simple joys of home and childhood.

Referral: The Early Days

As palliative care was in its infancy when Rachel House started, convincing doctors to refer patients to Rachel House was challenging. Through Rachel House, palliative care was introduced to the hospitals in Jakarta as a service to help manage the pain and symptoms of patients at the end of life or when prognosis was poor. Nurses in the wards were quickly won over to the concept of palliative care. They saw this as a way to help relieve the symptoms of their patients who were being discharged home, and as a layer of support for the families, especially when parents faced the anxieties of caring for an ill child at home. With the support of nurses from hospitals, Rachel House was increasingly invited to participate in discussions with the families of children with poor prognoses prior to discharge into the community. Advocacy for palliative care grew despite challenges within a setting where doctors were pressured to "fight till the end" because parents expected them to.

Palliative Care Knowledge: Changing Mindset and Culture

As Rachel House began caring for more patients, the ward doctors and oncologists began to show interest in learning more about palliative care. Advocating for pain control was a major hurdle to cross. In the early years of palliative care in Indonesia, pain management was not a priority. In the past, doctors in Indonesia had been taught that treating pain would mask the source of pain and confound the diagnostic process. Rachel House would receive children with late-stage cancer being discharged with weak analgesics, as morphine was rarely prescribed. Wound dressings of cancer patients were frequently changed without consideration for pain or the need for analgesia. Pain was accepted as part of the local culture and as part of the illness journey. Advocating for increased awareness regarding the need to address pain took time. Eventually, doctors began to see the need to manage pain and patients gained confidence that pain could be sufficiently controlled during the cancer journey.

Home-Based Palliative Care-Team Composition

When Rachel House first started out, palliative care was a concept new to Indonesia. The biggest question then was that of the team composition. At Rachel House, where the target patient population was children from marginalized communities who were faced with life-limiting and life-threatening illnesses, the goal was to provide care at home, hence the decision was made to develop a nurse-led home hospice team.

As the team matured, Rachel House was faced with the challenge of training nurses in critical thinking, clinical excellence, and leadership. The idea of a nurse-led team was novel to the local hierarchical healthcare system where doctors were the usual leaders of healthcare teams [4].

Role modelling by nurses trained in palliative care and experienced in providing community-based care was the most powerful tool, inspiring the wider nursing community to see potentiality above and beyond what they had been taught.

"Aha!" Moments

How can we encourage doctors and nurses to turn towards suffering of their patients, and respond?

Turning Towards the Suffering

During a ward round attended by several palliative care experts from Singapore at a local children's oncology ward in Jakarta, a palliative care physician stopped on the way out of the room to speak to the father of a child whose medical issues had just been discussed.

Dr. Rosalie Shaw, from Singapore, quietly asked for an interpreter as she knelt down in front of the man who was sitting quietly on the floor. Dr. Shaw asked how long he had been staying at the hospital and invited him to talk about the journey he and his daughter had taken to reach the hospital from their village. As the child's father spoke, tears started streaming down his face. He said, "I have been here for 3 weeks. This is the first time anyone has spoken to me and asked me about my journey."

At that moment, a sacred silence of communion came upon all present. Hearts were opened to realize that although this is the father of the child, no one had noticed he was there or engaged him in the discussion of his child's illness. Palliative care demonstrated to local hospitals that healing must embrace all facets of a child's life, addressing her emotional and spiritual needs as well as her physical ailments. And in matters of the social and emotional aspects of care, parents must be included in the realm of medical professionals' care as well as part of the care team to ensure the child's well-being [5].

Responding to the suffering of patients requires healthcare professionals to have the courage to care, to witness, and to respond. This is particularly critical in the setting of patients' homes. This lesson, gleaned at an early stage of Rachel House's journey, formed an integral part of its mission.

Birthday Joy

Aji[1] was an 8-year-old child with incurable cancer who was faced with a prognosis of only a few weeks. The availability of Rachel House's home care team meant that Aji could be cared for at home, braving the devastating symptoms he experienced in the last few months of his life, such as neuropathic pain, bedsores, constipation, loss of appetite, loneliness, and anger. His wonderfully caring mother had a "life-line" to home palliative nurses through a 24-hour-a-day telephone hotline. This allowed the family to be embraced by a team to guide them in providing care in a manner that would keep Aji comfortable. During the last 15 months of Aji's life, Rachel House arranged to celebrate his birthday surrounded by loved ones and visited by his favorite clown and celebrity idol.

It Takes a Village: Community-Based Approach

A wealth of resources exists within a community that is often untapped in the provision of medical care, particularly for children living with life-limiting, life-threatening illnesses and their families.

The Role of Kader[2] Women (Community Health Workers)

When we began our journey into the homes of the children referred to Rachel House, we came across neighbors who offered their concerns, shared their knowledge, and generously gave their time beyond our expectations. Soon, these neighbors, many of them women, became part of our care team and introduced us to the culture and wisdom of the community, extensive knowledge which we otherwise would not have been able to obtain, or which would have taken us much time to develop.

Training of "Kader" Women

What are the roles of these women?

1. To identify people in the community who are living with life-limiting illnesses and need assistance.
2. To connect them to available networks of assistance, such as food, transport, medications, or even simply to community members

[2]'Kader' is Indonesian for cadre; health cadres are frequently engaged to render non-clinical aspects of care in the Indonesian healthcare setting.

who can help clean their homes, wash their clothes, or cook a simple meal.

3. To provide assistance and help them navigate the often complex health system to access care.
4. To accompany and help provide care for these people living at home with life-limiting illnesses, and to provide respite to their caregivers.

These Kader women are now an integral part of the Rachel House team and an important part of the care we provide to our patients. They are not only powerful partners to our clinical team, providing deep and wise insights to the socio-emotional aspects of the lives of patients, shedding light on their needs and priorities, but just as importantly, act as soothing balm for the patients and their families providing them comfort during frightening and difficult times.

Case-Based Illustrations

The story of the grandmother of one of our patients, Allya,[1] clearly illustrates this. Allya is a child with complex medical needs. Being Allya's sole caregiver, her grandmother could not attend a wedding she was invited to as there was no one else to care for Allya, whose parents had died. Ibu Eny, one of our Kader women, not only offered to take care of Allya that evening, but also brought her make-up kit to ensure that Allya's grandmother was beautifully made up for the event. These women from the community allowed Rachel House to embrace patients and families holistically.

Another example is the day when Abi, a 5-year-old boy, went for his first metro ride with one of our community health workers. Abi's grandmother, his sole caregiver, was frail and too weak to take him to the hospital. So, Abi would have to go to the hospital with our community health worker instead, where he would be met by one of our nurses who would accompany Abi to meet his doctor. Abi was very attached to his grandmother and reluctant for the hospital visit without her. To coax Abi to attend his appointment, our community health worker, offered him a trip on the new Metro in the city as a reward for attending the hospital visit. Not surprisingly, a trip to the hospital is often complex and hugely negotiated requiring close teamwork between different members of the multidisciplinary team.

Key Learnings from Rachel House's Journey

1. **Caring for the Whole Person: An Empowered Team**

   Patients need to be cared for as a whole person. Palliation of physical pain and symptoms cannot be addressed separately from social, emotional, and economic aspects. Team members must be empowered with support of the organization and stakeholders to help alleviate these socioeconomic challenges, beyond the physical symptoms. This renders a sense of hope and mitigates against burnout and feelings of helplessness derived from working in a limited-resource setting. Close teamwork to overcome the multidimensional issues faced by patients helps to build strong solidarity amongst team members, and importantly, allows the humanity in each and every member to blossom. A powerful reminder that they are not just healthcare professionals, but to quote Ram Dass, "We are all walking each other home."
2. **Caring for the Child and Family Supported by the Community**

   A child's well-being is very much dependent on the primary caregiver's presence and capacity. Caregivers of the children need to be seen as part of the care team and their needs should be supported. Successful and effective care for children living with life-limiting illnesses at home can only happen when families are supported and communities are empowered to care for them. To be able to deliver this well, Rachel House has had to lean on the support of community members – the "Kader" women, including them as part of the care team.

References

1. Agency CI. Central Intelligency Agency – The World Factbook 2009. Available from: https://www.cia.gov/library/publications/the-world-factbook/geos/id.html.
2. Putranto R, Mudjaddid E, Shatri H, Adli M, Martina D. Development and challenges of palliative care in Indonesia: role of psychosomatic medicine. Biopsychosoc Med. 2017;11:29.
3. Rochmawati E, Wiechula R, Cameron K. Current status of palliative care services in Indonesia: a literature review. Int Nurs Rev. 2016;63(2):180–90.
4. Arisanti N, Sasongko EPS, Pandia V, Hilmanto D. Implementation of palliative care for patients with terminal diseases from the viewpoint of healthcare personnel. BMC Res Notes. 2019;12(1):217.
5. Jones BL, Contro N, Koch KD. The duty of the physician to care for the family in pediatric palliative care: context, communication, and caring. Pediatrics. 2014;133(Suppl 1):S8–15.

Part XXXIII

South Asia: Thailand

Network of Primary Palliative Care in Thailand: A Prototype Driven by Education

Srivieng Pairojkul

Background of Thailand's Health Security System

Over the last four decades, Thailand has made remarkable progress in social and economic development, moving from a low-income to an upper-income country in less than a generation [1]. According to the National Statistical Office, the total population of Thailand in 2018 was 66 million, with one-third residing in the Northeastern region. Life expectancy at birth was 73 years for males and 80.1 years for females. One-sixth of the population (11.3 million) are elderly [2]. Concerning health service accessibility, Thailand has been recognized as one of the countries with a successful health development [3]. The Ministry of Public Health (MOPH) is the key health authority responsible for planning, implementing, monitoring and evaluating health policy and service implementation. There are other autonomous health agencies that have been established through legislation, notably the Health Systems Research Institute (HSRI, 1992), the Thai Health Promotion Foundation (ThaiHealth, 2001), the National Health Security Office (NHSO, 2002), the National Health Commission Office (NHCO, 2007) and the Healthcare Accreditation Institute (HAI, 2009) [3].

Thailand's policy on universal health coverage (UHC) has made good progress since its implementation of the National Health Security Act in 2002 [4]. Ninety-nine percent of the population have access to health insurance under three schemes: Universal Health Insurance, the Social Security Fund and the Civil Servants Medical Benefit Scheme [3]. Every Thai citizen is now entitled to essential health services at all life stages. The benefits of the policy comprise essential services in preventive, curative and palliative care for all age groups. Extension of coverage to high-cost services, such as renal replacement therapy, cancer therapy and stem-cell transplants, has improved financial protection for patients. Well-coordinated district health systems enable individuals to seek care or referral at health units close to home. The resulting increase in service utilization has contributed to a low prevalence of unmet needs for outpatient and inpatient services [3]. Most health care services in Thailand are delivered by the public sector, which includes 1002 hospitals and 9765 health stations.

The public hospitals are operated by the Ministry of Public Health and are classified as:

- **Regional hospitals** are located in the center of the province, have a capacity of at least 500 beds and have a comprehensive set of

S. Pairojkul (✉)
Karunruk Palliative Care Center, Faculty of Medicine, Khon Kaen University, Khon Kaen, Thailand
e-mail: srivieng@kku.ac.th

M. Silbermann (ed.), *Palliative Care for Chronic Cancer Patients in the Community*, https://doi.org/10.1007/978-3-030-54526-0_47

specialists. As of 2018, there are 34 regional hospitals.

- **General hospitals** are located in province capitals or major districts and have a capacity of 200 to 500 beds. There are 86 general hospitals.
- **Community hospitals** are located in the district level and further classified by size:
  - Large community hospitals have a capacity of 90 to 150 beds.
  - Medium community hospitals have a capacity of 60 beds.
  - Small community hospitals have a capacity of 10 to 30 beds.

There are, in all, 723 community hospitals. Their capacity is usually limited to providing primary care, while referring patients in need of more advanced or specialized care to general or regional hospitals.

Primary Health Care System in Thailand

The Thai Ministry of Public Health tackles health inequity through three major policies: (1) Region-based health services system. This policy aims to facilitate better sharing of resources within each region including funding, human resources, information and medicines/technologies, and to strengthen referrals across care levels within regions toward more efficient services. For health care service there is a referral system which facilitates referring upstream and downstream between primary health units to community hospitals and to higher health facilities at provincial hospitals or regional hospitals (2). Health services development plans or 'Service Plans', which comprise primary and holistic health care as one of 15 Service Plans that all health facilities under the MOPH will use as their operation plan and for implementation. The goals of these primary care and holistic care Service Plans include care provision by family care teams and establishment of long-term community care and health promotion for the elderly, disabled and vulnerable groups (3). District health system (DHS) that calls for multisectoral collaboration in the community using strategic approaches called "U-CARE": Unity district health team; Community participation; Appreciation; Resource sharing and human development; Essential care provision. It is also believed that the DHS could become an active participatory model that can harmonize upstream and downstream processes of health service systems in Thailand [5].

Thailand Cancer Epidemiology

In 2018, cancer was the leading cause of death in Thailand, accounting for 19% of mortality, followed by ischemic heart disease (12%) and stroke (10%) [6]. The summary cancer statistics in 2018 were: Number of new cancer cases 170,495; number of cancer deaths 114,199; the top five most frequent cancers in males, excluding non-melanoma skin cancer, were liver, lung, colorectum, prostate and gall bladder, while in females were breast, cervix, uteri, colorectum, lung and liver [7].

In 2019, the Karunruk Palliative Care Center and the Thai Palliative Care Network conducted a multicenter point prevalent survey of palliative care in patients from 14 hospitals in Thailand and found that 18.7% met the criteria of life-limiting illness [8]. Fifty-five percent were patients with cancer, while 44.4% were patients who were defined as noncancer (Table 1). Only 17.3% of these palliative patients were under the care of the hospital palliative care program, reflecting the under-diagnosis and lack of awareness of the doctors.

The majority of palliative patients being treated by palliative care teams had cancers, as cancer patients have more access to palliative care services. Our point prevalence survey showed that 22.7% of cancer patients received palliative care consultation compared to 11.9% of noncancer patients. The cancer patients primarily received treatment at the regional hospitals, where there are cancer centers. When reaching the palliative phase they are usually referred to the palliative care team, who provide

Table 1 Point prevalence of palliative care patients in 14 hospitals in Thailand

Hospital Level	Hospital No.	All patients	PC Patients	% PC Patient	Cancer (%)		Noncancer (%)	
					No.	%	No	%
Super tertiary	2	1148	212	18.5	153	72.2	59	27.8
Tertiary	7	3216	631	19.6	315	49.9	316	50.1
Secondary	5	1399	236	16.9	73	30.9	163	69.1
Total	14	5763	1079	18.7	600	55.7	538	44.4

continuous care if they are in the city area, but if they are in the district area or in other provinces, they are referred to the palliative care team in the community hospital and will be under the care of the district team until death. Most cancer patients receive palliative care continuously by the community palliative care team and the majority of the patients in the northeast, the north and the southern part of Thailand die at home.

Palliative Care Development in Thailand

Access to Palliative Care

Palliative care was first recognized during the AIDS epidemic, but the care provided was mainly psychosocial and spiritual. Most programs were run by a nurse who was compassionate and provided spiritual care for the patients by organizing religious ceremonies for the patients and their families. These programs lacked elements of pain and symptom management, and rarely was there a doctor involved in the program. The active services were provided by faith- and religion-based facilities such as the Camillian Social Center, St. Clare's Hospice and Mercy Center, which also provided antiviral drugs and palliative care services. A Thai temple called Wat Phra Baht Nam Phu, located in the hills of Lopburi 120 km north of Bangkok, provided care for patients with late-stage AIDS who were rejected by their families. After the introduction and availability of antiviral drugs under the universal coverage policy, the AIDS epidemic subsided and palliative care was then confined to advanced-cancer patients. In 2012, Thailand's palliative care services were classified in the Group 3a, which is localized palliative care provision, but not yet reaching a measure with mainstream service providers [9]. Since palliative care services were not integrated into the Service Plan of the MOPH, there was no career path and no financial support or time allocation for the personnel. The services were run on volunteer basis. The situation had been perpetuated due to the lack of doctors' education.

The policy for palliative care developed very slowly, and it was in 2006 that the Healthcare Accreditation Institute included several palliative care indicators, including pain management and psychosocial/spiritual care into hospital accreditation. In 2009, the National Health Security Office provided support for hospitals to develop a palliative care network. Many provincial hospitals, the majority in the northeast of Thailand, had begun to develop a network with their community hospitals, but still there was no symptom management. At that time, Karunruk Palliative Care Center was the only center that provided multi-level training programs. In 2014, the Ministry of Public Health issued a health policy stating that by December 2014 every provincial hospital was required to have a full-time nurse (trained in PC) coordinating the hospital palliative care unit and this would increase to 300 community hospitals by September 2015. With the implementation of this policy, palliative education was in dire need. In 2016 we developed a strong network in Service Plan area 7, which was composed of four provincial hospitals and 62 community hospitals in the northeast region of Thailand, by implementing a training curriculum which offered multi-level training for professionals and received financial support from the National Health Security Office. The networks were so strong that palliative patients could be referred to care and die at their homes under the supervision of community networks. It was in 2016 when palliative care was integrated into the

MOPH Service Plan, which was a big leap in palliative care development. We received financial support from the Thai Health Promotion Foundation to create a community network in the northeast region of Thailand using our training curriculum and the lessons learned from the network development of Service Plan area 7. The northeast region comprises of one-third of the entire country's population. The networking process continued to extend to the northern and the southern regions of Thailand in 2018, under the collaboration between Karunruk Palliative Care Center and the MOPH and with funding from Khon Kaen University. In 2019, we started a network in the central part of Thailand and in 2020 are moving forward to Bangkok's metropolitan area. Palliative home care has been endorsed by the National Health Security Office since 2016 by providing e-claim for palliative home care, which has had a great impact on palliative home care services.

Palliative Education

Changing or developing appropriate attitudes and practices among healthcare professionals regarding end-of-life care is important for enhancing the system's development which can be achieved through training and exposure with practical sessions. In the past, most of the educational programs were provided by medical school-based hospitals at an annual conference, primarily focusing on psychosocial/spiritual care. There were barely any palliative care programs in public hospitals and, if there were, they were mostly run by nurses who volunteered their extra time with no support from the hospitals. The National Cancer Institute and regional cancer centers, both of which are under the MOPH, started a home-care program in 1998, with management of pain and supportive care as the main focus [10]. Most palliative patients, when being discharged from the hospitals, would be followed-up by the primary care team in the community who did not receive any palliative training.

Most medical schools had integrated palliative care education in their curriculums but with no practice sessions, and some medical schools did not have any palliative care unit at all; the education was then more likely based on opportunity. Most doctors graduated with only little knowledge of palliative care, not to mention the lack of skills in cancer pain management and the use of opioids. The nursing curriculum contained more topics related to palliative care, but mostly emphasized psychosocial/spiritual care, and pharmacists and social workers rarely received any training in palliative care. When training in palliative care, it is important to have an opportunity to practice, as symptom management and communication skills must be used in real contexts. In 2012, Phungrassami conducted a national survey on a number of palliative care-trained personnel, and there were only a handful of doctors trained through intermediate or long-term courses; of these numbers, 12 doctors had graduated from more than one year of training and six graduated from at least a one-month course. Most of them were in medical schools. Only 40 doctors graduated from a < 1-week course and all together only a total of 59 doctors were trained in palliative care [11]. Most personnel gained knowledge by attending a 2–3-day conference conducted by the medical schools. Other allied health personnel rarely received training in palliative care (Table 2). Education in palliative care is scaling up and urgently in need.

Implementation of Scaling up Palliative Care Education

Thailand has been recognized as a country with a strong primary care network. Ninety-nine percent of the population are covered through a universal health insurance. Integrating palliative care into its health care system will provide wide access to palliative services.

Our health care system has been established with an emphasis on community primary care and networking (Fig. 1). When patients are discharged from the hospital they are referred to the community network, which composed of district (community) hospital and their primary care units (PCUs), and each village has health volun-

Table 2 Numbers of palliative-care-trained personnel in the sample hospitals

Duration of training	Community hospital	General hospital	Regional hospital	Medical school hospital	Cancer centre	Other hospital	Total (%)
Doctors							
≥ 1 year	0	1	1	10	0	0	12 (8)
1 month – <1 year	1	0	3	2	0	0	6 (4)
1 week – <1 month	4	1	3	2	0	0	10 (7)
< 1 week	40	14	16	16	0	1	87 (59)
Unknown duration	14	11	4	1	2	0	32 (22)
Total	**59**	**27**	**27**	**31**	**2**	**1**	**147 (100)**
Nurses							
≥ 1 year	0	0	0	0	0	0	0 (0)
1 month – <1 year	9	10	4	18	4	4	49 (3)
1 week – <1 month	30	9	11	16	1	0	67 (4)
< 1 week	786	301	201	42	10	23	1363 (81)
Unknown duration	133	7	7	52	1	1	201 (12)
Total	**958**	**327**	**223**	**128**	**16**	**28**	**1680 (100)**
Other professionals[b]							
≥ 1 year	0	0	0	0	0	0	0 (0)
1 month – <1 year	0	0	0	1	0	0	1 (2)
1 week – <1 month	0	0	0	0	0	0	0 (0)
< 1 week	39	6	1	4	0	1	51 (78)
Unknown duration	10	2	1	0	0	0	13 (20)
Total	**49**	**8**	**2**	**5**	**0**	**1**	**65 (100)**

With permission from Dr. Temsak Phungrassami
[a]Some hospitals reported only that there were "many" such personnel; they did not provide exact numbers
[b]For example: pharmacists, social workers, or dentists

teers, who look after 10–15 households. Together they provide home care. This system has created an effective community network. If the patients need to go back to the hospital, they will be referred back to the provincial hospital by the community hospital team.

The Karunruk Palliative Care Center was established in February 2010. From the start of the center, apart from establishing the services in our hospital, the other important mission has been to establish palliative care networks through scaling up education. Our strategy is to implement scaling up training for every level of health personnel, strengthening services at each level, and, if possible, to provide training to a group of professionals in the same Service Plan area, which will help with networking (Fig. 2).

We have designed several multilevel training courses that match the needs of the palliative care personnel (Fig. 3). More than 10 years ago, we only offered a 3-day training program for nurses and in 2010 we started a 6-week Basic Certificate Course in Palliative Nursing with the help of Dr. Suresh Kumar, the Director of the World Health Collaboration Center in Long-Term Care and Palliative Care along with a volunteer palliative care nurse from Sydney Hospital.

To date, more than 174 nurses have graduated from this course and most of them work as coordinators for the palliative care programs in their hospitals. Five years later, many Faculties of Nursing started to offer a four-month Palliative Care Nursing course and hundreds of nurses graduated from this course, filling up the hospitals' palliative care units. As most of the palliative care units lack a doctor, the activities were psychosocial/spiritual activities and lacked effective symptom management. In 2014 we began an eight-week Basic Certificate Course in Palliative Medicine for doctors who were to work part-time for the palliative care units. Until now more than 160 doctors have graduated from this course and act as the key person for hospital palliative care units. Until now there have been only a few phy-

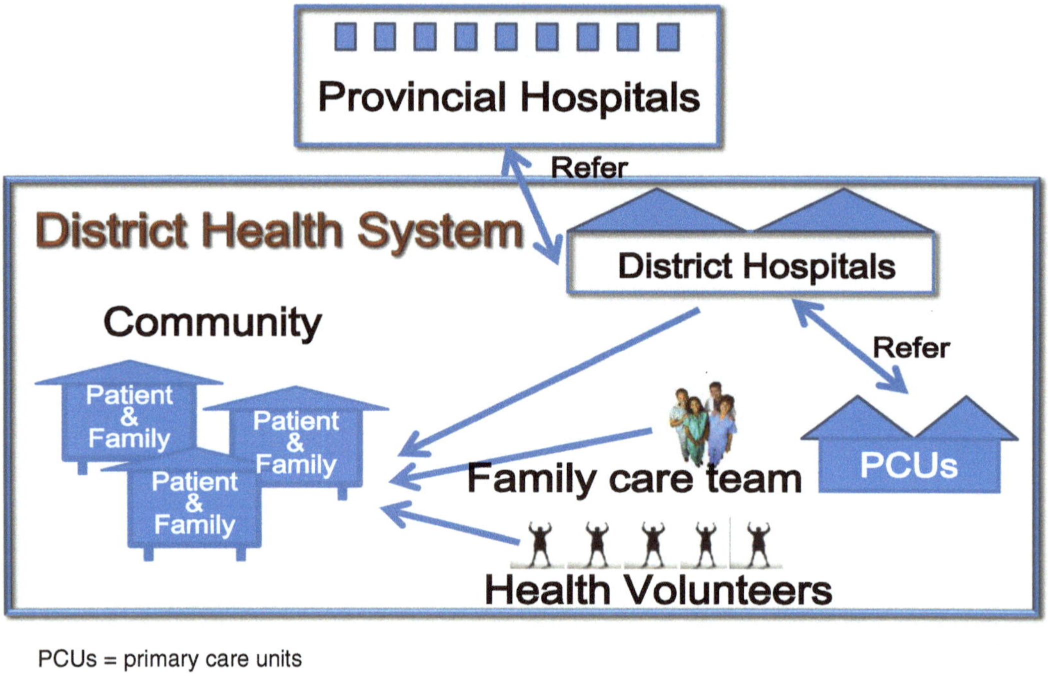

Fig. 1 Health Care Service Model in Thailand

Fig. 2 Strategy to Implement Palliative Care Education

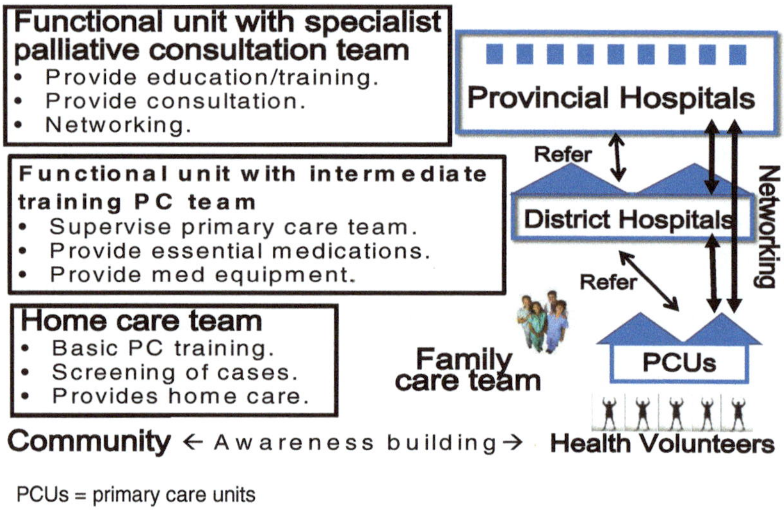

sicians working as full-time palliative specialists, as no structured career path has been established in the public hospitals. Most of the full-time palliative care specialists work in the medical school teaching hospitals. We also provide a short annual 40-hour training course for community doctors. In 2014 we started a four-week training course called "Clinical Palliative Care for Community Nurses." The curriculum included one week of theory training and three weeks of practical sessions. The first batch was all nurses who were responsible for palliative care programs in the community hospitals in Service Plan area 7, which is composed of four provinces and 67

Fig. 3 Karunruk multilevel training courses for palliative care personnel

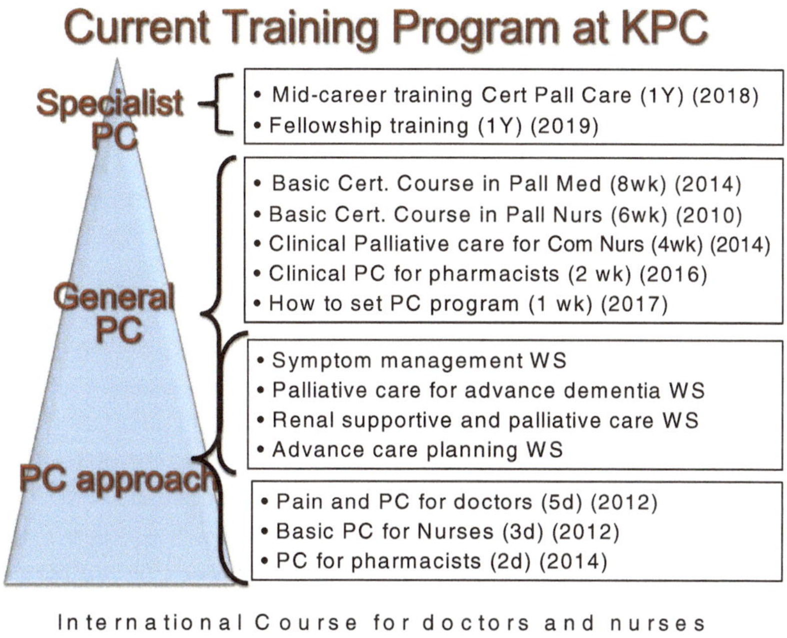

community hospitals. All the training and practical sessions were conducted by the Karunruk Palliative Care Center. We trained each province one at a time by supervising them in conferences, follow-up consultations and home care visits. After this training, we found that whenever we referred our palliative patients back to their homes, the community palliative care teams could all provide home care and continuous care until the patient's death. Dying at home was then possible as the community nurse could provide morphine subcutaneous infusion and take care of the patients in their final stages [4]. From evaluation data, this training program for community nurses proved very useful and became the essential part of community palliative care. As we had already trained nurses and doctors who serve as consultation teams in provincial hospitals, many of them are actively working as a multidisciplinary team providing care for palliative patients. In some hospitals they are skilled enough to help with the clinical training. In 2016 we implemented this four-week training course for all community nurses in Service Plan areas 8, 9 and 10, which included 25 provincial hospitals and 300 community hospitals. Service area 7, 8, 9 and 10 are the areas covering the northeast of Thailand, which holds one-third of the country's population. As a large number of personnel were trained, we used 15 provincial hospitals which have strong palliative care units as training sites for the practical sessions. With this strategy we could train a large number of nurses to fulfill the services at the community level. Later in 2018 we used this strategy to train community nurses in the north and in the south, and in 2020 training was arranged in the central part of Thailand. In total, more than 700 community nurses all around Thailand were trained in this four-week course. At least 90% of district hospitals have one nurse who has attended this four-week training course. In 2018 we began a Certificate Course in Palliative Care (Mid-career training), a one-year part-time training program. This course has been designed for doctors who graduated from our eight-week Basic Certificate Course in Palliative Medicine and six-week Basic Certificate Course in Palliative Nursing. They attend four one-week intensive courses, four workshops and one month of practicum at our center. In total, 29 doctors and six nurses graduated from this course and most of them direct the Regional Palliative

Table 3 Number of palliative care-trained personnel provided by the Karunruk Palliative Care Center between 2010–2019

Course	No. trained	Participants
Intermediate/long course		
For doctors		
Certificate PC (mid-career training) (1 year-part time) Basic certificate course in palliative medicine (8 weeks)	29 160	Doctors responsible for hospital PC program
Total	189	
For nurses		
Certificate PC (mid-career training) (1 year-part time) Basic certificate course for palliative nursing (6 weeks) Clinical palliative Care for Community Nurses (4 weeks)	6 174 747	Nurses responsible for hospital PC program in hospitals
Total	927	
For pharmacists		
Clinical palliative Care for Pharmacists (2 weeks)	249	Pharmacists who work in multidisciplinary PC team
Total	249	
Short course		
Pain and palliative Care for Doctors (5 days)	657	Community doctors
Basic palliative Care for Nurses (5 days)	2740	Community nurses
Basic palliative Care for Pharmacists	309	Community pharmacists
Palliative Care for Family Care Team (3 days)	1900	Community care team
Total	5606	
How to set quality hospital palliative care program	586	Palliative care team

Service Plan. Not until 2019 did we have fellowship training in palliative care. Initially there were only three medical schools that provided this fellowship training. The number of participants and types of intensive training courses conducted by the Karunruk Palliative Care Center during the years 2010–2020 are shown in Table 3, above.

Opioid Availability

Morphine consumption data reflects the quality of pain control provided. Thailand had a very low consumption with less than 0.1 mg per capita in the 1980s; consumption increased to 0.29 mg per capita in 1999 and to 1.16 mg in 2010 [12]. In 2012, per capita morphine consumption in Thailand was much lower than the global average of 6.28 mg [13].

A survey was performed by Thongkhamcharoen in 2012 on the situation of essential drug availability for palliative care in Thai hospitals [14]. Five hundred and fifty-five hospitals replied to the questionnaire (a response rate of 57%). Injectable morphine was the most available form of strong opioid in Thailand (96.9%). For the overall picture of oral morphine, immediate-released morphine was a less available form than the control-released form (32.2% versus 51.0%). The availability of immediate-released morphine in community hospitals was 24.7%, and 42.5% for control-released morphine. These findings reflected that more than half of the palliative patients needed to travel to a better care setting to acquire their opioid supply (Table 4.)

In 2016 the Karunruk Palliative Care Center conducted a questionnaire survey of pharmacists in Service Plan area 7 [15] (four provincial hospitals and 67 district hospitals); the response rate was 71%. The strong opioids available in their hospital formulary were as follows: morphine injection 91.5%, immediate-released morphine 78.8% and control-released morphine 90.6%. The figures were doubled compared with the sur-

Table 4 Numbers and percentages of opioid availability in different types of government hospitals

Drug list	*PH*	*CH*	*GH*	*RH*	*CC*	*MH*	*OH*	*Total*
Codeine	10	84	24	13	7	11	4	153
	90.9%	24.6%	55.8%	76.5%	100%	100%	50%	35.2%
Tramadol	12	387	48	17	7	11	10	492
	100%	98.7%	100%	100%	100%	100%	100%	99.0%
Methadone (immediate release)	6	36	13	11	1	7	2	76
	54.5%	10.7%	30.2%	64.7%	14.3%	63.6%	22.2%	17.5%
Immediate-release oral morphine	9	85	14	13	7	10	5	143
	81.8%	24.7%	31.1%	76.5%	100%	90.9%	55.6%	32.2%
Controlled-release oral morphine	8	149	35	16	7	10	6	230
	72.7%	42.5%	75.6%	94.1%	100%	90.9%	66.7%	51.0%
Injectable morphine	11	361	47	17	7	11	10	464
	100%	96%	100%	100%	100%	100%	100%	96.9%
Injectable fentanyl	8	102	40	15	5	9	8	187
	72.7%	29.8%	87%	88.2%	71.4%	81.8%	88.9%	42.3%
Transdermal fentanyl	7	15	11	14	7	9	6	69
	63.7%	4.4%	25.6%	82.4%	70%	81.8%	66.7%	15.8%

With permission from Dr.Rojanasak Thongkhumchareon
CC cancer center, *CH* community hospital, *GH* general hospital, *MH* medical school hospital, *OH* other hospital, *PH* private hospital; RH, regional hospital

Table 5 Perceived barriers to opioid availability from pharmacists' point of view

Perceived barriers		%
Significant concern in using opioids	Addiction	28.3
	Respiratory suppression	47.2
	Hastening death	25.0
	Abuse of drug	59.6
Perceived concerns of drug regulation	Strict hospital control policy	59.6
	Afraid of being punished if any problems occur	50.0
Barriers from the professional	Lack of knowledge & skills of the doctors	38.5
	Lack of knowledge & skills of pharmacists	34.5
	Lack of exposure to PC during training	62.3
	Concerning educational needs	98.1

vey in 2012. Concerning the problem of opioid procurement, the results were: limited stock 56.9%, delay in purchasing process 60% and problems with drug expiration 34.6%. The pharmacists' point of view concerning barriers to opioid availability are shown in Table 5. The most significant concern when using opioids is the issue of abuse. Strict hospital control policy is the primary concern of drug regulators, and palliative education is needed. We have started to train pharmacists from provincial and community hospitals and found that they are key in improving opioid availability.

One strategy to endorse opioid availability must include a government policy that directs the hospitals to include essential opioids into their hospital formulary, drug procurement and education of professionals. The Karunruk Palliative Care Center implemented an opioid availability program in 2016, in which there was an agreement among hospitals in the Service Plan area 7 to procure immediate-released and controlled-released morphine in their hospital formulary and training courses on palliative education for the hospital pharmacists. Knowledge sharing sessions among the pharmacists along with sessions with the Thai FDA was also included. This program resulted in an increase in the National Health Security Office opioid reimbursement in this Service Plan area, and lessons learned from the program had great influence on further program training for pharmacists. Doctor education still plays an important role in the prescription of opioids and must be implemented accordingly.

Toward Quality Improvement

Palliative care has been one of the National Service Plans since 2016. From the report of the Service Plan Inspection 2019, 97.3% of regional and general hospitals and 96.1% of community hospitals have a palliative care program [16]. The next step is to implement quality improvement. The Karunruk Palliative Care Center and the Thai Palliative Care Network developed a Quality Standards for Palliative Care in 2019, and it will be adopted by the Healthcare Accreditation Institute to be used as a guideline for the certification of excellent hospital palliative care programs [17]. This Quality Standards for Palliative Care could be used by the hospitals for self-evaluation and to implement quality improvement for their palliative care programs. We also conducted a workshop on "How to set a quality hospital palliative care program", emphasizing standard tools, quality indicators and a session on knowledge sharing. This workshop has been conducted in every region all over Thailand. In 2017, palliative care in Thailand was classified in Category 4a: Palliative care services at a preliminary stage of integration to mainstream health care services [18].

Conclusion

Thailand has made much progress in the development of palliative care service systems, as shown in the timeline (Fig. 4). The advocation to include palliative care as one of the Service Plans, along with the implementation of scaling up education for all professionals and multilevel training coupled with networking, plays a major role in the service development.

Thailand is moving forward to Category 4b: Palliative care services at an advanced stage of integration to mainstream health care services by way of improving access and quality improvement via wide certification of the hospital program, which could be facilitated by education, knowledge management and research activities.

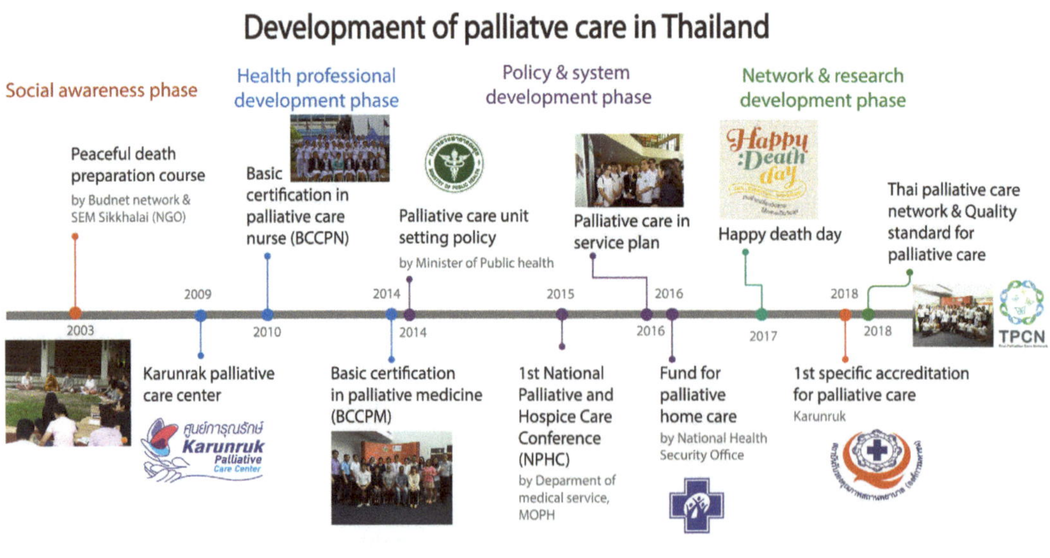

Fig. 4 Palliative care development in Thailand

References

1. World Bank. The World Bank in Thailand. https://www.worldbank.org/en/country/thailand/overview access Mar 5,2020 Access Mar 2020.
2. National Statistic Office. http://www.nso.go.th/sites/2014en Access Mar 2020.
3. Asia Pacific Observatory on Health Systems and Policies. The kingdom of Thailand health system review. Health System in Transition. 2015:5.
4. Tangcharoensathien V, Prakongsai P, Lim-wattananon S, Patcharanarumol W, Jongudomsuk P. From targeting to universality: lessons from the health system in Thailand. In: Townsend P, editor. Building decent societies: rethinking the role of social security in development. Hampshire: Palgrave Macmillan; 2009. p. 310–22.
5. Primary health care systems (PRIMASYS): case study from Thailand, abridged version. Geneva: World Health Organization; 2017. Licence: CC BY-NY-SA 3.0 IGO.
6. Strategy and Planning Division, Ministry of Public Health. Public Health Statistics AD. 2017. www. http://bps.moph.go.th/new_bps/sites/default/files/statistics60.pdf. Access Mar 2020.
7. World Health Organization. Global Cancer observatory. Thailand 2018. http://gco.iarc.fr/today/data/factsheets/populations/764-thailand-fact-sheets.pdf. Access Mar 2020.
8. Pairojkul S, Thongkhumcharoen R, Raksasattaya A, et al. Point prevalent survey of 14 hospitals in Thailand. In publishing process.
9. Worldwide Palliative Care Alliance. Global atlas of palliative care at the end of life. https://www.who.int/nmh/Global_Atlas_of_Palliative_Care.pdf. Access Mar 2020.
10. Wright M, Hamzah E, Phungrassami T, Bausa-Claudio A. Hospice and palliative Care in Southeast Asia: a review of developments and challenges in Malaysia, Thailand and the Philippines. New York: Oxford University Press; 2010. p. 87–133.
11. Phungrassami T, Thongkhamcharoen R, Atthakul N. Palliative care personnel and services: a national survey in Thailand 2012. J Pall Care. 2013;29:133–9.
12. Pain & Policy Studies Group. Availability of opioid analgesics in Asia: consumption trends, resources, recommendations (Monograph). pp. 6–7, 2002, university of Wisconsin Pain & Policy Studies group/WHO collaborating center for Pain Policy and Palliative care, Wisconsin.
13. Pain & Policy Studies Group. The Single convention on Narcotic Drugs implementation in Six countries: Albania, Bangladesh, India, Kyrgyzstan, Sri Lanka, Ukraine (Monograph). pp. 12, 2012, University of Wisconsin Pain & Policy Studies Group/WHO collaborating center for Pain Policy and Palliative care, Wisconsin.
14. Thongkhamcharoen R, Phungrassami T, Atthakul N. Palliative care and essential drug availability: Thailand National Survey 2012. J Pall Med. 2013;16
15. Sribulue P, Pairojkul. Survey of pharmacists' opinions on barriers of opioid availability in Thailand. APHC 2016, Singapore. Abstract.
16. Ministry of Public Health. Inspection guideline: Service Plan – Palliative care. 2019 report.
17. Pairojkul S. Quality standard for palliative care. Khon Kaen: Klung Nanathum Publishing; 2019. http://karunruk.org/home/index.php/component/content/article/91-content/135-quality-standards?Itemid=437
18. Clark D, Baur N, Clelland D, et al. Mapping levels of palliative care development in 198 countries: The situation in 2017. https://doi.org/10.1016/j.jpainsymman.2019.11.009.

Part XXXIV

Far East: China

Community Hospice Care for Cancer Patients in China

Lili Tang

Introduction

The concept of hospice care, mainly focusing on end-of-life care, was introduced in China in the late 1980s [17], but has developed slowly due to people's attitudes toward healing diseases at all costs, as well as the lack of systematic hospice and palliative care education and full-time professional staff. Things have changed in recent years, as more medical policies on hospice care have been carried out and an increasing percentage of the elderly population have advocated for the demand for hospice care at the end of life. In 2016, promoting hospice care in China was one of the topics in the two-week consultative forum of the 49th Chinese People's Political Consultative Conference. In February 2017, the National Health Commission of the People's Republic of China issued *basic standards of hospice care centers (trial), management standards for hospice care centers (trial), and guidelines for hospice care practice (trial).* In September 2017, five districts all around China had been chosen as experimental sites to carry out clinical hospice care, and another 71 sites were announced in 2019 [10]. According to the latest census data, the population of people over 60 years of age reached 178 million, accounting for 13.3% of the total population in China, and this proportion is expected to continue to rise [11]. The subjective concerns of the elderly include: how to live calmly and peacefully, to receive high-quality care for age-related diseases and organ function declining, and to die with dignity at the end of life, which reflects upon the medical care and humanistic care level in the country. Compared with "at all cost" treatment at the end of life, hospice therapy can not only improve quality of life for patients themselves but would also significantly reduce the meaningless expenditure of medical treatment and optimize allocation of medical resources.

The National Health Commission of the People's Republic of China has spent more effort to promote pilot work of hospice care all around China since 2017. The number of hospice care settings has increased during these years. But the national coverage rate of hospice care is still lower than that of developed countries. Additionally, the distribution of hospice care in the entire country is unbalanced: most hospices are located in cities with a higher level of medical care, with better and more convenient transportation. Hospice care education should be highlighted in post-graduate education and vocational training.

L. Tang (✉)
Department of Psycho-Oncology, Peking University Cancer Hospital & Institute, Beijing, China

M. Silbermann (ed.), *Palliative Care for Chronic Cancer Patients in the Community*,
https://doi.org/10.1007/978-3-030-54526-0_48

Hospice Care Models in China

At present, the service modes of hospice care in China include: (1) Family sickbeds – for patients registered at the hospital; physicians see the patients at home and document medical records regularly; (2) Hospice service – hospice care teams supported by the Li Ka Shing Foundation (LKSF) in the hospitals provide home care for the patients; (3) Community service – the team is composed of community physicians and nurses; each family with an end-of-life relative is equipped with one responsible physician and nurse.

Family Sickbed

In recent years, hospital beds at home, or family sickbed, has been the new model for community care services and have made great progress throughout the world [2]. Family sickbed refers to the sickbed set up on the spot by the medical unit for those patients who are able to receive adequate examination, treatment and nursing at the family home, which is the new medical service mode best suited for China's national conditions [7]. Born in the community, it is an integrated service with residents' health as the center, community as the scope, family as the unit, the elderly, weak, sick and disabled as the service focus, biological-psychological-social medicine model as the guidance, and general practitioners' door-to-door service as the means, aiming to improve patients' health level and quality of life [7]. The staff of hospitals or community health service institutions provide medical care service for those patients with special needs at home.

The first family sickbed in China was established in Tianjin in 1958, and over 73,000 sickbeds had been set up in Tianjin by 1988 [13]; but then many hospitals cancelled family sickbed setups and services. The development of family sickbeds stagnated and regressed. In recent years, however, family sickbeds were slowly rebuilt across the country.

The process for domestic family sickbed has three main forms: first, the family sickbed is arranged by second- and third-level hospitals, using the high-level diagnosis and treatment of large hospitals to carry out services; second, community health service institutions and secondary and tertiary hospitals cooperate to carry out and establish a consultation and two-way referral system, benefit sharing; and third, private hospitals or clinics provide such services [5].

Family sickbed has three main functions: to replace hospitalization of acute patients; to replace hospitalization for patients with chronic diseases; and to maintain patient access to health services at home or in the community in order to avoid excessive use of health facilities. Their fundamental purpose is to provide individuals with high-quality, timely, and cost-effective health services, so that patients can maintain a high degree of life autonomy and quality of life. Studies have shown that family sickbed effectively can reduce the high cost of hospitalization and the heavy burden of medical insurance and preserves limited health resources and medical human resources for operability, practicality, demonstration, sustainability, and medical access [14]. It improves the quality of cancer patients' lives at the end of life and, finally, patients die in a familiar environment surrounded by their family and friends. It also helps the care and bereavement process for family members go more smoothly [14].

Family sickbed as a complementary form of hospital beds, the main mode of community health services, has effectively improved efficient use of health resources, reduced the cost of medical treatment, and has met the growing health needs. It also reduced the stress of hospital-bed tension, and solved the problem of acquiring difficult medical care and hospitalization for some residents. This convenient, effective, and economical medical and health model has been gradually recognized by the society.

In China, the general family sickbed staff is composed of doctors and nurses from large hospitals or community health service institutions, which is a suitable structure. Nurses are often viewed as the primary resource of the family sickbed program, and they perform a variety of tasks and roles in their work. These tasks and roles include expert assistance, case management, preventive care, long-term care and short-term emergency care service preparation, working with physicians, overseeing informal health care delivery, mediating between family sickbed staff and patients, and acting as a liaison with the broader health system. Before these nurses take up their posts, they participate in a multidisciplinary and expert-led training program to ensure the quality of staff and the quality of care provided.

In view of the late start in understanding palliative care services, China lags behind in the popularization and the balance of service level; this family-oriented medical service mode has been more and more widely accepted and demanded by society. Family sickbed brings countless terminal cancer patients the safest, most comfortable and warmest humane overall care.

Hospice or Hospice Unit

Before the comprehensive implementation of the National Hospice Service Program (NHSP) founded by the Li Ka Shing Foundation (LKSF) in 2001, there were only a handful of hospice care institutions in China, with a slow development speed, because of the idea and understanding of the concept of hospice care, health policy, and medical management systems [8]. The establishment of the hospice research center of Tianjin Medical College in 1988 is regarded as the origin and symbol of the development of hospice care in China [4].

Later, hospices and hospice wards were set up in Beijing, Shanghai, Chengdu, and other big cities. The Shanghai Nanhui Nursing Hospital for Retired Workers was established in October 1988. It was the first hospice in China to take in retired workers with terminal diseases. This means that the beginning of hospice care services in China started in Shanghai, which is of epoch-making and milestone historical significance [8]. Beijing Songtang Hospice, the first hospice in Beijing, was established in 1989 [8].

The first Hospice Unit founded by LKSF to provide free home-based holistic care for patients with terminal cancer was set up in 1998 in Shantou. This Hospice Unit proved to be a feasible model for mainland China, and the NHSP was formed in 2001. By the end of July 2019, 38 Hospice Units were established and more than 30 Units are currently in operation, distributed throughout 31 cities of 29 provinces in mainland China and covering over 350 districts and counties. A total of over 200,000 patients have been served. Studies showed that it was a better choice for the patients with advanced cancer to receive home hospice services, and it avoids wasting medical resources and overtreatment [18].

The objectives and principles of NHSP include [6]: to improve the quality of life for patients and relatives; to provide “five domains of care”: whole person, whole family, whole course of illness, whole team, and whole community; to serve the patients in poverty with advanced cancer at home free of charge; to provide pain and other distressing symptoms control; to provide psychosocial, emotional, and spiritual assistance to the patients and their families; and to develop education and training in palliative care for society.

Each Hospice Unit has at least 2 physicians, 2 nurses, 1 social worker, 1 driver, and 1 clerk with a designated car. They provide free outpatient services, telephone counselling, home visits for poor people with advanced cancer and home services such as pain and other symptoms control, psychological and grief counselling, nursing instruction, and social support. They aim to improve quality of life of patients with advanced cancer, to ensure that they can live the final stages of their life with dignity. A study of 4732 patients with terminal cancer nationwide receiving Hospice Unit services showed that home-based hospice care is necessary and beneficial for cancer patients [15]. The study also found that providing nursing guidance, pain control, psychological counselling, and social information resources had a significant impact on the relief of family stress. The study also showed that compared with hospitalized patients, the psychological and financial burden on the families of patients receiving home-based hospice care is significantly lower.

Community Care

Community hospices are more easily accessed than hospice care centers in tertiary hospitals. From the time of the pilot project of hospice care promoted by the National Health Commission of the People's Republic of China in 2017, the number of community hospice units has increased. Community hospice service optimizes the utilization of medical resources. End-of-life patients, especially the advanced cancer patients, suffer from chronic disease, severe symptom burden, and have poor functionality. Community unit care is the best choice for them, as such patients' condition is critical with frequent fluctuations. The conjoined body of hospice care comprises home care, community wards, and tertiary hospitals, which can complement each other through a referral system. Patients with stable conditions can choose home care, where family members play the role of the main caregivers; doctors and nurses visit them regularly; when the condition changes and the caregivers cannot deal with it any longer, the patients are recommended to the nearby community hospice wards; referral to a tertiary hospital occurs when the patient is in critical condition.

Main Services in Community Hospice Care

Services are provided to those patients who show no response to the curative treatments. A multidisciplinary team will provide services such as symptom management, care for daily life functions, and psychosocial care. (1) Physicians provide management for symptoms such as: pain, dyspnea, cough, abdominal distention, edema, fever, insomnia, delirium and other common symptoms at the late stage of the disease, which can't be controlled by home care. (2) Care for daily life functions, mainly provided by nurses, include: bathing, movement, stoma care, pressure ulcer care, etc. (3) Psychosocial care, provided by professional psychologists/psychiatrists, or physicians/nurses who have received certification with enough psychology training, offer help with special psychosocial issues that can occur at the end of life, like depression and anxiety, losing life meaning, and death and dying anxiety. Additionally, after the patient passes away, care will be provided for the family members dealing with loss and grief.

Basic Settings in Community Hospice Care

According to the National Hospice and Palliative Care Organization's (NHPCO) Standards of Practice for Hospice Programs in China, community hospice care settings must guarantee the following requirements: (1) rational layout of the hospice inpatient department; departments should include ward rooms, nursing stations, treatment rooms, reviewing rooms, farewell rooms, offices for physicians, catering rooms, bathrooms and space for daily activities, and exercising. (2) staffing: at least 1 deputy chief (or higher ranking) physician, at least 1 physician for every 10 beds; at least 1 supervising nurse and at least 4 nurses for every 10 beds. Pharmacists, dieticians, psychologists/psychiatrists, physical therapists, traditional Chinese medicine doctors, and social workers volunteer, if necessary and available [9].

Challenges for Community Hospice Care

Development of community hospice care also incurs some challenges: (1) Lack of hospice knowledge among patients and family members: at the late stage of diseases, many patients and family members prefer to either stay at home or rush to nearby emergency departments of tertiary general hospitals when the patient's function fluctuates. Influenced by filial piety in traditional Chinese culture, elderly patients and adult children believe that sending late-stage patients with incurable diseases to receive hospice care means giving up on the patients and letting patients wait for death, which is considered "unfilial" and will be blamed by patients' other relatives, friends, or neighbors. So, those adult children either spare no effort in searching any possible curative treatments or prefer to conceal the accurate disease information and take the patient back home. However, attitudes have been changing over the years. High quality of life and natural death have increasingly become the care goal for both medical staff and patients/family members at the end of life. More attention should be paid to the dissemination of hospice care knowledge nationally. (2) The referral system is incomplete: if a more fluent referral system is coordinated between community hospice settings and tertiary hospitals, patients who are referred by physicians in tertiary hospitals will have more access to community hospice settings. This is an essential step based on the medical model of continuous medical care and whole-process care management [12]. (3) Community hospice wards also face operational pressure: hospice care is not covered by basic governmental health insurance in many cities, and these services follow other medical insurance's standards for charging, which are unsuitable for hospice care. At present, the revenues are not enough to support diversified development of community hospice wards, such as employing full-time multidisciplinary professionals. Cao et al. reported that the direct labor cost of community hospice service is much higher than what they are charging. Especially, the labor cost of free services, such as psychological and social services needed by patients, lacks a compensation mechanism [1].

Zheng et al. have suggested that, compared to the control group, end-of-life cancer patients who have received palliative and hospice care in community wards could significantly benefit in quality-of-life, physical/social/cognitive/emotional functions and common symptom burden like fatigue, pain, and insomnia [19]. Yang et al. [16] have reported that the utilization rate of community hospice wards is 65.2%, which revealed an increased level of acceptance among end-of-life patients and family members [19]. Chang et al. [3] have compared community hospice care and family sick beds and results showed that patients benefited more in total quality of life, symptom management, cognitive function at hospice wards and benefited more in role/social functions, saving in family sick beds [3]. Though facing many development challenges, opportunities also come into sight, as an increasing number of people have realized the importance of end-of-life and death quality. The government has begun to invest more resources to promote hospice services at all levels of medical institutions, and authorized medical experts and nongovernment social organizations are also trying to popularize the basic knowledge of hospice care.

References

1. Cao WQ, Shen TH, Miao J, Zhang DY, Wang XY. Study on the direct labor costs calculation of palliative Care Services in Community Health Service Centers Based on standardized technical labor value. Chin Primary Health Care. 2019;33(7):21–5.
2. Carpenter I, Gambassi G, Topinkova E, et al. Community care in Europe. The aged in-home care project (AdHOC). Aging Clin Exp Res. 2004;16(4):259–69.
3. Chang W, Sun L, Chen MJ, Sun XF. Comparison of the quality of life in patients with advanced cancer: based on two models of palliative care ward and home palliative care. Chin Medical Ethics. 2018;31(3):352–5.
4. He M, Cao Y, Wang Y, et al. Diversification reflection on palliative care in China. Chin Med Ethics. 2018;31(5):581–90.
5. Li S, Cao Y, Wang L, et al. Family sickbed is an important form of community health service. Appl J Gen Pract. 2004;2(3):189–90.
6. Li J, Davis MP, Gamier P. Palliative medicine: barriers and developments in mainland China. Curr Oncol Rep. 2011;13(4):290–4.
7. Ling J, Xie S, Lin S, et al. Practice and exploration of community family sickbed in Shenzhen. Chin Gen Pract. 2011;9(8):1243–4.
8. Liu J, Yuan M. The history, present situation, problem and prospect of hospice service system in mainland China. J Soc Work. 2016;2:34–49.
9. National Health Commission of the People's Republic of China. Notice of basic standards of hospice care centers (trial), management standards for hospice care centers (trial), 2017-02-03.
10. National Health Commission of the People's Republic of China. Notice on the second batch of pilot work of hospice care. 2019-05-20.
11. Population Census Office under the State Council of China, National Bureau of Statistics of Chine. Tabulation on the 2010 population census of People's

republic of China. Beijing: China Statistics Press; 2012.
12. Song YJ. A qualitative study on the referral experience of palliative care from general hospital to community hospital for cancer patients. Nanjing University. 2019–05.
13. Wang L, Schneider JW. Home care for the chronically ill elderly in China: the family sickbed in Tianjin. J Cross Cult Gerontol. 1993;8(4):331–48.
14. Wang P, Wang Y, Li F. Study on the standardized operation mode of palliative care in family sickbed of cancer patients. Hubei J Tradit Chin Med. 2011;33(11):23–5.
15. Xu L, Lu L. Analysis of influencing factors of hospice care on family stress relief effect of terminal cancer patients. Med Philos. 2018;39(2B):92–3.
16. Yang FJ, Wang LS, Wu J. Discussion on the current status of the soothing treatment room resources in Xuanqiao community, Pudong new area, Shanghai. Chin Primary Health Care. 2019;33(9):98–100.
17. Zhang XM, Hu XY. Developing situation, existing problems and prospects of palliative care in China. Chin J Mod Nurs. 2016;22(34):4885–8.
18. Zhang Y, Liu S, Li J, et al. Cost-benefit analysis between home and hospital hospice palliative Care Services for Patients with advanced Cancer. Chin Health Econ. 2012;31(4):73–4.
19. Zheng JP. Exploring the effect of hospice car by nursing in community hospice wards. 2019 Shanghai International Nursing Conference. Shanghai. 2019-09-24.

Part XXXV

Far East: Japan

The Role of the Home-Visit Nursing System in the Treatment of Terminal Cancer Patients in Japan

Tomoko Majima, Junko Kusunoki, and Tomoko Otsuka

Background

Trends for Cancer Patients in Japan

The National Cancer Center recently calculated the 5- and 10-year survival rates for cancer at 32 cooperating facilities. As a result, the overall 5-year relative survival rate for all clinical stages was found to be 67.9% in 2019, a gradual improvement from 62.3% in 1999 [16]. This suggests that advances in chemotherapy, radiotherapy, and early detection techniques have contributed to this change. Improved survival rates and more patients living in the community while receiving cancer treatment and radiation therapy also means more need for employment support for cancer patients, as well as more support for the growth and development of the younger generation, and that support has become a priority policy issue in Japan. Since younger generations of cancer patients are more likely to have problems such as marriage and employment, consultation services and peer support are needed.

Where patients spend the end of their lives has also shifted over time. In 1951, 82.5% of all deaths were at home, compared to 9.1% in hospitals. By 2009, hospital deaths had increased to 78.9% [13]. An international study [10] showed Japan had higher rates of hospital deaths than other countries, such as Sweden (42%) and the Netherlands (35.3%). This study points out that the reason for the low proportion of home care in Japan, even at the end of life, are people's high expectations for treatment, nuclear families, and a lack of mutual support in the community. However, survey results have shown that many people want to spend their last days at home.

According to a general survey conducted in 2018 [14] on health care awareness at the end of life, 69.2% of respondents indicated that, during terminal stage cancer, they would like to spend their time at their home. Data on doctors (69.4%), nurses (68.0%), and caregivers (69.3%) showed similar results. Thus, these findings show a gap between ideal end-of-life care and reality.

In the past, medical and nursing care systems in the community were built as support for elderly individuals and people with mental disabilities. Today, cancer patients in the terminal stage are also included. This system is called the community-based comprehensive care system [18]. The community-based comprehensive care system provides housing for the elderly, medical care, nursing care, rehabilitation, health/welfare, preventative care, and living support. This is to allow elderly people to continue to live in their own communities. Additionally, the cooperative systems of local medical facilities, home-visit

T. Majima (✉) · J. Kusunoki · T. Otsuka
Graduate School of Nursing, Chiba University, Chiba, Japan
e-mail: junjun@faculty.chiba-u.jp; t-otsuka@chiba-u.jp

M. Silbermann (ed.), *Palliative Care for Chronic Cancer Patients in the Community*,
https://doi.org/10.1007/978-3-030-54526-0_49

nursing stations, and home care support establishments have been created in various places to support patients and their families residing at home. Patients are transferred to long-term care hospitals or their homes after treatment is completed, and end-of-life care is provided in a familiar environment. This is expected to become increasingly common in the future.

In order to change where medical treatment is provided and care for patients in their homes, it is necessary for patients and their family members to understand the patient's medical condition and consider a location for medical treatment. Furthermore, when choosing a care environment, it is necessary to accept the condition that a full recovery cannot be expected and discuss this with family members. However, there are some situations in which patients and their families cannot fully discuss this topic.

Transitional Nursing Care from the Acute Care Hospital to the Community

Transitional care models have been developed to assist chronically ill patients and the elderly after hospital discharge [15]. In these models, support is provided by advanced practice nurses. Further, transitional care models have been used in cancer treatment. Enderlin et al. [4] compared several transitional care models, and showed that all models included patient-centered care and cost savings. Almost all models also included discharge planning, guidance, medication confirmation, early detection of potential problems, written discharge instructions, and improved patient outcomes. In addition to medical care, cancer patients need a wide range of support to live in the community [2]. Moreover, nurses have an important role in helping patients locate these resources and providing support [3].

In Japan, hospital nurses provide information when patients' social resources are insufficient due to the nuclear family [20] Thus, it is necessary to understand the background of patients and their families to provide the appropriate social resources. To highlight this, here's an example of nursing support provided for a patient who received chemotherapy and radiotherapy in an outpatient setting, following breast cancer surgery:

The patient was a woman in her 40s who worked part time. She lived with her husband, a 7-year-old, and a 4-year-old. She was diagnosed with breast cancer in 200X. She received preoperative chemotherapy and a breast partial resection + axillary lymph node dissection. The doctor recommended adjuvant radiation therapy and endocrine therapy. She was reluctant to receive postoperative adjuvant therapy, because none of her family members had experienced cancer treatment. She also had concerns regarding the side effects of treatment and anxiety about going to the hospital when she needed to resume work and pick her children up from daycare.

Therefore, the patient consulted with the nurse in charge, who introduced the patient to the discharge planning nurses. The discharge planning nurses referred the patient to the Community General Support Center, the family support center, and a support group for post-operative breast cancer patients.

The Community General Support Center consults patients regarding housework, such as cleaning and washing, and the Family Support Center consults patients regarding methods of pick-up and drop-off for their children. By receiving advice and consulting from nurses, she was able to find community support, not just help family members, and had a better idea of what to expect when visiting the hospital for radiation therapy. She also gained new, accurate knowledge by interacting in the support group with survivors her age and those with similar cancer experiences. Further, she gained more confidence and a better overview of the situations in her life. Additionally, patients were able to share their treatment experiences with other patients, reducing their anxiety and giving them the opportunity to think positively about the future.

Thus, she received support from nurses (ward nurses, discharge planning nurses), medical doctors (breast surgery, radiology), Medical Social Worker, the Community General Support Center, the Family Support Center, and support groups for post-operative breast cancer patients.

Visiting Nurses and Nurses' Support for Cancer Patients at the End of Life

In Japan, there were more than 1100 institutions that employed home visiting nurses in 2019 [19]. Visiting nurses provide care through long-term care insurance or medical insurance.

Fukui et al. [5] showed five categories for home-visit nursing agencies based on the type of service delivery system by cluster analysis. The five categories were: nurse-centered (560, 10.9%), rehabilitation-centered (211, 4.1%), psychiatric-centered (360, 7.0%), urban-centered (1784, 34.5%), and rural-centered (2246, 43.5%) home-visit nursing. Nurse-centered care provided 24-hour home-visit nursing care for patients who are highly dependent on medical care. Okamoto et al. [17] conducted an interview with 11 family members who took care of terminally ill cancer patients at home and analyzed the data inductively. The interview was conducted with the aim of listening to the content and evaluations of care provided by visiting nurses. As a result, the following six categories were identified: "patient's palliative care was good," "24-hour home team support provided relief," "home care support was helpful," "decision support for home care was helpful," "saved by regretless end-of-life care," and "suffered from inadequate care." These results indicated that care provided by visiting nurses and caregivers is important to home-based care for terminal cancer patients and their family members. At the end of life, patient symptom management is important, and inappropriate medical decisions or inadequate intervention can affect patients and their families.

Watanabe et al. [21] clarified the type of support provided by visiting nurses for terminally ill cancer patients with dyspnea and their families. The survey was a self-administered questionnaire included the experience of caring for patients with dyspnea at the end of life and the content of nursing practice. Responses were obtained from 162 (effective response rate 90%) and responses of visiting nurses who had previours expericence with patients with dyspnea was compare to those who did note." Compared to other nurses, experienced nurses were shown to more frequently consult with a doctor regarding emergency response in advance, immediately visit the patient's home to provide care for dyspnea and listen to the patient's complaints. Additionally, experienced nurses frequently provided support to family members by explaining changes in medical conditions and providing materials such as pamphlets, explaining how to contact with a health provider after respiratory arrest, and accepting family members' anxiety about worsening conditions. This suggests that visiting nurses with more clinical experience have more options for supporting respiratory distress.

Akiyama [1] has been engaged in home-visit nursing since 1992, and has taken care of patients in their homes. She identified the following conditions as important for at-home patient care in Japan: (1) change how community residents view medical care (e.g., move away from the belief that hospitals will solve everything); (2) change the mindset of healthcare professionals (ending health care professionals' fixed concept that home care is impossible); (3) establish a regional medical cooperation system; and (4) enhance the nursing care system in the community. Furthermore, she discussed cases of home care not only for elderly individuals but also cancer patients. Additionally, Maggie's Center (originating in the United Kingdom) has been opened to systematically support cancer survivors and their family members. The following is the case of Mr. B, who completed cancer treatment, wanted complementary and alternative therapies, and was introduced to home-visit nursing:

Mr. B was 70-year-old man who lived at home with his wife. He had one son who lived in another prefecture. Mr. B was diagnosed with ascending colon cancer in 200X, underwent a right hemicolectomy, and received adjuvant chemotherapy and radiation therapy. However, Mr. B experienced fatigue, and his wife's friends recommended he begin complementary and alternative therapies. He was diagnosed with lung metastasis through a CT scan in 200X + 1 year, and chemotherapy was repeated. In 200X + 2 years, lymph node metastasis, as well as thyroid, lung, liver, and bone metastasis, were found. The primary nurse and his medical doctor requested a consultation from the palliative care team. Pain control with opioids began with the intervention of an anesthesiologist and a certified cancer pain management nurse.

The primary nurse, Mr. B, his wife, and his son, confirmed his intentions regarding future post-discharge treatment and where he would like to live after discharge. Mr. B and his family both wanted him to stay at home and hoped for complementary and alternative therapies. Therefore, the primary nurse consulted with his medical doctor, an MSW, and the discharge planning nurse to provide information to Mr. B regarding the clinic and the visiting nursing institution that could provide complementary and alternative therapies. Additionally, the primary nurse, physiotherapist, and occupational therapist gathered information regarding the home environment from Mr. B and his wife started rehabilitation with the aim of maintaining and improving Mr. B's activities of daily living after discharge.

In this case, alternative therapy was included as a support, based on the patient's voluntary wishes. Alternative complementary therapies in Japan are not strongly recommended in acute care hospitals; however, they are often the last hope for patients and their family members.

Complementary and Alternative Medicine for Cancer Patients in Japan

Complementary and alternative medicine (CAM) is defined as any medical treatment other than mainstream, modern Western medicine generally taught in medical schools, and includes ethnic therapies, diet and herbal remedies, health supplements, and music therapies, Manipulation, Qigong, etc.

The number of CAM users has increased worldwide in recent years. According to a survey by the Ministry of Health, Labor and Welfare, approximately 45% of cancer patients in Japan use CAM. The main purpose is to treat cancer and control its progression. It includes health foods and supplements, qigong, moxibustion, and acupuncture.

There are issues in Japan's efforts regarding CAM. First, in Japan, most CAMs—except Chinese medicine—are not covered by medical insurance. Therefore, the financial burden on the patient increases. According to the survey of Hyodo et al. [8], the average financial burden CAM places on patients is 57,000 yen per month, or 684,000 yen per year [8]. Currently, it is difficult to include CAM to what is covered by public insurance, due to the rising cost of medical care in Japan.

Second, many effects of CAM are not supported by scientific evidence. Many doctors in the Japanese health care system have a negative opinion on CAM's effects because of the importance of evidence [9]. At the same time, there are reports that 45.5% of patients do not consult their doctors when they use CAM [6].

Thus, there is a gap between physicians and patients regarding the implementation of CAM, and it is difficult for doctors and patients to communicate with each other. Therefore, it is highly possible that patients use CAM without consultations from doctors.

Many nursing studies have revealed the experiences of cancer patients and nurses in Japan using CAM. Cancer patients' reasons for using CAM have included the following [11]: "want improved natural healing power," "want to do what I can do for the disease," "want hospital treatment to proceed smoothly," and "want to rely on something." A reported 52.2% of nurses have experience conducting CAM consultations with patients [12], and 70% of nurses believe that CAM is holistic and can work both physically and mentally to enrich the patient's life [7]. Thus, nurses have indicated they may consider incorporating patient support for CAM use in the future. This indicates that cancer patients who use CAM view it as a source of hope for retaining their lives, and many nurses want to support such patients. In addition to solving the issues, it is urgent for society to create an environment where cancer patients can independently and safely use CAM.

Future Challenges

In Japan, patients want to experience their end of life in their homes; however, the rate of hospital deaths remains high. Therefore, systems for community-based medical care, such as comprehensive community care, have been developed. To transition from the hospital to the community, patients and their families need to understand the patient's condition and decision-making, and collaborate with health care professionals. Various models of transitional care have been introduced; however, regarding cancer, the role of advanced practiced nurses is expected in the current system. Thus, in the future, it will be necessary to understand and support health care professionals who want CAM for patients.

References

1. Akiyama M. End-of-life Care in Integrated Community Care as seen from the perspective of home nursing practice: from prevention to end-of-life care:helping people to keep living in the community until the very end. J Health Care Soc. 2015;25(1): 71–85.
2. Amano K, Baracos VE, Hopkinson JB. Integration of palliative, supportive, and nutritional cre to alleviate eating-related distress among advanced cancer patients with cachexia and their family members. Crit Rev Oncol Hematol. 2019;143:117–23. https://doi.org/10.1016/j.critrevonc.2019.08.006.
3. Boling PA. Care transitions and home health care. Clin Geriatr Med. 2009;25(1):135–48. https://doi.org/10.1016/j.cger.2008.11.005.
4. Enderlin CA, McLeskey N, Rooker JL, Steinhauser C, D'Avolio D, Gusewelle R, Ennen KA. Review of current conceptual models and frameworks to guide transitions of care in older adults. Geriatr Nurs. 2013;34(1):47–52. https://doi.org/10.1016/j.gerinurse.2012.08.003.
5. Fukui S, Yamamoto-Mitani N, Fujita J. Five types of home-visit nursing agencies in Japan based on characteristics of service delivery: cluster analysis of three nationwide surveys. BMC Health Serv Res. 2014;14:644–4. https://doi.org/10.1186/s12913-014-0644-8.
6. Narui H, et al. The advice patients want from medical professionals on alternative therapies. J Aomori Univ Health Wel. 2007;8(1):53–62.
7. Narui H, et al. Nurses' attitudes toward alternative cancer therapies. J Aomori Univ Health Wel. 2006;7(2):177–86.
8. Hyodo I, et al. Nationwide survey on complemental and alternative medicine in cancer patients in Japan. J Clin Oncol. 2005;23(12):2645–54.
9. Hyodo I, et al. Perception and attitude of clinical oncologists of complementary and alternative medicine. Cancer. 2003;97(11):2861–8.
10. ILC-Japan International survey on terminal care, March. 2012 ILC-Japan. www.ilcjapan.org/study/doc/summary_1101.pdf Japanese.
11. Ito Y, Arakawa U. Expectations of cancer patients adopting alternative medicine. Jpn J Cancer Care. 2000;5(4):326–34.
12. Ito Y. Awareness of alternative medicine. Jpn J Cancer Care. 2005;10(3):267–75.
13. Ministry of Health, Labour and Welfare: Annual trends in the number and composition of deaths by location of death https://www.mhlw.go.jp/toukei/saikin/hw/jinkou/suii09/deth5.html Japanes.
14. Ministry of Health, Labour and welfare: attitude survey on medical care in the last stages of life, https://www.mhlw.go.jp/toukei/list/dl/saisyuiryo_a_h29.pdf Japanes.
15. Naylor M, Keating SA. Transitional care. Am J Nurs. 2008;108(9 Suppl):58–63.; quiz 63. https://doi.org/10.1097/01.NAJ.0000336420.34946.3a.
16. National Cancer Center Japan: Diagnosis and treatment cases of all cancer association member cancer specialty medical facilities, 9th April. 2019., https://www.ncc.go.jp/jp/information/pr_release/2019/0409/press_release20190409_04.pdf Japanes.
17. Okamoto E, Miyamoto M, Hara K, Yoshida J, Muto M, Hirai A, et al. Integrated care through disease-oriented clinical care pathways: experience from Japan's regional health planning initiatives. Int J Integr Care. 2011;11(Spec 10th Anniversary Ed):e125–5.
18. Song P, Tang W. The community-based integrated care system in Japan: health care and nursing care challenges posed by super-aged society. Biosci Trends. 2019;13(3):279–81. https://doi.org/10.5582/bst.2019.01173.
19. The National Association for Visiting Nurse Service: 2019 Nursing Home Station Survey Results (Nursing Home Stations)., https://www.zenhokan.or.jp/wp-content/uploads/r1-research.pdf.
20. Usami S, Mine H, Yoshida S. Activities and evaluation of certified nurse specialist in transitional care. Off J Jpn Nurs Assoc. 2015;67(7):78–90.
21. Watanabe K, Ohtake M, Kobayashi J. The relationship between implementation of home-visit nursing support and experience of previous case of terminal cancer patients with respiratory distress and their family members. J Jpn Acad Nurs Home Care. 2019;7(2):44–52.

Part XXXVI

Far East: Korea

In Vivo Study of Laser Irradiation Techniques for the Treatment and Palliation of Lung Cancer Using Photodynamic Therapy

Necla Kenar and Hyun Soo Lim

Introduction

Lasers have been widely used to irradiate target tissue in photodynamic therapy (PDT), along with noncoherent light sources such as light-emitting diode (LED) and lamps [1–9]. Photodynamic therapy utilizes a fiber optic probe to deliver nonthermal laser light to cancer tissue, activating a previously injected photosensitizer and new minimally invasive procedure effective in treating lung cancer.

One of the major advantages of using lasers in PDT is the ability to easily deliver light to the desired tissue via an optical fiber with a very small diameter and different specialized shapes depending on the shape of the organ being treated [3–10]. Another advantage is that light emitted from lasers is nearly monochromatic, thereby allowing all of the laser energy to be delivered to the tissue at the wavelength corresponding to the absorption peak of the photosensitizer (PS). The use of diode lasers is more convenient because of their portability relative to vapor dye lasers. However, low penetration depth within tissue and thermal damage to the irradiated tissue are the most important challenges in PDT [11]. Penetration depth depends on the optical properties denoted by the absorption coefficient, scattering coefficient, and anisotropy factor of the tissue. Absorption and scattering coefficients also vary according to wavelength. Depending on optical properties denoted by absorption coefficient, scattering coefficient, anisotropy factor, and refractive index, the photon energy absorbed by tissue differs. These optical properties depend also on density, species, shape, and size of tissue components such as cells, cell organelles; proteins, enzymes, water, and oxy and deoxy-hemoglobin molecules; and the roughness of the surfaces of the air–tissue interfaces [12–14]. In addition, polarization states of the incident light to tissue affect the propagation of light in tissues [12]. After laser irradiation to tissue, the laser energy is absorbed and converted to heat energy in tissue, and temperature of tissue increases [13, 15, 16]. Heat transfer in the tissues irradiated by laser light depends on tissue mass density (ρ), blood mass density (ρ_b), specific heat of the tissue (c), specific heat of blood (c_b), the temperatures of tissue (T) and blood (T_b), thermal conductivity (k) of tissue, the blood perfusion rate (w_b), and the metabolic heat generation (Q_m) [15–23].

N. Kenar
Department of Physics, Faculty of Arts and Science, Kocaeli University, Izmit-Kocaeli, Turkey
e-mail: necla@kocaeli.edu.tr

H. S. Lim (✉)
Department of Electric and Electronic Engineering, Faculty of Technology, Sakarya University of Applied Science, Serdivan-Sakarya, Turkey

Department of Biomedical Engineering, School of Medicine, Chungnam National University, Daejeon, South Korea
e-mail: hyunlim@sakarya.edu.tr

M. Silbermann (ed.), *Palliative Care for Chronic Cancer Patients in the Community*,
https://doi.org/10.1007/978-3-030-54526-0_50

Based on the degree of heating, stepwise and selective thermal damage can occur. Depending on the duration and peak value of the tissue temperature achieved, different effects like coagulation, vaporization, carbonization, and melting can occur [13]. At 42–45 °C, hyperthermia begins and conformational changes and shrinkage of collagen occur; at 50 °C, enzymatic activity decreases; at 60 °C, denaturation of proteins, coagulation of the collagens, and permeabilization of membrane can be seen [13]. During the process of coagulation, temperatures reach at least 60 °C, and coagulated tissue becomes necrotic [13]. Collagen denaturation starts at 65 °C. Water in tissue boils at 100 °C at atmospheric pressure. At temperatures above approximately 100 °C, the tissue starts to carbonize, leading to blackening [13].

The wavelength of the laser and the light dose, also known as fluence expressed as energy per area, are the major laser parameters. The laser wavelength is chosen according to the absorption peak of the PS. The fluence value in the tissue is controlled by the laser irradiation time, or exposure time, on the basis of the power density. Different power densities with different irradiation times can be used to achieve a fixed fluence. For example, high power density and a short irradiation time would yield a particular fluence, while low power density would require a long irradiation time to achieve the same fluence. In other words, different power densities with the same irradiation time will create different fluence values.

Since PDT only destroys the cancerous tissue and normal tissue regeneration occurs quickly, we can use PDT as a tumor selective cancer therapy. A PDT treatment protocol for cancer includes three main steps: (1) administration of PS to the body, (2) uptake of PS into cancer cells, and (3) light exposure to the tissue area being treated. Effective PDT requires not only optimal light and PS doses, but also an optimal oxygen concentration within the tissue, although the presence of oxygen also has a cytotoxic effect through the production of singlet oxygen [23–29]. The main damage induced by PDT within the cancer cells occurs at PS locations in the presence of singlet oxygen ($^1O_2$) [30–33]. The mitochondria, endoplasmic reticulum, cell cytoskeleton, and plasma membrane are the main subcellular targets of PDT.

Lung cancer is one of the most common causes of cancer-related deaths worldwide. As it is seen from statistics published by The Global Cancer Observatory, GLOBOCAN, in March 2019, there have been 2,093,876 (11.6% of all cancers) new cases and 1,761,007 (18.4% of all cancer) deaths from lung cancer in 2018 worldwide [34]. The American Cancer Society emphasizes that approximately 228,820 new lung cancer cases and 135,720 deaths were estimated in the USA in 2020 [35].

Lung cancer can be treated with surgery and PDT [36–39], which has been used for the treatment of lung cancers in clinics since 1980 [36, 37, 40, 41]. PDT is safe and effective in palliation of inoperable advanced lung cancer [42, 43] and in early lung cancer patients who don't qualify for surgical resection. PDT is an attractive option in the treatment of early lung cancer in clinical practice [44–48] and can also be used as a palliative therapy in advanced non-small cell lung cancer patients with endobronchial obstructive lesions [49, 50]. In addition, PDT of A549 lung cancer cells using 5-aminolevulinic acid and a 632 nm diode laser with a 3.2 J/cm^2 energy density induced cell death in vitro [51]. Moreover, PDT using Photogem and a 635 nm diode laser, with a power density of 600 mW/cm^2, corresponding to an energy density of 180 J/cm^2, caused nonselective necrosis and has a thermal effect on normal lung tissue in an in vivo mouse model [52].

Comparative studies have revealed that continuous wave (CW) and pulse laser irradiation modes show different levels of thermal damage [53–58]. Recently, burst pulse mode, which uses a pulse mode but outputs the laser as a type of pulse flux radiation, such as radiation-start/radiation-stop, has shown promise in tumor destruction without thermal damage [59]. Results from previously published studies underline the importance of finding innovative solutions to improve the effectiveness of PDT and extend its use in clinics. Here, we examined healing and thermal damage in lung cancer tumors in an in vivo mouse model treated with PDT using pulse, burst pulse, and CW laser irradiation modes.

Now a minimally invasive therapy appears to offer a potential treatment for endobronchial non-small cell lung carcinoma (NSCLC), as well as endobronchial carcinoma in situ, or microinvasive NSCLC in patients for whom surgery and radiotherapy are not indicated. Photodynamic therapy utilizes a fiberoptic probe to deliver non-thermal laser light to cancer tissue in order to activate the PS drug injected.

PDT for non-small cell lung cancer (NSCLC) was first used in 1982 by Hayata et al. to achieve tumor necrosis and reopening of the airway [60]. PDT for lung cancer is particularly useful for patients with advanced disease in whom PDT is used as a palliation strategy [42, 61] and patients with early central lung cancer when patients are unable to undergo surgery [62, 63]. PDT is considered to be more specific and lesion-oriented compared to other available modalities and produces less collateral damage, and therefore fewer complications. Indeed, a randomized trial of PDT versus Nd:YAG laser therapy for obstructing NSCLC lesions showed equal initial efficacy for these treatments, with a longer duration of response noted for PDT [61]. PDT plus palliative radiation also appears to increase the time to bronchus reocclusion when combined compared with radiation alone [64]. In patients with early-stage lung cancer, PDT has been used to successfully treat patients for whom surgery is not feasible.

In one phase 2 study, 54 patients with 64 lung carcinoma lesions underwent porfimer-sodium-mediated PDT and showed an 85% complete response rate with a 6.5% local failure rate at 20.2 months [63]. Other studies have supported these excellent results, with complete response rates averaging 73% in studies totaling 359 patients [64–66].

Methods

Ten hairless 5-week-old mice were obtained from Hoshino Laboratory Animals (Japan SLC, Inc.) and allowed to adapt to conventional conditions for 1 week before experiments began. Tumors were generated in these mice using the Lewis lung carcinoma cell line LL/2 (CRL-1642TM) (American Type Culture Collection or ATTCC®, Rockville, MD, USA), which was established by implantation of primary Lewis lung carcinoma cells in the lung of a C57BL mouse. Prior to their injection into the mice, cells were stored in the vapor phase of liquid nitrogen and grown in Dulbecco's Modified Eagle's medium (DMEM) (Gibco, Cat. No. 12100–046) plus 10% fetal bovine serum (FBS), 10 mL of antibiotics/antimycotics (Gibco, Cat. No. 15240–062), and 3.4 g/L bicarbonate (Sigma: S-5761) at 37 °C and 5% CO_2 in air atmosphere. Mice were injected with Photogem (2.5 mg/1 mL saline solution), a hematoporphyrin derivative product in powder form from the Moscow Institute of High Chemical Technologies, as a PS.

The PDT diode laser system (Laxcell T3000; BioOptics Co. Ltd., Daejeon, Korea) operating in CW, pulse, and burst pulse modes with a TEM_{00} profile was used for irradiation. The optical output power at the end of optical fiber with a *numerical aperture (NA)* of 0.36 and a 600 μm core *diameter* was up to 1.5 W. The wavelength spectrum of the laser is shown below (Fig. 1).

Characteristics of the diode laser used at 15 °C in this study are shown in Table 1. More detailed information regarding the laser system design and irradiation modes can be found in the reference article authored by Lim [59].

Cultivated Lewis lung carcinoma cells diluted in trypsin or DMEM media were injected into each hairless mouse via a 26 G needle. The single cell suspension volume was adjusted to obtain 5×10^5 cells per mL for injection into the animals. The seventh day after the tumor cells were transplanted, changes in the size of the tumor and skin color were observed. At this time, the tumor had formed and was palpable (Fig. 2).

After tumor growth was confirmed, mice were divided into 2 groups: the control group (n = 1) and the target group (n = 9). A combination of ketamine/xylazine (K/X, 100/10 mg/kg) was intraperitoneally injected to alleviate any pain and difficulty prior to PDT treatment. Xylazine was used at 0.029 mg/mouse, and ketamine was used at 1.442 mg/mouse, while glucose solution (5%) was injected into the control group mouse.

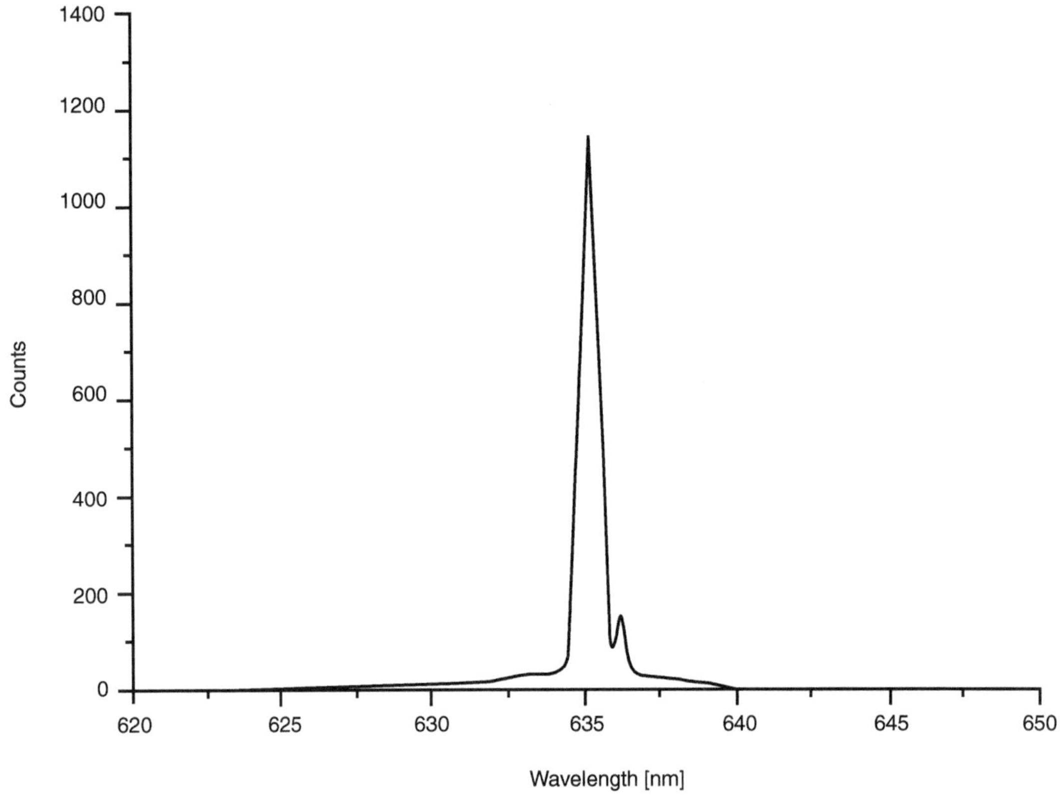

Fig. 1 Spectrum of laser from end of fiber

Table 1 Characteristic parameters of the diode laser used in the study at 15 °C

Laser characteristics (15 °C)	Symbols	Min	Typical	Max	Units
Center wavelength	λ_c		635		Nm
CW output power	P_o	1.5	1.5		W
Spectral width	$\Delta\lambda$		2	3	Nm
Temperature coefficient of wavelength	$d\lambda/dT$		0.2		Nm/C

Photogem (stored in the darkroom) was injected at 2.5 mg (1 mL) per kg through the tail vein of each mouse in the target group (Fig. 3a). Twenty-four hours after Photogem injection, 40 tumors (4 tumors per animal) that grew on the 10 experimental mice were exposed to the laser, 4 tumors on the control group and 36 tumors on the target group. Irradiated tumors on all the mice were chosen as shown in the Fig. 2. CW irradiation was applied to positions A and B shown in Fig. 2, pulse irradiation to position C, and burst pulse irradiation to position D in each of the mice. Laser light was delivered to the tumor using a surface illumination technique via a flat cut optical fiber.

Laser irradiation of tissue was performed at a dose of 100 J/cm^2 with a power density of 200 mW/cm^2 for the CW mode, 400 mW/cm^2 for the pulse mode, and 600 mW/cm^2 for the burst pulse mode, as shown in Table 2. Total surface light dose was controlled by exposure time. Light dose values for the photodynamic process were obtained using the following equations:

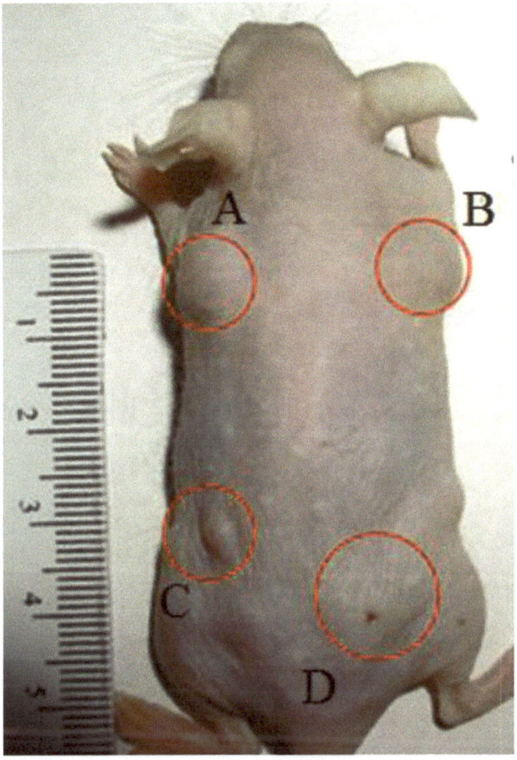

Fig. 2 Tumors at different sizes before PDT procedure

Table 2 Laser parameters used in this study

Irradiation mode	Power density (mW/cm^2)	Exposure time (s)	Energy density (J/cm^2)
CW	200	500	100
PL	400	250	100
BPL	600	166.7	100

$$Power\ Density = \frac{Power}{Spot\ Size} \quad (1)$$

and

$$Energy\ Density = Power\ DensityxExposure\ Time \quad (2)$$

Results

Changes in tissue color and a reduction in tumor size were apparent one week after irradiation. In the control group, tumor necrosis due to thermal damage was observed at all four positions irradiated by CW, pulse, and burst pulse modes. In the target group, after PDT treatment of 36 tumors, tumor necrosis occurred at 29 tumors, while only thermal damage occurred at the 16 of 18 positions irradiated by CW. Comparison of the images obtained after PDT treatment in the target group using different irradiation modes for different times showed a clear decrease in thermal damage in addition to an increase in healing for pulse and burst pulse irradiation modes relative to CW (Fig. 3a). Tumor and normal tissue necrosis due to an excessive rise in temperature were present at positions A and B.

As shown in the images in Fig. 3a obtained from target group after PDT treatment, the thermal damages in positions A and B are different even though they were exposed to the same CW laser irradiation with same energy density. According to tissue optics, it is an expected result. As mentioned in the Introduction, all biological tissues are optically inhomogeneous and spatial propagation of light and the thermal response in the tissue depend on both optical and thermal properties. In our experiments, mouse skin having multilayered anatomy of epidermis, dermis, and hypodermis has been irradiated by laser light [19]. Therefore, propagation of light in the skin tissue varies from point to point due to diversity in the thicknesses of these layers and in dermal collagen, elastic fiber, structural protein, water content, and the roughness of the surfaces of the skin layer, which affect the reflection and transmission of laser light [14, 19]. Furthermore, it has been shown that heat transfer in the tissue depends on thermal properties of tissue varying from point to point alike optical properties. Both optical properties and thermal properties are a function of blood and water content of tissues [20]. Water is a main component of skin tissue and has high thermal conductivity more than other skin components such as fat and protein [21]. Therefore, a change in the water content of skin tissue changes the thermal conductivity of skin tissue. As a result of osmotic pressure caused by blood perfusion, water content of skin tissue changes randomly and correspondingly the thermal conductivity of skin tissue varies randomly too [21].

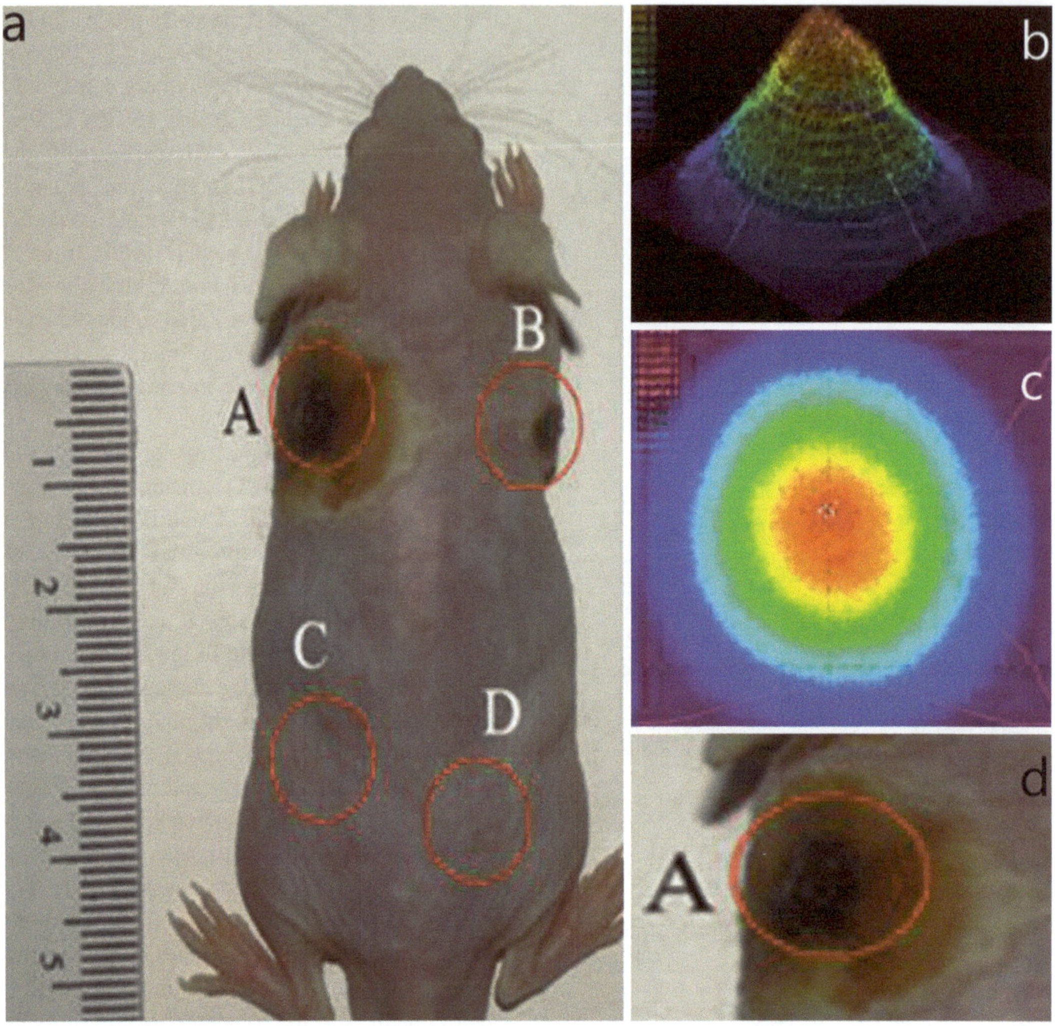

Fig. 3 Extensive survey and comparison of areas of the tumor after photodynamic process (**a**) tumor positions A and B irradiated by CW mode, position C irradiated by pulse mode, and position D irradiated by burst pulse mode; (**b**) 3D intensity profile of laser beam; (**c**) 2D intensity profile of laser beam used in the experiments; and (**d**) thermal damage present in area irradiated by CW mode

Tumor necrosis also occurred at positions C and D; however, thermal injury did not occur. Thermal damage of tissue, which depends on the increase in temperature, varies with the deposited energy per unit volume of tissue in unit time, which differs according to laser irradiation mode. Laser irradiations at the pulse and burst pulse modes diversely from CW provide opportunity for thermal relaxation to tissue as well. It is a cooling process where heat is conducted away from heated tissue by laser irradiation [22].

3D and 2D intensity profiles of the laser beam used in these experiments are shown in Fig. 3b and c, respectively.

The absorption of laser light contributes to the increases in temperature in the tissue. The incremental temperature rise generated by the laser radiation in the tissue in the absence of thermal diffusion is given by Eq. (3) [58, 59]:

$$\Delta T\left(r,z\right)=\frac{\mu_a F}{c_\upsilon}\exp\left(-\frac{2r^2}{w^2}\right)\exp\left(-\mu_a z\right) \quad (3)$$

where μ_a is the absorption coefficient of the tissue; F is the laser fluence at the surface of the tissue; c_v is the specific heat capacity of the tissue, and z is the axial coordinate perpendicular to the tissue plane. The temperature rise at any given radial position r can be calculated as Eq. (4) [58, 59]:

$$T(t) = T_{\max}(t)\exp\left(-\frac{2r^2}{w^2}\right) \quad (4)$$

where $T_{max}(t)$ is the time-dependent rise in temperature at the center of the laser spot.

The thermal damage rate due to temperature elevations in the tissue over time can be described by the Arrhenius equation, expressed as follows [60, 61]:

$$\Omega(r,t) = A\int_{\tau}^{0} e^{-E/RT(r,t)}dt = \ln\left(\frac{C(r,0)}{C(r,t)}\right) \quad (5)$$

where A is the frequency factor. E_a is the activation energy, R is the universal gas constant, and T is the temperature, C(r,0) and C(r, t), are the concentrations of undamaged molecules at the time of beginning (t = 0) and at t = τ, respectively.

According to Eq. (3), thermal tissue damage should increase as the temperature of the tissue increases, with a maximum occurring at the center of the laser spot, where the maximum increase in temperature occurs. The radial thermal damage profile observed experimentally in the tissue (Fig. 3d) has no Gaussian radial thermal damage profile due to tissues being inhomogeneous materials.

Furthermore, the measured 3D and 2D beam profiles of the laser used in these experiments (Fig. 3b, c) differ to the radial thermal damage profile shown in Fig. 3d.

The thermal damage in the tissue due to CW irradiation can be described by the absorbed energy per unit volume of tissue, ΔQ (J/cm^3), as shown in a previous study [59]. This previous study demonstrated that the average temperature increases in the in vitro pig muscle tissue per 10 J/cm^2 were 0.27 °C for the CW mode, 0.09 °C for the pulse (PL) mode, and 0.08 °C for the burst-pulse (BPL) mode, or $\Delta T_{CW} > \Delta T_{PL} > \Delta T_{BPL}$. These previous findings indicate that the different laser irradiation modes result in different absorbed energies per unit volume of tissue in the following order: $\Delta Q_{CW} > \Delta Q_{PL} > \Delta Q_{BPL}$. The burst pulse mode prevents thermal damage because of the excessive accumulation of optical energy in the laser, providing sufficient oxygen.

It has been demonstrated that the laser irradiation mode is a determining factor for efficient PDT. Laser-tissue interactions, such as photochemical and thermal interactions, in a mouse lung cancer model were investigated keeping the energy density constant, while varying the laser irradiation mode, power density, and exposure time. Despite the increasing intensity in the pulse and burst pulse laser irradiation modes, photodynamic effects were achieved without thermal damage due to the shortened exposure time relative to the CW mode. The advantage of pulsed and burst pulsed laser irradiation modes is that they involve a nonthermal process that avoids thermal diffusion into the tissue.

The current studies describe thermal effects of three different laser modes on photodynamic therapy in vivo. These macroscopic observable results show that pulse and burst pulse modes, with high power density and short irradiation times relative to CW, improve photodynamic reaction without thermal damage. All biological tissues are specific, and therefore effective PDT treatments require individual characterization of tissues, the studying and modeling of biodynamic process, and in vivo light–tissue interaction studies. It has been shown that pulse and burst pulse irradiation modes can be used at high power densities with shortened exposure times without thermal tissue damage, thus providing effective and safe photodynamic treatment by minimizing thermal damage and optimizing healing benefits. Although determination of the optimal dosimetry is pivotal for PDT application and better clinical outcomes, the pathological and histological evaluations under the microscope or cross-sectional views of each irradiated tissue are required as well. Here, the preliminary, non-quantitative (comparative) results of our research are presented. We also believe that more quantitative experimental data and quantitative and statistical analysis of the experimental data are required. So, before PDT, treatment planning should be done according to the optical and thermal properties of tissues. PDT is photochemical process. Thermal damage of tissues during PDT is undesirable.

In this chapter, we present the results based on the primary, observable, nonquantitative, and comparative practical experimental animal study. Our study was the first in vivo study showing comparisons of healing and thermal effects between irradiations modes. In this study, our aim was to examine whether there is a difference between thermal effects for different laser irradiation modes with same energy density after PDT.

New experiments should be planned including all modes and present more quantitative experimental data including parameters such as the pulse width, energy per pulse, average power, and repetition rate, etc.

Acknowledgments This research was supported by a grant from Academic Promotion Foundation of Chungnam National University of Korea (2015).

References

1. Mang TS. Lasers and light sources for PDT: past, present and future. Photodiagn Photodyn Ther. 2004;1:43–8.
2. Juzeniene A, Juzenas P, Ma LW, Iani V, Moan J. Effectiveness of different light sources for 5-aminolevulinic acid photodynamic therapy. Lasers Med Sci. 2004;19:139–49.
3. Wilson BC, Patterson MS. The physics of photodynamic therapy. Phys Med Biol. 1986;31:327–60.
4. Sterenborg HJ, van Gemert MJ. Photodynamic therapy with pulsed light sources: a theoretical analysis. Phys Med Biol. 1996;41:835–49.
5. Zhu TC, Finlay JC. The role of photodynamic therapy (PDT) physics. Med Phys. 2008;35:3127–36.
6. Wilson BC, Patterson MS. The physics, biophysics and technology of photodynamic therapy. Phys Med Biol. 2008;53:R61–R109.
7. Feather JW, Driver I, King PR, Lowdell C, Dixon B. Light delivery to tumour tissue through implanted optical fibres during photodynamic therapy. Lasers Med Sci. 1990;5:345–50.
8. Star WM. Light delivery and light dosimetry for photodynamic therapy. Lasers Med Sci. 1990;5:107–13.
9. Murrer LH, Marijnissen JP, Star WM. Light distribution by linear diffusing sources for photodynamic therapy. Phys Med Biol. 1996;41:951–61.
10. Hetzel FW, Brahmavar SM, Chen Q, Jacques SL, Patterson MS, Wilson BC, Zhu TC. The American Association of Physicists in Medicine, Photodynamic Therapy Dosimetry, AAPM Report No. 88, Medical Physics Publishing for the American Association of Physicists in Medicine. 2005.
11. Lenz P. Nonlinear optical effects in PDT. J Phys IV. 1994;4:237–40.
12. Tuchin V. Tissue optics light scattering methods and instruments for medical diagnosis. 2nd ed. Bellingham, Washington USA: SPIE Press; 2007.
13. Niemz MH. Laser-tissue interactions: fundamentals and applications. Berlin: Springer-Verlag; 2002.
14. Baranoski GVG, Krishnaswamy A. An introduction to light interaction with human skin. RITA. 2004;XI:33–62.
15. Welch AJ. The thermal response of laser irradiated tissue. IEEE J Quantum Electron. 1984;20:1471–81.
16. Welch AJ, van Gemert MJC. Optical-thermal response of Laser-irradiated tissue. New York: Plenum Press; 1995.
17. Zhou J, Chen JK, Zhang Y. Theoretical analysis of thermal damage in biological tissues caused by laser irradiation. Tech Science Press. MCB. 2007;4(1):27–39.
18. Shih TC, Yuan P, Lin WL, Kou HS. Analytical analysis of the Pennes bioheat transfer equation with sinusoidal heat flux condition on skin surface. Med Eng Phys. 2007;29:946–53.
19. http://ctrgenpath.net/static/atlas/mousehistology/Windows/integumentary/skin.html
20. Hamilton G. Investigations of the thermal properties of human and animal tissues. PhD Thesis, (Department of Physics and Astronomy, University of Glasgow, UK. 1998.
21. Tsai A., Investigation of variability in skin tissue intrinsic thermal conductivity measurements. Master of Science Thesis, Department of Electrical Engineering and Computer Science, Massachusetts Institute of Technology, US. 1995.
22. Choi B, Welch AJ. Analysis of thermal relaxation during laser irradiation of tissue. Lasers Surg Med. 2001;29:351–9.
23. Ochsner M. Photophysical and photobiological processes in the photodynamic therapy of tumours. J Photochem Photobiol B. 1997;39:1–18.
24. Juzeniene A, Nielsen KP, Moan J. Biophysical aspects of photodynamic therapy. J Environ Pathol Toxicol Oncol. 2006;25:7–28.
25. Mooreyzx JV, Westz CM, Whitehurstyz C. The biology of photodynamic therapy. Phys Med Biol. 1997;42:913–35.
26. Plaetzer K, Krammer B, Berlanda J, Berr F, Kiesslich T. Photophysics and photochemistry of photodynamic therapy: fundamental aspects. Lasers Med Sci. 2009;24:259–68.

27. Pervaiz S, Olivo M. Art and science of photodynamic therapy. Clin Exp Pharmacol Physiol. 2006;33: 551–6.
28. Agostinis P, Berg K, Cengel KA, Foster TH, Girotti AW, Gollnick SO, Hahn SM, Hamblin MR, Juzeniene A, Kessel D, Korbelik M, Moan J, Mroz P, Nowis D, Piette J, Wilson BC, Golab J. Photodynamic therapy of cancer: an update. CA Cancer J Clin. 2011;61:250–81.
29. Nowis D, Makowski M, Stoklosa T, Legat M, Issat T, Golab J. Direct tumor damage mechanisms of photodynamic therapy. Acta Biochim Pol. 2005;52:339–52.
30. Henderson BW, Waldow SM, Mang TS, Potter WR, Malone PB, Dougherty TJ. Tumor destruction and kinetics of tumor cell death in two experimental mouse tumors following photodynamic therapy. Cancer Res. 1985;45:572–6.
31. Chiaviello A, Postiglione I, Palumbo G. Targets and mechanisms of photodynamic therapy in lung cancer cells: a brief overview. Cancer. 2011;3:1014–41.
32. Ferreira SD, Tedesco AC, Sousa G, Zângaro RA, Silva NS, Pacheco MT, Pacheco-Soares C. Analysis of mitochondria, endoplasmic reticulum and actin filaments after PDT with AlPcS(4). Lasers Med Sci. 2004;18:207–12.
33. Tsai JC, Wu CL, Chien HF, Chen CT. Reorganization of cytoskeleton induced by 5-aminolevulinic acid-mediated photodynamic therapy and its correlation with mitochondrial dysfunction. Lasers Surg Med. 2005;36:398–408.
34. https://gco.iarc.fr/today/data/factsheets/cancers/15-Lung-fact-sheet.pdf
35. https://www.cancer.org/cancer/lung-cancer/about/key-statistics.html
36. Allison R, Moghissi K, Downie G, Dixon K. Photodynamic therapy (PDT) for lung cancer. Photodiagn Photodyn Ther. 2011;8:231–9.
37. Kim JO, Jung MK, Jung SS. Photodynamic therapy (PDT) in lung cancer. Tuberc Respir Dis. 2007;62:175–83.
38. Okunaka T, Kato H, Konaka C, Furukawa K, Harada M, Yamamoto Y. Photodynamic therapy of lung cancer with bronchial artery infusion of photofrin. Diagn Ther Endosc. 1996;2:203–6.
39. Okunaka T, Hiyoshi T, Furukawa K, Yamamoto H, Tsuchida T, Usuda J, Kumasaka H, Ishida J, Konaka C, Kato H. Lung cancers treated with photodynamic therapy and surgery. Diagn Ther Endosc. 1999;5:155–60.
40. Patrice T, Olivier D, Bourre L. PDT in clinics: indications, results, and markets. J Environ Pathol Toxicol Oncol. 2006;25:467–85.
41. Huang Z, Xu H, Meyers AD, Musani AI, Wang L, Tagg R, Barqawi AB, Chen YK. Photodynamic therapy for treatment of solid tumors – potential and technical challenges. Technol Cancer Res Treat. 2008;7:309–20.
42. Moghissi K, Dixon K, Stringer M, Freeman T, Thorpe A, Brown S. The place of bronchoscopic photodynamic therapy in advanced unresectable lung cancer: experience of 100 cases. Eur J Cardiothorac Surg. 1999;15:1–6.
43. Usuda J, Kato H, Okunaka T, Furukawa K, Tsutsui H, Yamada K, Suga Y, Honda H, Nagatsuka Y, Ohira T, Tsuboi M, Hirano T. Photodynamic therapy (PDT) for lung cancers. J Thorac Oncol. 2006;1:489–93.
44. Jang T, Kim HK, Oak CH, Jung MH. Photodynamic therapy in early lung cancer: a report of two cases. Korean J Intern Med. 2006;21:178–82.
45. Moghissi K, Dixon K, Thorpe JA, Stringer M, Oxtoby C. Photodynamic therapy (PDT) in early central lung cancer: a treatment option for patients ineligible for surgical resection. Thorax. 2007;62:391–5.
46. Lee JH, Jeon K, Koh WJ, Suh GY, Chung MP, Kim H, Kwon OJ, Han J, Um SW. Usefulness of photodynamic therapy in the management of early central lung cancer: a report of three cases. Tuberc Respir Dis. 2009;67:338–44.
47. Lee YS, Oh Y-M, Shim TS, Kim WS, An JS, Choi CM, Jang SH. The clinical outcomes of photodynamic therapy in early lung cancer patients. Tuberc Respir Dis. 2011;71:266–70.
48. Heo EY, Kim YJ, Yang SC. Fatal broncho-mediastinal fistula in a patient with non-small cell lung cancer after photodynamic therapy. J Lung Cancer. 2011;10:102–4.
49. Simone CB 2nd, Friedberg JS, Glatstein E, Stevenson JP, Sterman DH, Hahn SM, Cengel KA. Photodynamic therapy for the treatment of non-small cell lung cancer. J Thorac Dis. 2011;4:63–75.
50. Yoon SH, Han KT, Kim GN, Lee SI. Effect of photodynamic therapy in lung cancer. Tuberc Respir Dis. 2004;57:358–64.
51. Kim YS, Park JS, Jee YK, Lee KY. Photodynamic therapy induced cell death using ALA and 632 nm diode laser in A549 lung cancer cells. Tuberc Respir Dis. 2004;56:178–86.
52. Kang DW, Kwon SJ, Kim JO, An JY, Jung SS, Lim HS, Song KS, Lee YH, Kim SY. The histological changes of photodynamic therapy using 635 nm diode laser on normal tissues of C57BL/6 mouse model. J Lung Cancer. 2004;3:122–7.
53. Neckel CP. Comparative study on CW-mode versus pulsed mode in A1GaAs-diode lasers. Proc SPIE. 2001;4249:44–9.
54. Panjehpour M, Overholt BF, Sneed RE, DeNovo RC, Petersen MG. Comparison between pulsed and continuous wave lasers for photodynamic therapy. Proc SPIE. 1993;1881:319–24.
55. Barr H, Boulos PB, MacRobert AJ, Tralau CJ, Phillips D, Bown SG. Comparison of lasers for photodynamic therapy with a phthalocyanine photosensitizer. Lasers Med Sci. 1989;4:7–12.
56. Matthewson K, Coleridge-Smith P, Northfield TC, Bown SG. Comparison of continuous-wave and pulsed excitation for interstitial neodymium-YAG laser induced hyperthermia. Lasers Med Sci. 1986;1:197–201.
57. Ando T, Xuan W, Xu T, Dai T, Sharma SK, Kharkwal GB, Huang YY, Wu Q, Whalen MJ, Sato S, Obara

M, Hamblin MR. Comparison of therapeutic effects between pulsed and continuous wave 810-nm wavelength laser irradiation for traumatic brain injury in mice. PLoS One. 2011;6:1–9.

58. Karu TI, Ryabykh TP, Antonov SN. Different sensitivity of cells from tumor-bearing organisms to continuous-wave and pulsed laser radiation (λ = 632.8 nm) evaluated by chemiluminescence test II. Comparison of responses of human blood: healthy persons and patients with colon cancer. Lasers Life Sci. 1996;7:99–105.
59. Lim HS. Reduction of thermal damage in photodynamic therapy by laser irradiation techniques. J Biomed Opt. 2012;17:128001.
60. Hayata Y, Kato H, Konaka C, Ono J, Takizawa N. Hematoporphyrin derivative and laser photoradiation in the treatment of lung cancer. Chest. 1982;81:269–77.
61. Diaz-Jimenez JP, Martinez-Ballarin JE, Llunell A, Farrero E, Rodriguez A, Castro MJ. Efficacy and safety of photodynamic therapy versus Nd-YAG laser resection in NSCLC with airway obstruction. Eur Respir J. 1999;14:800–5.
62. McCaughan JS Jr, Williams TE. Photodynamic therapy for endobronchial malignant disease: a prospective fourteen-year study. J Thorac Cardiovasc Surg. 1997;114:940–6; discussion 946-947
63. Furuse K, Fukuoka M, Kato H, et al. A prospective phase II study on photodynamic therapy with photofrin II for centrally located early-stage lung cancer. The Japan lung Cancer photodynamic therapy study group. J Clin Oncol. 1993;11:1852–7.
64. Lam S, Muller NL, Miller RR, et al. Laser treatment of obstructive endobronchial tumors: factors which determine response. Lasers Surg Med. 1987;7:29–35.
65. Loewen GM, Pandey R, Bellnier D, Henderson B, Dougherty T. Endobronchial photodynamic therapy of Cancer 280 CA: a Cancer journal for clinicians photodynamic therapy for lung cancer. Lasers Surg Med. 2006;38:364–70.
66. Corti L, Toniolo L, Boso C, et al. Longterm survival of patients treated with photodynamic therapy for carcinoma in situ and early non-small-cell lung carcinoma. Lasers Surg Med. 2007;39:394–402.

Part XXXVII

Far East: Philippines

Community-Based Palliative Care for Chronic Cancer Patients in the Philippines

Maria Minerva P. Calimag

The Burden of Cancer in the Philippines

Cancer is the third leading cause of morbidity and mortality in the Philippines after diseases of the heart and the vascular system, and one in every ten registered deaths in the country is attributable to cancer [1]. It is a single disease in both children and adults that affects many different organs at various stages in a life course. Estimates of up to eight deaths per day for childhood cancer and up to 11 new cases and seven deaths occur every hour for adult cancer, resulting in approximately 110,000 new cancer cases and over 66,000 cancer deaths each year [2]. Furthermore, 189 of every 100,000 Filipinos are afflicted with cancer while 4 Filipinos die of cancer every hour or 96 cancer patients die every day [3].

The Philippines has the highest prevalence of breast cancer among 197 countries [4]. Among Filipino women, the five most common causes of age-standardized cancer mortality were breast, cervix uteri, colon/rectum, liver, and lung (including trachea and bronchus) cancer. Among Filipino men, the five most common causes of age-standardized cancer mortality were lung (including trachea and bronchus), prostate, liver, mouth and oropharynx, and colon/rectum cancer [4]. In comparison, the global age-standardized cancer mortality rates per 100,000 by type of cancer according to site for females were: breast (13.0), lung (11.2), cervix uteri (6.9), stomach (5.2), colon/rectum (4.6), and liver (4.6), and for males were: lung (27.1), liver (12.7), stomach (11.7), esophagus (8.3), and colon/rectum (6.4) [5]. Cancer incidence according to the site for Filipino females was: breast, cervix uteri, colon/rectum, lung, and ovary; and for Filipino males were: lung, colon/rectum, prostate, liver, and leukemia [4]. In comparison, estimated global age-standardized cancer incidence rates per 100,000 by type of cancer according to site for females were: breast (46.3), lung (14.6) cervix uteri (13.1), colon/rectum (10.1), corpus uteri (8.4); and for males were: lung (31.5), stomach (15.7), liver (13.9), nonmelanoma of skin (13.9), colon (13.1), rectum (10.0) [5].

The Philippines maintains its first reliable though limited local population-based cancer registry, the Philippine Cancer Society – Manila Cancer Registry, which is a member of the International Association of Cancer Registries. This was the first cancer registry in the Philippines, established in 1974 as one of the activities of the Community Cancer Control Program of the province of Rizal [6].

Systemic issues plague the Philippine healthcare system [7], which include excessive costs of

M. M. P. Calimag (✉)
Faculty of Medicine and Surgery, The Research Center for Social Science and Education and The Research Center for the Health Sciences, University of Santo Tomas, Manila, Philippines
e-mail: mpcalimag@ust.edu.ph

M. Silbermann (ed.), *Palliative Care for Chronic Cancer Patients in the Community*,
https://doi.org/10.1007/978-3-030-54526-0_51

healthcare; lack of healthcare professionals in critical areas like geographically isolated and disadvantaged area (GIDA), e.g., island provinces, mountainous terrains, and even just rural areas that are far from, or structurally excluded from, the cities; lack of infrastructure; mismanagement of resources especially in devolved healthcare systems; limited or no access to academic or continuing professional development among healthcare professionals; and, limited research into specific needs or limited knowledge about appropriate methodologies to use for specific research questions such as in palliative care [8].

Access to healthcare services is limited to a few cancer prevention and screening services. Many seek treatment during advanced stages of cancer and the most common barriers to early diagnosis and treatment are low-health literacy and the high costs of diagnosing and treating cancer in the Philippines. Because of poor access to health care, the many advances being made in cancer are still unattainable to many, especially for those who live below the poverty line. Another growing public health problem that needs to be addressed is the use of complementary and alternative medicine among cancer patients who dump anticancer drugs in favor of unproven herbal and dietary supplements [9].

The Philippine Cancer Control Program

In 1988, the first phase of implementation of the Philippine Cancer Control Program (PCCP) was conducted, providing the guidelines for the PCCP, specifying program policy and components and implementing guidelines and timetables. The PCCP is a comprehensive, systematic, organized and integrated approach towards the control of cancer through the utilization of primary, secondary (community level) and tertiary prevention in the different regions of the country. Supported by the six pillars of Epidemiology and Research, Public Information and Health Education, Prevention and Early Detection, Treatment, Training, and Pain Relief, the goal of the PCCP is to establish and maintain a system that integrates scientific progress and its practical applications into a comprehensive program that is intended to reduce cancer morbidity and mortality in the Philippines [10]. Ten years later, the Community-based Cancer Care/Control Network (CCCN) was begun in 1998, envisioned as a self-sufficient network of empowered communities sharing responsibility for total quality cancer care and control in the Philippines and its mission is to organize, integrate, and nurture such a network [11]. In 2000, the CCCN started to implement a registry software (CCCN Hospital Tumor Registry) for the different component hospitals of the Network and the DOH–PCCP.

History and Development of Palliative Care in the Philippines

Palliative care is a basic human right [12] and end-of-life is a public health issue [13]. The pioneering work of Cicely Saunders was instrumental in drawing attention to the end-of-life care needs of patients with advanced malignant disease [14]. The aim is to improve the quality of life of patients with life-limiting, complex, and chronic illnesses or those experiencing progressively debilitating diseases beyond any benefit from curative treatment. The World Health Organization (WHO) has highlighted the importance of palliative care in the developing world, yet many countries provide limited or no palliative care service.

The World Health Organization defined palliative care as "an approach that improves the quality of life of patients and their families facing the problems associated with life-threatening illness, through the prevention and relief of suffering through early identification and impeccable assessment and treatment of pain and other problems, physical, psychosocial, and spiritual" [15].

Internationally, three factors have influenced the shape of hospice-palliative care in Southeast Asia: the growth of palliative care development in the broader region of East Asia and Oceania; the activity of the pan-national Asia Pacific Hospice Palliative Care Network (APHN); and the paucity of funding from international donors. While the hospice concept was introduced into South Korea in East Asia as early as 1965, New Zealand and Australia in Oceania started their hospice at the close of the 1970s and the beginning of the 1980s, respectively. It was not until the 1980s that the movement started with Singapore in the Southeast Asia region. The movement toward palliative care and hospice care services in the Philippines began in the late 1980s for patients with cancer [16]. In 1991, the Philippine Cancer Society broke new ground when it established the country's first home care program for indigent, terminally ill cancer patients led by a multidisciplinary team made up of a doctor, a nurse, and a social worker [17].

This chapter discusses some of the important milestones in the evolution of Palliative Medicine, and the history and development of Community-Based Palliative Care in the Philippines. It explores some current issues concerning consistency in its implementation, and some likely prospects for its future advancement and expected expansion, from the perspective of one central question: "What constitutes the ethos of Community-Based Palliative Care in the context of the Philippine healthcare system and the family dynamics in Filipino homes?"

According to the 2006 mapping exercise of the International Observatory on End-of-Life Care, the Philippines is categorized under Group 3 in the 4-part typology depicting levels of hospice-palliative care development across the globe [10]. In 2011, a re-mapping exercise was done and two additional levels of categorization (groups 3a and 3b/4a and 4b) were included, and the Philippines is a part of Group 3a. In both instances, the Philippines was categorized together with other countries that have localized palliative care provision [16].

In the Philippines, institutional models of palliative care encompass the spectrum from basic, wherein palliative care needs are addressed in the community or primary health-care center setting by primary health-care providers, nurses, community health workers, volunteers, and/or clinical officers, to maximal, wherein palliative care is provided in inpatient palliative care beds in national hospitals, and the facility is staffed with trained professionals. Palliative care is available in about 45 medical centers in the country, based on information from the National Hospice and Palliative Care Council of the Philippines [17]. The Philippine Society of Hospice and Palliative Medicine, a specialty organization, was established in 2002 [18].

An emerging model of integrated palliative care delivery for the Philippines is the community-based palliative care (CPC). CPC's primary goal is to ensure that the administrative and funding models for palliative care are harmonious to the objective of minimizing disruptions to patients and their families and optimizing quality of life in every setting [19]. A Public Health Strategy (PHS) offers the best approach for translating new knowledge and skills into evidence-based, cost-effective interventions that can reach everyone in the population [20]. For public health strategies to be effective, they must be incorporated by governments into all levels of their healthcare systems; hence ownership by the community is assured because they are involved through collective and social action.

The community approach is the only realistic model for achieving significant coverage of care for two-thirds of the world's terminally ill patients. Meaningful palliative care requires a combination of socioeconomic, cultural, and medical solutions. Only by the active involvement of the community in addressing all three factors can palliative care reach all sufferers in need of it. Today there is an overemphasis on the medical approach, yet only by empowering the community and addressing the socioeconomic and cultural factors can balance in care be achieved. There are various models for community-based palliative care services: (1) services providing specialist advice and support for the family doctors and community nurses managing the patients; (2) services providing "hands-on" nursing and allied health services to patients at home, in cooperation with the patient's doctor; and (3) comprehensive services providing medical, nursing, and allied health care to patients and families at home [21].

In high-income countries, home-based care services are usually more resource-intensive than in low- and middle-income countries. They often operate from a specialist palliative care unit or hospice and sometimes provide round-the-clock coverage. In low- and middle-income countries, where patients usually prefer to die at home, home-based care is generally more acceptable and affordable than hospital care. Services are offered based on a needs assessment of patients and their caregivers, including essential drugs for the relief of pain and other symptoms and palliative care in a home-care package, as well as the provision of food for the patient and support for the patient's family (Logie and Harding, 2005) [22].

A variety of models of home-based palliative care are currently being implemented in low-resource countries. A popular approach in low-resource settings, where the number of people needing care is high and the number of nurses and doctors available to provide that care is low, is to provide care through community caregivers or volunteers who are supervised by a nurse trained in palliative care. Ideally, any model of home care will have strong links to an inpatient facility for patients requiring more intensive palliative care for symptom control or terminal care [23].

The story of the Hospice and Palliative Care Movement in the Philippines cannot be told without alluding to Dr. Josefina Bautista Magno, who broke ground in getting the medical profession to understand the need for pain relief and palliative care for terminally ill patients. She was a visionary who developed some of the first hospices in the United States while identifying advocates and galvanizing them to carry on the work in the hospices. She was instrumental in developing more than 8000 palliative care and hospice programs in over 100 countries. In 1994, she came back to the Philippines, mentored others and helped to establish hospices [24].

The Madre de Amor Hospice Foundation is a nonstock, nonprofit organization providing community-based hospice/palliative care service. It began in Los Baños in 1994 and currently covers 23 out of the 30 towns in Laguna [25]. There is a growing group of dedicated volunteers who devote their time and talent to the care of patients and their families. There are regular Volunteer Training Programs for interested volunteers and assist in setting up independent hospices in other communities (http://www.hospice.org.ph; interview with Dr. Ocampo).

The stories of volunteers resonate with images portraying a "journey of faith," a "mission of caring," finding the "heart of the hospice," and "cruisinginthelifeofangels."Onethemelingers–advocates and volunteers have experienced the pain of cancer by going through and surviving cancer or by journeying with and losing a loved one to cancer. The Foundation itself was borne out of a need felt after the founders suffered the loss of a daughter to cancer (http://www.hospice.org.ph; interview with Dr. Ocampo). "…the presence of a community of people who are there to help you and your family go through that journey mattered a lot" opined Dr. Rhodora Ocampo, Executive Director of Madre de Amor and Secretary of the Foundation [26].

The Hospice Unit at the University of the Philippines – Philippine General Hospital (UP-PGH) was started earlier in 1997 and the Fellowship training for physicians started in 2001. In the same year, the Section of Supportive, Hospice and Palliative Medicine (SHPM), under the Department of Family and Community Medicine, was organized by Dr. Catherine Krings. Today it is still the only fellowship training program in the country for doctors wanting to specialize in Hospice and Palliative Medicine. A similar initiative was started at the University of Santo Tomas (UST) under the Department of Anesthesiology in 1997 (interview with Dr. Corazon R. Arcangel, Palliative Care Specialist and Past Chair of Anesthesiology at UST Hospital) [27] with the guidance of Dr. Josefina Magno, who was an alumna of UST. Both institutions offer home care services for free to indigent patients.

The family is the basic social and economic unit of Filipino kinship. Although the family is important in many cultures, the central role that the family plays in the lives of its members in the Philippines is unusually significant, with family being rated the most important source of happiness [28]. In times of illness, the extended family provides support and assistance [17]. Important values that might affect interactions between providers and patients and families in the context of terminal illness include strong respect for elders, a strong reliance on family as decision-makers in case of illness, and strong expectations of care by the family [29].

Coupled with this is one's deep attachment to their family and friends, who reciprocally provide the love, concern, and care needed to meet the psychological requirements of everyday life despite uncertainties. Unlike in many cultures, Filipino families are supportive of one another in times of both greatness and doom [10]. According to Cordero et al. as cited in Ngelangel et al. [30], "The Filipino family is an institution of security which protects its members from the exigencies of living. The members are bound to help each other... they protect members against all kinds of misfortunes...." In these changing times, particularly culturally, we hope that this unique Filipino culture stands the test of time in supporting the Filipino in times of greatness and doom, in times of health, and psychological and social illness. The recommendation is for the continued awareness and positive practice of such Filipino values among Filipinos within the family, schools, the workplace, and the community.

Culture, traditions, beliefs, and religion play an important part in every Filipino's life and death. Moreover, the family is central and carries significant importance especially in healthcare decisions. Families are generally very involved in caring for their loved ones who are dying and equally expect healthcare providers to do the same. These are the hospice/palliative care activists who, against all odds, continuously try to improve their patients' quality of life and provide them with elements of dignity [31]. The ethical code also acknowledges the caregiving role of the Filipino family. The lack of professional end-of-life care means the dying become dependent on the support of their relatives and this may lead them to assume a passive role both within the family and concerning their illness. Authoritative individuals take decisive roles and medical decisions are decided in an extended-family context that includes parents, grandparents, siblings and in-laws. The changing context of palliative care over the last decade highlights the importance of recent research on home-based family caregiving at the end of life, whereby a comprehensive review of quantitative research (1998–2008) in this area was undertaken [32].

Back then, and up until now, however, palliative care is synonymous with pain control and hospice care with death and dying. Twenty-nine years later, thirty-six palliative care organizations of which twenty-two provide home care services all over the country, are listed in the Global Directory of Palliative Care Services and Organizations as members of the International Association for Hospice and Palliative Care [33]. The Philippine Society for Hospice and Palliative Medicine, a member of the Asia-Pacific Hospice Palliative Care Network, is taking on the role of advocating for the integration of all government and private initiatives regarding the implementation of palliative care services in the country.

Many community-based hospice organizations usually make free-of-charge provision for patients who are admitted to their programs. The home care program naturally sits well among Filipinos because its close-knit family structure allowed family members to default towards the culturally- ingrained task of caring for their sick and dying at home. In many programs, pain is managed concurrently with mobilization of the family support system. The last service offered is bereavement care for the family.

Future Directions

Integrating Palliative Care into the Undergraduate Medicine and Nursing Curriculum and Graduate Residency Training Programs

There is a need to fully integrate Palliative Care into the Undergraduate Curriculum of Medicine and Nursing. Dr. June Michael Razon, President of Hospice Philippines, shared his dream: "I am hoping that these young ones will become advocates of Hospice and Palliative Care themselves and soon serve their communities equipped with the knowledge and competencies of a Palliative Care Provider" (interview with Dr. June Michael Razon, January 23, 2020) [34].

Palliative care concepts and principles are part of the curriculum in major medical and nursing schools in the Philippines, and palliative care training programs are delivered to health providers and volunteers [35]. In 2016, hospice and palliative care were integrated into the Family Medicine Residency as a foundation course. Several hospitals provide training programs accredited by the Philippine Society of Hospice and Palliative Medicine, for interested diplomates in family medicine who want to pursue a subspecialty path in palliative and hospice care.

Improving Access in Resource-Constrained Settings

In 2016, recognizing the need to provide research-based recommendations for symptom management, clarification of treatment goals, support of coping and distress management, and coordination of care from the time of a cancer diagnosis through the entire life-course spectrum of treatment, recurrence, and long-term survivorship or the end-of-life, the American Society of Clinical Oncology (ASCO) published an update to its Clinical Practice Guideline, "Integration of Palliative Care Into Standard Oncology Care" [36]. Moreover, cognizant of the differences in access to palliative care services across health-care settings, a follow-up document entitled "Palliative Care in the Global Setting: ASCO Resource-Stratified Practice Guideline Summary" [37] was released to provide expert guidance to clinicians and policymakers for implementing evidence-based palliative care in resource-constrained settings for practice in low- and middle-income countries.

The recommendations outlined help to define the most practical models of delivery of palliative care to patients and their caregivers, staffing requirements, as well as the roles and training needs of palliative care team members in various resource settings. They also include suggestions for palliative care models based on local resources; timing of implementing palliative care; workforce, knowledge and skills; the role of nurses in pain management; spiritual care; social work/counseling; and availability of opioid analgesics. Calimag and Silbermann [38] outlined the current challenges and evolving strategies in implementing palliative care services in the Philippines.

Promoting a Shift in Patient Care Model

The National Comprehensive Cancer Care Network Adult Cancer Pain Guidelines recommend taking a broader, multidisciplinary approach. A "multidisciplinary team approach" refers to a patient care model that includes experts from different disciplines, whereas an "interdisciplinary team approach" requires a more integrated and coordinated approach to patient care, where experts from different disciplines establish shared patient care goals for a more holistic approach to patient care. As in the Integration of Palliative Care Into Standard Oncology Care Guideline Update: "In this guideline, a family caregiver is defined as either a friend or a relative whom the patient describes as the primary caregiver; it may be someone who is not biologically related" and this guideline recognizes there are cultural variations in the definition of families/primary caregivers. Ferrel et al. [36] focus on palliative care as an interdisciplinary, coordinated delivery approach.

At this point, it becomes imperative to define the distinction between the terms interdisciplinary, multidisciplinary, and transdisciplinary. Multidisciplinarity contrasts disciplinary perspectives in an additive manner, meaning two or more disciplines each provide their viewpoint on a problem from their perspectives. Multidisciplinarity involves little interaction across disciplines. Interdisciplinarity combines two or more disciplines to a new level of integration, suggesting component boundaries start to break down. Interdisciplinarity is no longer a simple addition of parts but the recognition that each discipline can affect the output of the other disciplines.

The "Advocating for Clinical Excellence Project" takes the multidisciplinary definition a step further, saying that providers in a palliative care team should take a transdisciplinary approach [39]. This means that "members create a shared team mission, benefit from role overlap, and have integrated responsibilities, training and leadership." Transdisciplinarity occurs when two or more disciplines' perspectives transcend each other to form a new holistic approach. The outcome will be completely different from what one would expect from the addition of the parts. Transdisciplinarity results in a type of xenogenesis where output is created as a result of disciplines integrating to become something completely new. A transdisciplinary team is an essential component of palliative and end-of-life care. The transdisciplinary approach to palliative care involves incorporating nursing, social work, spiritual care, and pharmacy in an acute care setting. A transdisciplinary team has a shared team vision for care and recognizes integrated responsibilities, training, leadership, and decision-making [40].

The role of nurses in palliative care in the Philippines abides by the principles of the dignity-conserving care model [41]. The Ruth Foundation for Palliative and Hospice Care (TRF) has organized annual ELNEC-Core training from 2012 to 2016. Much of this work has been developed and overseen by Rumalie Corvera, MD, DPAFP, FPSHPM, DipPalMed, and Ayda Nambayan, Ph.D., RN, who has taught palliative care to over 400 nurses. In 2016, Dr. Nambayan served as the core faculty consultant on the first ELNEC-Pediatric Palliative Care course in the Philippines. Dr. Corvera continues to do outreach work with the Ruth Foundation, having made free home visits to 471 patients and families as of January 2016 [42].

Fortifying the Community-Based Palliative Care Model Through Legislation

To make morphine more widely available, President Gloria Macapagal Arroyo signed Proclamation 2016 in March 2010, declaring that the National Hospice and Palliative Care Council be a conduit of the DOH in the nationwide distribution of morphine to patients of its accredited members [43].

The Department of Health Administrative Order 0052 series of 2015 issued December 21, 2015, set forth the National Policy on Palliative and Hospice Care in the Philippines [44].

There are also several legislative initiatives to institutionalize a national integrated cancer control program and palliative and hospice care into the Philippine healthcare system. On July 11, 2019, House Bill No. 2010 "An Act Integrating Palliative and Hospice Care into the Philippine Health Care System" was filed in the Lower House [45]. Its counterpart, Senate Bill No. 2150, was filed in the Upper House on January 15, 2019 [46]. The passage of the bill on palliative and hospice care would decongest government hospitals and stop the draining of public hospital resources intended for indigent patients because it would encourage the development of home-based palliative and hospice care programs at the grassroots level, which would increase the poor's access to quality health service.

In February 2019, two landmark Philippine laws impacted on cancer care in general and on palliative and hospice care in particular. On February 14, 2019, Republic Act 11215, or the National Integrated Cancer Control Act, was signed into law. The Act intended to institutionalize an integrated multidisciplinary, multisectoral, nationwide cancer control and management for all types of cancer, for all genders and ages. The Act shall serve as the framework to integrate all cancer-related activities of the government to achieve a progressive and sustainable increase in its response capacity, as well as build expected future needs and requirements [28]. Article IV Section 19 provides for Health Education and Promotion in Communities fortifying government support for the communities. Article V Section 21 provides for PhilHealth benefits for Cancer, further specifying that: "It shall also develop innovative benefits such as support for community models of care to improve cancer treatment journey and reduce costs of care, including stand-alone chemotherapy infusion centers, ambulatory care, community- or home-based palliative care and pain management and community-based hospice facility." Furthermore, Article VI Section 24 provides for Palliative Care and Pain Management Medicines, whereby: "The DOH shall ensure sufficient supply of medicines for palliative care and pain management that are available at affordable prices" [47].

On February 20, 2019, Republic Act 11223 or The Universal Health Care Act of the Philippines was signed into law, whereby palliative and end-of-life care services to patients with life-threatening diseases will be covered by PhilHealth. Under the proposed allocative health policy, "every Filipino shall be granted immediate eligibility and access to preventive, promotive, curative, rehabilitative, and palliative health services" [48].

The Philippine healthcare system will not only work on curing and preventing sickness, but it will also promote people's well-being, especially when they are enduring intense pain and suffering from chronic diseases. This measure guarantees the right of Filipinos to quality health care throughout their life cycle. The Universal Health Care Bill is a step forward in ensuring that every Filipino family can be given proper care and assistance during the most challenging stages of illness. Notwithstanding these challenges, and in the face of enormous need, hospice-palliative care activists strive to improve the quality of life of their patients.

Acknowledgments Arcangel, Corazon R., is an Anesthesiologist and Palliative Care Specialist; Past Chair, Department of Anesthesiology and Founder of UST Hospital Hospice, University of Santo Tomas Hospital. Interviewed October 21, 2019.

Ocampo, Rhodora is an Otorhinolaryngologist and Palliative Care Specialist, Director of the Madre De Amor Hospice and Secretary of the Madre de Amor Hospice Foundation. Interviewed January 14, 2020.

Razon, June Michael, is a Palliative Medicine Specialist whose passion includes end-of-life care, hospice home care and palliative care training. Before going into Palliative care, he was a Family and Community Medicine practitioner and was part of the Medical Affairs Team of two multinational pharmaceutical companies. Interviewed January 23, 2020.

References

1. Department of Health. Palliative care and hospice Philippine report. 2008;1–98. Available from: http://www.doh.gov.ph/sites/default/files/health_programs/Palliative and Hospice Report Philippines.pdf.
2. International Agency for Research on Cancer (IARC). 2012.
3. Department of Health. Philippine cancer control program [Internet]. Available from: https://www.doh.gov.ph/philippine-cancer-control-program.
4. Kimman M, Norman R, Jan S, Kingston D. The burden of cancer in member countries of the Association of Southeast Asian Nations (ASEAN). Asian Pac J Cancer Prev. 2012;13:411–20.
5. Bray F, Ferlay J, Soerjomataram I, Siegel R, Torre LA, Ahmedin J. Global cancer statistics 2018: GLOBOCAN estimates of incidence and mortality worldwide for 36 cancers in 185 countries. CA Cancer J Clin. 2018;68(6)
6. International Association of Cancer Registries. [Internet]. [cited 2019 Feb 5]. Available from: http://www.iacr.com.fr/in-de x.php? opti on=com _com-profi l - er&task=userProfile&user=985&Itemid=498.
7. Philippine Health System at a Glance [Internet]. [cited 2019 Dec 20]. Available from: https://www.doh.gov.ph/sites/default/files/basic-page/chapter-one.pdf.
8. Calimag MMP. Palliative care research: issues and challenges in developing and resource-constrained countries with focus in Southeast Asia. In: Silbermann M, editor. Palliative care: the role and importance of research in promoting palliative care practices reports from developing countries, vol. 3. New York: NOVA Medicine and Health; 2019.
9. Jermini M, Dubois J, Rodondi PY, Zaman K, Buclin T, Csajka C, et al. Complementary medicine use during cancer treatment and potential herb-drug interactions from a cross-sectional study in an academic centre. Sci Rep. 2019;9(1):1–11. Available from: https://www.ncbi.nlm.nih.gov/pmc/articles/PMC6434040/pdf/41598_2019_Article_41532.pdf.
10. Ngelangel CA, Wang EHM. Cancer and the Philippine cancer control program. Jpn J Clin Oncol. 2002;32(suppl 1):S52–61.
11. Ngelangel CA, Tanael SB. From Luzon to Mindanao: networking communities against cancer. Manila: community-based cancer care network–DOH. 1998.
12. Brennan F. Palliative care as an international human right. J Pain Symp Manag. 2007;33(5):494–9.
13. De Lima L, Pastrana T. Opportunities for palliative care in public health. Annu Rev Public Heal. 2016;37:357–74.
14. Clark D. From margins to centre: a review of the history of palliative care in cancer. Lancet Oncol. 2007;8(5):430–8.
15. Sepúlveda C, Marlin A, Yoshida TUA. Palliative care: the world health organization's global perspective. J Pain Symptom Manag. 2002;24(2):91–6.
16. Wright M, Wood J, Lynch T, Clark D. Mapping levels of palliative care development: a global view. J Pain Symptom Manag. 2008;35(5):469–85. Available from: https://www.researchgate.net/publication/5607822_Mapping_Levels_of_Palliative_Care_Development_A_Global_View.
17. Wright M, Hamzah E, Phungrassami T, Bausa-Claudio A. Hospice and paliative care in Southeast Asia: a review of developments and challenges in Malaysia, Thailand and the Philippines. Oxford: Oxford University Press; 2010.
18. Tsuneto S. Development of palliative medicine in Asia. Textbook of palliative medicine and supportive care. Florida: CRC Press Taylor Francis Group; 2015. p. 71–7.
19. Kamal AH, Currow DC, Ritchie CS, Bull J, Abernethy AP. Community-based palliative care: the natural evolution for palliative care delivery in the U.S. J Pain Symptom Manag. 2013;46(2):254–64.

20. Stjernswärd J, Foley KM, Ferris FD. The public health strategy for palliative care. J Pain Symptom Manag. 2007;33(5):486–93.
21. World Health Organization. Planning and implementing palliative care services: a guide for programme managers. World Heal Organ [Internet]. 2016;9–17. Available from: http://www.who.int/about/licens-ing/copyright_form/en/index.html.
22. Florence D, Davis RM. Palliative treatment of cancer in resource poor settings: traditional medicine perspective. J Pharmacogn Phyther. 2015;7(5):73–9.
23. Spruyt O. The status of palliative care in the Asia-pacific region. Asia Pac J Oncol Nurs. 2018;5:12–4. Available from: https://www.ncbi.nlm.nih.gov/pmc/articles/PMC5412150/pdf/APJON-4-127.pdf.
24. Newman L. Josefina Bautista Magno: a leader of the hospice movement in the United States and internationally. Br Med J. 2003;753. Available from: https://go.gale.com/ps/anonymous?id=GALE%7CA108879794&sid=googleScholar&v=2.1&it=r&linkaccess=abs&issn=17592151&p=AONE&sw=w.
25. Ocampo R. The Madre de Amor Hospice Foundation [Internet]. Webpage. 2019 [cited 2019 Nov 25]. Available from: http://www.hospice.org.ph.
26. Ocampo R. Interview. 2020.
27. Arcangel CR. Interview. 2019.
28. Virola R, Encarnacion JO, Pascasio MC. Improving the way we measure progress of society: the Philippine happiness index among the poor and the unhappy. 2011;4985–4990.
29. Coolen PR. Cultural relevance in end-of-life care cultural competency in clinical practice. 2012.
30. Ngelangel, CA, Ramiro LS. Quality of life in the health care of Filipinos – focus on cancer patients. In: Maximizing the quality of life of the elderly through better health [Internet]. National Academy of Science and Technology Philippines; 2006. p. 65–71. Available from: https://nast.ph/images/pdf files/Publications/Monograph Series/NAST Monograph Series 10.pdf#page=75.
31. Nambayan AG, Lu H. Palliative care in the Philippines. In: Ferrell BR, et al., editors. Oxford textbook of palliative nursing. 5th ed. Oxford: Oxford University Press; 2015. Available from: https://oxfordmedicine.com/view/10.1093/med/9780199332342.001.0001/med-9780199332342-chapter-81.
32. Stajduhar KI, Funk L, Toye C, Grande G, Aoun S, Todd C. Part 1: home-based family caregiving at the end of life: a comprehensive review of published quantitative research (1998–2008). Palliat Med. 2010;24:573–93.
33. International Association for Hospice and Palliative Care. Global Directory of palliative care services and organizations [Internet]. 2019 [cited 2019 Dec 21]. Available from: https://hospicecare.com/global-directory-of-providers-organizations/search/?idcountry=53.
34. Razon JM. Interview. January 23, 2020.
35. Gorospe EC, Bausa AB. Integrating volunteers in palliative care: the Philippine experience. J Palliat Care. 2006;22(4):297–9.
36. Ferrell BR, Temel JS, Temin S, Alesi ER, Balboni TA, Basch EM, et al. Integration of palliative care into standard oncology care: American society of clinical oncology clinical practice guideline update. J Clin Oncol. 2017;35(1):96–112.
37. Osman H, Shrestha S, Temin S, Ali ZV, Corvera RA, Ddungu HD, et al. Palliative care in the global setting: ASCO resource-stratified practice guideline. J Glob Oncol. 2018;4:1–24.
38. Calimag MP, Silbermann PM. Current challenges and evolving strategies in implementing cancer and palliative care services in the Philippines. 2019;2(2):257–263.
39. Otis-Green S, Yang E, Lynne L. ACE project ~ advocating for clinical excellence: creating change in the delivery of palliative care. OMEGA. 2013;67(1–2):5–19.
40. Gray B. Enhancing transdisciplinary research through collaborative leadership. Am J Prev Med. 2008;35(2):S124–32.
41. Doorenbos AZ, Perrin ME, Eaton L, Abaquin C, Balabagno AO, Rue T, Ramos R. Supporting dignified dying in the Philippines. Int J Palliat Nurs. 2011;17(3):125–30. Available from: https://www.ncbi.nlm.nih.gov/pmc/articles/PMC3140826/pdf/nihms308500.pdf.
42. Malloy P, Takenouchi S, Kim HS, Lu Y, Ferrell B. Providing palliative care education: showcasing efforts of Asian nurses. Asia-Pacific J Oncol Nurs. 2018;5(1):15. Available from: https://www.ncbi.nlm.nih.gov/pmc/articles/PMC5763433/.
43. Republic of the Philippines. Proclamation No. 2016. Official Gazette. 2010.
44. Department of Health. National Policy on Palliative and Hospice Care in the Philippines. Administrative Order 0052. 2015.
45. Representative Alfred Vargas. Integrating Palliative and Hospice Care into the Philippine Health Care System [Internet]. Philippine Congress; 2019. Available from: http://www.congress.gov.ph/legisdocs/basic_18/HB02010.pdf.
46. Senator Maria Lourdes Binay. Integrating Palliative and Hospice Care into the Philippine Health Care System [Internet]. Senate of the Philippines; 2019. Available from: http://senate.gov.ph/lisdata/2932125922!.pdf.
47. Republic of the Philippines. Republic Act 11215. Official Gazette. 2019.
48. Senate of the Philippines 18th Congress. Angara: Palliative, End of Life Care to be covered by PhilHealth under Universal Health Care Bill [Internet]. Press Release. [cited 2019 Oct 28]. Available from: https://www.senate.gov.ph/press_release/2018/1031_angara1.asp.

Part XXXVIII

Oceania: Australia

Australian Palliative Care for Chronic Cancer Patients in the Community

Tim Luckett, Meera Agar, and Jane Phillips

Australia's Changing Demography and the Growing Demand for Palliative Care

Australia is typical of high-income countries in that many people with advanced cancer are living for increasingly extended periods due to treatment advances. This includes people living with stable disease, those whose disease continues to respond to ongoing anti-cancer treatment, and those with incurable progressive disease who will either be off treatment or receiving treatment with palliative intent.

Many people with chronic cancer are also living with multi-morbidity that confers complex care needs. Australia's ageing population and societal changes also mean that more people are living alone and families are geographically dispersed, resulting in fewer people being available or willing to act as informal carers for older family members. These changes are increasing the demand for formal palliative care, which is outstripping resources and driving policy reform towards finding innovative ways of organising and delivering care.

Australia's Health System

Australia is a federation of states and territories ('jurisdictions'), and responsibility for healthcare is shared between these two tiers of government. Australia's universal healthcare insurance system was implemented in 1973 and is augmented by a private insurance scheme.

Australia was ranked second among 80 countries in the most recent Economist Intelligence Unit Quality of Death Index, behind the United Kingdom [1]. This index rated Australia highest in the world for human resources and affordability of care, and within the top three countries for all other criteria except community engagement (measured by public awareness of palliative care and availability and training for volunteer workers).

Australia has well-developed palliative care policy, including a National Palliative Care

T. Luckett (✉) · J. Phillips
IMPACCT – Improving Palliative, Aged and Chronic Care through Clinical Research and Translation – Faculty of Health, University of Technology Sydney, Sydney, NSW, Australia
e-mail: tim.luckett@uts.edu.au; jane.phillips@uts.edu.au

M. Agar
IMPACCT – Improving Palliative, Aged and Chronic Care through Clinical Research and Translation – Faculty of Health, University of Technology Sydney, Sydney, NSW, Australia

South Western Sydney Clinical School, University of New South Wales, Sydney, NSW, Australia

Ingham Institute for Applied Medical Research, Sydney, NSW, Australia
e-mail: meera.agar@uts.edu.au

M. Silbermann (ed.), *Palliative Care for Chronic Cancer Patients in the Community*,
https://doi.org/10.1007/978-3-030-54526-0_52

Strategy [2] and jurisdictional frameworks, as well as an established specialist palliative care service structure [3]. Palliative care service planning is increasingly taking a population- and needs-based approach, and assumes that the degree of specialist palliative care service involvement should increase with complexity of patient need in partnership with primary (i.e. non-specialist) palliative care providers such as general practitioners (GPs) and community nurses (see Fig. 1) [3].

Unlike some other countries, people in Australia can access palliative care concurrently with curative treatment, and access to opioids for people with advanced disease remains good despite national initiatives aimed at curbing over-prescribing to people with chronic non-cancer pain [4].

However, the growing complexity within the Australian health system and more people living with multi-morbidity means that *integration* of care is becoming increasingly challenging and important. There is a need for better *coordination* of services and providers to ensure patients experience care as *continuous* rather than fragmented [5]. This includes not only healthcare services but other sectors that can address needs relating to social care, accommodation, transport and financial support, for example.

In Australia, primary care is largely funded by the national (Commonwealth) government, whereas hospital care (including inpatient palliative care units and hospices and outpatient/ambulatory services) is largely funded by the jurisdictions. Community specialist palliative care service models are more varied, with some funded by the Commonwealth as community care, some funded through hospitals in a close relationship with inpatient and outpatient services and still others funded by non-government organisations with jurisdictional and/or Commonwealth government subsidy.

Residential aged care facilities, while partly funded by government, are largely privately run, and constitute a separate sector with variable links to the healthcare system. However, it is worth noting that only around 15% of deaths in residential aged care are from cancer [6] – about half the proportion of deaths from cancer in the general population [7].

Understanding the ways in which different services are organised and funded is important because these factors drive their respective areas of responsibility and the ease and manner in which they work together. For example, electronic health records have historically varied between states and territories, and even among local health districts within these. Only recently have attempts to improve interoperability between these different healthcare systems begun to show promise, in concert with a new national patient-held record called My Health Record [8], which at the time of writing this chapter was just beginning to gather momentum.

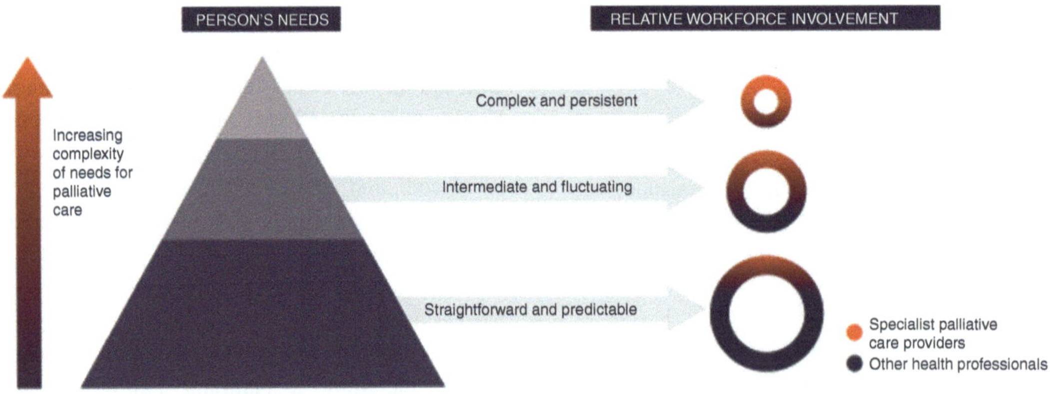

Fig. 1 Alignment of need for palliative care against workforce capability (Palliative Care Service Development Guidelines [Palliative Care Australia 2018, p. 11] [3])

Around half of all Australians choose to have private health insurance to have more choice about their healthcare providers, shorter wait times and access to services and therapies beyond those available through the universal healthcare system [9]. A proportion of people will elect to receive their cancer and/or end of life care within the private healthcare system. However, only a small number of private inpatient palliative care services/units operate across Australia, with most operating within the public healthcare system.

Historical Context of Australian Palliative Care in the Community

Australia has a documented history of providing formal palliative care dating back to the 1780s when the country was first colonised by the British [10]. Christian non-government organisations played a major role during the first phase of palliative care development in Australia. The second phase of development emerged in the late 1970s, largely as a counter -revolutionary movement driven by community concerns about the unnecessary suffering of people dying of advanced cancer. Over the past three decades, palliative care has evolved rapidly and more so since the implementation of Australia's first National Palliative Care Strategy in 2000 [11], with greater focus on a needs-based model of palliative care. As of 2012, Australia had 226 services providing specialist palliative care to people with a variety of life-limiting illnesses [12].

Ensuring Palliative Care in the Community Is Accessible

A major focus of recent Australian policy has been on increasing access to palliative care in the community *for the right people, at the right time* [3].

The Right People

The 'right people' include people with non-malignant diagnoses as well as cancer because Australian palliative care has traditionally focused only on those with malignant diagnoses but there is an increasing recognition that other life-limiting illnesses confer similar burdens and needs. From a social determinants perspective, the 'right people' also include population subgroups with recognised barriers to access, including people living in rural areas and from lower socio-economic backgrounds, as well as those from minority groups such as people from culturally and linguistically diverse communities and especially Aboriginal and Torres Strait Islander peoples.

Improving Access for Rural and Remote Australians

Australia is the world's sixth largest country but has a population of less than 26 million people [13]. Large parts of the country lack the number of people required to render specialist services economically viable from a health systems perspective. Specialist services are therefore delivered either on a 'fly-in-fly-out' basis (i.e. where a palliative medicine specialist from a metropolitan centre provides a clinic and/or consultancy within a hospital during a 1–2-day visit) or via telehealth (which can include nursing as well as medical services). In some larger regional and rural centres, a smaller specialist team, often comprising one or a small number of specialist nurses but no medical practitioner, provides a single-discipline service. Fortunately, advances in technology are enabling not only video link-up to facilitate assessment and 'difficult conversations' regarding prognosis and advance care planning, but also readier access to medical records.

In more remote Australia, even GPs and community nurses may be sparse. In these regions, there is an increasing emphasis on trying to leverage community social capital to develop the capacity of informal care networks to provide basic palliative care and support [14].

Improving Access for Aboriginal and Torres Strait Islander Peoples

Improving cancer-related prevention, screening, diagnosis, treatment and palliative care for

Aboriginal and/or Torres Strait Islander people is a major priority for Australian national policy and practice [15].

Like most first nation peoples around the world, Australian Aboriginal and Torres Strait Islander peoples are disadvantaged in socio-economic and health terms compared to the colonising majority. Life expectancy for Aboriginal and/or Torres Strait Islander people is some 10 years less than other Australians, and the prevalence of nearly all chronic diseases is higher [16]. Incidence of many cancers is higher (especially for lung cancer), and diagnosis is typically later and associated with limited access to services, leading to worse outcomes. Unfortunately, palliative care is no exception, with national data from 2010 to 2015 suggesting that only 1% of specialist palliative care patients self-identified as Aboriginal and/or Torres Strait Islander, compared to 3% of the general population [17]. The higher prevalence of disease, barriers to accessing services and poorer outcomes for Aboriginal and/or Torres Strait Islander people are rooted in social determinants stemming from ongoing colonisation.

Efforts to increase access to healthcare and outcomes for Aboriginal and/or Torres Strait Islander people have focused in large part on improving cultural safety. Where possible, this has consisted of care being delivered by Aboriginal Community Controlled Health Services (ACCHS), which are best placed to take a strengths-based approach to ameliorating the social determinants of health through connection to country, language and culture. However, while there is a growing Aboriginal and/or Torres Strait Islander workforce, there remains a need for healthcare to be provided by other health professionals for the majority of cases in many specialties, including palliative care. In these cases, twelve key processes have been identified for providing effective palliative care for Aboriginal and/or Torres Strait Islander patients, families and communities (Fig. 2) [18]. Working in collaboration with an Aboriginal Health Worker or Liaison Officer is especially recommended to minimise risks to cultural safety.

The Right Time

Emphasis on delivering palliative care in the community at the 'right time' has emerged following recognition that most patients prefer to be cared for at home rather than in hospital and that many hospitalisations could be avoided if needs were addressed more proactively before they escalate to a crisis. This imperative has potential to deliver a 'win-win' by enabling patients to spend as much of their remaining life as possible in their preferred place, whilst also saving the health system unnecessary expenditure on inpatient care.

Efforts to improve timely palliative care have partly focused on encouraging earlier referral to specialist palliative care by raising awareness among health professionals and the public that such services are not only focused on the last days of life. As explored in the rest of this section, efforts have also focused on ensuring palliative care can respond rapidly and is available out of hours when people need it.

Ensuring Care Can Respond Rapidly

As in other high-income countries [19, 20], Australian policy and practice has increasingly recognised that patient needs can change quickly, and that services need to respond to these rapidly to stabilise problems and put in place a plan for them to avoid and address a future re-escalation, with ongoing support as required. While care of this kind is sometimes delivered by a dedicated specialist palliative care team, more recent models have taken up the challenge of coordinating care from across specialist and non-specialist services, tailored to the needs of the individual patient and family. A brief description of two such models is presented as follows.

1. The 'pop-up' model of palliative care
   In a pop-up model, a specialist palliative care service provides 'just-in-time' training to build capability in local non-specialist health providers who are brought into a collaborative network in a 'bespoke' way as

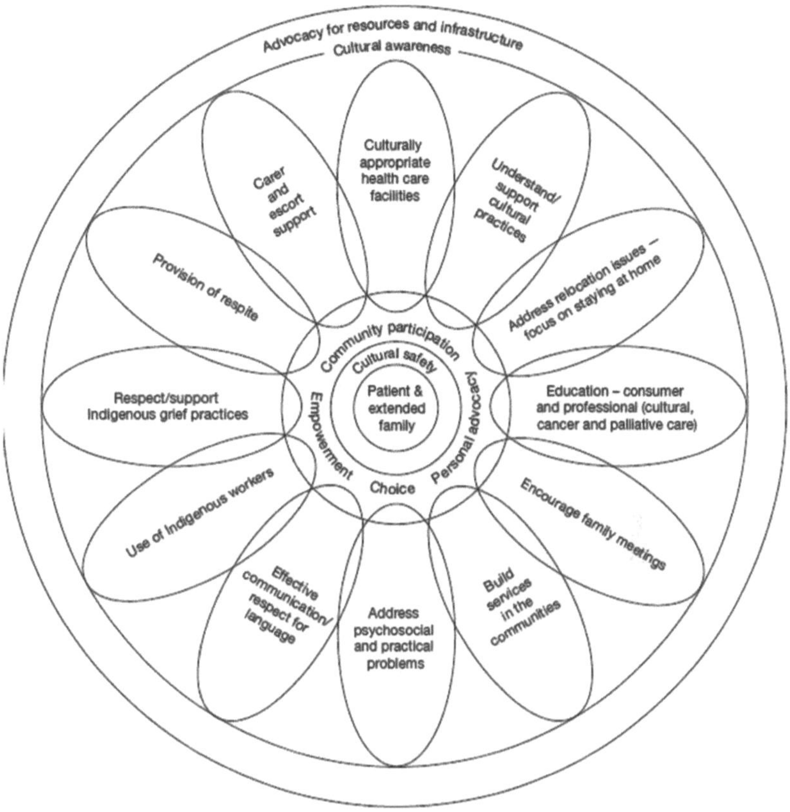
Advocacy for resources and infrastructure
Cultural awareness
Culturally appropriate health care facilities
Understand/ support cultural practices
Address relocation issues – focus on staying at home
Education - consumer and professional (cultural, cancer and palliative care)
Encourage family meetings
Build services in the communities
Address psychosocial and practical problems
Effective communication/ respect for language
Use of Indigenous workers
Respect/support Indigenous grief practices
Provision of respite
Carer and escort support
Community participation
Cultural safety
Personal advocacy
Choice
Empowerment
Patient & extended family

Fig. 2 'Living Model' for Aboriginal and Torres Strait Islander palliative care (McGrath, 2010, p. 62 [18])

required [21]. This approach is especially useful in regional or rural areas where specialist services are scant and local health providers have limited experience of providing care of the kind required [22]. The pop-up model of palliative care was originally developed in paediatrics because, thankfully, children rarely die of life-limiting illness so health professionals receive little opportunity to develop related skills.

A case study of a patient managed through the pop-up model is available online [23].

2. PEACH Program
While a pop-up model may be the only option where no existing networks and capacity are available, a rapid response model is likely to work better if there are established relationships between providers, with governance and communication systems in place. The PEACH (Palliative Extended and Care Home) Program is an example of this kind of model, operating in a lower socio-economic area of one of Australia's largest cities, Sydney. In this model, medical governance and case management remain with the primary care team, but specialist palliative care nursing support and personal care are provided on a contractual basis by a private nursing provider. PEACH provides high-intensity care for up to 7 days, including not only nursing care but also personal care and support for activities of daily living (e.g. shopping, cooking) to enable family carers to spend more time with the patient. Whilst relatively expensive for a community service, the PEACH Program shows promise of being cost-effective from a health system perspective by reducing hospital bed days [24].

A hypothetical case study of a patient who received support from the PEACH Program is provided in Box 1.

Box 1 Hypothetical case study of a patient receiving support from the PEACH program

Patient name: Mrs Jenny Nguyen

Age and gender: 64-year-old woman

Diagnoses: Metastatic non-small cell lung cancer and diabetes mellitus

Cultural background: Australian of Vietnamese origin

Living situation: Lives in metropolitan Sydney with her daughter (primary carer) and son-in-law

Mrs Nguyen is in hospital with pneumonia and has only partially responded to antibiotics. Her imaging results show progressive disease and new brain metastases. She has expressed a wish to spend the last days of her life at home, and her clinical team think it likely that she has only days to live.

The PEACH Program allows the hospital team to rapidly put the required support needed for a discharge within 24 hours, including arranging medication in the home, hospital bed and communication of care plan to her GP and community palliative care team. There is additional support from a specialist palliative care evening visit to monitor and adjust clinical management, and provide carer support.

Both of the above models share in common an emphasis on facilitating:

- Symptom management, including timely access to restricted medicines such as opioids
- Timely access to equipment at home (e.g. a hospital bed)
- GP involvement
- Support of informal carers

Ensuring Access to Care Out-of-Hours

Access to out-of-hours care in the community remains among the greatest challenges faced by Australian palliative care. Few Australian GPs or specialist palliative care physicians offer home visits even within-hours, and specialist palliative care community nurses usually only work during business hours on weekdays. Without the right support for escalating symptoms and carer distress, people may feel they have no choice but to present to the Emergency Department. Palliative Care Australia (2018) has recommended that the minimum level of access to specialist services should be 24/7 telephone support [3], and this is now available for parts of the country either at a state/territory or local health district level. However, patients in most parts of Australia who require hands-on specialist palliative care out-of-hours will have only private healthcare options available, with even these being limited to nursing rather than medical support Currently, the state of Victoria leads Australia in being the only jurisdiction to have an out-of-hours palliative care framework that requires access to both medical and nursing support [25].

Importantly, an emphasis on out-of-hours access should not be interpreted as reducing the imperative for proactive care planning and support for self-management.

Summary and Conclusion

This chapter has summarised the current state of palliative care in the community in Australia, highlighting challenges and progress made in enabling access to the right people at the right time. Australia performs well from an international perspective, but especially requires improvement in enabling palliative care for its rural and Aboriginal and Torres Strait Islander populations, and ensuring out-of-hours access.

References

1. The Economist Intelligence Unit. The 2015 Quality of Death Index: ranking palliative care across the world lien foundation; 2015.
2. Australian Department of Health. National Palliative Care Strategy 2018. Canberra: DOH; 2018.
3. Palliative Care Australia. Palliative Care Service Development Guidelines. Melbourne; 2018.
4. Campbell G. How is Australia responding to the pharmaceutical opioid problem? UNSW National Drug and Alcohol Research Centre [Internet]. 2019.

Available from: https://ndarc.med.unsw.edu.au/blogs/ms-morgaine-wallace-steele.
5. World Health Organization. Continuity and coordination of care: a practice brief to support implementation of the WHO Framework on integrated people-centred health services. Madrid: WHO; 2018.
6. Australian Institute of Health and Welfare. Cause of death patterns and people's use of aged care: a pathway in aged care analysis of 2012–14 death statistics. Canberra: AIHW; 2018.
7. Australian Institute of Health and Welfare, Australasian Association of Cancer Registries. Cancer in Australia: in brief 2017. Canberra: AIHW; 2017.
8. Makeham M. My health record: connecting Australians with their own health information. Health Inf Manag J. 2019;48(3):113–5.
9. Lewis S, Willis K, Franklin M. Explainer: why do Australians have private health insurance? The Conversation [Internet]. 2015. Available from: https://theconversation.com/explainer-why-do-australians-have-private-health-insurance-38788.
10. Phillips J, Ingham JM, Macleod R. Development of palliative care in Australia and New Zealand. In: Bruera E, Higginson I, von Gunten C, editors. Textbook of palliative medicine and supportive care. 2nd ed. Boca Raton: CRC Press; 2016. p. 94–105.
11. Australian Department of Health. National Palliative Care Strategy 2000. Canberra: DOH; 2000.
12. Australian Institue of Health and Welfare. Palliative care services in Australia 2012. Canberra: AIHW; 2012.
13. Australian Bureau of Statistics. Australian demographic statistics. Canberra: ABS; 2019.
14. Rosenberg JP, Horsfall D, Leonard R, Noonan K. Informal caring networks for people at end of life: building social capital in Australian communities. Health Sociol Rev. 2015;24(1):29–37.
15. Cancer Australia. National Aboriginal and Torres Strait Islander cancer framework. Surry Hills: Cancer Australia; 2015.
16. Australian Health Ministers' Advisory Council. Aboriginal and Torres Strait Islander health performance framework 2017 report. Canberra: AHMAC; 2017.
17. Woods JA, Newton JC, Thompson SC, Malacova E, Ngo HT, Katzenellenbogen JM, et al. Indigenous compared with non-indigenous Australian patients at entry to specialist palliative care: cross-sectional findings from a multi-jurisdictional dataset. PLoS One. 2019;14(5):e0215403.
18. McGrath P. The living model: an Australian model for Aboriginal palliative care service delivery with international implications. J Palliat Care. 2010;26(1):59–64.
19. Bainbridge D, Seow H, Sussman J. Common components of efficacious in-home end-of-life care programs: a review of systematic reviews. J Am Geriatr Soc. 2016;64(3):632–9.
20. Seow H, Bainbridge D. A review of the essential components of quality palliative care in the home. J Palliat Med. 2018;21(S1):S37–44.
21. Mherekumombe MF. From inpatient to clinic to home to hospice and back: using the "pop up" pediatric palliative model of care. Children. 2018;5(5):26.
22. White K, Wilkes L, Yates P, Cairns W, Kristjanson L, Monterosso L. Development of a model for palliative care in rural and remote communities: the "pop-up model" 8th National Rural Health Conference; Alice Springs, Northern Territory, Australia 2005.
23. NSW Paediatric Palliative Care Programme. Pop-up case study 2016 [Available from: https://www.nswppcprogramme.com.au/Portals/18/Documents/2016-May-Pop-up-case-study.pdf.
24. McCaffrey N, Agar M, Harlum J, Karnon J, Currow D, Eckermann S. Is home-based palliative care cost-effective? An economic evaluation of the Palliative Care Extended Packages at Home (PEACH) pilot. BMJ Support Palliat Care. 2013;3(4):431–5.
25. Victorian Department of Health. After-hours palliative care framework. Melbourne; 2012.

Part XXXIX

Oceania: New Zealand

Palliative Care for Chronic Cancer Patients: Global Approaches and Future Applications New Zealand

Catherine D'Souza

New Zealand

New Zealand is an Island country in the South western Pacific Ocean. Because of its remoteness, it was one of the last lands to be settled by humans. It has 2 main Islands; the North and South Island and 600 smaller Islands.

New Zealand ranks highly in comparison with other nations in terms of national performance, including health [1]. New Zealand's population is around 5 million [2], the majority of which is urban but with a significant population living rurally, some in remote, hard-to-reach locations.

Life expectancy for New Zealanders is 84 years for females, and 80 years for males [3].

Palliative Care in New Zealand

Palliative care in New Zealand grew from the grassroots up. Communities, NGOs, religious organisations and health workers sought to provide better care for the terminally ill. The first physical hospice inpatient units were opened in Wellington, Auckland and Lower Hutt in 1979. Now there are hospices in virtually all large towns and cities and 1 in 3 people who die are supported through the hospice movement [4].

In 2001 the Ministry of Health released the NZ Palliative Care Strategy aiming to establish "a systematic and informed approach to the provision and funding of palliative care services." Inequalities exist throughout the provision of Palliative Care and these "include access for Māori, Pacific peoples, isolated communities, children, the very old, those with non-malignant disease, as well as those with special needs: asylum seekers/refugees, people in prison, and those with mental illness" [5].

Place of Death

The majority of people who know they are dying and express a preference wish to die at home [6]. However only a limited number achieve this [7]. This is often due to inadequate symptom control necessitating a hospital/hospice inpatient admission or prolonged stay [8]. People who are dying often cannot take medications orally. Even when 24-hour home-based services are available, it can take a considerable time for a nurse to reach a home and provide subcutaneous medication for symptom control.

C. D'Souza (✉)
South Canterbury Hospice and District Health Board, Timaru, New Zealand

Cameroon Baptist Convention and Hospice Africa, Bamenda, Cameroon

M. Silbermann (ed.), *Palliative Care for Chronic Cancer Patients in the Community*,
https://doi.org/10.1007/978-3-030-54526-0_53

Lay Carers

Lay carers provide a substantial amount of the care required by someone dying at home [9]. This can be a positive experience for carers, but can also place a great burden and feeling of insecurity for the carer [10].

New Zealand palliative care teams have adopted protocols whereby family members and carers can give subcutaneous medications at home. With a significant number of New Zealanders living in remote and hard-to-access rural locations, the ability of carers to give medications in this way alleviates the need for a long wait for PRN/as required subcutaneous medication to be given. Even in urban settings it can take considerable time for community nurses to travel to administer medication. Currently in the UK, trials are looking at feasibility, acceptability, recruitment rates, attrition and selection of the most appropriate outcome measures of home administration of subcutaneous medication given by lay carers at the end of life [11]. This is, however, an unusual practice worldwide.

The practice of allowing subcutaneous medication delivery by carers for palliation grew organically. Some carers are understandably nervous about their responsibility in giving the medications [12] but the practice has been highly valued by care givers. Carers are willing to give these medications as it not only allows patients to be at home but also gives the possibility of providing immediate symptom relief. They feel empowered and have a sense of pride and achievement in their caring role [13].

Formal educational packages can be used, which have been found to support carers in this process [14]. However professional opinion on the safety of this method is still variable [14].

Safety concerns have been addressed by some services drawing up risk assessment guides and exclusion criteria. This goes in some way to remove excessive risk of diversion or inappropriate administration of medication.

An Example of Inclusion and Exclusion Criteria

Inclusion Criteria

- The patient is an adult with a palliative diagnosis and is experiencing symptoms that may require subcutaneous medication administration. This may be regular or as required medication.
- The patient and/or carer have consented to administer subcutaneous medication and have been assessed as having the capability (physical and mental capacity) to do so.
- There is agreement from the multi-professional team (minimum General Practitioner (GP) and Case Manager) that it is appropriate for the patient and/or carer to administer subcutaneous medication.
- The patient and/or carer have successfully completed the necessary training and are considered competent by a healthcare professional and feel confident to administer subcutaneous medication.
- It is suitable for a staff member, if acting as a carer and not an employee, to administer injectable CDs provided they meet all of the other criteria that would apply to any carer.
- Both patient and carer are aged 18 years or over.

Exclusion Criteria

- The patient or carer who would like to administer the medication is under the age of 18 years.
- The patient or carer willing to give the subcutaneous medication has been assessed and lacks the capability (physical or mental capacity) to do so.
- The patient or carer who would like to administer the medication has a known history of substance misuse. There are concerns relating to substance abuse involving the patient or carer or persons who may have access to the home environment.

- There are safeguarding concerns in relation to the patient or relevant carers who may be willing to administer medication.
- Failure to adhere to the protocol and agreed plan of management [15].

Most palliative units that work with carers giving subcutaneous medication at home have a risk assessment policy which evaluates the safety from the patient's and carer's perspectives. Most also use a formal training package with videos and pictorial guidance.

Practicalities

When carer-administrated subcutaneous medication is being set up, first a prescriber will prescribe medications to be given regularly and PRN/as required. The team will need to ensure there are adequate supplies in the house and are restocked if they become low. Medication may include a syringe driver providing symptom control medication given over 24 hours subcutaneously.

An indwelling needle with a luer lock (twist on and off mechanism) is inserted subcutaneously and covered with a dressing. All PRN medication is drawn up in plastic luer lock syringes, labeled clearly and left in separate bags with instructions on each syringe, each bag and on paper. For example, the label might read: 2.5 mg morphine for pain or breathlessness, to be given up to every hour.

Written information about the medication, how to call for help and troubleshooting guide should be provided to the care giver. Twenty-four-hour advice should be available, at a minimum phone advice. The carer should be provided with a written record, for them to record when medication is given and why.

A nurse will visit the home daily, asses the patient and check on the wellbeing of the carers. The nurse will then reinstate a syringe driver if it is being used. They will check the subcutaneous site is still clean and not inflamed. The nurse will assess how many extra doses of medication have been given by the carer and draw up enough subcutaneous boluses for the next 24-hour period.

If the nurse and/or carer feels that the dose needs to be changed or the patient needs to be assessed, they will call upon the prescriber to review the patient and the doses.

Conclusions

Carer-administered subcutaneous medication delivery in dying patients cared for at home has been found to be safe, effective and acceptable to carers. It can aid in the delivery of good symptom control at the end of life for those dying at home.

References

1. https://www.socialprogress.org/index/global. Retrieved 2020.
2. Population clock. Statistics New Zealand. Retrieved 2020.
3. NZ life expectancy among world's best. Stuff.co.nz. Fairfax NZ. Retrieved 2020.
4. https://www.hospice.org.nz/what-is-hospice/facts-figures/. Retrieved 2020.
5. New Zealand ministry of health. New Zealand palliative care strategy. 2001.
6. Hoare S, Morris ZS, Kelly MP, Kuhn I, Barclay S. Do patients want to die at home? A systematic review of the UK literature, focused on missing preferences for place of death. PLoS One. 2015;10(11):e0142723.
7. Productivity Commission. Introducing competition and informed user choice into human services: reforms to human services, report no. 85. Canberra; 2017. Available from: http://www.pc.gov.au/inquiries/completed/human-services/reforms/report/human-services-reforms-overview.pdf.
8. Gerrard R, Campbell J, Minton O, et al. Achieving the preferred place of care for hospitalised patients at the end of life. Palliat Med. 2011;25(4):333–6.
9. Zapart S, Kenny P, Hall J, Servis B, Wiley S. Home-based palliative care in Sydney, Australia: the carer's perspective on the provision of informal care. Health Soc Care Community. 2007;15(2):97–107.
10. Hov R, Bjørsland B, Kjøs BØ, Wilde-Larsson B. A sense of security in palliative homecare in a Norwegian municipality; dyadic compari-

sons of the perceptions of patients and relatives – a quantitative study. BMC Palliat Care. 2020; 19(1):7.

11. Poolman M, Roberts J, Byrne A, et al. CARer-ADministration of as-needed subcutaneous medication for breakthrough symptoms in homebased dying patients (CARiAD): study protocol for a UK-based open randomised pilot trial. Trials. 2019; 20:105.
12. Israel F, Reymond L, Slade G, Menadue S, Charles MA. Lay caregivers' perspectives on injecting subcutaneous medications at home. Int J Palliat Nurs. 2008;14(8):390–5.
13. Anderson BA, Kralik D. Palliative care at home: carers and medication management. Palliat Supportive Care. 2008;6(4):349–56.
14. Healy S, Israel F, Charles M, Reymond L. An educational package that supports laycarers to safely manage breakthrough subcutaneous injections for home-based palliative care patients: development and evaluation of a service quality improvement. Palliat Med. 2012;27(6):562–70.
15. https://leedspalliativecare.org.uk/wp-content/uploads/2019/05/Guidance-for-Patient-or-Carer-Administration-of-Subcutaneous-Medication-Palliative-Care-.pdf. Accessed Jan 2020.

Index

M. Silbermann (ed.), *Palliative Care for Chronic Cancer Patients in the Community*,
https://doi.org/10.1007/978-3-030-54526-0

D

E

Kolibri 360 GmbH
Ferdinand-Jühlke-Straße 7
99095 Erfurt, Deutschland
produktsicherheit@kolibri360.de